Therapeutic Breathwork

Christiane Brems

Therapeutic Breathwork

Clinical Science and Practice
in Healthcare and Yoga

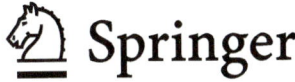 Springer

Christiane Brems
Department of Psychiatry and Behavioral Sciences
Stanford School of Medicine
Stanford, CA, USA

ISBN 978-3-031-66682-7   ISBN 978-3-031-66683-4   (eBook)
https://doi.org/10.1007/978-3-031-66683-4

This Springer imprint is published by the registered company Springer Nature Switzerland AG
The registered company address is: Gewerbestrasse 11, 6330 Cham, Switzerland

If disposing of this product, please recycle the paper.

This book is dedicated to all who breathe.

*May we inspire one another to save
this earth;*

*to protect its resources and honor its
treasures;*

to return it to a pristine state

with clean water to drink and

pure air to breathe for all beings.

Preface: The Book's Journey into Breathwork

To do anything well you must have the humility to bumble around a bit, to follow your nose, to get lost, to goof. Have the courage to try an undertaking possibly doing it poorly. Unremarkable lives are marked by the fear of not looking capable when trying something new.—Epictetus

Preface Overview: A Journey Through the Forest and into the Weeds

Thank you so very much for picking up my book on human breath and breathing. I appreciate that you are holding this book in your hands or looking at it online, whether you have already purchased it or are just pondering it. This volume has been a labor of love. It has brought me joy and heartache in the process of putting it together. This book has had a very long lifespan already. It started out as a training manual a few years ago; and, in many ways, it has existed even long before it went on paper. The journey of this work, in many ways, started more than six decades ago, when I was a young child who had a hard time breathing, who grew up driving my family crazy because almost from birth I was coughing constantly. This book started way back then, when my parents worried about my respiration and had to take actions that were quite extreme to try to support my healthy breathing and growth. This book continued to find life as I moved through my years as a university student, who often had a hard time catching my breath given the demands of life and study in a foreign country (and language); who sometimes could not breathe because I was too afraid to be authentically myself in the settings and places where I was supposed to develop my professional pathway and persona. This book was already with me, when I felt professionally compelled to conceal a central practice that helped support my health and resilience, namely yoga. Yoga's movement, breathwork, and contemplative practices, its deep grounding and ethics, and its encouragement of a lifestyle of discipline have guided my personal life and my professional journey. It has given me purpose and meaning, direction, and guidance. This book already existed but was very much expanded when its contents and wisdoms guided me through my journey with cancer. It existed during moments of joy in my own life and during moments of awareness, awe, joy, and insight of my students and patients. This book is permeated by all the work over the decades with psychotherapy patients, who breathed with me, and more recently with yoga students, yoga clients, and yoga teacher trainees who share life force with one another. This book has been a long time coming, and it is my true joy to offer it to you in this moment. Unfortunately, this book is like me: incomplete, imperfect, flawed, and despite many years (well, decades …) in the making, still not really finished and far from certain about whether it fully captures everything it means to be. Let me explain. ☺

No Book Is Ever Finished…

Everything in life changes. This is one of the most basic philosophies of yoga and Buddhism, so dear to my heart. This is one of the most basic philosophies that all of us as humans can feel wholly in our bodies, our vitality, and our minds. No thought we ever think comes to a full completion. Nothing we have ever learned does not at some point have to be unlearned and relearned. Nothing that we ever do comes to a full stop—it reverberates. We may call it done at some point, but the effort lives on. No human being is ever fully finished and refined. We transform at least until the moment of death, and who knows what happens after that. This book is the same way. Just because you are holding it in your hands now does not mean that it was finished at the moment I handed it over to my wonderful publisher. It was a moment of trepidation, a moment of letting go, of knowing that there were still things to be said, that there were still edits to be made, that there were still contents to be refined, and that there were still mistakes to be found. So forgive me for sharing this unfinished product with you and allow me to encourage you to help me finish this book by giving me your feedback, your comments, your opinions, and your suggestions for refinements. Who knows, maybe someday another version of this book will appear on all of our shelves that will be a bit more finished, but still not done.

No Book Is Ever Perfect…

Nothing in life is perfect. Some things are simply less flawed than others. Perhaps we are really not meant to be perfect. If we were perfect, then what would give us direction, meaning, or purpose? What would invite us into open-hearted compassion and open-minded reflection? No human being is perfect; no collective is perfect; no society is perfect … why would our books be otherwise? There will be errors. There will be reflections of my own misperceptions and misunderstandings. I have tried as hard as possible to ground my work in science and experience; to base my conclusions in observations of my clients and patients, my friends and my family, and even my own experiences. But these are still just my perceptions, and my perceptions are flavored by my own background, biopsychosociocultural context, struggles, and joys. What seems so right to me in this moment may turn out to be so wrong tomorrow. Therefore, please forgive me for the imperfections in this book. And please know that I see this book as a project to continue to refine, to try to perfect, and to cherish even with its imperfections. To paraphrase Shunryu Suzuki, *each of us is perfect the way we are ... and we can all use a little improvement.*

No Book Is Ever Up To Date...

I heard an amazing statistic somewhere not too long ago. My apologies to the author of this fact, I cannot remember who you are in this moment. But your claim stayed with me. It asserted that the amount of knowledge and information about medicine *doubles every 73 days.* This is a frightening statistics... but it is also very freeing. For me, it came at just the right moment. As I was working on this book, I felt as though I could never relax into any of my assertions. There were always new studies, new books, new insights, new reactions by patients, new understandings reflected by students, and changes in my own experience of something. I felt constantly out of date and compelled to learn more. (I am sure some of my friends would say that I *am* constantly out of date. And they would be right.) I do not, I cannot, stay up on everything—no matter how compelled I feel always to learn more, to evolve. I am not current on most things in life. I try, but I fail all the time. This book is no different. It is as up to date as I could coax it to be by the time it needed to be turned over to the publisher. But I am sure there are new findings and ponderings already. So, please forgive me for facts that I have left out and for science that already has evolved beyond what I claim in these pages. Please be an inquisitive reader and do your own research. Let the book inspire you and then go out and find a new study that has already disproven me. Do please know that I did my best, that what I am writing in these pages is my understanding of the art and science of breathwork as I understand and appreciate it, right up until this very moment that I am writing this sentence.

No Book Can Be all Things to all People...

I know a lot of people. Some may like me; some may not; some are still undecided. Some just cannot figure me out; some think I am pedantic; others think I am too willing to call something good enough. Some think I am a deep thinker; others may find me superficial. You may end up having all of these thoughts about this book. No book can cover everything in exactly the way that a reader wants to read it. We are all too unique in how we learn, in how we think, in how we respond and react to new learning; we all have different opinions and attitudes, and so many diverse experiences, needs, and preferences. We are all from different biopsychosociocultural contexts and, simply for that reason, we have different needs, different desires, and different ways of being in the world. I know some of you will be disappointed in this book. Others may go so far as to say they like it. Maybe a few of you will actually celebrate it, learn deeply from it, and enjoy it. I hope all of you will get some use out of it. I have tried as hard as I could to please as many of you as possible, based on my experience with my students, clients, colleagues, and friends over the years.

I apologize to those of you who may be put off by the occasional redundancy in the book. Please know it is intentional. There are some things that needed to be said multiple times in various contexts to really be driven home in terms of their complexity and lack of straightforwardness. Some of you will be annoyed by my need to always capture not just the forest but also the trees … and my desire not only to look at each tree but also to present a bird's eye view of the whole forest. I have always been this way. I want to understand the big picture; and then I like to get into the weeds. I hope you follow me into the forest that is this book and are open to exploring some excruciating details more than once, finding some information in multiple places, hearing a lot of "that depends on context," and being encouraged over and over again to learn this information and then to apply it in your own unique and idiosyncratic way, based on the needs of the students and clients in front of you. I cannot help myself—I am driven to giving you suggestions and invitations, but in the end you have to decide what this book and its information means to you and how you will apply artfully with your own patients and in your own life, as you engage some of this material in the context of your own self-care and wellbeing.

No Book Can Say It All...

And now on to my final point. This book could have easily been a thousand pages long. I have not said it all. I said many things that (thanks to skillful editing by my husband and colleague) are no longer in these pages. Kind-hearted editing has taken them out, letting me know that I am going too far into the weeds. So, I apologize to you for things that are missing, things that maybe I have removed and should not have, things that I never thought to include and that are now leaving a gap in your experience of this material. Let me know what I have missed, what should have been there. Also feel free to let me know what I could take out, if the book dares to evolve over time.

> The importance of breathing need hardly be stressed. It provides the oxygen for the metabolic processes; literally it supports the fires of life.
> But breath as "pneuma" is also the spirit or soul.
> We live in an ocean of air like fish in a body of water. By our breathing we are attuned to our atmosphere. If we inhibit our breathing we isolate ourselves from the medium in which we exist. In all … mystic philosophies, the breath holds the secret to the highest bliss.—Alexander Lowen in The Voice of the Body

How this Book Is Structured…

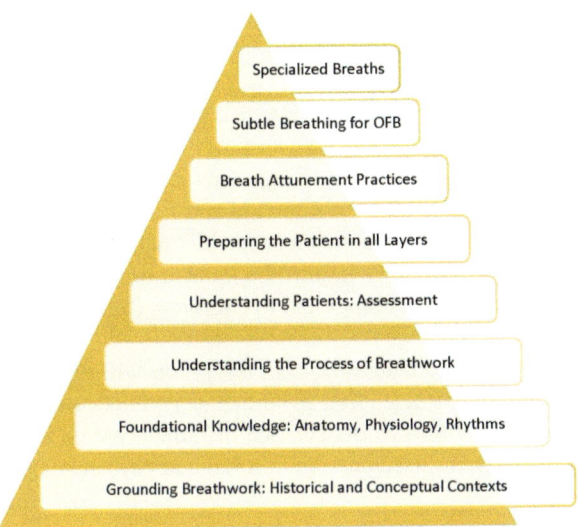

Before delving into the specifics of the book, it helps to understand the book's structure as forming a pyramid, with each tier of the pyramid building on and integrating the prior tiers, leading the reader to a full understanding of how to implement breathwork into their personal and professional lives. Chapter 1 serves as the backdrop—creating a historical and conceptual context for breathwork and its pyramid-based structure. Chapters 2 to 4 build the base or first tier of the pyramid, the solid foundation of scientific knowledge that is necessary for every clinician to engage in auspicious breathwork. Chapter 5, the second tier of the pyramid, presents a clear understanding of the process of breathwork, attending to creating ideal environments, procedures, and relationships. The third tier, offered in Chap. 6, consists of understanding each patient from their unique perspective, using assessment procedures and tools to tailor breath interventions specifically to them. Chapter 7 builds the next tier in the pyramid, consisting of careful patient preparation for breathwork, attending to all of their layers of experience. The fifth tier in the pyramid is established in Chap. 8, which consists of strategies for breath observation and awareness. Such careful breath attunement optimally prepares patients for actual breathing practices. Chapter 9, representing the next tier in the pyramid, offers instruction for subtle breathing practices to help patients cultivate optimal functional breathing that allows them to move through life with resilience and coherence. Finally, the top tier and the smallest part of the pyramid (covered in Chaps. 10 and 11) offers specialized breathing practices, those that may have a very particular purpose or application. Although these specialized practices often make up the bulk of *pranayama* books in yoga, they make up the smallest part of this book. They are simply the icing on the cake. Each chapter starts with a figure showing its place in the pyramid to help the reader appreciate the meaning of the chapter in the overall context of integrated holistic breathwork. I hope you appreciate the symbolism of the pyramid. It was a joyful way to structure the book in this way, and I hope it helps you in your journey through this volume and into breathwork beyond reading about it.

Why You may Want to Read this Book...

I was not going to offer you a narrative overview of the book in this preface. I simply invite you to flip to the table of contents and maybe to read the opening paragraphs in each chapter to help you get a sense of where the book hopes to take you. I always skip narrative overviews in introductions or prefaces and do what is recommended to you. But then I felt compelled to conform. ☺ So here we go—following is a quick overview of the pages to follow (feel free to skip it—but do check out the table of contents and flip through the chapters). You will notice that the content is offered in four distinct parts, leading from the art and history of breathwork (in the context of yoga and beyond) to the science of human breath and breathing, to the application of the art and the science in tailored and person-centered practices.

Part I: Breathwork To Honor the Whole Human Being

With a single chapter, Part I explores the history of breathwork across the millennia. It introduces the idea that we all stand on the shoulders of giants and are deeply indebted to the wisdom of ancient and modern thinkers. From there, it moves on to explain the integrated holistic framework that underlies the breathwork offered in this book. Integrated holistic breathing practice is committed to accessibility, intentionality, beneficence, wholism, and integration. These principles are the very foundation of all the work book offers; they honor their deep roots in ancient wisdom and modern science. These principles are a deep reflection of who I am as a human being, a breather, a yogi, an educator, a scientist, and a clinician.

Part II: Breathwork Grounded in Science and Informed by Wisdom

Part II consists of three chapters that provide a broad overview of the science of breathing. Chapter 2 provides a thorough overview of breath anatomy, diving deeply into the respiratory system and biomechanics of breathing. It offers insights about how breath interacts with many anatomical aspects of what it means to be human. For example, it covers how posture can affect breathing and the difference in tongue placement can make to our wellbeing. Chapter 3 provides a thorough overview of breath physiology, exploring the fascinating biochemistry of breath. It provides a foundation for understanding respiration at multiple levels, especially internal and external respiration. It encourages breathwork teachers to be cognizant that breathing is not just something we do, but something that has the power to reshape the very essence of our wellbeing and capacity for thriving—from the inside out. Chapter 4 dives into rhythms and cadences of breath and elucidates its important link to our human nervous system, making important links to polyvagal theory. It proposes a paradigm for breathing based in the science of breathing. Finally, the chapter and section culminate in defining resilient and coherent breathing as the very foundation of human wellbeing and thriving (and the remainder of the book).

Part III: Breathwork Preparations To Create Intentionality, Beneficence, and Accessibility

With three chapters, Part III moves into the application of historical contexts and wisdoms as well as modern science to breath and breathing. Chapter 5 offers a paradigm for breathwork that is based in science and ancient wisdom. The offered conceptual model emphasizes that clinicians need to understand their clients fully to offer them tailored and person-centered breathwork. Chapter 6 offers strategies for assessment that help clinicians understand clients more deeply so that there can be full engagement with patients to help them thrive via enhancing breath and breathing. Assessments are wide-ranging and commensurate with information offered in the science chapters. Chapter 7 provides information to help clinicians guide patients into deeper motivation to engage in the complex breathwork that can support their thriving. It provides an overview of physical practices that can be helpful in supporting breathwork. These physical practices ideally accompany breathwork; some may need to precede it. Only through understanding the profound interaction between physicality, vitality (or breath), and emotionality clinicians can offer breathwork in a way that fully honors each client's individuality and context.

Part IV: Breathwork Strategies and Techniques for Integrated Holistic Practice

In its four chapters, Part IV offers specific breathing strategies. For some of you that may be the highlight of the book. I hope you will persevere and read the prior chapters. The specific breathing techniques offered in this part work most auspiciously if grounded in the larger integrated holistic paradigm offered throughout. Chapter 8 offers guidelines and hints about how to introduce patients to breathwork by first inviting them to become more attuned to how they are already breathing. Breath observation and awareness are key to beginning breathwork in the most auspicious way. From there, Chap. 9 provides thorough instructions for how to help patients move into optimal functional breathing in daily life, with significant focus on subtle breathing strategies. Finally, Chaps. 10 and 11 present a variety of specialized breathing techniques, most grounded in the yoga tradition and thoroughly supported by modern science. These techniques range widely from four-part breathing, alternate nostril breathing, breathing with sound, to breathing with force. For all techniques, many variations are offered that help create greater accessibility, clarify intentionality, lead to benefit from the practice, honor all layers of experience of each patient, and integrate a multitude of strategies.

And with that we have come full circle. The integrated holistic paradigm for breathwork is now yours to explore.

My Expression of Gratitude to You the Reader...

Thank you for reading this book in all its imperfections. If you know me, perhaps you will see, hear, and feel me in these pages. I am in there somewhere—sometimes more hidden, sometimes more openly present. I can tell you that my spoken voice is not like my written voice. So, if you know me really well, you may be surprised at times. I would like to say I am a little funnier and more open-hearted in person than in writing. But maybe that is just my delusion, one of my many misperceptions. 😊 Anyways, enjoy the journey through this forest—enjoy the bird's eye view from above, enjoy each tree, and maybe even enjoy the weeds. I am offering this writing to you with humility, gratitude, and a deep sense of appreciation that I have been given this opportunity to journey with you through the art and science of breathwork. I thank all of you who are holding this book in your hands, whether in paper or electronic form. I thank all of you who have been an important part of the journey. May you breathe well; may you breathe softly, gently, silently, and with your whole being. May the pulsation of life guide you in your journey as you breathe resiliently and coherently.

> For breath is life, and if you breathe well
> you will live long on the earth.—Sanskrit Proverb

P.S. *Dear Clinicians and Teachers,*

Many samples of the practices discussed in this volume are offered in one of my non-public YouTube playlists. Please feel free to access this exclusive playlist with the following link. As needed and appropriate, you may share individual video links from this playlist with your patients and students. https://www.youtube.com/playlist?list=PLzvkZpUGjwIGxil7eP9j41Zw4PALDm6yx.

Additional breathing-related practices are accessible in my public playlists on the YogaXTeam YouTube channel. These playlists are being updated regularly. The most relevant playlist is about a variety of breathing practices and can be accessed via the following link. https://www.youtube.com/playlist?list=PLzvkZpUGjwIFmpZVzy_25k4Zr4GHm75Y5.

With gratitude,

Stanford, CA, USA   Christiane Brems

Acknowledgments: It Takes a Community

There are two ways to live your life: One is as though nothing is a miracle, the other is as though everything is a miracle.—Albert Einstein

My life has been full of miracles—mostly miracles in the form of people who came into my life at the right time and in the best possible way. I owe all of you a larger debt of gratitude than I can ever repay. I have done my best to be worthy of your kindness, compassion, and teachings. This book is yours as much as it is mine. Your wisdom, compassion, and inspiration infuse every page.

Allow me to start with my profound indebtedness and deep caring for my colleague, friend, and role model, Dr. Laura Roberts, Chair of the Department of Psychiatry and Behavioral Sciences at Stanford School of Medicine. Laura, you came into my life in the last millennium! (Yes, this likely "outs" both of us for our age and—hopefully—associated wisdom.) ☺ Since that time, you have inspired me through your actions and commitments; encouraged me through your belief in the basic goodness of human beings; and been a confidante, friend, compassionate other, and loving and kind presence. Most recently, it was you, Laura, who opened not only your heart, but also a door. You took a chance on my vision to bring yoga—and its many integrated practices—into healthcare. You gave a home to YogaX, a collective dedicated to helping create access to yoga for those who need it most and are often excluded. Since 2019, YogaX has had the privilege to train healthcare providers to become yoga professionals who integrate the practice into their lives and clinical practice. All of us associated with YogaX owe you a deep debt of gratitude, Dr. Roberts.

Speaking of YogaX, my deepest gratitude goes to the YogaX community—colleagues, trainees, alumni and alumnae, affiliates, friends, students, and the larger circles of people who share the joy of yoga with us. The YogaX community is a precious gift to all of us. It has provided us opportunity to bring yoga into settings where it often is needed but not accessible. We are grateful to be part of a greater movement, shared by the International Association of Yoga Therapy and Yoga Alliance, that is promoting recognition of yoga as a therapeutic discipline, deeply honoring its salutary and wholesome roots and finding ways to integrate it proactively and thoughtfully into modern healthcare.

Deep appreciation and ever-lasting gratitude also goes to my many teachers on the path to self-discovery. Klaus, my very first yoga teacher when I was just a wide-eyed youth—you started me on this journey and I cannot thank you enough. I may have forgotten your last name (it was after all 50 years ago), but your impact on my life is as palpable today as it was back then. Lynne Minton—you are an eye-opening inspiration, a yogi in the truest sense of the word, and a wonderful mentor as I started my journey into teaching yoga. Monica Devine, Sarahjoy Marsh, Judith Hansen Lasater, and Christopher Wallis—you inspired me and guided me in the most meaningful ways. Marty Rossman—you gave me the gift of guided imagery; Patrick McKeown— you shared your profound wisdom and belief in the Buteyko method; Stephen Porges—you imparted your insights into polyvagal theory. Your collective depth of knowledge and commitment left indelible marks on my work and my life. Many Buddhist teachers have deeply inspired and transformed me although I never met them in person—thank you, Yongey Mingyur Rinpoche, Joseph Goldstein, and Lama Tillmann Borghardt. My commitment to diversity, equity, and accessibility was shared and nourished by two beloved (late) colleagues—indigenous psychologist Robert Morgan and Yupik healer Rita Blumenstein (once an elder on the International Council of 13 Grandmothers). You remain in my heart always. All of you have shaped me as a human being, teacher, clinician, colleague, and partner. I am filled with gratitude to each and every one of you.

I am forever grateful to you, my students and clients, who may have taught and changed me most of all. I am grateful to you for sharing your wisdom, insights, vulnerabilities, faith, courage, hearts, and experiences. Nothing in life taught me more than being a part of your journeys and witnessing your resilience, joy, and learning. I have learned more from you than I could have ever hoped for. I am filled with the deepest gratitude and love for all of you. You have enriched my life in endless ways that will be with me always. To my "students" (well, you are really my teachers as much as I am yours) who have shared the journey through cancer—my weekly time with you has been nothing short of miraculous. You have shown the strongest spirit, deep capacity for mutual compassion and caring, and enormous resilience in the wake of intense suffering.

I am filled with gratitude and love for all of my German family, especially my father Bernard Brems, my sister Gabriele Strubel, and brother-in-law Floh Strubel. You are my roots. We may be thousands of miles apart; yet whenever we meet, whenever we talk, whenever we are in one another's thoughts, the distance is gone. We are connected in spirit—always. I am deeply thankful for your presence in my life—Ich danke Euch allen von ganzem Herzen.

Finally, I am most profoundly and eternally grateful for my intrepid, compassionate, patient (beyond belief), supportive, loving, funny (thanks for the strong core muscles), and unwavering partner, Mark Johnson. You are the love of my life, my best friend, my most trusted human being, and my inspiration. You have helped shape my way of being in the world more than anyone. You constantly rekindle my faith and my joy; you help me feel whole. The greatest miracle in my life was crossing paths with you nearly 40 years ago and having shared a road ever since.

Thank you all!

Chris

One moment can change a day, one day can change a life and one life can change the world.—The Buddha

Contents

About the Author

Christiane Brems directs YogaX in the Department of Psychiatry and Behavioral Sciences, Stanford School of Medicine where she is a Clinical Professor. YogaX is an innovative special initiative providing therapeutic yoga education for healthcare professionals, yoga teacher training, and community services with emphasis on integrating therapeutic yoga into healthcare. Dr. Brems is a licensed and board-certified clinical psychologist (ABPP); registered yoga teacher (E-RYT500); and certified C-IAYT yoga therapist, Interactive Imagery Guide, and Buteyko Method Breathing Instructor. She is professor emerita at the University of Alaska Anchorage, where she held leadership positions, including Director of the Center for Behavioral Health Research and Services, Director of the Ph.D. Program in Clinical-Community Psychology, and Interim Vice Provost for Research. She is professor emerita at Pacific University Oregon, where she served as Dean of the School of Graduate Psychology. Dr. Brems is a professor, researcher, and clinician with interest in yoga, health promotion, and rural healthcare delivery. Her research has been funded by the NIH, CDC, and SAMHSA, among others. Dr. Brems has shared her work in the peer-reviewed literature, technical reports, and books, including the *Comprehensive Guide to Child Psychotherapy*, *Dealing with Challenges in Psychotherapy and Counseling*, *Basic Skills in Counseling and Psychotherapy*, and others.

Part I

Historical and Conceptual Context for Breathwork

Creating a Context for Breathwork

1

Yoga psychology sees the mind and breath as bound together in the frame of the human body. There is no mind without breath, no stillness in the body without stillness in the mind, and no stillness in the mind without settled breath… The practice of waking up the mind and body and the practice of stilling the mind and body go hand and hand in what is referred to as the royal path of yoga.

Michael Stone in the Inner Tradition of Yoga

1.1   Overview: Breathwork in Context

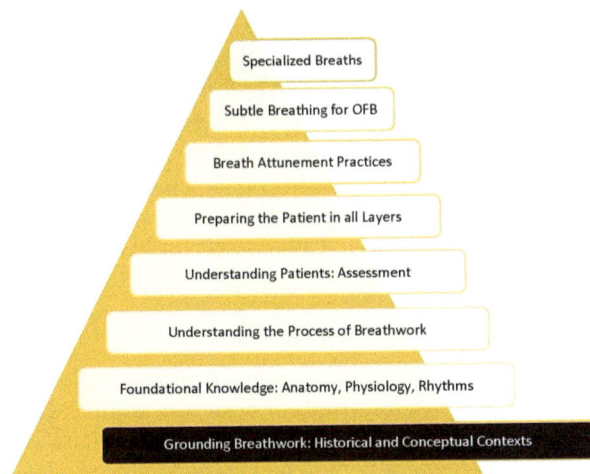

Specialized Breaths

Subtle Breathing for OFB

Breath Attunement Practices

Preparing the Patient in all Layers

Understanding Patients: Assessment

Understanding the Process of Breathwork

Foundational Knowledge: Anatomy, Physiology, Rhythms

Grounding Breathwork: Historical and Conceptual Contexts

C. Brems, *Therapeutic Breathwork*,
https://doi.org/10.1007/978-3-031-66683-4_1

Breath is life, breath is the bridge between body and mind, breath reflects our inner world, breath absorbs our outer experiences, breath can support us or fail us, breath binds us together. Breathing is essential and therefore largely automatic. It tends to come to our attention when there is difficulty or challenge—when we cannot catch our breath, when we hyperventilate, when we are congested, when we are afraid. We do not have to learn how to breathe—the breath comes naturally. However, sometimes our breath presents or reflects challenges, difficulties, illness, and worry. It is in the moments when breath becomes a struggle that we take note and begin to wonder. It is in these moments, when learning something about how we breathe, can support greater health and well-being in our bodies, our vitality, even our thoughts and emotions. This is these moments in which breathwork—learning about healthful and nourishing breathing—can become life-changing. This chapter provides an overview of the history of breathwork and presents an integrated and holistic context for learning how to work with breath and breathing to increase health, vigor, and resilience, and to foster greater fortitude, persistence, and compassion. This chapter explains that breathwork is not a practice to be engaged in free of the greater context that shapes our human lives and experiences—that breath and breathing are linked to our circumstances, our relationships, our work, our communities, even our planet. It provides an integrated holistic context for breath, breathing, and breathwork that attends to accessibility, beneficence, intentionality, wholism—honoring all layers of our human experience, and integration—drawing on all available resources to deepen and enhance the experience of living a human life.

1.2   Breathwork in a Historical Context

Breath, like most human experiences, is both simple and complex. Breath is with us from the moment we are born to the moment we die. It is with us every minute of every day, embedded in every experience and reflected in every action. Our first breath is likely a very jolting breath and, of course, energizing and vitalizing. Our last breath is likely subtle and muted as vitality and life gently leave our bodies; or, perhaps, that final breath is sudden, outside of our awareness, as life and vitality end abruptly. For some of us, breath feels natural and is simply there, often outside of our awareness. For others, breath is labored and difficult and grabs our attention with a fear for our lives. Many of us recognize at an intuitive level that breath represents more than inhalations and exhalations, as it imbues us with vitality, provides feedback about our state of mind and body, helps us release tension, and supports us in a nourishing and enlivening way. This realization points to the subtler dimensions of breath called *life force* based on ancient wisdom traditions (i.e., *chi* in Chinese medicine; *Prana* in yoga; *pneuma* in ancient Greece) or the wise *combination of affect and arousal* in the language of modern science. This force, energy, or vitality lies within us, as well as outside of us, around us, and in others—a combination of personal and collective vital forces that connect us to our greater community of sentient beings (and perhaps beyond).

1.2.1 A Modern Context for Breathwork

Breath, and the life force it represents, have many manifestations and patterns and are truly an endless subject of interest and influence. It is not surprising that breath has been pondered, contemplated, talked about, and eventually written about for millennia. Ancient thinkers and practitioners, as much as we are today, were fully aware of the central role of breath and vitality. Almost every ancient spiritual or contemplative tradition has addressed breath and breathing. These explorations have created overlapping concepts and practices, as well as highly unique ways of addressing breath and breathing historically. Of great interest in current times, are traditions of breathwork that arose from ancient Buddhism and yoga. In Buddhism, the focus on breath and breathing is generally directed to breath observation and breath awareness. Yoga offers additional complexity. It too honors and values observing the breath and becoming aware of how breath and vitality move through us. Additionally, yogic tradition offers practices that seek to alter or enhance the breath and its rhythms. Yoga traditions treasure subtle, soft smooth, gentle, and muted breathing. In fact, it is said that ancient yogis declared life to be measured not in days, but in breaths. It stands to reason from that assertion that the slower, softer, and gentler we breathe, the longer our lives may be. Of course, this notion has been impossible to measure; however, modern science has produced compelling data that support the idea that stable, coherent, and slow-paced breathing may be more helpful to us than vigorous or forceful breathing, especially in circumstances of rest and daily life. Certainly, some circumstances require an active breath, adapted to the level of effort and exertion. Unfortunately, in current times labored breathing and overbreathing have become more common than they are helpful, manifesting even when energetic demands are met best by slower and subtler breathing.

Our current culture of overbreathing [1] has many causes and conditions and involves many factors and forces. Not the least of these forces have to do with the types of environments and experiences we have created. Biopsychosociocultural factors that affect how we breathe and how we experience our vitality range widely in their characteristics and in their influence on the breath. In some places in the world, strong influences on breath arise from the political reality that there is no air clean enough to breathe without unwholesome consequences. In other places, social and socioeconomic influences on breath and breathing are related to stressors that strain mental and emotional well-being. Overly challenging, controlling, demanding work circumstances can lead to stress breathing that becomes so habitual that it settles itself into our nervous system and tissues in a relentless way. Experiences of complex trauma can embed themselves in our nervous system, causing permanent changes in our affect and arousal in response to typical stimuli in the world. Some factors that affect our breath may be biological, such as sudden exposure to an environmental or food-based allergen that causes dysregulation, perhaps even discontinuation, of the breath.

Causes and conditions that affect breath and vitality can arise situationally, acutely, or chronically and can either support or dysregulate our breathing. Often, we are not aware that this is happening, as we are out of tune with our physical, energetic, and affective consciousness. This lack of attunement to our inner world prevents us from noticing our own distress patterns and interferes with our capacity to access ready strategies for helping us come back into physical and energetic equilibrium (both with regard to arousal level and affective reactivity). For these reasons, modern breathwork is finding its place in healthcare and mental healthcare as a strategy for grounding and recovery. Breathwork in the context of healthcare (broadly defined) can serve care providers' own self-care and well-being and provide a range of helpful interventions for clients, patients, or students. However, because of its complexity, breathwork is most effective and conducive to success if applied in a tailored, strategic, informed, and intentional manner. Contrary to popular belief, breathwork is not as simple as applying random breathing techniques in a room full of people in a yoga studio or gym. Each of those human beings is likely to have a different breathing pattern as well as different life factors and conditions that affect their breath, moment to moment, in diverse and idiosyncratic ways. These human beings in their diversity need approaches that reflect their unique context and varied experiences.

The relationship between context and experience with breath is not a one-way street. It is not even a two-way street. It is more akin to the complex tangle of the streets of London. There are so many locations to turn toward, so many ways to reach to the same place, innumerable ways to get lost, too many options to choose wisely all the time, opportunities to be lost *and* found, side streets that end up being dead ends, detours that end up being the most amazing discoveries, etc. The metaphor could continue. If we, as healthcare providers or yoga teachers, are interested in applying yoga in healthcare, if we want to be breathing guides, we need to untangle the complexity of breath and breathing for ourselves and with each patient. We need to understand the context in which breathing patterns arose and in which each new breath continues to arise; we need to understand the conditions in which the breath affects each and every aspect of our own and our clients' way of being and relating. We need to understand and honor the complexity of breath and breathing, and we need to understand how to work with breath and breathing in intentional and beneficial ways that are tailored to our patients' needs. We need to understand breathwork, and breathing interventions, on a multitude of levels, an understanding that can trace its roots in ancient wisdom and its branches in modern science. Ancient wisdom and spiritual traditions have transmitted—across the ages and across practitioners—profound breathing strategies for transformation, evolution, and growth. Modern science has offered refinements by providing data that help illuminate which practices serve and do not serve in particular circumstances and under particular conditions with specific human beings. The integration of ancient wisdom about breath and breathing with modern science about breathwork applications creates a tailored and wise approach to guiding students, clients, and patients into the world of breath, breathing, and breathwork in a skillful, wholesome, and auspicious manner.

The journey into the many complexities of breath and breathwork is not always easy, but it deeply honors the biological, psychological, social, and cultural contexts and experiences of breathers as well as clinicians who may help guide them into new experiences of breath and breathing. The paradigm of breath complexity offered in this volume is deeply grounded in ancient wisdom traditions that honor breath and life force (including, but not limited to, Buddhism and yoga) as well as in modern neuroscience, interpersonal neurobiology, physiology, anatomy, and psychology. As we start our journey into the science of breath and breathing, our explorations may seem somewhat dry as we look at the breath from an anatomical and physiological perspective; sometimes, they may be startling and eye-opening as we explore breath rhythms and nervous system adaptations that develop over the course of life; sometimes, our explorations may offer empowerment, pointing out ways in which we and our patients can breathe to reverse unwholesome patterns and ways in which household energy. We begin our journey with a very brief look at how breath and breathing have appeared across the millennia in various wisdom and contemplative traditions.

1.2.2   Tracing the Lineage of Breathwork from Antiquity to Modernity

The following brief historical overview simply serves to remind us that breathwork is not new; it did not emerge in the 1900s or in the era of COVID-19. It simply was brought to the forefront of our attention while we were struggling with our breath during the recent pandemic that took too many lives. It is not surprising that books on breath and breathing rose to success during the COVID-19 crisis. However, breathwork has been an important part of human life for more than two millennia. It is important to remember this fact and to appreciate that each form of breathwork tells a story about the specific context in which it was created. There is no right or wrong story or approach; there are many stories reflecting the unique circumstances in which particular types of breathwork developed, were practiced, and were taught. Some causes and conditions may still apply today; others may be obsolete. Certain kinds of breathwork that are adaptive in one context may no longer apply in newer contexts. Conversely, and perhaps curiously, some breathwork that has been developed in modern times may only serve to reflect and perpetuate the already agitated and overly energized and exhausted organisms that we have become.

Breath and Breathing in Ancient and Pre-Modern Yogic Traditions
Not surprisingly, given its grounding in ancient histories and a variety of human contexts (from philosophy, to healing arts and science, to spiritual practices), breathwork encompasses a diverse array of techniques aimed at harnessing the power of breath to promote physical health, mental well-being, and spiritual growth. From the ancient Vedic texts of India to the philosophical reflections on breath and breathing of ancient Greece, from Taoist traditions of China, to contemplative practices of Buddhism, the significance of breath and breathing to coping, healing, and thriving has been recognized and explored through various conceptualizations and applications of breathwork. Following is a very cursory journey through the rich history of breathwork, tracing the most relevant spiritual roots, philosophical underpinnings,

and practices developed in a variety of contexts across time. This history is offered to acknowledge that modern breathwork is nothing new—it stands on the shoulders of the ancients who recognized the importance of breath and breathing before the advent of objective research methods and modern technologies to measure the physical, vital, mental, and emotional impacts of breathwork. This history is also not complete or comprehensive; it is likely to suffer from grave omissions that hopefully can be filled by resources dedicated specifically to exploring the historical evolution of breath and breathing. The following exploration is an acknowledgment, not a history of the ancient tapestry of breathwork.

Roots of breathing practices are deeply anchored in a long history of Eastern spiritual traditions and philosophical or healing contexts worldwide since at least 700 BCE when breathwork references first emerged in the *Brihadaranyaka Upanishad* of India. In ancient India, breathwork was deeply intertwined with spiritual practices concerned with accessing higher states of consciousness and self-realization. The Vedas, the oldest scriptures of Hinduism, contain hymns about the vitality or life force (*Prana*) that moves through everything and the specific life force that is embodied in breath and breathing (lowercase *"prana"*). From these ancient explorations of breath and breathing, the yogic concept of pranayama emerged, which is typically translated as *control or regulation of breath* to harness and conserve vital energy to support physical, mental, and spiritual well-being. Ancient breathwork, or *pranayama*, became deeply embedded in the spiritual practices of yoga, as elucidated in many ancient and premodern sacred texts, including, but not limited, to the *Brihadaranyaka Upanishads, Bhagavad Gita, Maitrayanaiya Upanishads, Yoga Sutras of Patanjali,* and *Hatha Yoga Pradipika*. These texts contain detailed instructions on various breathing techniques aimed at purifying the body, vitalizing energy, calming the mind, and awakening higher states of consciousness.

The *Brihadaranyaka Upanishad*, one of the oldest texts in the Vedic tradition, holds profound insights into the nature of existence, consciousness, and the practice of yoga. Its earliest explicit reference to pranayama may date back to at least 700 BCE, stating *"One should indeed breathe in (arise), but one should also breathe out (without setting) while saying, Let not the misery that is dying reach* me" (translation by John Wells; http://darshanapress.com/Brihadaranyaka%20Upanishad%20Book%201.pdf, p. 71). The *Brihadaranyaka Upanishad* thus explores the significance of breath as a physiological act *and* a spiritual practice. The text emphasizes the importance of both inhalation and exhalation, highlighting the cyclical nature of breathing and, as such, encapsulates the aspiration for liberation from suffering and the transcendence of the cycle of birth and death. The breath's cyclical process is seen as mirroring the rhythms of existence, in which every beginning is followed by an end, and every end paves the way for a new beginning. By acknowledging both aspects, this perspective on breathing invites practitioners to align with the natural flow of life, transcending fears of death or suffering.

The *Brihadaranyaka Upanishad* suggests that through the practice of pranayama, humans can move beyond physical existence to realize deeper, spiritual dimensions of being, allowing them to gain access to higher states of consciousness and the experience of union or unity. The notion that we can realize immortality through proper breathing suggests that the true essence of self, according to this ancient text, is eternal and transcendent. Simply by attuning to subtle energies of breath and breathing, human beings can recognize their interconnectedness with one another and the cosmos. *Pranayama*, from this perspective, provides a portal into the union of individual consciousness with the universal life force, a profound sense of interconnectedness that transcends boundaries between self and the divine.

Further addressing breath and breathing, the *Bhagavad Gita* is a sacred Hindu scripture that is part of the Indian epic *Mahabharata*, dating fifth to second centuries BCE. In a dialogue between Prince Arjuna and the god Krishna (Arjuna's charioteer and spiritual guide), the text addresses profound philosophical, moral, and ethical dilemmas. Chapter 4 of the *Bhagavad Gita*, titled "The Yoga of Knowledge," looks at various paths of spiritual practice, including the concepts of sacrifice (*yajna*) and regulation of breath as a means to attain higher states of consciousness and control over the senses. Verse 29 specifically highlights the significance of breath control in spiritual practice. It describes different methods of offering the breath as a sacrifice, symbolizing *control* and *regulation* of life energy (*Prana*) for spiritual purification and enlightenment. It states:

> Still others offer as sacrifice the outgoing breath in the incoming breath, while some offer the incoming breath into the outgoing breath. Some arduously practice *prāṇāyām* and restrain the incoming and outgoing breaths, purely absorbed in the regulation of the life-energy. Yet others curtail their food intake and offer the breath into the life-energy as sacrifice. All these knowers of sacrifice are cleansed of their impurities as a result of such performances. (Translation by Swami Myundananda; https://www.holy-bhagavad-gita.org/chapter/4/verse/29-30)

As such, the text suggests various approaches to pranayama, beginning with the merging of exhalation and inhalation—a metaphor for harmonizing the breath cycle that symbolizes an integration of opposing forces or dualities within oneself. Other practices focus on the incoming breath, merging it into the outgoing breath, in a slightly different approach to achieving unity and balance, implying more activating energy. Various other techniques of breath control and regulation include consciously manipulating breath to regulate the flow of *Prana* (life force) throughout the body, thereby calming the mind and gaining mastery over the senses. From the perspective of the *Bhagavad Gita*, pranayama cleanses impurities in the practitioner's physical, mental, emotional, and spiritual realms. Such purification allows for alignment with higher truths and ultimately leads to self-realization and spiritual evolution. Unfortunately, concepts of purification that emerge in the *Bhagavad Gita* have been abused in modern times as justifications for enormous atrocities of genocide, making reference to the *Bhagavad Gita* highly problematic and controversial.

The *Maitrayaniya Upanishad*, dated to approximately the fourth century BCE, is another significant text within the Upanishads, ancient India's collection of philosophical and spiritual texts. This particular Upanishad is known for its elucidation of a complex framework for spiritual practice, a frame that places great importance on pranayama. The *Maitrayanaiya Upanishads* confirm pranayama as a method for harnessing and directing *Prana* (life force) to achieve physical health, mental clarity, and spiritual enlightenment. Relevant to the current context, *Maitrayaniya* Sections. 6.18–6.30 emphasize pranayama as being most appropriately situated in a broader framework of six component practices (most are familiar to modern yogis in the lineage of Patanjali's 8-limbed path, which is elucidated below):

- *Pranayama*: control of breath
- *Pratyahara*: withdrawal of the senses from external stimuli, directing attention inward
- *Dharana*: concentration, focusing the mind on a single point or object
- *Dhyana*: meditation, the uninterrupted flow of awareness toward a chosen object or concept
- *Tarka*: reasoning or contemplation, engaging the intellect in reflective inquiry or creative exploration
- *Samadhi*: union or absorption, the state of complete integration and transcendence, often described as the culmination of spiritual practice

The inclusion of pranayama in this listing of spiritual practices underscores the importance of breathwork in the process of spiritual self-realization and liberation. However, it also underscores that pranayama is not practiced in isolation, but is optimally embedded in a system of practices. This concept of practice integration is encountered repeatedly over the centuries; it also is the approach to breathwork described in this book. We encounter the clearest call for practice integration in the *Yoga Sutras of Patanjali*.

The *Yoga Sutras of Patanjali*, believed to have been compiled between the second and fifth centuries CE, is a foundational text of yoga philosophy, outlining integrated yoga principles and practices in 196 concise sutras (or aphorisms). Central to the *Yoga Sutras is Patanjali's* elucidation of eight limbs of yoga, with pranayama being the fourth limb, following the ethical practices of yoga (Limb 1 or *yama*), practices of discipline and life purpose (Limb 2 or *niyama*), and physical practices (Limb 3 or *asana*). *Pranayama* is an essential prerequisite for the inner practices of yoga, namely, withdrawal or guarding of the senses (Limb 5 or *pratyahara*), concentration (Limb 6 or *dharana*), meditation (Limb 7 or *dhyana*), and absorption (Limb 8 or *samadhi*). Relevant to the context of breathwork, Patanjali described *pranayama* as the regulation of inhalation, exhalation, and breath retention, leading to the preservation of vitality and life force, as well as increasing mental clarity and focus. Given the continued relevance of the *Yoga Sutras of Patanjali* and the 8-limbed approach to yoga practice, a more detailed exploration of the eight limbs of yoga and their interdependence and co-practice with pranayama or breathwork is presented later in this chapter.

The *Hatha Yoga Pradipika*, a seminal text attributed to the sage Swami Swatmarama and believed to have been written in the mid-1300s, can be understood as one of the earliest comprehensive manuals detailing the application of hatha yoga, including *pranayama*. *Pranayama*, as prescribed in the *Hatha Yoga Pradipika*, is not only a practical set of recommendations about how to breathe but emphasizes yet again that breathing practices need to be woven into a larger framework of yogic practices to achieve health in all aspects of self—physical, vital, mental, emotional, and relational. The text emphasizes the integration of physical postures, breathwork, and contemplative (or inner) practices to facilitate overall resilience and well-being. While the manual outlines a variety of specific breathing strategies, such as alternate nostril breathing, breath retention, and subtle breathing, these practices are not to be used in isolation but rather in an integrated and complete context. The integrated approach advocated in *Hatha Yoga Pradipika* highlights the interconnectedness of all layers of human experience within the relational contexts of human existence. It emphasizes the need to deepen our understanding of being in the world, of our reactivities and needs, suggesting that we grow and transform through freeing ourselves from pattern locks and habits in all realms of existence. The focus on integrating a variety of tailored and meaningful practices to support health and resilience is a strong foundation for the type of breathwork that is offered in this book, called integrated holistic breathwork (described in detail later).

Breath and Breathing in Other Ancient Traditions

In Taoist traditions, breathwork is known as *qigong* or *chi kung* and has played a central role in the pursuit of longevity, vitality, and spiritual cultivation. Taoist thinkers viewed the breath as a bridge between the material and immaterial realms, with breathing techniques designed to harmonize and refine the flow of vital energy (or *chi*, the Taoist equivalent to *Prana*) within the body. Numerous breathing practices have been developed and applied to circulate and refine vitality, fostering physical health, emotional balance, and spiritual enlightenment. Ancient Greek philosophers, including Socrates and Plato, contemplated the nature of breath and its significance to human existence. These important thinkers explored the role of breath in sustaining life, regulating emotions, and attaining self-mastery. Their concept of *pneuma* or breath encompassed the physical act of breathing as well as the animating principle (or life force) that was perceived as permeating the cosmos. Western philosophers, while clearly aware of the importance of breath and life force, did not document specific breathing practices.

Breathwork has also been explored in the context of Islam, with scholars exploring connections between breath, health, and consciousness in medical and philosophical works. For example, Avicenna, in the "*Canon of Medicine*," emphasized the importance of breath in maintaining physical health and balance and preserving overall well-being. Islamic mystics or Sufis have been reported to practice forms of breath control as a means of purifying the heart, quieting the mind, and drawing closer to the divine. While some ancient Taoist and Sufi breathing practices are still used in their original context, they have less prominence in modern Western breathwork than yogic pranayama traditions. Thus, we will not explore these practices in any greater detail.

Yogic Breathwork in the Modern Era

Teachings from ancient yogic texts have laid a foundation for modern yoga practices that are integrated rather than unidimensional (although unfortunately, many modern Western yoga practices have unduly reduced themselves to physical practices). Wisdom-based yoga practices emphasize the integrated nature of postural or movement work; breathwork; concentration and meditation; awareness, self-inquiry, and insight; and ethical and purposeful lifestyle commitments. Influential modern-day yogis have further refined the understanding and application of *pranayama* in contemporary contexts, often profoundly influenced not only by ancient text, but also by modern thinkers and research. A few examples of modern breathwork teachers from the integrated yogic tradition are introduced here, followed by an overview of other modern breathwork providers who are less linked to ancient yoga and yet often offer techniques and strategies that are linkable to or derived from ancient yogic practices (although without formal acknowledgment). Any omissions of important breathwork guides are unintentional and do not mean to diminish their importance or influence.

B.K.S. Iyengar, renowned for precise alignment-based postural yoga, emphasized the importance of pranayama as a means to refine the mind and body [2]. *Pranayama* is integrated into a broader practice of yoga, often following a period of posture practice. Iyengar's *pranayama* techniques typically involve specific breath ratios, controlled inhalation, controlled exhalation, and breath retention practices, all contextualized within a greater yoga practice that fosters awareness of body alignment and energetic pathways. Iyengar yoga emphasizes yoga as a lifestyle that deeply honors inner practices as well as yoga's ethical foundations [3].

Richard Rosen offers a contemporary perspective on pranayama rooted in traditional integrated teachings. His approach emphasizes simplicity and accessibility, making pranayama practices adaptable for modern practitioners. Rosen teaches a graduated approach to pranayama that builds on careful foundations of physical and emotional preparedness. He encourages foundational breathwork with a focus on cultivating mindfulness and steady breath rhythm before diving into more advanced and complex breathing practices. His meticulous books [4, 5] that take readers through carefully sequenced breathwork and physical preparation have had a profound impact on yogic breathing, as taught in the context of Western yoga asana classes. The books remain helpful and meaningful references for yoga students, and even yoga teachers.

Robin Rothenberg, a yoga therapist and Buteyko breathing coach, explores pranayama from a personal and subtle perspective of breath and breathing [6]. Her approach honors the deep wisdom roots of yoga. Drawing on her training in the Buteyko method in addition to yoga traditions, she emphasizes subtlety in breathing, guided by breath awareness and mindful exploration of breathing patterns to support healing and self-regulation. She offers thoughtful variations and approaches to deeply rooted pranayama practices that emphasize diaphragmatic breathing, attention to exhalation, and exploration of breath rhythms. She acknowledges the profound influence of breath on the nervous system and investigates the subtle dimension of breathing as represented in the yoga traditions that honor the chakras. She is a modern breath guide who offers an integrated pranayama experience.

Iyengar, Rosen, and Rothenberg are examples of yoga teachers who embed pranayama in a greater context of wisdom- and history-guided yoga practice. They clarify that breathwork is only one of many steps in the yogic journey. As such, they are deeply influenced by ancient wisdom. Many modern yoga studio practices, on the other hand, offer breathwork as an aside, not as an essential practice to the overall immersion in yogic wisdom. Breathing is a by-product of or support for movement; other aspects of the ancient traditions (such as lifestyle, ethics, and inner practices) are often left out altogether. It is beyond the scope of this book to explore how reducing yoga to a physical practice came to be. Others have begun this exploration, and the reader is referred to their work [7, 8].

Western Breathwork in the Modern Era

Buteyko Method

Turning now to developments in breathwork in the twentieth century, the *Buteyko Method* offers a set of breathing guidelines developed by Konstantin Buteyko in 1950s Russia. It focuses on correcting dysfunctional breathing patterns, particularly overbreathing or hyperventilation, which Buteyko believed to be a root cause of various health issues. The method emphasizes nasal breathing, reduced breathing, and breath retention to support healthy levels of CO_2. In contrast to other modern breathing methods that incorporate hyperventilation or extreme breathing practices, the Buteyko Method advocates for gentle, controlled breathing techniques aimed at restoring natural breathing patterns. Rather than emphasizing forceful inhalations or rapid breathing, it prioritizes the regulation of breath volume.

Patrick McKeown has played a significant role in popularizing and expanding upon Buteyko's work and has become the current expert in the field of breathing re-education. He has greatly elucidated the physiological mechanisms behind the method's effectiveness, having dedicated himself to providing evidence-based explanations for its benefits. McKeown [9, 10] has refined and expanded the repertoire of breathing exercises and techniques within the method, along with structured programs and protocols to guide individuals through the process of retraining their breathing habits. His work has demonstrated how Buteyko techniques can enhance athletic performance, alleviate stress and anxiety, transform asthma, improve sleep quality, and promote overall well-being. By making the method accessible through books, online courses, and workshops, McKeown has empowered individuals worldwide to take control of their breathing habits and optimize their health. Many of his principles and practices are embraced in this book.

Various Other Modern Breathwork Systems

Western interest in breathwork as a wellness practice grew beyond yoga, promoted (among others) by Wilhelm Reich, Stanislav Grof, and Wim Hof. While their breathing practices are not of great importance to the context of this book, it is helpful to be aware of their existence, as they have influenced some modern yoga teachers and breathing guides in a manner that may not be fully useful to their students or patients. Thus, a few of these Western systems are explored here, not as examples of integrated systems of breathwork, but as examples of how breathwork can arise out of a specific context or intention. While such practices have great meaning and utility *in their specific contexts*, if they are removed from their original intention and thoughtlessly applied in new contexts, they may have the potential to do harm.

Wilhelm Reich, a psychiatrist and psychoanalyst, developed breath-oriented psychotherapy techniques in the 1930s and 1940s. His work focused on the relationship between body and mind, emphasizing the importance of releasing physical and emotional tension stored in the body to promote mental health and well-being. Reich developed breathing-oriented psychotherapy techniques as part of his broader exploration of the mind-body connection and the role of energy in psychological well-being [11]. His work, influenced by his background in psychoanalysis and bioenergetics, aimed to address emotional blockages and restore energetic balance in the body through specific breathing exercises. Reich believed that emotional trauma and repressed feelings could manifest as physical tensions and blockages in the body, leading to various forms of psychological distress and physical illness. He theorized that by accessing and releasing these emotional blockages, individuals could experience profound psychological and physical healing.

Reich's techniques were designed to help individuals become aware of their breath and its connection to emotions and bodily sensations. They involved a combination of deep, diaphragmatic breathing, mindful awareness of bodily sensations, and gentle movement exercises to encourage the release of emotional energy trapped in muscular tensions. Through these practices, individuals can gradually unravel layers of emotional armor and access buried feelings, leading to a sense of catharsis and relief. Overall, Wilhelm Reich's development of breath-oriented psychotherapy techniques represented a pioneering effort to integrate the principles of psychoanalysis with somatic approaches to healing. By focusing on the breath as a pathway to accessing and releasing emotional blockages, Reich offered a holistic framework for promoting psychological well-being and restoring energetic balance in the body.

In the early 1970s, Stanislav Grof explored breathwork as a catalyst for psychospiritual transformation via what he termed Holotropic Breathwork [12]. In his method, clients lie down in a comfortable space and engage in continuous, deep, and fast breathing intended to increase the flow of oxygen and energy in the body. Influenced by Grof's research on LSD-assisted psychotherapy, rapid breathing is intended to activate innate healing and self-exploration mechanisms. The altered states induced by this type of breathwork are meant to facilitate access to the unconscious mind, the release of repressed emotions, and the recovery of memories, including those related to past trauma. The cathartic emotional release, profound insight, and spiritual experiences offered by this method are most likely to be realized in the presence of a carefully trained facilitator who creates a safe and supportive environment to help participants navigate challenging or intense experiences that may arise.

Last, beginning in the 1980s, the Wim Hof Method [13] emerged and gained significant attention and momentum in the early twenty-first century. This method combines specific breathing exercises, cold exposure, and mindset techniques to improve physical and mental well-being. Breathwork involves three phases, beginning with a series of hyperventilation breaths, followed by breath retention, and ending with breath recovery. The three-step process is repeated for several cycles. Although the Wim Hof Method has gained popularity and has been endorsed by many practitioners for its potential health benefits, it needs to be approached with caution, especially by individuals with underlying health conditions. The focus on hyperventilation, especially in combination with breath holding, can present great challenges and has the potential to cause harm.

1.3   Breathwork in an Integrated Holistic Context

In contemporary practices to promote health, well-being, and resilience, breathwork continues to evolve as a powerful tool for stress reduction, emotional release, and personal growth. Breathwork history reveals a profound exploration of human breath as a gateway to physical vitality, mental clarity, and spiritual awakening. Across cultures and ages, from the ancient wisdom of India and China to modern Western innovations, breathwork continues to inspire human beings on their journey toward well-being and self-transformation. As we breathe, we connect not only with the rhythms of our own bodies but also with the deep energetic connection we have with all sentient beings. Given this book's deep honoring of ancient wisdom traditions and their support by modern science, we now explore the type of breathwork that serves as the basis for this book. We begin with a definition of the integrated holistic context that serves as the foundation for the breathing practice promoted in this book, blending ancient wisdom and modern science to arrive at an application of breathwork that honors accessibility, intentionality, beneficence, wholism, and integration.

1.3.1   Definition of the Integrated Holistic Framework

An integrated holistic approach offers a vision that honors the deep cultural traditions of transformative practices, such as yoga and Buddhism, that date back thousands of years. It integrates modern neuroscience with ancient psychologies and practices to demonstrate the profound wisdom in the original teachings that we are relearning and rediscovering every day. The integrated holistic framework underlying all practices offered in this book embraces inclusiveness, access, diversity, health, well-being, and resilience for everyone. It is a practice of and for the community; it honors interdependence and co-regulation. Integrated holistic work embraces an honoring of traditional practices—practices, grounded in the eight limbs of yoga, that are physical only to prepare practitioners for more important interior practices (such as concentration and meditation) and interpersonal applications of a thoughtful and deliberate code of ethics, lifestyle, and discipline [14, 15]. This *integrated holistic approach* combines body, emotion, mind, spirit, and community through a comprehensive lifestyle with implications for individual and collective well-being [3, 16, 17]. It promotes self-compassion, introspection, and community that lead to insights that alter human physiology and anatomy and—perhaps more importantly—emotions, cognitions, behaviors, and relationships. Integrated holistic practices are accessible to anyone who can breathe without assistance, almost anywhere, for little to no cost [18, 19]. They motivate practitioners to adhere to a complete practice that honors all human needs and experiences, more so than a unidimensional posture practice, and free from Western stereotypes that tend to limit who engages with yoga or other types of transformative work [18].

The integrated holistic framework, as defined by Brems [20, 21], includes five foundational principles that intertwine and create meaning. The integrated holistic approach encourages whole-hearted and open-minded commitment to practices that:

- Reflect intentional lifestyle choices on behalf of *personal and collective* well-being, health, and resilience, deeply grounded in a commitment to live ethically and compassionately in the world
- Create profound health and mental health benefits, individually and collectively, via a diverse set of practices that facilitate many mechanisms of change and that, first of all, do no harm
- Invite everyone into the practice, creating accessibility, equity, advocacy, inclusion, and engagement at the individual and collective—all within a context of affiliation, of deeply appreciated and carefully crafted community
- Emphasize and honor human complexity and our deep grounding in relationships and communities
- Offer a multitude of practices and approaches derived from ancient wisdom and modern science, cooperatively delivered in a manner that invites self-agency, empowerment, and discerning personal choices

Each of these important aspects of integrated holistic practice (summarized in Table 1.1) deserves more attention and definition. These principles are reflected in every chapter and offered guidelines or practice throughout this book. Understanding this background for the intentionality and beneficence of the book's offered approach to breathwork perhaps can help cultivate motivation and patience during the journey through this lengthy treatise.

Table 1.1 Integrated holistic practice: Definition and commitment

- *A practice of intentionality*—Commitment to making the world a better place; to living and practicing with intention, purpose, and meaning; to helping all beings develop meaningful goals and life purpose
- *A practice of beneficence*—Commitment to facilitating mechanisms of change that do no harm and lead to positive health and mental health outcomes
- *A practice of accessibility and affiliation*—Commitment to creating communities of healing that honor and practice diversity, inclusion, equity, advocacy, engaged action, and personal as well as collective empowerment
- *A practice of wholism*—Commitment to honor human complexity, biopsychosociocultural contexts, interconnection, and community
- *A practice of integration*—Commitment to offering a diversity of integrated practices, carefully tailored to the individual and collective needs of all humans

1.3.2 Commitment to Intentionality

The basis of any dedicated practice is the setting of a clear intention, termed *sankalpa* in Sanskrit. The Sanskrit word *kalpa* means vow; the Sanskrit root word *san* refers to the highest truth. Thus, setting a *sankalpa* means that we vow to orient our practice to the search for truth; we resolve to search for the deeper meaning of our individual and collective lives; and we commit ourselves to a deeper search for purpose.

Intentions signal commitment and dedication; they anchor us to a deeper meaning so that we can stay with our practice when it becomes challenging—which it inevitably does. Intentions infuse actions with volition and motivation. They set in motion thought, speech, and behavior that pervade the outcomes and impacts of our actions. However, intention and impact must not be confused—we can have a positive conscious intention that may be flavored by unconscious processes, resulting in a negative impact.

Intention setting is best woven into any practice, psychology, and philosophy from beginning to end. It is a bit like values clarification in that we figure out where we want to place our intention, what we truly desire, and to what we want to dedicate ourselves. We can set intentions in many different ways, including for an individual practice session, for practices across a lifetime, or for a particular timeframe. Intentions are—in a way—a focus (*drishti* in Sanskrit) for life—a focal point for our attention and concentration that orients our thoughts, speech, behaviors, and relationships.

Intentions are useful tools that help set a direction toward a particular goal—a goal that we hold loosely while enjoying the journey and what unfolds, rather than clinging to a particular outcome. Intentions are not like New Year's resolutions that we set to fix something that is broken or to correct the error of our ways. Instead, intentions are orienting principles that help us stay the course even when life becomes tough, when we are tempted to give up, or when doubt rears its head.

Intentions are an important step or stage in committing to any practice, but especially to practices with deeper meaning, as we aspire to a more enlightened and compassionate way of being in the world. Intentions in this sense are aspirations—a very different type of commitment than concrete goal-setting. They are central to personal life commitments toward living an ethical and inspired life. They contain within them a commitment to do no harm, to be gentle and kind, and to be of service; they encourage us to live with an open heart. If we are serious about cultivating and integrating intentions, we may choose to start and end each day with a review of our open-hearted commitment to them. For example, we cultivate a gratitude practice; a conscious vow to live the day with awareness, compassion, and/or insight; and a daily recommitment to our intention as we move into our day. We may end each day with a review of the day to assess if we were true to our intentions; a review of our commitment to awareness, compassion, and insight; or a gratitude practice for the gifts of the day.

Intentionality creates lifestyles out of practice; it is a commitment to ourselves, our loved ones, our communities, our world of sentient beings, our environment, and our planet. It brings to our lives a clarity of purpose that is larger than our own small world and selfish perspectives. It instills a passion for making the world a better place, for being engaged and feeling responsible for the betterment of society and the earth. Intentionality creates growth and change; clarity and wisdom; a way of living that is of value, includes service, encouraging us to move beyond habit into discernment; and a way of creating awareness, compassion, and insight. Practices grounded in compassionate intentions that honor beneficence make us better people on the outside and inside. They prompt us to be loving, kind, compassionate, joyful, equanimous, and generous—first with ourselves and then with others; they remind us that we have a greater connection and interdependence than we may even be able to fathom.

1.3.3 Commitment to Beneficence

As suggested in the last sentence of the prior paragraph, intentionality requires beneficence. Only intentions guided by principles of doing no harm will create healthful and wholesome outcomes that benefit the individual and everyone in their biopsychosociocultural context. Research has provided ample evidence that yoga-based movement and breathing practices, in their many manifestations, are helpful for a variety of challenges and for many types of individuals [22, 23]. The synergy of the multitude of embodied mindfulness practices has a profound impact on several human systems that greatly affect day-to-day functioning, wellness, and resilience in times of stress, busyness, challenge, and demand [24]. Integrated holistic breathing, movement, and inner practices optimize autonomic control, regulate endocrine (e.g., decreased cortisol and increased gamma-aminobutyric acid) and immune functions, shape adaptive emotional and behavioral responses, and lessen reactivity (as evidenced by less widespread arousal, enhanced vagal tone, improved relaxation response, and increased cardiac variability). They facilitate optimal physiological conditions [25], enhance executive functioning and working memory, increase pain tolerance, and enable adaptive emotions and behaviors by helping practitioners maintain a positive attitude, find new ways of dealing with old inputs, and make accurate discernments in times of stress and challenge [25, 26]. Integrated holistic practices increase resilience in body, emotion, and mind and bring about self-regulation that supports adaptive responsiveness to meet the needs of the environment, body, emotions, and mind. These benefits arise because these practices affect and integrate both top-down and bottom-up pathways in the human brain for coping with internal and external demands, while they recalibrate the nervous system and maintain homeostasis in the body and mind.

Breathing, movement, and contemplative practices based in an integrated holistic paradigm, especially breathing and interior practices, create bi-directional feedback and feedforward loops in the brain that result in greater accuracy of input detection and interpretation, and greater resilience and self-regulation in emotional, mental, relational, and behavioral responses [24, 27, 28]. For example, coherent and slow-paced breathing and movement stimulate the basal ganglia cortico-thalamic circuits that help humans unlearn maladaptive behaviors and allow for extinction learning. Simultaneously, mindfulness practices, often using the breath as a mindful focus, create greater connectivity of the caudate with other (higher and lower) brain regions, facilitating new, goal-directed, flexible learning and behavior [29, 30].

Breathing strategies restore balance to the nervous system by supporting autonomic nervous system styles (and, commensurately, unconscious cognitive expectations or predictions) that place the organism in a calm, relaxed, interpersonally engaged space (i.e., ventral vagal neural platform). This effect is important because the poly-vagal system regulates allostatic load or the "ability of an organism to maintain stability/homeostasis through change by actively adjusting to both predictable and unpredictable events" [30] (p. 13).

Yoga-inspired breathwork offers many tools that decrease allostatic load by offering behavioral choices, emotional flexibility, and cognitive reappraisal and restructuring. Resilience in body, emotion, mind, and behavior facilitates a ventral vagal response and promotes successful, integrated (bottom-up and top-down) self-regulation. Allostasis is dependent on the capacity to take self-regulatory action based on accurate internal [31] and external [32] sensory pathways to bring the organism back into balance. Much of what embodied mindfulness and awareness facilitates is exactly that—it prepares the practitioner to take appropriate and adaptive action in response to accurately perceived demands and needs. Mindfulness, which is central to many therapeutic breathing practices, encourages an accurate perception of sensory input from internal bodily systems and environmental stimuli through conscious awareness of neuroceptive, interoceptive, exteroceptive, and proprioceptive stimuli. In other words, integrated holistic practices encourage conscious and accurate processing of sensory inputs from inside and outside the body to support self-regulation, bidirectional feedback, and adaptive behavior in support of successful allostasis (ongoing change in the service of stability). They facilitate meta-awareness and in-the-moment lived experience of interoceptive, neuroceptive, exteroceptive, and proprioceptive inputs and thus help integrate information across top-down and bottom-up systems, a process that is largely coordinated by the insula [25, 28, 29, 33].

Not surprisingly, as will be amply documented and detailed in the many pages that follow, breathwork of all types has been linked to many positive outcomes and benefits. Table 1.2 previews the many benefits of breathwork—a long listing that nevertheless is

Table 1.2 Documented benefits of breathwork practices

Mental and emotional benefits
- Reduce stress and anxiety
- Boost mood
- Improve emotional regulation
- Relieve depression
- Improve sleep
- Enhance focus
- Hone concentration
- Increase self-awareness

Physical benefits
- Lower blood pressure
- Boost energy levels
- Improve respiratory function
- Support immune system function
- Reduce menstrual discomfort
- Help manage seizures
- Improve heart rate variability
- Reduce pain and pain perception
- Enhance digestion
- Reduce muscle tension
- Ameliorate asthma
- Enhance blood sugar management

General well-being
- Promote relaxation
- Increase resilience
- Boost creativity
- Enhance mindfulness
- Improve self-care
- Support recovery from illness or injury

not exhaustive. With each new research study that emerges, more evidence is offered for the many advantages of mindful, interoceptively-based breathwork that integrates the wisdom of the ages and the subtle additions of modern science.

1.3.4 Commitment to Accessibility and Equity

In the integrated holistic paradigm, all breathing and mindfulness practices are accessible to everyone, with appropriate variations and adaptations to individual needs. Lifestyle, breathing, and inner practices are accessible to all bodies; yoga postures and embodied movement come in many forms that are inviting to nearly everyone, particularly with openheartedness about using adaptations and variations that are individually tailored and compassionate. While Western postural yoga practice is often (and counter to ancient yoga) forceful, energetic, and focused on physical beauty and fitness, all embodied practices can be varied and adapted to fit individual practitioners. Widespread stereotypes about yoga shapes and movement falsely suggest that the practice is for the fit, the young, the slim, and the flexible. This misleading and stereotypical perception of yogic practices creates unnecessary barriers for the very individuals who could benefit most from integrated holistic practices, namely, those who are experiencing health challenges or who are subjected to chronic stress [34–36]. However, integrated holistic posture and breathing practices are carefully adapted to individual patients' needs by destigmatizing the use of supportive props, such as blocks, straps, bolsters, blankets, pillows, and chairs, to invite human beings of all shapes, ages, sizes, states of health and mobility, and experiences to participate fully and reap the benefits of mindful self-expression and self-exploration [37]. Properly varied and adapted, nearly all students, clients, or patients, even those with significant physical challenges and limitations, can experience the benefits of integrated holistic movement and breathing practices.

Accessibility and affiliation mean that these practices are meant to be shared; they are practices for everyone, carefully crafted to be patient-centered. Sadly, we frequently hear stories from clients and patients who have shunned these valuable practices because of perceptions such as "yoga is not for guys," "Yoga is not for women my age"; "I am too old… too big… too stiff … too lazy … too *whatever*"; "I am not fit enough"; "I don't fit in"; and "Yoga conflicts with my religion." Some individuals who could have benefitted have tried *conventional* Western yoga and given up—they stopped going to class when they felt like an outsider, the only one who could not keep up, the only one who did not seem to know what to do, the only one in their demographic. Some gave up because they had pain or physical challenges and did not know how to work within their limitations; some did not know how to move into and out of a pose safely; and some were afraid that they would be the only ones left lying on the mat at the end of a pose or class because they could not hear the teacher. Some gave up because they were hurt in class or by a teacher, had strong emotions emerge without support, or were upset about something that was said or done in class. All these patients gave up because of the failure of the teacher or clinician to make the practice accessible to the individual client, student, or patient.

Even among those who regularly practice yoga, some have confided that they have encountered teachers whom they perceived as having pushed too hard, made painful adjustments, failed to offer props, been too demanding, had no understanding of their unique social and cultural circumstances, and had no experience with older people, men, individuals with physical limitations, or people with emotional or mental challenges. Some talked about being bothered by having to look at themselves in a mirror, feeling uncomfortable about their clothes or their body, or feeling left out when they cannot access a pose that everyone else in the room seems to do with ease. As integrated holistic teachers or clinicians, we need to understand, appreciate, and address these concerns. Most of us are well-intended and thoughtful about preparing for movement, breathing, or meditation sessions. That said, we likely all have left students or patients behind in our instructions and offerings. We can all do better; we can all become more mindful to make yoga more accessible, especially in settings where people are already served who could benefit from the practice, including healthcare and mental healthcare settings.

As clinicians or yoga teachers who want to bring breathwork (and its associated movement, lifestyle, and contemplative or mindfulness practices) into healthcare and mental healthcare, we embrace solutions for bringing our offerings to everyone. We can embrace the broad principles shown in Table 1.3; we can offer the type of intentional, beneficial breathwork that is the subject of this book.

Table 1.3   Guidance for making practices and offerings accessible and affiliative

- We can emphasize the psychology and philosophy of the offered practice, integrating emotional supports and mental coping strategies in a context of movement and breathwork practice that is easy and accessible to most, if not all
- We can offer movement practices in preparation for breathwork that honors varying levels of skill, physicality, emotionality, and psychological needs
- We can demonstrate multiple expressions or variations of physical shapes or movements, giving our clients the opportunity and permission to choose what is right for their bodies at the moment
- We can offer accessible movement and breathing practices that are adaptable, inviting, and realistic for the average, non-stereotypic patients
- We can use props for every pose and every person, demonstrating all shapes or movements with props, encouraging the use of props, and inviting our clients to be advanced practitioners by honoring their bodies and using the proper supports for a safe practice
- Our language can become clearer, our voice crisper; our words can be chosen to be more inclusive and inviting
- We can invite humor and lightness into the practice without making fun of anyone
- We can signal openness to input and feedback when we have excluded a patient, always checking in about how an offering was received and reverberated in the patient's body
- We can offer practices without expectations for a particular outcome, adapting and flexing with client needs as they emerge
- We can normalize the reality that everyone has different needs and seeks different benefits and that our practice, environment, and relationship-building deeply honor diversity, equity, and inclusion
- We can communicate our profound commitment to welcoming everyone, being clear about our scope of practice, and about realistic goals for each patient
- We can embrace and promote active advocacy and engage in local activism

As clinicians committed to breathwork, movement, and lifestyle commitments of integrated holistic practice, we need to collaborate with as many people as possible to transcend current stereotypes about who can practice yoga-based movements, breathwork, and mindfulness and who (i.e., everyone) is welcome. We can choose to become part of the change that will carry these practices into more lives. We can commit to making efforts to understand and honor the biopsychosociocultural contexts of our clients and patients and to offer environmental and relational cues of safety and understanding for all. This may mean that our work at times has to become political and has to challenge institutionalized, systemic, and structural racism; White supremacy; and the fantasy that we are all one and the same. We need to understand that there is indeed diversity and great variation in how we experience and feel safe (or not) in the world. A practice of inclusion, accessibility, and equity is political, open-hearted, and open-minded. It is a practice of values, engaged action, and a commitment to make the world a better place for everyone.

1.3.5 Commitment to Wholism

Integrated holistic practices acknowledge and work with all aspects of the human experience, honoring the mind as much as the body, breathing as much as calming of the nervous system, individuals as much as the collective, stillness as much as movement, and effort as much as ease. Such practices assess and address the needs and resources of *whole people at all their layers* (or *koshas*, in Sanskrit): body, breath, mind, heart, and spirit—grounded in community and a complex interpersonal setting (or matrix) of biological, psychological, social, and cultural influences. Integrated holistic practice is therefore particularly well-suited for applications in healthcare and mental healthcare settings, as well as in under-resourced and underserved communities.

Integrated holistic clinicians and teachers always remember that our physicality is only the tiniest tip of the iceberg—the real work in sessions and offices happens energetically, emotionally, and mentally. We understand and are in the physical world first; hence we grow and evolve from there. Embodied movement teaches us to understand, acknowledge, and inhabit our bodies—not deny, repress, or dissociate from them. We learn to understand our physical reality and how to rest in equanimity regardless of what happens in the body. Alongside the work with the body, we work with breath and energy, mind and emotions, and ultimately, we move toward a deep understanding of our human connection to a greater web of life, awakening perhaps to a new level of consciousness.

Holistic Systems

Holistic systems consider the interaction of all living beings to create an environment for the maximum benefit of all. They do not focus on specific components or features, instead being dedicated to the understanding, well-being, and support of the entire system in all its multidimensional complexities. Nothing is ignored; nothing is left out.

Teaching and learning approaches that embrace wholism integrate all human traits, attending to the physical, energetic, mental, emotional, behavioral, relational, and psychological aspects of all who are coming together for the purpose of learning.

Holistic approaches to healthcare, education, politics, environmental policy, gardening, and so on encourage personal and collective responsibility, accountability, duty, well-being, welfare, security, health, and happiness.

Wholism Avoids Reductionism and Embraces Complexity

Working from an integrated holistic paradigm avoids reductionism and invites us to embrace wholism. It embraces the complexity of human life and growth while resting in the simplicity of a well-designed practice or clinical intervention. Just like a spiderweb, offerings to patients weave together many intricate strands with great attention and purpose. The result is a complex structure that is beautiful to behold in its seeming simplicity and genuine clarity.

Reductionism hones in on select aspects of clients without honoring their full history, experience, and complexity. It may hone in on the physical aspect, treating a single symptom or using a single intervention. It may hone in on perceptions of people as unidimensional or stereotypes that fail to see each patient's unique expressions, needs, or contexts. Reductionist healthcare interventions, educational approaches, recommended physical activities, endorsed nutritional styles, or breathwork are all too often prescribed based on generalizations that are exclusive to certain populations, restricting access to and utility of the "standard of care" or universal approach. Reductionism tends to exclude and frighten, as opposed to include and invite.

Wholism is the opposite of reductionism; it is the honoring of complexity, of critical analysis and thinking, of embracing the role of a guide when providing education, healthcare, and other human interactions. From a holistic paradigm, clinicians provide services tailored to each client, as well as their circumstances and context, with deep caring and wisdom, and informed by intentionality, beneficence, and accessibility. A holistic paradigm that avoids reductionism is the perfect approach for embodied movement and therapeutic breathing practices in healthcare and mental healthcare settings. It can help transform challenges faced in modern healthcare by treating the whole person, rather than symptoms.

Wholism Honors All Human Layers of Consciousness

Wholism makes a point of seeing the entirety of each human being regardless of presenting concern, context, or relationship. Patients are seen and acknowledged in all their many layers of experience and consciousness, namely, body, vitality (breath, arousal, affect, and energy), mind (thoughts, beliefs, attitudes, emotion), heart (connection, community, and relationship), and belongingness. From this perspective, humans have multiple ways of being conscious of themselves as they live and interact in the real world of daily life. In modern language, we refer to this complexity as the many layers of human experience. Ancient yogis conceived of the self as layered—composed of several aspects or components that make up our consciousness (a consciousness to which we refer as our *self*). In Sanskrit, these layers are called *koshas*, which can be loosely translated as "sheaths."

The word "*kosha*" is translated as layer or sheath of the self in most Western translations. However, the koshas are perhaps better understood as layers or stages of consciousness, awareness, or experience. They are our human way of experiencing ourselves in the tangible world. In reality, each layer of self is a construct, giving us a false sense of separation. However, each aspect of human experience is an opportunity—a way to build relationships, share experiences, be in community, and provide support and interventions. The word *koshas* is occasionally used in this text because no English translation can quite capture the complexity of the concept. Each *kosha* has a separate and distinct function while also being completely integrated and interdependent with the others. All layers of experience are with us (if only as seeds) from birth to death—yet each takes on particular significance and reaches maturation during different stages of our lives and development. In other words, the layers of human experience develop and become important neurosequentially. Specific meanings and expressions of each *kosha* depend on the circumstances we face as we move through life and relationships. Table 1.4 offers a summary of the five layers of experience.

Wholism Recognizes Interdependence and Embeddedness in Community

Human development, which can be considered synonymous with development along the lines of the *koshas*, is profoundly influenced by and dependent upon a multitude of individual, relational, and contextual factors that are utterly interpersonal and interdependent. Human development depends on being solidly and

Table 1.4 The five *koshas* or layers of consciousness

Layer of experience	Definition	Translation
Annamaya kosha	Embodied self or physical experiences	*Anna* = food
Pranamaya kosha	Energetic or affective self or vital experiences	*Prana* = life force
Manomaya kosha	Verbal and social self or mental and emotional experiences	*Mano* = mind
Vijnanamaya kosha	Decentered, wisely intuitive self, or experience of wisdom	*Vijnana* = wisdom
Anandamaya kosha	Joyfully connected self or experiences of being connected to a greater web of life	*Ananda* = bliss, joy

supportively anchored in a greater web of life, especially in a web of loving, joyful, kind, and compassionate humans. Human newborns cannot survive outside of a caretaking human matrix of relationships that support their physical survival, emotional needs, and mental growth [38, 39]. This interpersonal matrix [40] and its influence has been thoroughly documented in the developmental psychology literature and is unquestioned in the importance of its influence.

In the integrated holistic model [41], development is viewed as a lifelong process of refinement and emergence, shaped by individuals' experiences in and interactions with their context and environment. Development thus defined resembles evolution [42] and results in the acquisition of behaviors, useful skills, shaping of new responses, un- and re-learning habits, and expansion of awareness [43, 44]. In this model, development is utterly dependent on the context in which it occurs. How bodies, energy and vitality, mind and emotions, and ways of being in relationships develop, grow, and transform is strongly affected by the context that surrounds us, including relationships we experience, environments in which we grow up and grow old, cultural forces that bring us advantages or disadvantages, social and sociopolitical pressures we feel, and educational and career or job opportunities that emerge or fail to emerge. All have profound and long-lasting effects on how we grow, emerge, and evolve in all layers of self, in our relationships, in our families, and in our communities.

This integrated holistic model of understanding human development and human existence and experience is premised on continual change, emergence, and evolution that optimizes and integrates learning and experience over time, constantly transcending and improving upon prior learning and conditioning [38, 39, 45–47]. The empowering premise that humans are subject to and agents in their own lifelong growth is consistent with findings from modern neuroscience and psychology as well as yogic perspectives on human development.

Ancient traditions and modern sciences recognize that humans change, emerge, and grow in the context of their embeddedness in an interpersonal matrix and need to be understood from the unique developmental and contextual embeddedness at any moment in time. All are equally optimistic, by virtue of their developmental focus, that there is an inherent capacity of humans to transcend their current state, to improve with experience and discipline, and to evolve continually, and ultimately to embrace their human interconnection, interrelation, and interdependence—along with the responsibilities that emerge from this recognition of connection. The context in which development and healing occur is relational, collective, and biopsychosociocultural in nature.

Four dimensions are defined and understood from an integrated holistic lens. They are *biological, psychological, socioeconomic/sociological*, and *cultural/familial*, or *biopsychosociocultural* [48]. Biopsychosociocultural contexts are in and of themselves ever-emerging, always changing, and in flux. This adds complexity, ambiguity, uncertainty, and volatility to our understanding of ourselves and our clients. In other words, our human experience is always grounded in a volatile, uncertain, complex, and ambiguous (VUCA) world. The biopsychosociocultural paradigm invites clinicians to gain an in-depth understanding of clients' (and their own) webs of life, webs of relationships, and greater connections. It reminds us that sources of challenges, difficulties, and presenting concerns, even overall life experience, are always relational and embedded in a greater context. It leads to recognition of the importance of having an understanding of biopsychosociocultural contexts that have had and continue to have a bearing on the development and experience of human beings.

Wholism Specifically Applied to Breathwork

True to wholism, integrated holistic breathwork adapts itself to the human complexity and biopsychosociocultural individuality of its practitioners. A key consideration in learning and applying anatomy, physiology, and psychoemotional well-being principles to breathwork is the understanding that there are large individual variations in how anatomy and physiology are expressed in the breath. How patients breathe and function is affected by highly individual factors that may challenge them to work at their own edges of comfort in ways that seem less than obvious. Following is a review of some of these factors of uniqueness to foreshadow the carefully adapted and tailored work that can be offered through integrated holistic breathing practices.

Biological factors of uniqueness: We are enormously bio-individual, unfathomably unique. This makes understanding the anatomy and physiology of breathing (and movement, for that matter) a central key to teaching breathwork well—we cannot teach to the average body; we cannot teach to the norm. We have to teach the patients in front of us. This means that general breathwork cues have to be tempered with bio-individuality cues, with the acknowledgment that each breathing practice needs to be created and experienced from the inside out, not formed and perceived from the outside in.

In that context, it is helpful to remember that anatomical charts and models show average bodies; we as actual humans, however, do not exist that way in nature. Each human being has different lungs, noses, and rib baskets— different structures. Just as we differ in blood pressure, weight, height, skin tone, age, background, culture, and education, so do we differ in organ shapes, cavity depths, locations of body structures, angles of bony protrusions, and so much more. Similarly, many *physiological variables* must be factored in when we ask people to breathe and move. Blood pressure, blood sugar, digestive symptoms, lung health, and hormonal states are just a few examples that can alter how we breathe, move, and function. Table 1.5 offers more examples.

Acute or chronic injuries can influence what is or is not possible for an individual and can be compensated for by using props and creativity to make the offered practice accessible. Specifically, inflammation (and hence swelling) post-injury or post-stress (including emotional or psychological stress) can result in decreased mobility especially in fascia (via the myofibroblasts in the contracting fascia). *Sleep and restedness*, chronic or acute, can affect how we move and breathe and how our energy can be used. Relatedly, the time of day for breathwork can make a large difference with regard to energy level and what type of breathing practice may be most healthful. *Nutritional patterns* and status can affect how well we can function

Table 1.5 Physiological influences on breath and breathing

- Blood sugar levels may affect physical and respiratory capacity, even concentration
- We may get light-headed from postural orthostatic tension syndrome or orthostatic hypotension. We may not safely go upside down because of high blood pressure or glaucoma
- What we have eaten (e.g., foods to which we are sensitive or that are highly processed) may affect our breathing rhythms, making us more prone to hyperventilation
- Level of hydration (overly hydrated or poorly hydrated) affects flexibility or mobility [49] which, in turn, may affect the breath via rib basket flexibility or rigidity
- We may be tighter or more flexible depending on hormones such as estrogen (e.g., higher estrogen levels have been associated with increased flexibility, even laxity in ligaments; lower estrogen levels may be related to less muscle mass and bone loss, with implications for aging), and relaxin (a hormone that relaxes all ligaments in the pelvis, possibly throughout the body; this can result in injury from overstretching), and from effects of the menstrual cycle on thermoregulation, water retention, and energy
- How we sleep may affect the breath, as well as being influenced by the breath. Our breathing is more dysregulated when we are not rested

physically, related to movement, energy, and stamina (e.g., an 81-year-old client who suddenly started feeling weak during practice, which could have been mistaken for "normal aging"; however, it turns out she failed to eat breakfast before the session; once she took time to eat and started her practice a bit later, she was fine).

Psychological factors of uniqueness: Emotional and mental factors influence how patients present for breathwork. Just as anatomical and physiological factors affect shapes and breathing practices that we can ask students to engage in, so too can psychological issues set boundaries and edges around what is possible for them energetically and vitally. The following influences can be explored in how we approach breathwork with our patients and what types of interplay between breath and movement may be possible:

- Affective and arousal states—polyvagal states and gunas
- Emotional influences—trauma history, fears, attachments, grief, depression, helplessness
- Mental influences—mental habits, mental sets, beliefs, attitudes, coping styles and resilience
- Cognitive capacity—jargon, intelligence, educational level, language skills

Social and socioeconomic factors of uniqueness: Many social and sociological factors are present in people's lives that affect their relationship with their bodies and breath. Current social circumstances may limit access to healthful movement and optimal breathing.

- *Use of modern conveniences*: Our social environment has evolved such that it no longer encourages and supports spontaneous movement and gentle breathing. In fact, if anything, work settings and educational demands can create stressful environments that result in significant hyperventilation and energetic exhaustion.

- *Quality of environments of care*: Availability of props, cost of breathwork, lack of access to insurance or inadequate reimbursement options, and lack of interaction or coordination of care with other care providers.
- *Quality of air and noise levels*: Restriction of access to safe and natural outdoor spaces, especially for urban dwellers, that would support healthful breathing of clean air; noise levels in the environment that interfere with quiet breathing practice or mindful presence.
- *Neighborhood safety and crime*: Access to outdoor life in neighborhoods that invite breathing and moving in safe and welcoming environments, safety of the practice space, and accessibility of practice space (e.g., lack of transportation to access the only breathwork instructor in town).

Cultural factors of uniqueness: Cultural and familial factors may influence how we relate to movement and physical activity, as well as to seeking healthcare and breathwork.

- *Stereotypes about yoga-based services*: Perceptions that pranayama is only for a select few, as well as many other stereotypes about who, what, how, why, and when as related to yoga practices.
- *Stereotypes about breathing and movement in general*: If movement and breathwork are framed as exercise and exercise is just another burden of modern life, motivation may be low.
- *Attitudes about breath, movement, and physicality*: Family and cultural values may affect attitudes about the meaning and value of physical activity, optimal breathing, and sleep or nutritional habits.
- *Attitudes about psychological and physical intervention for health and mental health concerns*: Family and cultural values may affect attitudes about the meaning and value of meditation, breath and energy work, guided imagery, and other emotional or psychological interventions.
- *Attitudes about spirituality*: (Mis)perception of yoga-based practices as a religion that may be incompatible with personal religious or spiritual beliefs; perceived conflicts between yoga-based breathework and one's own religion.

The layers of self-experience or consciousness are influenced by many variables in our environment. They are adaptive to outer and inner influences and provide wonderful and multiple portals into intervention. If we understand that our patients present with a multitude of layers, we have the option of beginning to relate with them from the place where they are suffering most tangibly or where they perceive the greatest likelihood of relief from their symptoms. As all layers are related, breathwork can begin with an exploration of how the breath reverberates in the body, in patients' vitality (their arousal or affect), or their thoughts and emotions (maybe they simply have a misunderstanding about how to breathe most appropriately). Chapter 5 presents a deliberate model of conceptualization that makes clinical use of the understanding of the koshas and the various ways in which we can connect to our patients. Table 1.6 provides an overview of the five layers (*koshas*) of

Table 1.6 Panchamaya Kosha: A model for human complexity

Definition	Developmental concepts	Intervention notes
Annamaya Kosha = embodied self or physical experience ("*anna*" = food)		
Anatomy and physiology; development and maintenance of physical health and allostasis; recovery from illness/disease, embodiment; recognition of physical habits and preoccupations	Movement is necessary for many developmental lines, including language development, social engagement, memory consolidation, and embodied self-development; gunas and polyvagal states begin in this layer	Emphasize how the body senses, metabolizes, moves, and functions; physical inputs and outputs are autonomously managed via the brain stem; movement is strongly linked to the dopamine system
Pranamaya Kosha = energetic or affective self or vital experience ("*prana*" = breath; "*Prana*" = life force)		
Breath, energy, vitality, affect, blood flow, electrical impulses, neurochemical transmissions, and more; energetic and physical layers inseparably/ jointly process signals from inside (neuroception, interoception, proprioception) and outside (exteroception) of the body	Ties strongly to the limbic system and interoceptive network (including salience and default mode networks); sensations now also carry a feeling tone (vedana in Sanskrit) that is positive, negative, or neutral; this prepares us for the emergence of affective predilections (i.e., kleshas in Sanskrit: Attachment, aversion, ego, confusion, fear) and attachment styles	Explore how we feel energetically and affectively; link to the affective reactivity; link to a shared experience of connection, codependent arising, co-regulation, and interdependence; work with shared vibration, communal affect and arousal, shared tranquility and peace; prana vayus come into play and are explored to regulate energy
Manomaya Kosha = verbal and social self or mental and emotional experience ("*mano*" = mind)		
Perceptions, thoughts, labels, and emotions arise from mental interpretations, and expressions of acquired personality; encompasses (emerging and always evolving) perceptual and cognitive understanding of the world, including perceived roles in communities and relationships	Develops out of the capacity for representational learning, as mediated by language development; memory encoding via the hippocampus leads to explicit declarative memories that help us remember the past and predict the future → brain becomes a prediction "machine"	Gain clarity about habitual reactivity and can transform habit into conscious choice; recognize mental biases and cognitive habits (vrittis, especially as flavored by the gunas and kleshas); explore and transcend physical, affective, cognitive, emotional, and relational samskaras
Vijnanamaya Kosha = decentered, wisely intuitive self or experiences of wisdom ("*vijnana*" = wisdom)		
Innate intelligence, talents, traits, and natural inclinations (or innate temperament) meet emerging/growing wisdom and deeper understanding, leading to conscious recognition of interdependence, that there is no solo self, no self at all—But only a relative self that helps us navigate life	Conscious awareness of this kosha requires having achieved cortical and hemispheric integration; our brains need to have matured and become capable of holistic processing of experience; we become the observers of our own (inner) reactions and outer responses to the world and in relationship	Perceive roles and responsibilities with more clarity; recognize human responsibility to invite joy, lovingkindness, compassion, and equanimity; apply ethics and morality with discernment and a lens that includes complexities and contexts that might easily be missed; live our highest intentions for the collective

(continued)

Table 1.6 (continued)

Definition	Developmental concepts	Intervention notes
Anandamaya Kosha = joyfully connected or experiences of being part of a greater web of life ("*Ananda*" = bliss, joy)		
A joyful and connected self emerges and leads to the realization of co-regulation and interdependence, as well as deep inner, unconditional joy, and awakened living	Union and bliss emerge as duality is transcended—The subject (i.e., what we may perceive as our *self*) now includes everything there is and is decentered, hence altruistic and compassionate	Understand deeply that there is a greater connection and coexistence that transcends each of us individually; brahma viharas guide intention, thought, speech, and action

human experience as defined in yoga psychology. This overview serves to highlight the complexity of humans and the opportunities for intervention presented by this wholistic approach to breathwork and yoga.

1.3.6   Commitment to Integration

Integrated holistic breathwork integrates methods, tools, and strategies based on the traditional limbs of yoga as well as new tools that have emerged as useful via scientific exploration. From an integrated perspective, no single practice is raised above the rest. Practice begins with the understanding that wisdom- and yoga-inspired clinical work is primarily a practice of mindfulness in all the many layers of our modern and ancient conceptions of self (or experience). Mindfulness begins in the body, as we tune into personal needs, tailor our physical activity, attune to inner sensations, and develop interoceptive awareness of how our body responds to different demands and actions. Mindfulness encompasses the breath, to help us find attunement to how we move energy through our body; how the breath enlivens our experience; how affects and arousal arise, are experienced, and dissipate; and how we perceive safety in our environment via neuroception. Mindfulness moves toward cultivating awareness of the fluctuations in the mind to help transcend and transform mental and emotional habits that support or impair our psychological growth and transformation, flavor our breath, affect our relationships and communities, and color our understanding of how life unfolds and interconnects.

From mindfulness of body (sensation), breath (affect and arousal), and mind (perceptions, cognition, memory, thoughts, emotions, interpretations, attitudes, opinions, etc.), slowly wisdom emerges and guides us toward an appreciation of life as a journey of connection, transformation, growth, and perpetual change. We move toward an understanding that when we find the gap between stimulus and response, we give ourselves the gift of conscious choice, and novel ways of being, reshaping our lives and relationships. Of course, we do not practice with a goal in mind—we simply realize the journey's potential and open our hearts and minds toward perhaps becoming wiser, more equanimous, compassionate, and joyful. We engage in the practice altruistically, for the benefit of our greater community and world.

As noted above, ancient or traditional yoga consists of eight sets of ancient practices called *limbs of yoga* [3, 50], grouped into four categories based on modern research [28, 51]. In the first category, the integrated holistic journey guides us along a varied path of practices that begins with a commitment to and grounding in *ethical practices* (yoga's Limb 1) that encourage us to strive to live peacefully, truthfully, and with a sense of abundance, joy in moderation, and non-possessiveness. It includes a commitment to purposeful living that embraces *life-choices* of simplicity, contentment, impassioned practice, self-reflection, and dedication to a greater purpose (yoga's Limb 2). On the foundation of these ethics and life-choices, in the second category, we integrate a *physical practice* (yoga's Limb 3) that is mindful, easeful, compassionate, and committed to enhancing our capacity to perceive ourselves accurately, especially in our bodies and energy. The third category adds *mindful breathing* (Yoga's Limb 4) to physical practice integrating feedback mechanisms that calm our nervous system, help regulate physiological arousal and emotional reactivity, and enhance emotional and psychological resilience.

As we get to know our body and vitality with greater accuracy and honor our physical and energetic needs with compassion, we turn to the fourth category as our practice moves inward. We allow time for the mind to become quiet—we settle into the *inner practices* (yoga's Limbs 5, 6, and 7), which include breath attunement practices. Guarding the senses from constant (over)stimulation, we develop the capacity to recognize how our mind works, how we can transform its fluctuations, and how we can become more peaceful and rest in stillness. We develop the capacity to become concentrated and achieve a single point of focus and ultimately, we move into a spacious awareness that forges new neural pathways, creating neuroplasticity, increased decisional control, spaciousness, peacefulness, and loving responsiveness to ourselves and others.

What emerges perhaps spontaneously along the path of integration is a sense of being grounded and integrated in community, a sense of belonging to the earth, a desire to connect and preserve, and a *joyful connection* (yoga's Limb 8) to something greater, a transformation of suffering. We emerge with a sense of compassion, joy, equanimity, and lovingkindness. We emerge with a sense of integration and of being whole again. Integrated holistic practice offers a journey *inward* so that ultimately we can journey outward—it is an exploration that invites us to know ourselves more deeply in all our layers so that we may become a positive force in our communities and in the lives of others. We move inward to move outward—and the breath is with us every step of the way.

Table 1.7 offers an overview of the yoga-based practices that are integrated with therapeutic breathwork. *This integration greatly facilitates auspiciously tailored breathwork.* Many patients cannot simply jump into complex breathing practices. Some need to become more comfortable in their body to access their energy and vitality through the breath. Others may need to develop the skills to move into the concentration or mindfulness that is necessary to meet their own vitality, as exemplified by the breath. Others need to develop self-compassion before they can allow themselves to alter their breathing, as they do not understand the harm they may be doing to themselves with their current breathing patterns.

Table 1.7 Eight limbs of yoga and sample intervention strategies derived from each limb

Limb	Description	Sample therapeutic strategies
Yama	Life choices for ethical living	• Creating safety in the therapeutic relationship and environment • Inviting self-compassion, honesty, and moderation • Committing to ethical and empathic intentions, speech, thoughts, and actions
Niyama	Life choices for purposeful living	• Values clarification • Developing motivation for change • Developing discipline and commitment • Setting intentions and finding purpose
Asana	Physical postures ("taking a seat")	• Attunement (e.g., body scan) and mindful movement practices to invite somatic and somatosensory awareness • Physical practices for strength, mobility, and/or stability • Movements that are balanced and balancing • Movements that revitalize, tonify, and energize • Movements that calm, ground, and bring peace or calm • Practices that invite recognition of physical samskaras • Physical routines [e.g., healthful nutrition, mindful eating, proper hydration, physical activity in nature (hiking, swimming), dancing, referral to medical care]
Pranayama	Breathing exercises ("freeing the breath")	• Breath attunement practices to invite attention and awareness • Optimal functional breathing practices • Balancing or stabilizing breathing practices • Vitalizing or uplifting breathing practices • Calming or grounding breathing practices • Practices to nourish vitality (e.g., restorative practices) • Practices that invite recognition of breath, arousal, or affect-related samskaras • Energetic routines (e.g., sleep hygiene, rest and recuperation, music, chanting or singing, referral to mental healthcare)
Pratyahara	Drawing inward ("guarding the senses")	• Practices to cultivate awareness of mind states and emotional predispositions (e.g., guided imagery) • Practices that reduce sensory stimulation (e.g., breaks from watching the news; creating a quiet and calm environment, decluttering the home)
Dharana	Concentration and attention	
Dhyana	Meditation and awareness	• Practices to cultivate awareness of mental and emotional samskaras • Practices that explore action and relationship patterns • Practices that cultivate mental resilience and enhance coping • Practices for working with emotional, behavioral, and relational reactivity • Mental and emotional routines (e.g., journaling, puzzles for cognitive flexibility, changing up routines like taking a different route to work, time in nature, referral to talk psychotherapy)

(continued)

Table 1.7 (continued)

Limb	Description	Sample therapeutic strategies
Samadhi	Awakening to joy and connection	• Cultivation of compassion, lovingkindness, and joy (e.g., maitri meditation) • Practices for the cultivation of wisdom and insight (e.g., journaling) • Practices that invite taking responsibility for own and others' health, resilience, and thriving (e.g., random acts of kindness)

1.4 Where We Go from Here

The word *pranayama* can be traced to very interesting and illuminating etymological roots that can deeply inform breathwork from multiple perspectives. The Sanskrit word *prana* has complex meanings, including breath, life force, and vital energy. It is derived from the root words *pra*—which means "*forth*" and *an* which can be translated as "*to move or breathe.*" These roots suggest the deeper meaning of the word: breath and life force are brought forth by and bring forth life and movement; they are vital and dynamic. They move energy through humans as well as through the entirety of the universe. The current convention is to use the lowercase p in the word *prana* when it refers to breath, and to use the uppercase P in the word *Prana* when it refers to life force. This convention is followed in this book. The Sanskrit word *yama* is typically translated as control or restraint. Thus, most Western translations of the full word pranayama are typically breath control. When an "*a*" is placed in front of a Sanskrit word, it is meant to denote the *opposite* of the word that follows. When the word that precedes "*a*" ends in an *a* (as in the word prana), only one "*a*" is used to link the two words.

This view of the linguistic roots of the word can lead to two different definitions or emphases of the word and the practice of *pranayama*. First, and most typically in the Western world, the word *pranayama* can be interpreted as *prana-yama*, which would mean breath control or restraint (by interpreting the *a* in the middle of the word as being the ending of the word *prana* as opposed to contributing its own separate meaning). Second, the complete word may be interpreted as *pran(a)yama*, where "*a*" is linked to the word *yama* to denote its opposite, turning restraint into freedom. According to this interpretation, the word pranayama can now be interpreted to mean the *freeing* of the breath [52–54].

We cannot know for certain if the ancients preferred one meaning over the other or if both meanings of the word are implied. However, in the lineage of integrated holistic yoga-based practice embraced in this book, both meanings are embraced and used deliberately for the sequencing of breathwork. In the integrated holistic approach to breathwork, we start our work with patients with *freeing the breath* in beginning practices and add control of the breath only if necessary and in the context of more advanced practices with a particular purpose or intention. The combination of freeing and restraining the breath may seem strange. However, interestingly, integrating the more ancient writings about pranayama *and* modern science about breathing helps us understand the utility of this integrated concept quite clearly. In fact, the integrated viewpoint makes it likely that the play on words—*pran(a)yama* and *prana-yama*—may have been intentional all along to clarify that integrating these two ways of addressing breathing creates the most tailored ways to make a breathing practice whole and integrated, as well as accessible and intentional in a person-centered way.

We free the breath in the sense that we moderate our expenditure of energy invested in breathing—making the breath as light and subtle as possible to preserve energy and vitality. We do not strain to expel the breath hard or to draw it in forcefully; we do not try to exhale the breath fully (which is not possible anyway, as we will see in Chap. 2) or to inhale fiercely or completely. Instead, we set the breath free to follow its natural rhythm—the rhythm that preserve energy yet bring enough air into and out of the body to bring oxygen to our tissues as needed given our state of being and doing, and to carry the most healthful amount of carbon dioxide away to allow for optimal oxygen uptake. We restrain the breath to bring more health and well-being to our breathing, especially if modern life has resulted in dysfunctional breathing patterns (causes of which are rampant in modern life, including stress, sleep deprivation, nutritional choices, and inadequate amounts of exercise and movement). Short breath pauses, tailored cadences, and other ways of shaping the breath are recommended by ancient yogis and are garnering research-based evidence as useful ways to improve health and well-being.

As will be explored in detail in the chapters that follow, modern breathwork practices place (too) much emphasis on *deep breaths, full breaths, big breaths*, and similar invitations. Although such cuing may be meant to invite a free-flowing breath, cuing breathing in this way often creates the opposite. As we will explore, encouraging deep, full, or large breaths often results in excessive volumes of breath being inhaled and exhaled, unhelpful biomechanics, dysregulated biochemistry, anxious states of mind, and emotional reactivity.

Integrated holistic breathwork is dedicated to breathing for overall health, well-being, and resilience, with possible effects on immune, digestive, cardiovascular, pulmonary, and hormonal health. It is a breathing practice for physical health and fitness, contributing to healthful movement (in exercise and daily life) that supports strength, balance, mobility, stability, and coordination. Integrated holistic breathing practices enhance functional capacity and quality of daily living—creating optimally functional breathing that contributes to ideal oxygenation of tissues, lung health, balanced biochemistry for gas exchange, and even optimal posture and athletic endurance and performance. Integrated holistic work pays attention to safe practices that support healthful breathing biomechanics, biochemistry, and rhythms, without suggesting fragility or vulnerability. Indeed, the work—because it is person-centered and specifically adapted to each individual—is empowering and invites breathing practitioners to take charge of their breath health and overall well-being by teaching them principles they can apply in daily life and special circumstances. It is psychoeducational, empowering, and flexible.

Integrated holistic breathwork is *pranayama* defined as both freeing and restraining the breath. It is wholistic in that it addresses and is tailored to needs in all layers of human experience and consciousness. It is rarely taught in and of itself, instead being most auspiciously embedded in a context that integrates it with movement (Limb 3) and introspection and attentive presence (Limbs 5–7), with non-violence, truthfulness, moderation, and non-attachment (Limb 1), and with dedication, intention, clarity of purposes, discipline, and the joy of contentment (Limb 2). Breathwork thus practiced can help induce clarity of vision and access to deep joy and connection (Limb 8). It is a practice that is accessible to all by being tailored to individual needs and context; developed and carried out with intention and specific purpose, yet with the openness of mind and heart and non-attachment to particular outcomes; and with a deep faith in its potential benefits.

We will now move into the science of integrated holistic breathwork, starting with journeys into breath anatomy (Chap. 2) and physiology (Chap. 3). Scientific aspects of breath and breathing are then rounded out by exploring breath rhythms and the breath's profound connection to the human nervous system (Chap. 4). Once the science of the breath has been explored, Chaps. 5, 6, and 7 shift attention to integrated holistic preparations for breathwork. Chapters 8, 9, 10, and 11 offer a toolbox of breathing practices that, resting on the strong foundation that was established, can now be offered in a patient-centered, tailored, compassionate, and practical manner.

Our body is much more nearly perfect than the endless list of ailments suggests.
   Its shortcomings are due less to its inborn imperfections than to our abusing it.—Albert Szent-Györgyi

References

1. Nestor J. Breath: the new science of a lost art. Riverhead Books; 2020.
2. Iyengar BKS. Light on pranayama. HarperCollins; 2013.
3. Iyengar BKS. Light on life. Rodale; 2006.
4. Rosen R. The yoga of breath: a step-by-step guide to pranayama. Shambala; 2002.
5. Rosen R. Pranayama beyond the fundamentals: an in-depth guide to yogic breathing. Shambala; 2006.
6. Rothenberg R. Restoring prana: a therapeutic guide to pranayama and healing through the breath for yoga therapists, teachers, and healthcare practitioners. Singing Dragon; 2020.
7. De Michelis E. A history of modern yoga. Continuum; 2004.
8. Singleton M. Yoga body: the origins of modern posture practice. Oxford University Press; 2010.
9. McKeown P. The breathing cure. Humanix; 2021.
10. McKeown P. Oxygen advantage: the simple, scientifically proven breathing techniques for a healthier, slimmer, faster, and fitter you. William Morrow; 2015.
11. Reich W. Character analysis. 3rd ed. Orgone Inst. Press; 1949.
12. Grof S, Grof C. Holotropic breathwork. 2nd ed. State University of New York Press; 2023.
13. Hof W. The Wim Hof method: activate your full human potential. Sounds True; 2020.
14. Brems C, Colgan D, Freeman H, et al. Elements of yogic practice: perceptions of students in healthcare programs. Int J Yoga. 2016;9:121–9. https://doi.org/10.4103/0973-6131.183710.

15. Freeman H, Vladagina N, Razmjou E, Brems C. Yoga in print media: missing the heart of the practice. Int J Yoga. 2017;10:160–6. https://doi.org/10.4103/ijoy.IJOY_1_17.
16. White G. Yoga beyond belief. North Atlantic Books; 2007.
17. Feuerstein G. The psychology of yoga: integrating eastern and western approaches for understanding the mind. Shambala; 2013.
18. Dittman KA, Freedman MR. Body awareness, eating attitudes, and spiritual beliefs of women practicing yoga. Eat Disord. 2009;17:273–92. https://doi.org/10.1080/10640260902991111.
19. Ross A, Friedmann E, Bevans M, Thomas S. National survey of yoga practitioners: mental and physical health benefits. Complement Ther Med. 2013;21:313–23. https://doi.org/10.1016/j.ctim.2013.04.001.
20. Brems C. Ancient wisdom and modern science of yoga: a companion for 200-hour yoga teacher training for healthcare and allied healthcare settings. Santa Barbara, CA: Self-published. 2024. p. 670
21. Brems C. A yoga stress reduction intervention for university faculty, staff, and graduate students. Int J Yoga Ther. 2015;25:61–77. https://doi.org/10.17761/1531-2054-25.1.61.
22. McCall MC. How might yoga work? An overview of potential underlying mechanisms. J Yoga Phys Ther. 2013;3(1):1. https://doi.org/10.4172/2157-7595.1000130.
23. Riley KE, Park CL. How does yoga reduce stress? A systematic review of mechanisms of change and guide to future inquiry. Health Psychol Rev. 2015;9:379–96. https://doi.org/10.1080/17437199.2014.981778.
24. Sullivan MB, Moonaz S, Weber K, Taylor JN, Schmalzl L. Toward an explanatory framework for yoga therapy informed by philosophical and ethical perspectives. Altern Ther Health Med. 2018;24(1):38–47. https://www.ncbi.nlm.nih.gov/pubmed/29135457
25. Taylor AG, Goehler LE, Galper DI, Innes KE, Bourguignon C. Top-down and bottom-up mechanisms in mind-body medicine: development of an integrative framework for psychophysiological research. Explore J Sci Heal. 2010;6:29–41. https://doi.org/10.1016/j.explore.2009.10.004.
26. Schmalzl L, Crane-Godreau MA, Payne P. Movement-based embodied contemplative practices: definitions and paradigms. Front Hum Neurosci. 2014;8:205. https://doi.org/10.3389/fnhum.2014.00205.
27. Sullivan MB, Erb M, Schmalzl L, Moonaz S, Taylor JN, Porges S. Yoga therapy and polyvagal theory: the convergence of traditional wisdom and contemporary neuroscience for self-regulation and resilience. Front Hum Neurosci. 2018;12:67–82. https://doi.org/10.3389/fnhum.2018.00067.
28. Gard T, Noggle JJ, Park C, Vago DR, Wilson A. Potential self-regulatory mechanisms of yoga for psychological health. Front Hum Neurosci. 2014;8:770. https://doi.org/10.3389/fnhum.2014.00770.
29. Gard T, Taquet M, Dixit R, Holzel B, Dickerson B, Lazar S. Greater widespread functional connectivity of the caudate in older adults who practice kripalu yoga and vipassana meditation than in controls. Front Hum Neurosci. 2015;9:137. https://doi.org/10.3389/fnhum.2015.00137.
30. Schmalzl L, Powers C, Blom EH. Neurophysiological and neurocognitive mechanisms underlying the effects of yoga-based practices: towards a comprehensive theoretical framework. Front Hum Neurosci. 2015;9:235. https://doi.org/10.3389/fnhum.2015.00235.
31. Craig AD. How do you feel? An interoceptive moment with your neurobiological self. Princeton University Press; 2014.
32. Witkiewitz R, Roos CR, Colgan DD, Bowen S. Advances in psychotherapy evidence-based practice. Hogrefe; 2017.
33. Tsakiris M, Jiménez AT, Costantini M. Just a heartbeat away from one's body: interoceptive sensitivity predicts malleability of body-representations. Proc R Soc B. 2011;278(1717):2470–6. https://doi.org/10.1098/rspb.2010.2547.
34. Brems C, Justice L, Sulenes K, et al. Improving access to yoga: barriers to and motivators for practice among health professions students. Adv Mind Body Med. 2015;29(3):6–13. https://www.ncbi.nlm.nih.gov/pubmed/26026151

35. Justice L, Brems C, Jacova C. Exploring strategies to enhance self-efficacy about starting a yoga practice. Ann Yoga Phys Ther. 2016;1(2):1–7. https://austinpublishinggroup.com/yoga-physical-therapy/fulltext/aypt-v1-id1012.pdf

36. Sulenes K, Freitas J, Justice L, Colgan D, Shean M, Brems C. Underuse of yoga as a referral resource by health professions students. J Altern Complement Med. 2015;21:53–9.

37. Vladagina N, Freeman H, Razmjou E, et al. Media images of yoga poses: increasing injury instead of access. Paper presented at: 144th Annual American Public Health Association Meeting and Exposition; October 2016.

38. Cozolino L. The neuroscience of psychotherapy: healing the social brain. 3rd ed. W.W. Norton & Company; 2017.

39. Cozolino L. Why therapy works: using our minds to change our brains. W.W. Norton & Company; 2015.

40. Stern D. The interpersonal world of the infant. Basic; 1985.

41. Brems, C. Yoga for mental health: Cultivating emotional resilience and mental fortitude. Santa Barbara, CA; 2024. p. 250.

42. Wilber K. Integral psychology. Shambhala; 2000.

43. Grant A. Think again. WH Allen; 2021.

44. Wimbarti S, Self PA. Developmental psychology for the clinical child psychologist. In: Walker CE, Roberts MC, editors. Handbook of clinical child psychology. Wiley; 1992. p. 33–46.

45. Badenoch B. The brain-savvy therapist's workbook. Norton; 2011.

46. Badenoch B. Being a brain-wise therapist: a practical guide to interpersonal neurobiology. W.W. Norton and Company; 2011.

47. Siegel DJ, Payne BT. Whole-brain child: 12 revolutionary strategies to nurture your child's developing mind. Scribe Publications; 2012.

48. Brems C, Rasmussen CH. A comprehensive guide to child psychotherapy and counseling. 4th ed. Waveland; 2019.

49. Clark B. Your body, your yoga. Wild Strawberry Productions; 2016.

50. Hartranft C. The yoga sutra of Patanjali: a new translation with commentary. Shambala Classics; 2003.

51. Ward L, Stebbings S, Sherman K, Cherkin D, Baxter GD. Establishing key components of yoga interventions for musculoskeletal conditions: a Delphi survey. BMC Complement Altern Med. 2014;14(196):1. https://doi.org/10.1186/1472-6882-14-196.

52. Farhi D. Bringing yoga to life. HarperCollins Publishers; 2005.

53. Farhi D. The breathing book: good health and vitality through essential breath work. Holt; 1996.

54. Maki B. The Yogi's roadmap: the Patanjali yoga sutra as a journey to self-realization. CreateSpace; 2013.

Part II

Science of Breathwork

Understanding the Anatomy of Breath and Breathing

2

> *Breath reflects physical sensation; physical sensation reflects breath*
> *Pain may lead to disrupted breathing; choppy breathing can create physical suffering*
> *Breath responds to posture; posture responds to breath*
> *Slouched posture may result in constricted breathing; labored breathing can distort posture*
>
> *Christiane Brems*

2.1 Overview: Breath in the Body

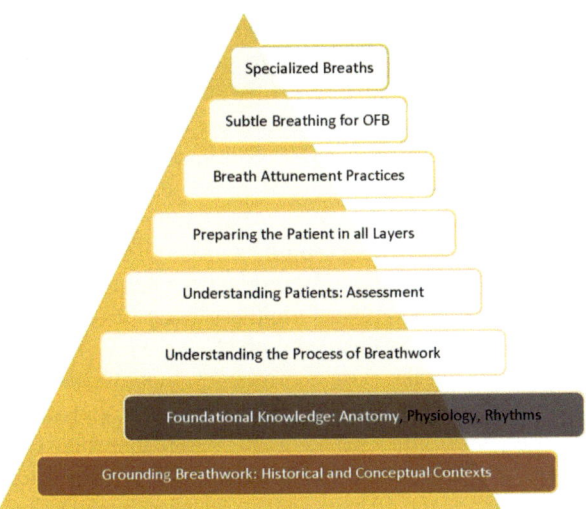

Specialized Breaths

Subtle Breathing for OFB

Breath Attunement Practices

Preparing the Patient in all Layers

Understanding Patients: Assessment

Understanding the Process of Breathwork

Foundational Knowledge: Anatomy, Physiology, Rhythms

Grounding Breathwork: Historical and Conceptual Contexts

C. Brems, *Therapeutic Breathwork*,
https://doi.org/10.1007/978-3-031-66683-4_2

As noted in Chap. 1, the original Sanskrit word *prana* has a multitude of meanings, including breath, life force, and vital energy. It is derived from the root words *pra*—which means "*forth*" and *an* which can be translated as "*to move or breathe.*" These roots suggest the deeper meaning of the word: breath and life force are brought forth by and bring forth life and movement; they are vital and dynamic; they move energy through humans as well as through the entirety of the universe. *Prana*—as breath, energy, and life force—penetrates us in a variety of ways. Of interest in this chapter is its relationship with the physical body, known in yoga psychology as *annamaya kosha*. Our physical layer moves and pulses with the breath, is imbued by its energy, and houses its vitality. The physical self comes alive because of the breath and dies when the breath ceases to move through it. The relationship between body and life force is essential to the human capacity to move, learn, play, communicate, build relationships, and be in community. *Prana* expresses itself in the body as movement, and we can access our vitality through witnessing how the body dances with the breath. The simple exercise of placing our hands on our belly or lower rib basket can put us in touch with how *prana* moves our physical being and how its vitality vibrates, pulses, and enlivens us.

To understand the energy and vitality of breath in its relationship to *annamaya kosha*, it is important to understand the aspects of physical being that are most tangibly related to breathing—our respiratory anatomy and physiology. Most notably, and where we will start in this chapter, breath dances with a variety of physical structures in our respiratory system and beyond.

Breathing, so obviously essential to life, is known biologically as respiration or pulmonary ventilation. As these alternate labels indicate, breathing is the inhalation (or inspiration) and exhalation (or expiration) of air into and out of the lungs to facilitate the carefully calibrated exchange of gases at the cellular level and to sustain life. Each breath cycle is meant to increase tissue levels of oxygen and decrease levels of carbon dioxide. To summarize this process, oxygen (O_2) is necessary for the survival and proper functioning of all tissues in our body, including and especially the brain, and for the production of cellular energy (via ATP production in the mitochondria). O_2 is absorbed into the bloodstream from our breath at the alveoli of the lungs. From there, it is carried (via hemoglobin in the red blood cells) first to the heart (via the pulmonary circulatory system) and then throughout the body via systemic circulation, propelled by the pumping action of the heart. As elaborated upon in Chap. 3, carbon dioxide (CO_2) is a byproduct of metabolism and energy production in the mitochondria. It is returned via the venous system to the heart and from there to the lungs, where it is exchanged with O_2 at the level of the alveoli. The flow of air to the lungs begins at the nose and mouth. Once the air has traveled through the conducting zone of the airways (i.e., the nose, mouth, and more), the lungs work with the heart and the rest of the circulatory system to distribute O_2-rich blood to the cells and to return oxygen-poor and CO_2-rich blood back from the cells to the lungs. CO_2-rich air travels out of the airways and is released from the nose or mouth into the atmosphere.

2.2   Anatomy of Respiration

2.2.1   Overview of the Respiratory System

Anatomically speaking, each breath requires the collaboration of the thoracic cavity, abdominal cavity, and diaphragm. The thoracic cavity houses the heart and lungs and is open to the top of the body via the nose and mouth. It changes shape and volume during breathing to adjust to atmospheric pressure changes created by the movement of the diaphragm. The abdominal cavity houses the stomach, liver, gallbladder, spleen, pancreas, kidneys, bladder, and large and small intestines. It only changes *shape* during breathing, not *volume*, unlike the thoracic cavity, which changes in both shape and volume. The change in shape in both the thoracic and abdominal cavities is driven by the movement of the diaphragm downward and upward during breathing and is explored in detail below.

The respiratory system (Fig. 2.1) includes many structures and related functions. An overview follows, traced via the general movement of air through the system,

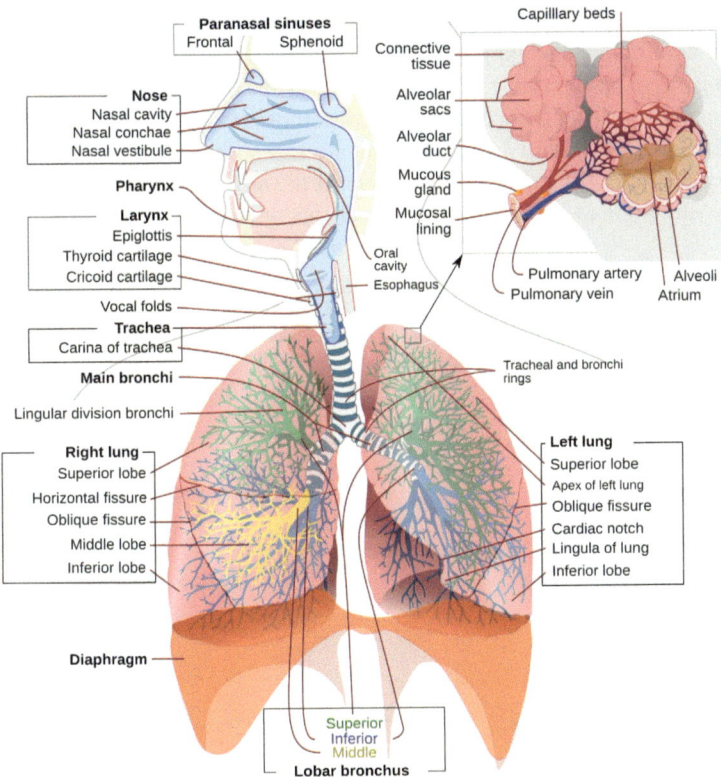

Fig. 2.1 Overview of respiratory system. (Data source: https://commons.wikimedia.org/wiki/File:Respiratory_system_complete_en.svg; public domain)

starting with the entry points at the nostrils and ending with a discussion of ancillary structures (muscles and bones) that affect the respiratory system directly—either biomechanically, biochemically, or both.

Nose and Nasal Cavity

The nasal cavity is the uppermost portion of the respiratory tract and the first point of contact between the air to be inhaled and the body. The nasal cavity is the inner portion of what we may generally call the nose; technically, the *nose* per se is the outer structure. The nose proper is similar to the tip of an iceberg. It is a tiny portion of the nasal structure. The bulk of the nasal cavity is behind the nose and covers a large inner area, all the way to the throat and roof of the mouth.

The nose proper is the prominent feature on our face; that is, the nose is the only external part of the respiratory tract and a tiny portion thereof. Many other structures fashion the inner portion of the respiratory tract (more below). The nose is shaped by bone and cartilage. Alar cartilage forms the apex of the nose (dorsum) and the wings of the nostrils (ala nasi). The septum, which divides the two nostrils (nares), is also made of cartilage. Nasal, maxillary, and frontal bones shape the root of the nose.

The nasal cavity (Fig. 2.2) is the inner portion of the nose, from the nostrils to the pharynx—the large base of the nasal iceberg. The entire nasal cavity is lined with mucous membranes that support immune health (by trapping pathogens) and nasal cleansing. The nasal cavity is divided into two sides, starting with the septum between the nostrils and continuing into the sinuses. The floor of the nasal cavity is also the roof of the mouth and can be palpated by sliding the tip of the tongue from the inner top of the upper teeth back toward the soft palate at the throat. This is a good way to begin to appreciate the dimensions of the nasal cavity. The nasal cavity

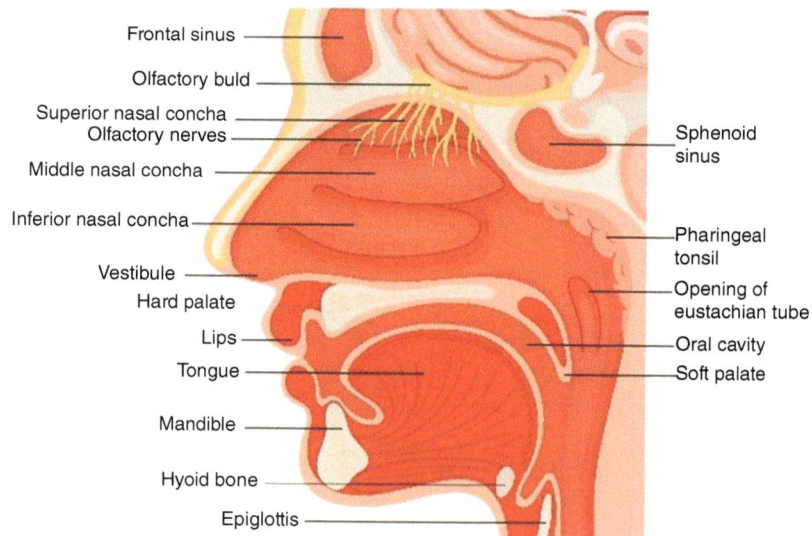

Fig. 2.2 Nasal cavity. (Data source: istock.com)

has three primary chambers: the vestibule, respiratory segment (or section), and olfactory segment.

- *The vestibule* is basically the internal portion of the nose itself. The nostrils are lined by tiny hairs, called cilia, that filter dust and other small particles from the air that enters the nose. Blood vessels are also present in the nostrils and help warm the air upon inhalation. The upper airway is rewarmed by exhalation, as air exiting the body is warmer than air entering it.
- *The respiratory segment* of the nasal cavity includes all passages through which air travels on its way from the start of the nostrils to the pharynx. Each side of the respiratory segment has three turbinates (nasal conchae: upper, middle, and lower), essential for preparing inhaled air for the lungs. Turbinates are shell-shaped structures composed of blood vessels, bone, and highly vascularized tissue. They can change size by swelling from engorging with blood; in other words, they are erectile tissue (in fact, they are related to other erectile tissues in the body and may engorge when those other tissues engorge, resulting in nasal obstructions that have been endearingly called honeymoon rhinitis). The engorgement of the turbinates can restrict airflow. Natural variation in nostril dominance has been documented in humans [1]. We tend to breathe primarily through one side of the nose—a laterality that switches on average every 1.5–2.5 hours (although the range can be as wide as 30 minutes to 8 hours). This laterality is due to alternating engorgement of the turbinates on one side of the respiratory segment of the nose and then the other. It is very typical for us to notice that we are breathing significantly more through one nostril and that this predominance switches every so often. We return to this fact when we explore the practice of alternate nostril breathing.
- Below the turbinates in the respiratory segment are passageways that lead deeper into the airway connecting to the paranasal sinuses. The paranasal sinuses surround the respiratory section of the nasal cavity and drain into it, ultimately draining out of the nostrils. As an aside, it is interesting to note that the lacrimal (or tear) ducts also connect to the nasal cavity and drain into it when we are not crying. When we cry, well, we know what that drainage looks like.
- Air then travels through the back of the throat (the glottis has to be open) to the front pharynx (which also passes food from the mouth to the esophagus—that is why we can sometimes confuse the channels) into the larynx past the vocal cords to the trachea (the larynx, or voice box, is the upper portion of the trachea).
- *The olfactory segment* houses the smell (or olfactory) receptors of lesser interest to the mechanics of breathing but is sometimes extremely important as a risk assessment device. Strong survival reflexes can create substantial positive or negative changes in breathing, depending on what smell is perceived. For example, if a smell is registered by the olfactory receptors that are interpreted by the brainstem as dangerous, we have an immediate reflex to hold our breath. If a smell is registered that is interpreted as soothing, the breath may slow down, becoming gentle and light. It is also useful to note that smell greatly contributes to taste; a congested nose (often due to mouth breathing) greatly impairs the sense of taste.

Inhaling and exhaling through the nose is *optimal for respiratory health* (unless there is an urgent or emergent reason to breathe through the mouth) due to the intricate cleansing, moistening, warming, and preparatory process of the air that starts there. A few specifics follow here, and additional details about nasal breathing are provided later.

- Cilia in the nostrils prefilter the largest particles out of inhaled air (expelling them with the next exhalation). Mucous membranes excrete a sticky, salty substance that contains lysosomes that kill bacteria, providing further cleansing (i.e., removal of pathogens and particles) and wetting of inhaled air. The combined action of cilia and mucus behaves like a conveyor belt that moves filtered impurities and debris from the nose into the stomach at a rate of ½ in./min.
- The mazelike conchae (or turbinates) in the nostrils move the inhalation similar to a turbine by providing resistance to air traveling in, which, in turn, increases O_2 uptake and maintains lung elasticity. The turbinates slow, pressurize, and purify air that enters the nose at a rapid rate of 5 miles/h.
- The nasal cavity contains complex structures, including the paranasal sinuses and an intricate network of blood vessels, that warm, moisten, and cleanse inhaled air before it reaches the lungs.
- The nasal passages also excrete nitric oxide, a superstar gas that further sterilizes the air and—when carried into the lower airway—enhances gas exchange, dilates blood vessels, and significantly increases the efficiency of each breath cycle.
- The inner portion of the nose has the capacity to be cleansed and remoistened by the exhalation. This does not occur if exhalation occurs through the mouth, contributing to dried-out mucous membranes and stuffy noses.
- The nose (rather than the mouth) is also the most healthful passageway for exhalation. This is so because exhaling through the nose expels particles in the nasal cilia (trapped during filtration during inhalation). Additionally, exhaled air has been warmed by its journey through the body and serves to re-humidify and warm the nasal cavity for the next inhalation.
- Additionally, from a yogic perspective, exhaling and inhaling through the nose is more healthful than mouth breathing for energetic reasons. The flow of air through the nose is believed to stimulate the third eye according to ancient yoga traditions. This perceived stimulation may be related to the energetic "buzz" created by nitric oxide that accompanies nasal, but not oral, breathing.

Mouth or Oral Cavity

As a part of the respiratory system, the mouth (Fig. 2.3) is the emergency backup system for breathing, in case nasal breathing is not possible (e.g., during severe congestion or due to an external force that closes the nostrils). The mouth is *not* meant for breathing as a matter of course. The passage of air through the mouth for purposes of breathing does not provide the many advantages offered by the nose (i.e., there are no structures to filter, moisten, cleanse, sterilize, slow, or otherwise enhance

Fig. 2.3 Oral cavity. (Data source: https://commons. wikimedia.org/wiki/ File:Illu_mouth.svg; Creative Commons Attribution 1.0)

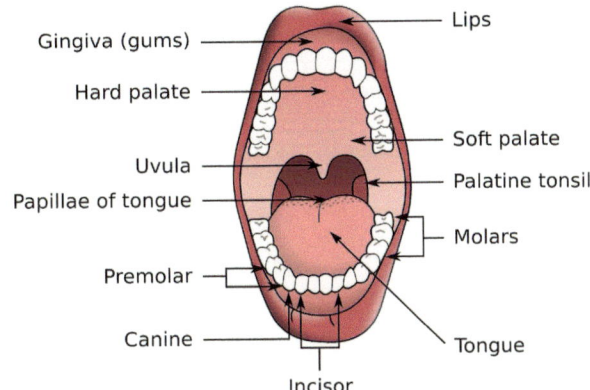

the airstream). The mouth is not an essential part of the respiratory system—it truly is an emergency backup to be used for short (acute) periods. Of all the structures in the oral cavity, the tongue has the most important connection to healthful respiration. If placed against the upper hard palate, touching the backs of the upper teeth, the tongue supports the ideal spinal alignment necessary for efficient breathing mechanics. Poor placement and restricted movement of the tongue, on the other hand, contributes to oral and shallow breathing, or poor respiratory biomechanics.

- The oral cavity consists of lips and cheeks, as well as mucous membranes that line them; tongue; upper and lower gums; hard (anterior roof) and soft (posterior roof) palates, and glottis. Another main structure in the oral cavity are the teeth.
- The mouth is an integral part of the digestive tract—as such, its specialty is dealing with food, not breath. The mouth (well, the teeth with support from the tongue) masticates food and begins the digestive process. The tongue supports swallowing.
- Related to its digestive function, the tongue helps taste food and drink entering the mouth. It contains five types of taste buds, scattered along the surface of the tongue, that can detect five types of tastes or flavors: sweet, sour, salty, bitter, and umami or savory. Taste also depends on smell and when the nose is congested, the capacity to taste is impaired—another reason to keep the nose decongested.
- The mouth is specifically designed for speech, using air to create sound. Speech is a collaboration of the tongue, lips, and teeth controlling airflow from the throat to produce sounds. However, while speaking involves airflow and affects breathing, it is not essential to respiration (although it can interfere with breathing).

Nevertheless, many people use their mouths for breathing—generally to their profound disadvantage. The preference for nasal breathing—as opposed to mouth breathing—is addressed in detail below.

Fig. 2.4 Respiratory tract. (Data source: National Cancer Institute; https://commons.wikimedia.org/wiki/File:Illu_conducting_passages.svg, public domain)

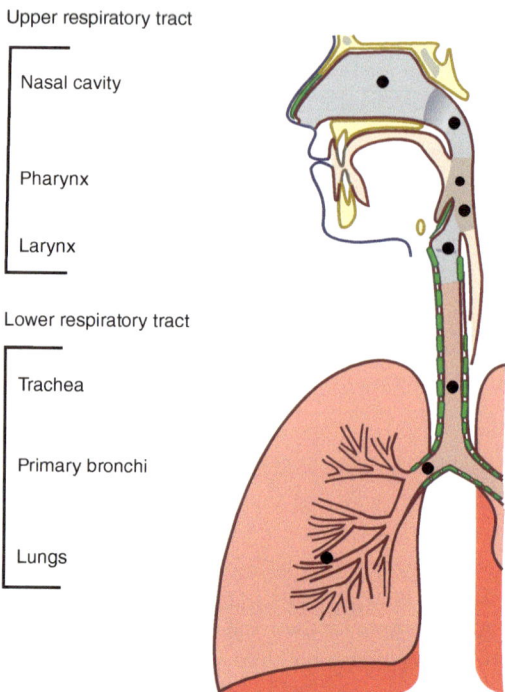

Upper respiratory tract

Nasal cavity

Pharynx

Larynx

Lower respiratory tract

Trachea

Primary bronchi

Lungs

Pharynx

The pharynx, part of the respiratory tract (Fig. 2.4), is a passageway in the throat, delivering air from the nose (or mouth) to the trachea. "The pharynx is a crossroads for the passage of air and food" [2] (p. 71). It has three portions, namely, laryngo-pharynx, oropharynx, and nasopharynx.

- The laryngopharynx is the point at which the pharynx overall divides into the larynx and esophagus. It is a potential central meeting point of food, water, and air that enter either through the mouth or nose.
- The oropharynx is the middle part of the throat. It is a passageway for food and air that enter through the mouth and contains the muscles that allow us to swal-low. Its primary function is to transport food from the mouth to the esophagus, which is situated posterior of the trachea and just anterior of the spinal column. The glottis closes the nasopharynx when we swallow food to prevent it from going down the wrong way, from moving into the trachea. This explains why we cannot breathe and swallow at the time (go ahead and try).
- The nasopharynx delivers air to the larynx which, in turn, conducts air into the trachea. The nasopharynx is closed (hopefully) when we eat to prevent food from entering the larynx. When this closure fails, we cough and choke reflexively to prevent food from entering the airway. When this process is unsuccessful, food

Fig. 2.5 Conducting passages. (Data source: Medical gallery of Blausen Medical. WikiJournal of Medicine 1 (2). DOI: https://doi.org/10.15347/wjm/2014.010. ISSN 2002-4436. Creative Commons Attribution 3.0)

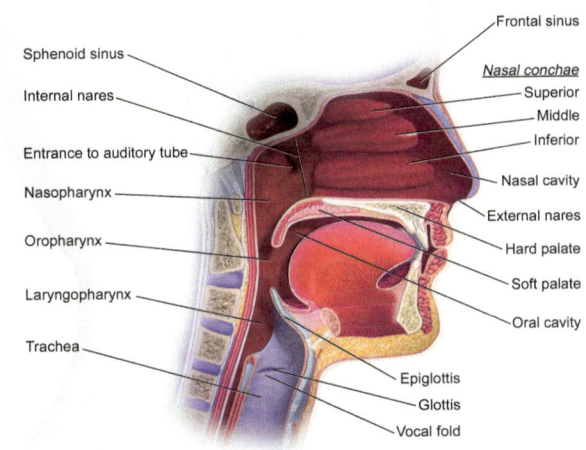

The Upper Respiratory System

particles can reach the lungs and can become the cause of infections. The complete closure of the nasopharynx in the presence of food is facilitated by mindful and slow eating. Functions of the muscles in this region reportedly become less effective with age, termed presbyphagia, resulting in more risk for food being misdirected (Fig. 2.5) [3].

Trachea

The trachea is connected to the nasopharynx via the larynx. It is the conduit that connects the throat to the lungs via bronchi and bronchioles. The trachea is a rigid tube with cartilage rings to maintain its diameter when pressure drops in the lungs. Without this cartilage, the passageway would collapse into itself each time we exhale.

- During activation of the sympathetic nervous system (e.g., during fight or flight), the trachea's diameter increases to facilitate faster and more voluminous air movement. During parasympathetic nervous system activation, the trachea's diameter decreases—and muscles relax. Airflow becomes light, gentle, and calming.
- The trachea has mucus cells that further trap air particles and special cilial cells (called the mucociliary elevator) that transport trapped particles to the pharynx, from where mucus-borne particles can be swallowed or spit out.
- The trachea splits into two large passageways at its bottom—the main bronchi. The bronchi connect the trachea (in fact, the entire upper airway) to each set of *lungs* (Fig. 2.6).

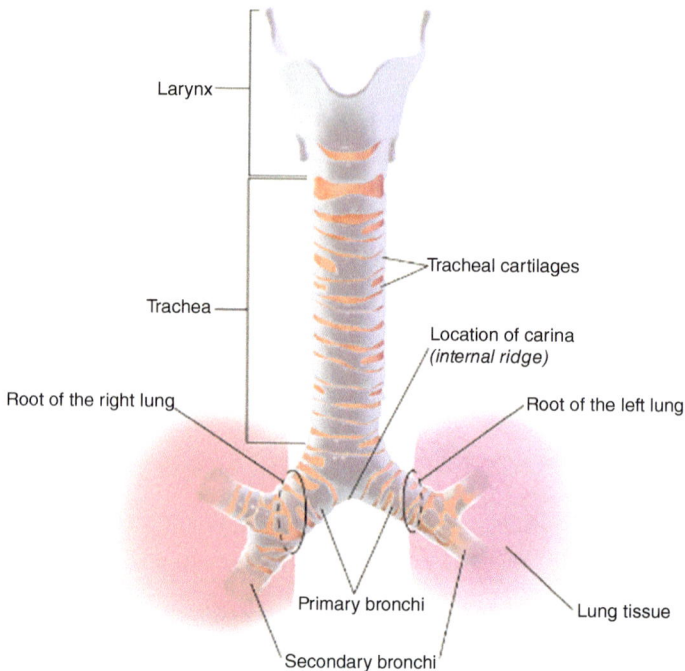

Larynx

Trachea

Root of the right lung

Tracheal cartilages

Location of carina
(internal ridge)

Root of the left lung

Primary bronchi

Lung tissue

Secondary bronchi

Fig. 2.6 Anatomy of the trachea. (Data source: Medical gallery of Blausen Medical 2014. WikiJournal of Medicine 1 (2). DOI: https://doi.org/10.15347/wjm/2014.010. ISSN 2002-4436. Creative Commons Attribution 3.0)

Lungs

The lobes of the lungs constitute the organ that houses the gas exchange that defines breathing. There are three lobes in the lung on the right side and two lobes on the left side. The "missing" third lobe on the left makes room for the heart, which shares the left side of the chest cavity in a space called the cardiac notch. Since the heart takes up space in the front body, approximately 60% of lung tissue is in the back body. The lungs mold themselves around the heart and into the chest cavity they inhabit. When they are healthy, they are bright pink; when they are diseased, they lose their vibrant color, shrink back, and show evidence of scarring and pockmarking by toxic deposits [4].

The pleural membrane surrounding the lungs prevents air from escaping this important respiratory organ. The lung is wrapped by an inner surface called the visceral pleura. The thoracic cavity is wrapped by the outer surface of this membrane, called the parietal pleura. Between the two surfaces is the pleural space (often called a cavity, although it is actually not a "cavity"). The pleural space contains a thin layer of fluid (only approximately 6–12 mL in the average adult) that creates a vacuum to seal the pleurae together and to give the lungs the opportunity to glide along the parietal pleura of the thorax to move and change shape with each inhalation and exhalation. This construction means several things:

- First, this means that as the ribs move, so do the lungs. When the ribs expand, the lungs inflate/expand. Of course, this depends on the size of the rib basket—the lungs cannot inflate any further than the rib basket and the diaphragm can move out of the way. This aspect of our anatomy limits the total lung capacity we have and creates bioindividuality for how much air can move in and out of our lungs.
- The structure of the pleural membranes ensures that the lungs remain inflated with air; therefore, due to the increasing or decreasing amount of air during respiration, these membranes have enormous elasticity to change shape and volume as needed.
- Finally, the vacuum in the pleural "cavity" holds the lungs firmly in place inside their space in the rib basket, and, as long as nothing penetrates the lungs from the outer world, breath will flow. However, if an object were to pierce the lungs (and pleural membrane), the lungs collapse and breathing becomes impossible as air intrudes into the space between the lungs and chest wall.

The lungs (Figs. 2.7 and 2.8), of course, are the location where oxygen is removed from the air to pass it into the bloodstream and carbon dioxide is passed to the alveoli to be expelled through the nose or mouth. The lungs are the destination of air that has traveled through the upper airway toward the lungs' far reaches; they are also the recipient of waste gas from the body to release it outward through the same airways into the atmosphere. *Bronchi and bronchioles* are essential structures inside the lungs for transporting air to and from the structures in the lungs that support gas exchange. Gas exchange proper occurs through the blood-gas barrier between the

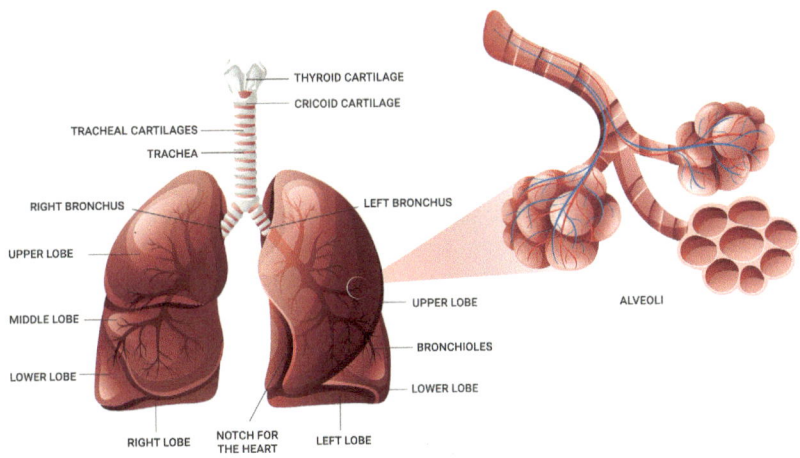

Fig. 2.7 Lobes of lungs with bronchi, bronchioles, and alveoli. (Data source: istock.com)

Fig. 2.8 Lung lobes and rib basket. (Data source: Lungs and chest wall, at https://anatomytool.org/content/cenveo-drawing-lungs-and-chest-wall-english-labels, by Cenveo, Creative Commons Attribution 4.0)

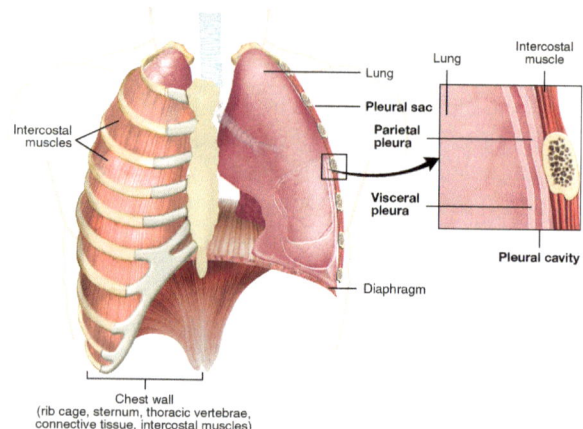

alveoli and the capillaries (explored below) and relies on partial pressure differences in the concentrations of O_2 and CO_2 in capillaries versus alveoli. Interestingly, lungs are largely comprised of nothing other than air. After the exhalation, air comprises 50% of the lungs; after the inhalation, 80%. Air intake into the lungs (i.e., alveoli) is facilitated by the creation of a vacuum in the lungs via the muscles of respiration. The important biomechanics of this process are discussed below.

Bronchi and Bronchioles

Both sets of lungs are deeply penetrated by bronchi and bronchioles to transport inhaled air to the alveoli (for gas exchange) and back to the nose or mouth for expulsion. The bronchi, at the cranial end of the lungs, split many times into smaller and smaller pathways, dividing into lesser bronchi or bronchioles. The trachea, bronchi, and bronchioles are often described as an upside-down tree: the trachea is the trunk, the bronchi are the two main branches, and the bronchioles are the many limbs that split off from the branches.

- Like the trachea, bronchi are cartilage-supported airways that split into secondary and tertiary bronchi. Ultimately, they bring forth bronchioles, the transitions between the strong and resilient airways above and the tiny alveoli below.
- Bronchioles extend deeply into the lungs and split into increasingly small structures, such as the increasingly tiny branches of the metaphoric upside-down tree. They are some of the smallest airways in the respiratory tract. Their main function is the distribution of oxygen-rich inhaled air to the gas-exchanging zone of the lungs and carbon-dioxide-rich exhaled air out of the lungs to the upper airways.
- Bronchioles are lined with particle-trapping mucus and mucociliary cells to further cleanse inhaled air. They also warm and moisten inhaled air.
- Bronchioles are wrapped in smooth muscle, and unlike bronchi, they contain no cartilage. They rely on smooth muscle action to change their diameter. Smooth

muscles that wrap them tamp down on the bronchioles, keeping these channels small until activity requires more air. At that time, the smooth muscles wrapping these tiny airways relax. This action serves to increase the bronchiolar diameter, which allows for more voluminous and faster airflow. As explained in the context of the trachea, diameter adjustment, in this case of the bronchioles, is an autonomic nervous system process that occurs outside of our awareness. In the case of the bronchioles, sympathetic nervous system activation increases the diameter (muscles contract); parasympathetic nervous system activation decreases it (muscles relax).

- The terminal or respiratory bronchioles end in *alveoli*, which look like a honeycomb at the end of the bronchiole terminal. Gas exchange occurs only at this level in the respiratory tract.

Alveoli

At the far ends of the smallest bronchioles, alveoli are the structures where gas exchange with capillaries occurs. Even in the alveoli, additional air cleansing takes place to ensure the cleanest possible air for gas exchange. There are 500 million alveoli, each wrapped with capillaries, to create approximately 50–100 m^2 of surface area available for gas exchange. The majority of alveoli inhabit the outer third of the lungs, similar to leaves on a tree. While typically pictured like grapes on a vine, they actually press up against each other, sharing their tender walls, to create a honeycomb structure.

Alveoli (Fig. 2.9) are lined with pneumocytes that help keep alveolar ducts open for clear airflow. The alveolar wall—only one cell thick—connects to capillaries at the blood-gas barrier on the outer surface of each alveolus. This is the junction where oxygen/carbon dioxide exchange occurs. Capillaries that enwrap alveoli are so tiny, that the red blood cells that pass by them to facilitate gas exchange have to do so single-file. This arrangement and scale maximizes how much gas can be exchanged and creates enormous efficiency. According to Han [5], it means that in

Fig. 2.9 Alveoli and gas exchange between alveoli and capillaries. (Data source: istock.com)

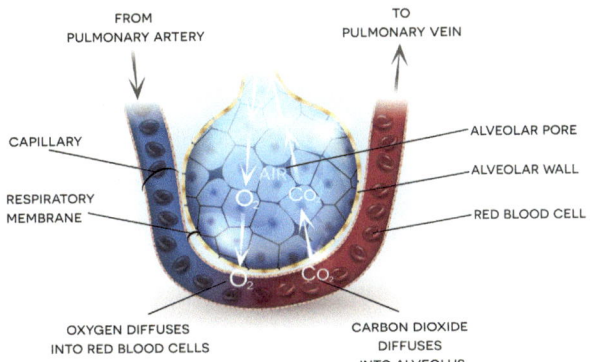

FROM PULMONARY ARTERY

TO PULMONARY VEIN

CAPILLARY

RESPIRATORY MEMBRANE

ALVEOLAR PORE

ALVEOLAR WALL

RED BLOOD CELL

OXYGEN DIFFUSES INTO RED BLOOD CELLS

CARBON DIOXIDE DIFFUSES INTO ALVEOLUS

"the span of 45 seconds, the lungs are able to process the body's entire volume of blood ..., with nearly every red blood cell passing through the tiniest of alveolar capillaries" (p. 8). Alveoli are filled with oxygenated air; capillaries are filled with deoxygenated air; the pressure difference between capillaries and alveoli facilitates the influx of O_2 into the capillaries and the outflux of CO_2 into the alveoli.

- Inhalation releases O_2 from the alveoli into the capillaries. Here, O_2 attaches to hemoglobin—one O_2 molecule per each of four hemoglobin molecules. This process happens in each of 25 trillion red blood cells, each of which houses 270 million hemoglobin molecules. Oxygenated blood then travels through the pulmonary vein to the heart, and from there is pumped throughout the body, making a full-body circuit about once every minute. In the presence of the right conditions (which includes the presence of an optimal amount of CO_2 in the blood), O_2 is released from hemoglobin and delivered to all body tissues, including the brain.
- Blood collects accumulated CO_2 while it is being pumped through the body to release O_2. Deoxygenated blood returns to the heart and from there to the alveoli via the pulmonary artery. Exhalation releases CO_2 into the alveoli, from which air makes its journey back through the airways and out through the nose or mouth.
- The focus in this chapter is on respiratory biomechanics; details about the biochemistry of gas exchange follow in Chap. 3.

Bones Involved in Respiration

Although seemingly counterintuitive, bony structures can and do contribute significantly to variations in breathing rhythm and ease. Thus, explanations about a few bones and their potential role in respiration are helpful and enlightening. The main organ involved in respiration, the lungs, is anchored inside the thoracic cage (or rib basket; Fig. 2.10) The ribs themselves are anchored posteriorly to the thoracic spine

Fig. 2.10 Overview of rib basket numbering. (Data source: istock.com)

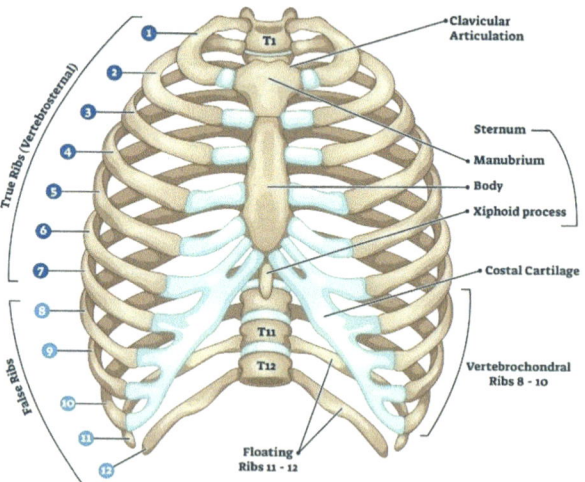

and anteriorly to the sternum (or breastbone). Excessive hyperkyphosis (or curvature) in the thoracic spine, for example, is correlated with tight pectoralis and intercostal muscles, as well as tight hip flexors. This tightness can draw the rib basket inward, which limits mobility in the thoracic spine, resulting in restricted breathing ability and breath volume. In other words, resilience, stability, and mobility of the rib basket are key components of respiratory health. The degree of mobility in the rib basket, especially along various sections, greatly affects the type of breathing and respiratory capacity. Ribs 1–5 (high in the chest) play an important role in breathing that involves movement in the upper chest. These ribs largely protect the lungs and heart. Ribs 6–10 (mid-thorax) play an important role in breathing that is driven primarily by the diaphragm (e.g., breathing low into the abdomen). These ribs protect the organs.

The rib basket contributes to pressure changes in the lungs. It contracts outward (via external intercostal muscles) to help create a greater vacuum that invites the inhalation; it contracts inward (via internal intercostal muscles) to increase pressure on the lungs to support the exhalation. Interestingly, the rib basket and its movements can change significantly across the lifespan, with different orientations in space and changing levels of resilience [6]. These changes include a stiffening of costal cartilage with age that can restrict ease of breath and respiratory capacity due to less movement in the rib basket. Stiffening in the inhalation position of the rib basket (barrel chest or low ribs jutting outward and up) is especially common. This stiffening interferes with complete exhalation and decreases the efficiency of gas exchange [7]. It interferes with optimal diaphragmatic movement, especially its relaxation upward during the outbreath.

Rib orientation for older children and adults is such that rib movement during breathing goes outward and upward (often likened to the movement of a bucket handle). Rib orientation upon birth is very different from rib orientation as we grow older, with a significant change in how the ribs move during breathing. This difference contributes to the strong belly breathing that is natural in babies. This movement is much less natural later in life and breathing instructions that adults should emulate the breath movements of babies may therefore be somewhat misguided [8]. Sex differences in the orientation of ribs are necessary to accommodate physical changes that occur during pregnancy [6]. Rib orientation to accommodate pregnancy directs breath higher into the chest, making biologically female bodies more likely to chest- rather than belly-breathe. However, individual variations in anatomy may overpower such sex difference. Observation of the individual is more important than drawing sex-based conclusions.

Although the pelvis does not play a direct role in respiration, it can have significant indirect effects. For example, a chronic habit of tucking the pelvis (posterior rotation of the pelvic girdle) can interfere with freedom of movement of the diaphragm (via its fascial connection to the hip flexors) and hence the breath [7]. In that sense, assessing pelvic alignment can be helpful. The relationships among pelvic positioning, rib basket positioning and resilience, and spinal alignment with the breath are attended to in detail in the section related to posture and breathing.

Muscles Involved in Respiration

At least three sets of muscles support respiration, namely, diaphragm, intercostals, and core muscles. The undisputed primary driver of the mechanics of respiration is the diaphragm. Its complex biomechanical function is explored in great detail in the biomechanics section below. It is supported to varying degrees and utility by chest and neck muscles as well as ancillary muscles along the spine and in the abdominal (including pelvic) regions. We first explore the anatomy of respiratory muscles; then, we turn to the biomechanics of their complex interrelationships.

Diaphragm

The diaphragm is a thin musculotendinous sheet of skeletal or striated muscle that molds itself to surrounding organs (i.e., heart, lungs, stomach, liver, spleen, and kidneys) and creates the separation between the thoracic and abdominal cavities. The diaphragm is double-dome shaped—one dome under the right and one under the left lobes of the lungs. Coulter [2] describes its shape as that of an umbrella that is deeply indented to accommodate the spinal column; Rothenberg [9] compares it to a parachute. Both metaphors are useful for understanding the upward doming of the diaphragm that can and does change shape at the central axis during breathing.

The diaphragm has three portions: a central tendon, costal portion (toward the rib basket), and crural portion (toward the lumbar spine). The *central tendon* makes up the top surface of the dome and is attached only to the diaphragm's costal and crural portions. In other words, it is a tendon in name only—it does not actually attach to bone; rather, it floats freely. The diaphragm's *costal portion* constitutes its largest portion and faces the rib basket. Its muscle fibers fan out from the central tendon and attach to the rib basket along its lower perimeter. The diaphragm's *crural portion* has muscle fibers that attach to the lumbar spine. The left and right crus are divided by the opening that accommodates the aorta. These two crura merge with the fascia to connect to the anterior longitudinal ligament along the lumbar spine (crus = singular; crura = plural). The crus tendons are also tied fascially to the quadratus lumborum and psoas. These linkages create reverberations of the breath throughout the lower back and hips; they can contribute to stability along the axial body.

Complex fascial and tendinous connections of the diaphragm give it and its surrounding (connected) structures great freedom of movement. Specifically, the central tendon (i.e., the dome's surface), base of the rib basket, and lumbar spine can move independently of each other as well as in unison. This provides many options for how the breath can move through the body in varying positions and in the face of varying obstructions (e.g., different structures move depending on whether we are lying on our bellies or on our backs, determined by which body parts have space to move in a given position; similarly, pregnancy requires different movements during breathing). This reality contributes to the fact that breath affects posture and posture affects breath, a relationship very relevant to breathwork and movement practices (more on this topic later).

The diaphragm (Fig. 2.11) spans the torso's entire circumference and is attached to the base of the rib cage and lumbar spine in an almost circular fashion. It has strong fascial connections caudally (toward the feet) to several sets of muscles (e.g., abdominal muscles, psoas complex muscles, and quadratus lumborum, among

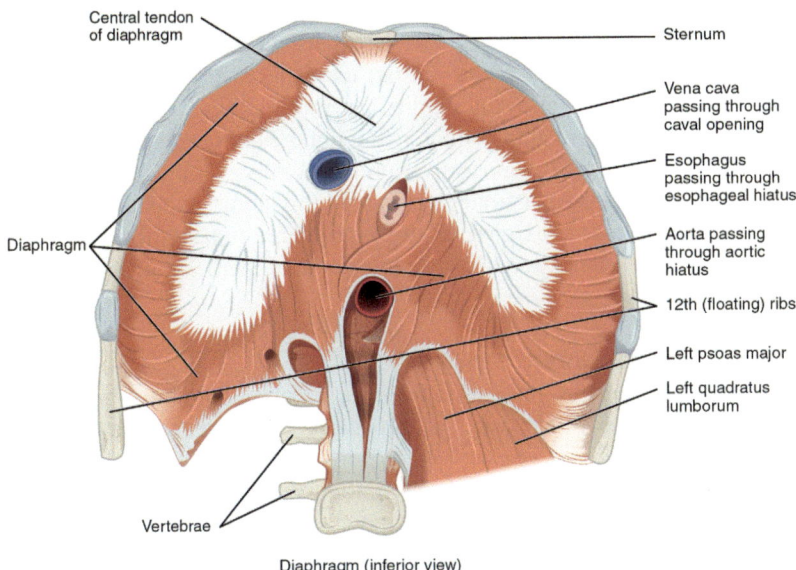

Diaphragm (inferior view)

Fig. 2.11 Anatomy of the diaphragm. (Data source: The Diaphragm at https://anatomytool.org/content/openstax-anatphys-fig1117-diaphragm-english-labels, by OpenStax, Creative Commons Attribution 4.0)

others) and organs (such as stomach, liver, spleen, pancreas, and kidneys, even the upper portion of the intestines). Cranially (toward the head), the diaphragm has strong fascial connections to the heart. With every breath, fascial connections are expressed in various ways. For organs, this connection means that as we breathe, the heart, stomach, liver, and so on receive a gentle massage. For muscles, it creates a complex connection between core strength, spinal stability, pelvic stability and mobility, and movement of breath, as stimulated by the diaphragm. The connection of the diaphragm caudally and cranially also means that our heart is connected to our abdominal organs and vice versa. This connection upward and downward, including via openings in the diaphragm for various blood vessels and nerves, means that breathing, especially force and biomechanics of breathing, can profoundly affect heart rate, blood pressure, digestion, and signaling of stress via the vagus nerve [10]. Everything is indeed connected to everything else.

Several major structures have to pass through the diaphragm by virtue of its placement between the thoracic and abdominal cavities. The inferior vena cava returns blood to the heart and passes through the caval opening of the diaphragm. The descending aorta passes through the aortic opening as it carries blood from the heart to the organs; this opening is shared by the descending aorta and thoracic duct, the main vessel of the lymphatic system. The esophagus passes through the diaphragm at the esophageal opening to allow food to transition from mouth to stomach. The vagus nerve shares this opening as well. It is no surprise that scientific literature points to a close relationship between the diaphragm and vagus nerve, with breathing having direct implications for autonomic nervous system states, such as sympathetic arousal, ventral vagal ease and connection, or dorsal vagal collapse [11]. The close link of the diaphragm to the vagus nerve, along with its innervation by the phrenic nerve, aids in somatosensory feedback that is relayed back and forth between the diaphragm and autonomic nervous system. Generally, gentle and relaxed diaphragmatic breathing counters the fight-flight response, initiating restful parasympathetic nervous system activation, especially when combined with slow stretching or other relaxation strategies. Forced breathing involving the chest muscles, on the other hand, is a signal for the vagus nerve to take off the brake and for the sympathetic nervous system to become predominant. These relationships are explored in detail in Chap. 4.

External and Internal Intercostal Muscles

Many anatomists consider intercostal muscles (Fig. 2.12) to be primary breathing muscles; others consider them accessories because they cannot move the chest independently of the diaphragm. Intercostals support the diaphragm in creating expansion and stabilization in the rib basket. The *internal* intercostal muscles run between adjacent ribs, starting more laterally on the cranially located ribs and moving outward (medially) to connect to the adjacent more caudally located ribs. They lie interior of the external intercostal muscles (as the names suggest). When the internal intercostal muscles contract concentrically, they actively support the diaphragm in creating an exhalation by drawing the ribs closer together and slightly downward. During quiet breathing, however, they do not contract concentrically (i.e., they do not shorten) but simply contract isometrically. They do not change the shape of the rib basket in this situation, but simply help the ribs not to collapse inward during the inhalation. The *external* intercostal muscles also connect to adjacent ribs, but in the opposite direction as the internal intercostals. They support the inhalation; to do so, they contract to lift and expand the rib basket—again in unison with the diaphragm, not independently.

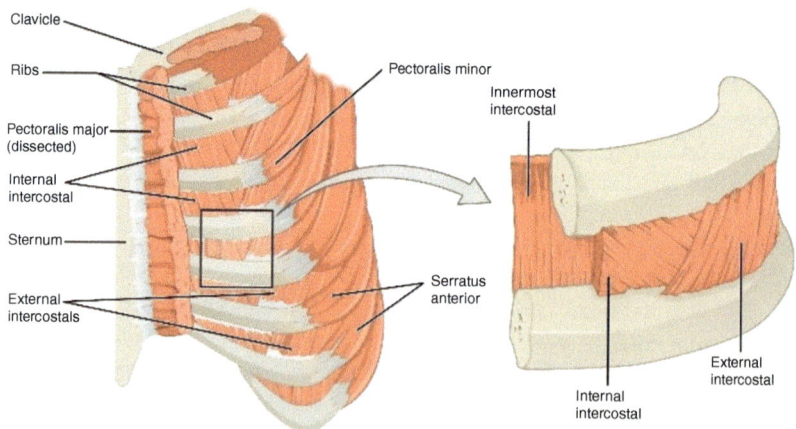

Fig. 2.12 Anatomy of the intercostal muscles. (Data source: Thorax at https://anatomytool.org/content/openstax-anatphys-fig1118-thorax-english-labels, by OpenStax, Creative Commons Attribution 4.0)

Core Muscles, Psoas Complex, and Quadratus Lumborum

Core muscles, including hip flexors and stabilizers, are listed by many anatomy and yoga resources as breathing-related muscles. All interact with breath but are not muscles of necessity for all forms of breathing. In fact, natural breathing does not recruit these muscles specifically. Of course, any muscles with attachments to the rib basket or fascial connections to primary and accessory breathing muscles have the potential to affect the breath and vice versa. The core muscles (*rectus abdominis, transverse abdominis, external obliques, and internal obliques*) collaborate with the diaphragm to help stabilize the spine and optimize posture (especially the transverse abdominals and obliques, as explored below). They support deep exhalations, but may only engage very naturally or lightly (if at all) during natural breathing. In fact, excessive contraction can get in the way of the inhalation. Core muscles are also important for spinal stability and posture; they have a strong two-way relationship with the diaphragm and the psoas complex in the pelvis. Following are some anatomy basics about these sets of muscles; their more complex movement relationships with breath are covered in the biomechanics section below.

Short Journey into the Abdominal Muscles

The abdominal muscles have to be understood in the context of the abdominal cavity. The abdominal cavity can change shape, but not volume (unlike the thoracic cavity, which can change both shape and volume). It is lined with a membrane called the parietal peritoneum. The peritoneum secretes moisture to ease the movement of the organs and holds the organs in place via folds called the mesentery.

The abdominal muscles are completely integrated with the skin, superficial fascia, diaphragm, and the parietal peritoneum. They consist of flat muscles (that have fibers in crossing directions and entwine at the midline as the linea alba, a strong, flat band of connective tissue at the front of the abdominal cavity) and vertical muscles. They are arranged to make a cross (transverse abdominis runs horizontally, and the rectus abdominis runs vertically) and an X (external obliques make up the two top portions of the X, and internal obliques create the two bottom portions of the X). All are centered on the navel. Lasater [7] describes that the *"abdominal muscles create a 'basket weave' effect on the front of the body and wrap around the sides of the body, so that when we stand erect or lift things or bend in all directions or walk, we are able to maintain our upright postures. The abdominals 'hold us together' in a sense..."* (p. 115). Myers [12] says that all roads in the abdomen lead to the umbilicus. He perceives the navel as a mechanical and emotional crossroads.

The core muscles are part of the abdominal wall, which creates a firm boundary and protection for the viscera; assists in forceful exhalation; contributes to stabilization of the torso, spine, and pelvis; and helps increase or maintain intrabdominal pressure (such as in childbirth and during coughing, sneezing, vomiting, laughing, etc.). The abdominal muscles' primary function is the stabilization of the trunk, spinal column, ribs, and pelvis. Stabilization means that these muscles act to stabilize a part of the body while another part moves, making the movement in the active part of the body easier and more efficient through the stabilization of the parts that need not or should not move (e.g., lift the neck while supine—notice how the abdominal muscles stabilize the ribs and pelvis). The abdominals are strengthened via postures focused on stabilization (e.g., boat pose [navasana]; table top with one arm lifted and slowly moving the weight of the torso forward step-by-step). The stabilization function of the abdominals is less effective or powerful when the low back is arched, stretching the abdominals. The abdominals also fire any time we have to stabilize the trunk against gravity.

Stabilization of the torso occurs developmentally; by the age of 6 months, babies have enough strength in the torso from their core muscles to sit upright. Stabilizing the ribs and pelvis is one of the abdominals' major jobs in sitting, standing, walking, and all daily activities and yoga postures. They draw the ribs toward the pelvis and the pelvis toward the ribs to create a sense of core integration through their origins and insertions along the ribs and pelvis. They work entirely in conjunction with the diaphragm and the pelvic floor. All these muscles are part of a strong anatomy train called the deep front line.

Short Exploration of the Psoas Complex—Main Operators of Hip Flexion

The psoas complex consists of hip flexors, spine flexors, and side-benders. The main functions of the psoas complex are flexion at the hips, flexion in some lumbar joints, and side-bending of the trunk. It also contributes to core stability and walking/breathing rhythms. The psoas complex and diaphragm are intimately connected [12]. There are fascial and muscular connections so that movement (or restriction) in the psoas affects the diaphragm and movement in the diaphragm affects the psoas. The psoas complex includes several important muscles and is fascially connected to the sartorius in the thighs and the quadratus lumborum (QL) in the low back. With the diaphragm, core muscles, and pelvis floor, the psoas complex is part of the deep front line (set of fascially-connected muscles deeply embedded and supporting movements in the front of the body, from feet to head).

Psoas major flexes the hips and helps sidebend the trunk (origin: T12–L5 vertebrae; insertion into the lesser trochanter). *Psoas minor* flexes the lumbar joints (origin: T12–L5 vertebrae; insertion into the lateral pubic bone). *Iliacus* flexes the hip (origin: iliac crest; insertion with psoas major into the lesser trochanter). All these psoas complex muscles are connected to the *sartorius,* which flexes the hip and externally rotates it, as well as when in flexion, flexes and internally rotates the knee (origin: anterior superior iliac spine (ASIS); insertion: medial superior tibia). *Quadratus lumborum* stabilizes the pelvis and spine; it helps sidebend the lumbar spine (origin: iliac crest; insertion: inferior border of the last rib).

The psoas complex and quadratus lumborum (QL) are primary muscles for pelvic stability and mobility. They are related to breathing in that they collaborate with the diaphragm to support the coordination of walking and breathing. They have strong fascial connections to the diaphragm and, as such, become relevant to breathing especially if they have pathologies (e.g., such as tight psoas muscles due to excessive sitting or less-than-optimal posture). The fascia that connects the diaphragm, psoas complex, and QL also reaches cranially to the pericardium of the heart. In that sense, all these areas become important for respiration. The core muscles, psoas complex, and posture as a whole strongly impact the zone of apposition, the region within which the diaphragm can descend and ascend freely inside the ribcage. The zone of apposition plays an important role in the relationship between posture and breathing, as explored below.

Pectoralis Major and Minor, Scalenes, and Sternocleidomastoid Muscles
These muscles are high in the chest or neck and may be supportive during active breathing. They are accessory and not necessary (in fact, often counterproductive) for quiet natural breathing. They are mostly recruited during times of strain and exercise. They are *at times* considered primary because some humans use them as such. However, this is not an ideal function for these muscles because their activation signals stress, even the need for fight or flight, to the autonomic nervous system, triggering a sympathetic nervous system response by releasing the vagal brake.

2.3   Biomechanics of Breath

Breathing depends on the ability to change the shape and volume of the chest and on the elasticity of the lungs. All muscles of the chest that contribute to changes in the shape of the chest might therefore be considered respiratory muscles, some primary, some accessory, and some recruited only under certain circumstances (e.g., during stress or exertion). Breathing depends on posture, flowing more freely in optimal alignment and being potentially impaired by collapsed or overly braced postures. In that sense, all muscles involved in standing and walking may be considered accessory breathing muscles. There is little agreement among anatomists about which muscles are primary, secondary, accessory, or recruitable to support breathing. However, *one* agreement is that *the* primary muscle of respiration is the diaphragm, biomechanically supported by intercostal muscles, abdominal and pelvic floor muscles, psoas complex, and several sets of (much smaller and weaker) accessory muscles (such as scalenes, sternocleidomastoid, and pectoralis minor muscles). All these deeply fascially connected muscles collaborate to create the movement of breath, stabilize the spine, and coordinate (stabilize and mobilize) the pelvis.

2.3.1   Role and Movement of the Diaphragm and Fascially Connected Muscles in Respiration

To review, the diaphragm is undisputedly the primary muscle of respiration and creates the separation between the thoracic cavity (in some yoga circles called the *air body*) and the abdominal cavity (in some yoga circles, the *water body*). The way it is designed to facilitate breathing is nothing short of amazing. The diaphragm is not attached to the lungs but simply touches their inferior or lower edge and creates surface friction. This primary breathing muscle is tethered only to the lumbar vertebrae and bottom of the ribs, with origins at several thoracic (T7–T12) and lumbar (L1–L3) vertebrae (via the right and left crus tendons), low ribs, and inner portion of the xiphoid process, and insertions at the central tendon. The diaphragm is absolutely unique in the way it moves.

When breath is resting (i.e., gently suspended at the exhalation's conclusion) or exhaled, the diaphragm's domes are relaxed and press up gently against the lungs via their inherent elasticity. During the inhalation, the diaphragm contracts and flattens (i.e., the centers of its domes move downward, and the edges move outward and upward), increasing the diameter and vertical height of the rib basket and thoracic cavity. Partway during inhalation, the diaphragm's insertions and origins switch, with the anchored and nonstationary end of the muscle becoming the moving end and vice versa (the only muscle in the body that does this). This transition is necessary to facilitate the *downward* movement of the diaphragm and the *outward* movement of the low rib basket.

This design is unique and ingenious; it provides enormous freedom of movement to the diaphragm so that it can facilitate breathing in any position that the body may be taking on, including positions that limit the movement of any part of the body involved in breathing, such as the abdomen, mid- to lower back, and chest. The movement of the diaphragm and its accessory muscles varies depending on whether we are standing, sitting, lying prone or supine, or walking. Thus, movement of breath can be experienced in different places of the body depending on how we are moving or positioned. Regardless of position, the downward and upward and/or inward and outward movements of the diaphragm and rib basket together change the pressure in the lungs, creating a vacuum during the inhalation (inviting air into the lungs) and increasing pressure in the lungs during exhalation (supporting the movement of air out of the lungs).

Understanding the Movements of Breath Traveling Through the Body
Breathing depends on movement and movement reflects the breath. Similarly, breath affects posture and posture affects breath. In many contexts, including yoga and meditation, cuing, or talking about the breath revolves around the up and down movement of the diaphragm. Unfortunately, how many clients hear this description is as strictly chest and belly movement. This is reinforced by the frequent focus on feeling the belly rise and fall with the inhalation and exhalation. Although none of this is incorrect, it *is* incomplete. The movement of the diaphragm and related structures (via attachment points and fascia) is not just up and down, but also in and out to the sides. The movement of the low ribs and resilience in the rib basket, when optimal, is upward and outward with the inhalation and downward and inward with the exhalation. The abdomen does not just rise and fall with the breath; it travels outward and inward to both sides as the breath comes and goes. It is helpful to cue and talk about all these directions—up and down; and in and out. The inward and outward movements are as, if not more, important and greatly contribute to breath health. We do not want a heaving chest; we want a resilient rib basket.

Experiencing this combination of movements can be helpful in understanding diaphragmatic breath:

- Sit in a comfortable position.
- Wrap the thumb and index fingers around the low waist (just above the hip bones), with fingers pointing forward and palms parallel to the floor.
- Breathe in and notice—the hands likely are being pushed outward to the both sides by the inhalation.
- Breathe out and notice—the hands release inward toward the center as the exhalation travels out.

The diaphragm's movement (Fig. 2.13) massages the heart and stomach, assists with lymphatic flow, and plays a supportive role in expulsive actions—including vomiting, sneezing, coughing, urination, defecation, and "pushing" during childbirth—by increasing pressure in the abdominal cavity in conjunction with the abdominal muscles. The psoas complex and diaphragm are intimately connected so that movement (or restriction) in the psoas affects the diaphragm and movement in the diaphragm affects the psoas. Walking connects the psoas complex and diaphragm

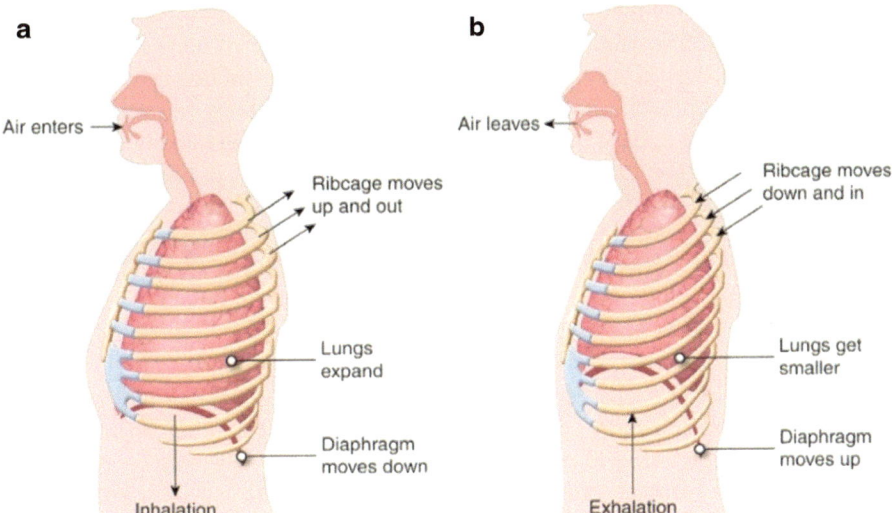

Fig. 2.13 (**a**) Movements of the diaphragm in breathing (inhalation). (Data source: Diaphragm, rib cage and lungs during inhalation, at https://anatomytool.org/content/cenveo-drawing-diaphragm-rib-cage-and-lungs-during-inhalation-english-labels, by Cenveo, Creative Commons Attribution 4.0). (**b**) Movements of the diaphragm in breathing (exhalation). (Data source: Diaphragm, rib cage and lungs during expiration, at https://anatomytool.org/content/cenveo-drawing-diaphragm-rib-cage-and-lungs-during-expiration-english-labels, by Cenveo, Creative Commons Attribution 4.0)

in dynamic stability. As the legs alternate, one side of the psoas tugs on the diaphragm and then the other—back and forth with each step (stable on one side; loose on the other). This relationship links movement and breath, and it may have as much or more to do with pelvic and core stability and mobility as the abdominal muscles.

The diaphragm contributes to core stability [13, 14], and has important connections to the abdominal muscles. As noted above, when co-contracted with the abdominals, the diaphragm helps with expulsive actions. However, this co-contraction can also have negative effects, potentially resulting in shallower breathing and impaired inhalation, if engaged in an inappropriate manner, with excessive force, or with poor timing. Specifically, while abdominal muscles can help with *forceful* exhalations, they are not involved in quiet or natural breathing (contrary to common belief and cuing in yoga classes). In fact, they can interfere with breathing when strongly contracted. The notable movement in the abdomen during breathing is initiated by movement of the diaphragm and its slight displacement of abdominal organs—there is no need for the abdominal muscles to help this process during quiet, natural breathing.

Movement of the diaphragm during breathing also activates the thoracic pump to support the cardiovascular system. Negative pressure in the thoracic cavity and intra-abdominal pressure, created during the inhalation by the diaphragm's downward contraction, not only facilitates airflow into the lungs, it also results in compression of the vena cava, supporting blood being drawn into the right atrium of the heart. Changes in pressure that occur with the exhalation, via the diaphragm's upward relaxation toward the thoracic cavity, help propel blood out of the heart and into the body and lungs. The more natural the diaphragm's range of motion, the more its action supports the cardiovascular system; the less range of motion in the diaphragm, the less it supports the pumping action of the heart. Without unrestricted support from the diaphragm, the circulatory system does not work at maximum efficiency, resulting in increased stress on the system. Given the volume of blood pumped each and every minute (our blood makes one full circuit through the body every minute) and each and every day (the heart circulates approximately 2000 gallons of blood per day), any increase or decrease in stress placed on the heart can accumulate quickly.

2.3.2   Biomechanics of Different Types of Breathing

Biomechanics of breathing can be elucidated further by exploring various *types of breathing* that can unfold from the action of primary and accessory breathing muscles. The types of breath presented here are closely linked to muscles that work alongside or instead of the diaphragm. While these most commonly recognized types of breath are discussed separately, it is helpful to remember that they are not always distinct; they often overlap. While all these types of breath can be differentiated and easily observed in ourselves and our clients, not all are of equal quality, utility, or functionality. Some may be helpful in particular situations; others are hardly ever beneficial to health, and yet all are common ways of breathing. Natural diaphragmatic breathing optimally supports a functional, wholesome, and natural breath.

Thoracic Breath

This breath largely involves the upper chest muscles with little to no recruitment of the diaphragm. The chest muscles are not truly viewed or supposed to be used as primary breathing muscles. However, reality is different from the ideal. Many individuals engage in chest—or thoracic—breathing because this breath is autonomically associated with stress or anxiety. Thoracic breathing relies on the actions of the pectoralis, scalene, and sternocleidomastoid muscles; it also engages the intercostals. It moves the breath biomechanically into the upper chest, moving air into the much narrower space of the lungs higher in the rib basket. Movement in the diaphragm is minimal, often due to the overly-braced (tensed) or overly-collapsed (slumped) posture associated with this type of breathing (and with stress—hence the connection between high chest and stress breathing). Over time, the diaphragm loses elasticity and tone, becoming less resilient and sending signals to the nervous system that there is a sense of threat or danger.

The abdominals are often unfavorably engaged in thoracic breathing, as are the psoas complex muscles. The low ribs may flare out or draw in excessively and further impair the diaphragm's natural movement. The individual may be gasping for air, taking big breaths, but not getting the benefits of all this air as gas exchange in lungs and tissues becomes inefficient, with more voluminous breaths being drawn than necessary and yet with less successful gas exchange at the tissue level. Finally, without significant diaphragmatic movement, we miss its massaging actions, supportive recruitment of abdominal and pelvic muscles, and supportive action of the intercostals. Thoracic breathing can be recruited in challenging situations that require sympathetic nervous system arousal, such as situations requiring actual physical fight or flight. Accordingly, thoracic breathing can show up in two ways—empowering or constricting.

Empowering Thoracic Breath—Braced

Thoracic breath can feel empowering when it supports an open chest (e.g., in a slight backbend) while standing to allow the lungs to *inflate* more fully. An empowering thoracic breath is not a breath for supine or prone positions; however, it can be helpful when engaged to meet a specific short-term empowering, activating need or purpose [2]. The focus of this breath is on taking voluminous inhalations, which makes it a strong and vitalizing breath that may serve well when there is a need for immediate and powerful action, including physical fight or flight. Even in these functional moments, however, thoracic breathing can make the individual vulnerable to overbreathing, especially if empowerment is not needed to support vigorous physical action (such as running or fighting) or if this type of breath is engaged habitually [9].

Empowering thoracic breath stimulates the sympathetic nervous system, increasing heart rate and blood pressure, as well as interfering with digestion and elimination—all helpful when we have to run to save our lives, but not supportive of our health if engaged chronically. Posturally, thoracic breath is associated with an overly lifted, posteriorly rotated rib basket, flattened lumbar spine and mildly posterior pelvis, braced abdominals, and braced psoas complex muscles [15]. Although this conveys a short-term sense of vigor and power, in the long term, this posture and these biomechanics interfere with functional movement and optimal breathing.

Constricted Thoracic Breath—Collapsed

Thoracic breath is constricting when it is performed because of a closed chest and slumped posture that impedes the flow of air into the lungs. In this case, the rib basket is not flared out, but rather is drawn in and collapsed. The lumbar spine is rounded, without its natural lordotic curve; the thoracic spine may be overly kyphotic. The pelvis is rotated posteriorly [9, 15]. This collapsed posture and constricted thorax create an anxious and shallow breath that moves high up into the torso, perhaps all the way to the clavicles (which may turn it into *clavicular breathing*). It is emotionally challenging and often associated with significant distress, anxiety, even panic. It may be associated with a state of dorsal vagal collapse (i.e., a sense of giving up, of hopelessness) in the autonomic nervous system. Constricted thoracic breathing is a significant challenge for human physiology if used habitually.

Paradoxical Breath

This is another breath that relies heavily on high chest muscles to move air. In addition to being biomechanically thoracic, paradoxical breath is accompanied by *reverse diaphragmatic movements*, in which inhalation causes the diaphragm to move upward and exhalation results in its downward movement. For this reason, paradoxical breath has also been called reverse breathing, and is always a breath that involves and signals sympathetic nervous system activation. Paradoxical breath can be noted by the reverse movement of the abdomen moving inward upon inhalation and outward upon exhalation (although this may be subtle). It can also be noted when client seem utterly confused—because it is counter to their experience—when we cue opening the heart with inhalation and drawing inward with exhalation. Their experience is the opposite.

Paradoxical breath is a startled, shocked breath that causes a jolt of adrenaline to be released. In a way, it is a braced thoracic breath taken to an unhealthful extreme. For example, if we jump into a lake with unexpectedly icy cold water, the breath that follows is almost always paradoxical. With startled (panicked) inhalation, the intercostal muscles enlarge the rib cage, and the abdominal wall moves in rather than out. The abdominal organs and diaphragm are lifted upward toward the lungs by the force of the strong and reactive contraction of the intercostal muscles. This extremely upregulating breath that shocks us into a sympathetic nervous system response can become chronic and is correlated with anxiety and panic. Paradoxical breathing that has become chronically linked to anxiety or panic slowly erodes organ and endocrine health due to constant sympathetic nervous system hyperarousal and no "breaks" to reset, to restore the body physiologically, to digest properly, to find ease and relaxation. The body might stay in fight-or-flight mode with little opportunity for rest, recuperation, healing, and relaxation.

Abdominal Breath

Abdominal breathing relies *largely* on the diaphragm, with little if any recruitment of intercostals, no recruitment of high chest muscles, and little interaction with abdominal or pelvic muscles. The latter is due to the fact that this type of breath happens only if we are seated or lying on our backs (supine). It is not a natural breath for standing, walking, or moving. Thus, abdominal breathing is most often used in the context of restorative yoga and meditation. There are two forms of abdominal breathing: supine and seated. A hybrid abdominal breath combines these two forms by using a propped supine position in which the torso is sloped upward, in between lying flat on the ground and sitting upright. Nasal breathing typically accompanies abdominal breathing, as it is crucial for optimal recruitment of the diaphragm.

Supine Abdominal Breath

Abdominal breath while lying on our backs is based (nearly) entirely on diaphragmatic movement. In a supine position, inhalation requires moderate effort, while exhalation is more, though not completely, relaxed yet active (there is a need for eccentric lengthening of the diaphragm in the supine position). The intercostal muscles simply isometrically stabilize, but do not elevate or expand the chest or low rib basket. The abdominal muscles are relaxed. The diaphragm's movement inferiorly pushes abdominal organs down and hence requires the abdominal wall to move outward. Because in a supine position, the abdominal organs ride higher than when standing or seated (i.e., pulled lower by gravity), the exhalation is fuller (moves more volume of air). This can be a very relaxed and relaxing breath. It is not a breath that is likely (if it is even possible) while standing or moving [2].

Seated Abdominal Breath

Abdominal breathing while seated is *mostly* based on diaphragmatic movement. In a seated position, the exhalation is completely relaxed (or passive) or relaxed, yet active. The intercostal muscles contract isometrically to stabilize the chest, but the chest does not expand. Abdominal organs are shifted lower into the abdomen due to gravity; this lowered placement of organs (compared to supine abdominal breathing) results in less expiratory lung volume (less air is moved out). Seated abdominal breathing can rely on a more relaxed exhalation than supine abdominal breathing and is preferred for meditation due to its greater calming or soothing effect on the nervous system. A partly reclined seat (e.g., on an inclined bolster) is a compromise between supine and seated abdominal breathing and invites a deep sense of relaxation or ease.

Natural Diaphragmatic Breath

Natural diaphragmatic breathing is the most natural way to breathe; it engages the diaphragm and intercostal muscles in a gentle rhythmic manner. It collaborates, as needed, with abdominal and pelvic muscles, supporting stability and mobility of the spine and pelvis; it massages the heart and abdominal organs, as well as moving lymph. Natural diaphragmatic breath moves low into the abdomen, including the lowest ribs; it does not (typically) move high into the rib basket, chest, or clavicles. Suppleness in the rib basket supports this breath as the low ribs need to be able to move out/upward and in/downward, with the inhalation and exhalation, respectively. As is true for abdominal breathing, nasal breathing typically accompanies diaphragmatic breathing because of its role in optimal diaphragmatic recruitment. As we will explore below, nasal breathing has many biomechanical and biochemical advantages.

Diaphragmatic breathing is an integrated holistic expression of healthy biomechanics, biochemistry, cadence, and subtle energies and, thus, an optimally functional breath with many advantages and benefits. In this chapter, the focus is on the *biomechanics* of this breath. We return to this type of breathing again in the contexts of biochemistry, breath rhythm, and subtle dimensions of breathing. Additionally, this breath is the ideal basis for all breathing or *pranayama* practices. It is, of course, worth noting that all types of breath involve the movement of the diaphragm—it is, after all, the primary breathing muscle. However, *natural diaphragmatic breath* is labeled in this way to reflect that this is the most natural way to breathe, as it creates and maintains optimal anatomical, physiological, autonomic, and psychoemotional conditions.

Biomechanics of Natural Diaphragmatic Inhalation

The biomechanics of diaphragmatic inhalations unfold as follows, much in line with the biomechanics overviewed above in the context of primary and accessory breathing muscles. The diaphragm contracts and flattens toward its attachments on the lumbar spine upon inhalation. The centers of the diaphragm move caudally; its edges move cranially. The diaphragm moves downward but never beyond the caudal rim of the ribs, staying with a range of motion that allows its costal section to stay in direct contact with the inner lining of the rib basket. If the diaphragm were to descend lower, it would reach an area where it could no longer move freely and smoothly because it would move past the slippery surfaces of the chest cavity. The portion of the body beyond which the diaphragm cannot descend is called the *zone of apposition*. The zone of apposition is key to a healthy posture that supports healthy breathing. We will return to this concept.

Helpful YouTube Resources about the Biomechanics of Respiration by Ninja Nerd
https://youtu.be/RnWVCE9KdR8 = Biomechanics of Respiration | Half Head Anatomy
https://youtu.be/uYm4l_alVV0 = Respiratory | Mechanics of Breathing: Inspiration | Part 1
https://youtu.be/LewPdsjzEic = Respiratory | Mechanics of Breathing: Inspiration | Part 2
https://youtu.be/-oVL0CDduAY = Respiratory | Mechanics of Breathing: Expiration | Part 3

For either quiet or forceful breathing to be optimal, the lungs must be elastic. Elasticity in the context of anatomy is the ability of an anatomical structure to recoil to or recover its original shape, size, or length after being or having stretched or contracted. For muscles, this means they return to their original shape and length after lengthening or when relaxed. For the lungs, this means that they want to recoil to their original shape and position in the rib basket after inspiration.

In optimal diaphragmatic breathing (quiet breathing), a pressure change occurs in the lungs relative to the atmosphere: upon inhalation, negative pressure is created in the lungs (as the diaphragm moves downward and air streams in); upon exhalation, pressure in the lungs increases (as the diaphragm moves upward and air streams out). In other words, pressure changes in the lungs are key to the flow of breath. This is the reason why geographic altitude affects breathing. Atmospheric pressure decreases with altitude (due to changes in gravitational forces as we climb or fly higher), making air lighter. This means less outside pressure supporting the flow of breath into the lungs, leading to more labored breathing during high-altitude climbing or training. Therefore, it is more difficult to breathe at high altitudes and easier to breathe at low altitudes.

The downward movement of the diaphragm during inhalation creates a vacuum in the lungs (a pressure difference from the atmosphere) and allows the lungs to expand as air is sucked in by the lower pressure that was created. According to Boyle's law (i.e., pressure and volume of gas in a contained space are inversely proportional), as the pressure in the thoracic cavity decreases (negative pressure compared to the atmosphere outside of the body), volume (of air in the lungs) increases and air travels in.

The downward movement of the diaphragm causes the abdomen to expand in 360° as organs must move to make room for the diaphragm to descend into the lower abdominal cavity. In the process, the centers of each diaphragmatic dome press on the internal organs of the abdominal cavity (pancreas, spleen, liver on the right, stomach on the left—that is why it is harder to breathe when your stomach is very full or while pregnant). The centers of the domes can descend only so far before the pressure of the organs stops the diaphragm. At this stopping point, *the origin and insertion of the diaphragm flip* and now the edges of the diaphragm pull upward cranially on the low ribs to expand the *low* rib basket to make room for more air to travel in. This is often called the bucket handle expansion of the ribs. It is mostly caused by the diaphragm, supported by intercostals as needed. If the intercostals do activate, they have a supporting role, not a primary role in the movement of the low rib basket. Inhalation decreases tension on the crus tendons (and thus the lumbar spine to which it is attached). The internal intercostal muscles relax upon inhalation, allowing the slight outward movement of the low ribs. The external intercostal muscles co-contract or isometrically contract along with the diaphragm to ensure that the low ribs do not move too far outward.

Pulmonary stretch receptors in the smooth muscles of the bronchi, bronchioles, and trachea perceive the stretch that occurs as the lungs expand during inhalation. They relay this information to the ventral respiratory complex (VRC) in the medulla and the pons via the vagus nerve. The VRC analyzes the signal received from the stretch receptors and triggers the Hering-Breuer reflex to begin to slow respiration as the lungs become increasingly stretched. The Hering-Breuer reflex prevents the lungs from overinflating, especially during large inhalations. When maximum stretch is perceived, the VRC begins to send inhibitory signals to the inspiratory muscles, namely, the diaphragm and external intercostal muscles. This means that the inspiratory muscles, at that point, stop contracting and relax into their original shape, in effect ending the inhalation.

Biomechanics of Natural Diaphragmatic Exhalation

Relaxation of the inspiratory muscles consequently reduces the volume in the thoracic cavity, as the diaphragm relaxes up against the lungs and external intercostals relax the rib basket inward and downward. The decreasing volume (as per Boyle's Law) increases pressure in the lungs and the air begins to travel out via the exhalation. Thus, while even quiet *inhalation* requires active engagement of the diaphragm and (minimal) of the external intercostals, quiet *exhalation* is passive, initiated because of feedback from baroreceptors to the medulla. Passive expiration (as occurs during quiet breathing) depends on the lungs' tendency to resist being stretched, that is, on the lungs' elasticity and inclination to recoil to their original shape. When the lungs recoil, they automatically draw in the rib basket because of the connection of the visceral pleura to the parietal pleura. The shift from inhalation to exhalation occurs when intrapulmonary ("inside the lungs") pressure increases to be equal to atmospheric ("outside the lungs") pressure. This creates a gap in the breath at the top of the breath.

To recap, on exhalation, discontinuation of diaphragmatic contraction facilitates elastic recoil of the lungs. There is no active muscular contraction in the diaphragm upon exhalation. Elastic recoil of the lungs and relaxation of the diaphragm are followed by upward movement of the centers of the diaphragmatic domes toward the lungs as the diaphragm returns to its dome shape. According to Boyle's law, as the pressure in the thorax increases (positive pressure compared to the atmosphere outside of the body), volume of air in the lungs decreases, and air travels out. The exhalation thus increases tension on the crus tendons (and therefore on the lumbar spine). The external intercostal muscles relax and the rib basket can return to its original shape. The internal intercostal muscles either isometrically or concentrically contract on the exhalation, and low ribs move inward to their starting position and to stabilize the low portion of the rib basket.

Natural Diaphragmatic Exhalation

Chest breathing can be likened to the forceful up and down movement of a piston, resulting in great force and intensity. Not surprisingly, it is associated with anxiety, even panic, and stimulates the sympathetic nervous system.

Natural diaphragmatic breathing, on the other hand, can be likened to the pulsing movement of a jelly fish as it moves gracefully through water. This movement is rhythmic, efficient, and gentle. Not surprisingly, it supports ease and well-being and is associated with the stimulation of the parasympathetic nervous system, allowing the vagus nerve to put the brakes on sympathetic arousal.

The exhalation can be gently supported by resilient contraction of the transverse abdominis and the internal and external obliques, the three deeper of the four layers of abdominal muscles. This gentle contraction results in a slight movement inward of the abdominal wall, creating intra-abdominal pressure that supports diaphragmatic recoil, thus assisting the outbreath. It can support caudal movement of the low ribs, helping with creation of stability. Contraction of the abdominal muscles needs to be balanced—not too strong and not too weak—to create support for a natural exhalation. Too much contraction (especially if it persists during the inhalation) becomes counterproductive. Recruitment of the abdominal muscles reverberates into the pelvic floor muscles, which lift toward the center of the abdomen, assisting with the energetic movement of the diaphragm and its accessory muscles as we breathe out. This movement of the pelvic floor muscles is a great way to support their resilience and health (Fig. 2.14).

Fig. 2.14 Summary of biomechanics for diaphragmatic respiration. Data source for inhalation image: https://commons.wikimedia.org/wiki/File:Inhalation_diagram.svg; public domain; data source for exhalation image: https://commons.wikimedia.org/wiki/File:Expiration_diagram.svg; public domain)

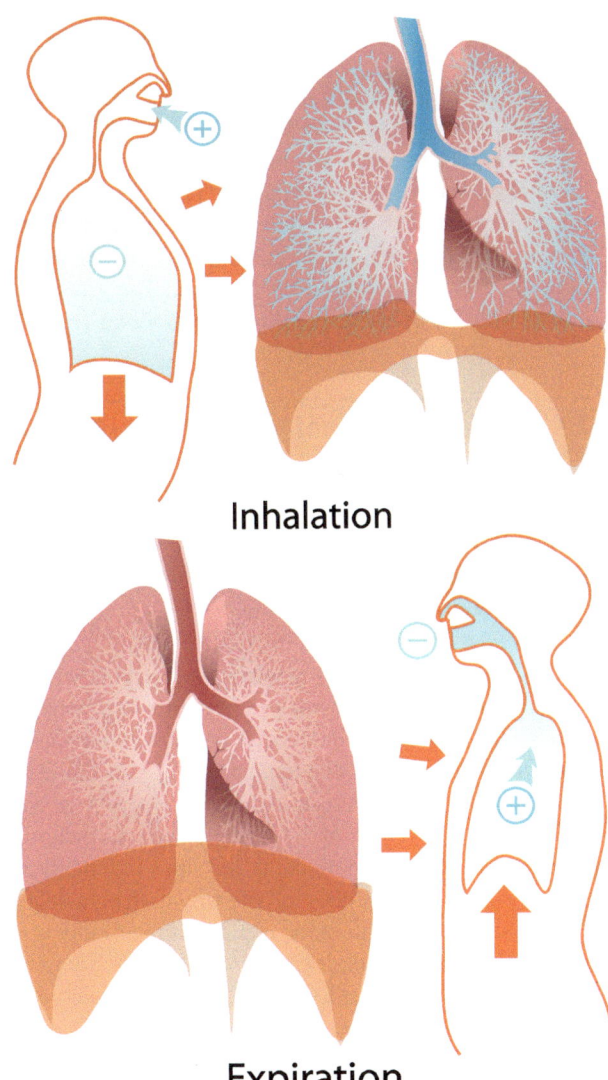

Inhalation

Expiration

Quiet Versus Forced Breathing

In teaching and engaging in breathing practices, it is important to differentiate between quiet breathing and forced breathing. *Quiet* exhalation requires no muscular contraction. During *forced* exhalation, non-respiratory muscles become active to support (or press in or up against) the relaxed diaphragm. The internal intercostal muscles assist, drawing ribs inward and upward. The transverse abdominis and obliques fire up to create an inward and upward action that compresses the relaxed diaphragm against the lower border of the thoracic cavity and lungs, compressing the space available to the lungs (thus increasing pressure) and forcing additional air to travel out.

During *quiet* inhalation, the major muscle that contracts is the diaphragm, possibly supported minimally by external intercostal muscles. During *forced* inhalation, internal intercostals become more active and forceful in expanding the rib basket outward and upward. These muscles may be joined by contraction of the scalenes, sternocleidomastoid (SCM), and pectoralis major muscles. The SCMs move the sternum outward and upward (in a type of action that resembles the movement of a handle on a water pump). The scalenes lift the top ribs upward; the pectoralis minor muscles draw several ribs high in the chest outward. All these actions increase the size of the thoracic cavity, which reduces intrapulmonary pressure more than sole action of the diaphragm. The greater pressure differential compared to atmospheric pressure permits even more air to travel in.

2.4   Biomechanical Interactions of Posture and Breathing

The breath and the posture are intimately connected.
When one is correct, the other is automatically correct.—Sri K. Pattabhi Jois

Several intuitive and some not-so-intuitive aspects of how we hold and move our bodies are strongly related to the flow of breath, affecting volume, location, sound, and texture. Free breathing is an interplay of many factors. First, there is the wonderfully unique ability of the diaphragm to switch origin and insertion—that is, to move downward into the abdomen with a contraction and, when it meets resistance, to use the contraction to help the intercostal muscles move the low rib basket outward and up (bucket handle effect). The amazing design of the diaphragm provides great biomechanical flexibility for breathing. We can breathe in with expansions that make room for the growing volume of the lungs in many directions. The movement can be downward toward the abdomen, out to the sides into the flanks, into the back body, or—in a pinch—high into the chest all the way to the clavicles. We need this ability to allow the lungs to expand within the reaches of the thorax in various ways to ensure that we can draw enough breath, regardless of the body's position, shape, or movement. If we could only breathe in the low belly, how would we breathe when lying firmly prone on the floor? How would we breathe while slumped lazily onto a couch?

However, just because we can breathe high into the chest while being slumped over or tired, this does not mean that all ways and orientations of breathing are of equal benefit. Chest breathing—while it may save our life when we encounter an icy cold pool of water—is not as wholesome as a habitual or day-to-day breath. As discussed above, thoracic breathing has many disadvantages over natural diaphragmatic breathing (essentially breathing into the midriff); most disadvantageously, it restricts the diaphragm's elastic range of motion. However, the reality is that we encounter many individuals (perhaps some of us included) who have developed breathing patterns that move the air habitually high into the chest. Often, such a habit is difficult, if not impossible, to break simply by cuing the individual to breathe differently. More importantly, we need to change the physical posture (i.e., the anatomy) that has developed around, or even caused, less-than-optimal breathing patterns and rhythms.

Many postural influences on the breath center in their impact on how the rib basket moves, and, in response, the range of motion available to the diaphragm. The diameter of the low ribcage is strongly related to the zone of apposition (the space inside the rib basket within which the diaphragm can descend and ascend freely, without hitches or glitches). If the lower rim of the rib basket flares significantly, the diaphragm's domes are not able to move as freely as they could with optimal arrangement and resilience of the low ribs. If we imagine the diaphragm, as Porter [15] suggests, as a parachute, if we stretch the perimeter of the parachute in 360°, the dome of the parachute flattens. If, on the other hand, we pull inward in all directions on the perimeter of the parachute, without the ability of the dome to make up for this drawing-inward in height, the parachute loses lift.

Extending this analogy to the diaphragm means that the domes will not recoil into the lungs as much if— posturally—the low ribs are flared out. The inability of the low ribs to move downward and inward limits the diaphragm's ability to recoil fully upon exhalation (the top of the parachute stays flat). This scenario leads to inadequate exhalations and continuous hyperinflation of the lungs. On the other hand, if excessive engagement of core muscles draws the low rib basket inward tightly, at the same time lifting abdominal contents upward, the inhalation cannot flow freely as the diaphragm's descent is restricted (the parachute loses lift).

Drawing inward of the low ribs and restriction of diaphragmatic movement can also result from excessive and habitual slumping—how many humans these days sit habitually for hours, as they use electronic devices. Slumping (dropped—overly anteriorly rotated—rib basket and chest, with a flexed spine, especially a hyperkyphotic thoracic spine) impedes diaphragmatic up-and-down movement. It creates shallow breathing that becomes rapid and dysregulated, signaling to the nervous system that something is not quite right.

Other common postural patterns that affect diaphragmatic action arise from the positioning of the pelvis and the commensurate relationship with the psoas complex and core muscles. A tucked tailbone (pelvis with posterior rotation) interferes with breathing due to the diaphragmatic connection to three of the lumbar vertebrae (flattening the lumbar spine), the effect on the thoracic spine (exaggerating its kyphosis), and the bracing that occurs in the psoas complex and core muscles. The diaphragm can move freely only with a relaxed and elastic psoas complex, which, in turn, requires a relaxed and dynamically stable posture, whether we are sitting, standing, lying prone or supine, or moving. When psoas complex muscles are braced (tightened or contracted excessively concentrically or eccentrically) either to overly rotate the pelvis anteriorly or posteriorly, natural and free diaphragmatic movement is impaired. Additionally, somatic nervous system signals are relayed to the brainstem that suggest danger—a cue either to get ready to fight or flee or a signal to collapse in fear. These somatic signals take off the vagal brake and move us into self-defense mode, and commensurately dysregulated breathing.

Ironically, many yoga and exercise teachers still cue tucking (posterior rotation) the tailbone in many different shapes, in some of which tucking is not helpful. Even more unfortunately, many of their students hear this as a suggestion that they should take off the mat, as they confuse it with core strength and stability. However, the bracing and lack of resilience involved in pelvic tucking and tilting actually bring *tightness* to the core (*not strength*—an enormous difference). A tight core can further interfere with natural diaphragmatic breathing.

2.4.1 Healthy Posture for Wholesome Breathing

For optimal breathing, it is helpful to find the most natural, dynamically stable, elastic, and resilient posture in all positions and movements that are possible in our bodies, whether in the context of breathwork, yoga, or daily living. Natural alignment of bones, muscles, and connective tissues, including fascia, brings strength without tightness, stability balanced with mobility, relaxation without laxness, ease balanced by effort, and action balanced by wisdom. Although a full discussion of postural health is beyond the purpose of teaching breathwork, it is important for breathing instructors to understand the basics of healthful postural alignment due to its profound relationship to breathing. Healthfully aligned posture and movement are resilient, dynamic, and stable. They support anatomically optimal breathing by encouraging diaphragmatic breathing that resonates naturally into the lower rib basket and abdomen.

In standing, a healthy and stable posture arises from being anchored in grounded feet, strong ankles, and resilient knees aligned with hip and shoulder joints. The pelvis is the foundation of strength and resilience for the entire spine above it—regardless of whether standing or seated. A resiliently anchored pelvis that can support a resilient and dynamic spine is in its neutral position, neither tucked posteriorly nor tilted (excessively) anteriorly. An anchored pelvis invites the spine to move with the pelvis as a dynamic unit that is adaptable and resilient—neither braced nor collapsed. In its natural curves, a spine invites diaphragmatic breathing that unfolds optimally at the mid-torso with gentle outward and upward movement of the abdomen and low rib basket.

For natural curves of the spine to emerge (inviting healthy breath anatomy), the base of the body is anchored (whether seated, standing, or walking), and all vertebrae (along the spine's full length) are stacked at all three joints that connect any two vertebrae (two facets of the transverse processes and one vertebral body of each vertebra), forming a tripod of weight transfer for maximum stability [8]. The spine is essentially a kinetic chain, the curves of which are supported by the intervertebral joints, as well as the wedge shape of the intervertebral discs, which have greater anterior thickness in the spine's lordotic sections (i.e., lumbar and cervical) and greater posterior thickness in its kyphotic (i.e., thoracic) parts.

The spine atop an anchored pelvis is elongated; it rests stably *yet dynamically* in its natural curves. What are these natural curves that support optimal breathing? They come in two shapes—*lordotic* (or concave into the back) or *kyphotic* (convex back). At birth, the spine is fully kyphotic. As we learn to walk, our lumbar and cervical spines become lordotic, and the thoracic spine and sacrum remain kyphotic. These curves develop to provide us with the *"freedom of movement"* and *"power of stability"* necessary to be bipeds—to walk upright on two legs rather than on four legs [7] (p. 1). These curves are essential for a healthy alignment that supports free, natural breathing. It is important to understand these curves so that we do not inadvertently counteract them to create postural habits that interfere with breath and spinal health (Fig. 2.15).

Natural kyphosis is the primary convex curve with which we are born. At birth, it spans the full length of the spine. As we learn to walk and move in an upright posture, it remains expressed only in the thoracic spine and sacrum; lordosis (our secondary curves) develops in the lumbar and cervical spine. It is important not to flatten natural kyphosis. The thoracic spine has a soft convex curve, but some yogis and many individuals with unhealthy (overly braced) posture flatten this curve, distributing weight unhealthfully throughout the rest of the spine and altering the rib basket's shape and hence the breath's flow. Hyperkyphosis (too much of this curve) in the thoracic spine leads to excess lordosis in the lumbar and cervical spines, often

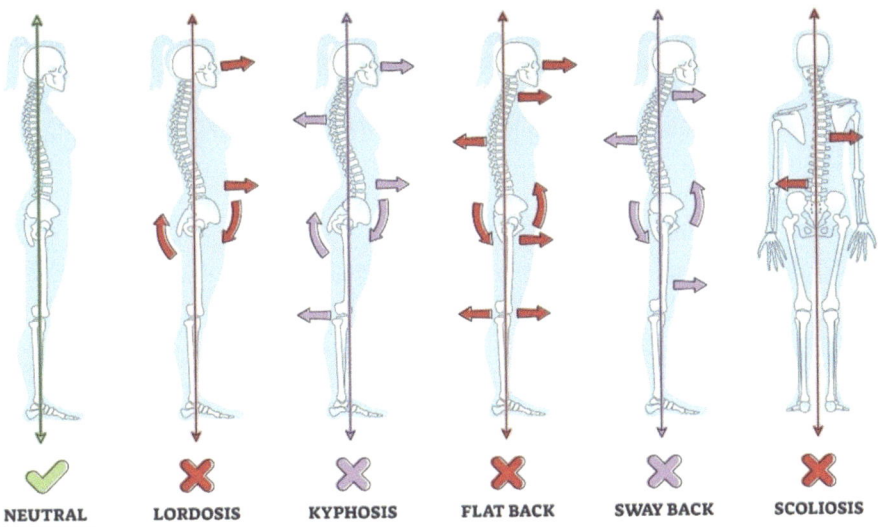

Fig. 2.15 Overview of spinal alignments. (Data source: istock.com)

with forward head posture. In this scenario, weight distributes poorly, resulting in more necessary muscular efforts to maintain stability. This overefforting can lead to pain; collapse in posture, compression, and lack of core integration; and weak core muscles with overworking back muscles. Hyperkyphosis is correlated with tight hip flexors (although it is not clear which is cause and which is effect) and tight pectoralis and intercostal muscles. This alignment can cause the ribs to be drawn inward and restricts ease of breath. The sacrum also needs to have a natural kyphosis and a proper 30° lumbosacral angle where the lumbar spine meets the sacrum. Over-tucking the sacrum and tailbone destabilizes the spine and SI joint. This is common due to excessive sitting and sitting without proper lumbar support.

Natural lordosis represents the developmental or secondary curve in the lumbar and cervical spines. Secondary developmental curves are more vulnerable to injury, dysfunction, and pain. They move sympathetically—when one flexes, so does the other (one can easily observe and experience this link between the lumbar and cervical curve and movement in a cat/cow flow). Natural lumbar lordosis is essential for holding and supporting the weight of the organs (which otherwise drop their weight into the pelvic floor). Excessive tucking of the pelvic girdle flattens lumbar lordosis. Too much lumbar lordosis causes disc and possibly nerve compression; it increases the lumbosacral angle and results in a forwardly tilted pelvis. Lack of natural lordosis can cause high amounts of pressure on lower lumbar vertebrae and discs (especially at L4-L5). Cervical lordosis is essential for carrying the weight of the head. Insufficient neck lordosis can lead to excessive compression of intervertebral discs and connective tissue, potentially resulting in headaches and backaches.

A natural spine is stable and at ease by creating the least amount of tension as well as good bilateral balance in joints, fascia, other connective tissues, and muscles. This type of stability is dynamic, not static; it is a constant adjustment to load factors such as compression, tension, torsion, and shear. We are always in motion, always readjusting to factors that affect posture, shapes, or movements—and, of course, breath. We are constantly rebalancing and readjusting to accommodate and meet various influences (examples shown in Table 2.1) to maintain stability and natural breathing.

Table 2.1 Factors influencing breath and stability

- Environmental influences, such as soft or uneven surfaces, temperature, humidity
- Muscular involvement, including muscles that are relaxed versus engaged, active versus passive movement, bracing versus collapsing, habit versus novel movement, and more
- Joint alignment, both healthy alignment and extant injuries or pathologies
- Other connective tissue issues, including form (that followed habitual function) that resulted in pattern locks in the fascia, ligaments, tendons, even bones
- Exteroceptive sensory inputs, such as visual distractions, nociception, noises, smells, inner ear balance, etc.
- Inner sensory inputs, such as proprioceptive and interoceptive inputs, even neuroception
- Nervous system inputs, such as neuroception, polyvagal states, fears, reactivity

Some have linked dysfunctional breathing and scoliosis (i.e., lateral spinal curvature). Habitual breathing into only one side of the lungs may contribute to the development of functional scoliosis. Scoliosis related to breathing patterns may be resolvable by changing dysfunctional breathing patterns. This particular practice was developed by Katharina Schroth and is used at Johns Hopkins (cf., https://www.hopkinsmedicine.org/health/conditions-and-diseases/scoliosis/schroth-method-for-scoliosis; retrieved on 1.11.2024).

Perhaps most unexpected is the role of the tongue in posture, movement, and respiratory health. The tongue is myofascially connected to a chain of muscles and fascia that runs from the feet, up the inner leg, through the pelvic floor, deep core, and up through the anterior neck to the base of the skull (called the deep front line [12]). The tongue is connected to many important postural and respiratory muscles, including the psoas major, quadratus lumborum, and diaphragm [10]; it also has a strong connection to the hyoid muscles, which contribute to head and cervical and thoracic spine alignment. It is fascially connected to all structures along this chain as well as to the lungs and the muscles of the jaws and throat. Placement and movement of the tongue can therefore have profound effects on posture [16], movement [17], balance [18], and respiratory efficiency [19, 20]. These effects can be explained, as can all postural reverberations through our body's biotensegrity, via strong fascial connections along the deep front line, jaws, and throat. For example, with regard to movement and posture, poor tongue placement can result in misalignment in the neck and throat; this in turn affects cervical and thoracic spinal alignment [21], which in turn affects breathing. Tongue dysfunctions that alter the placement or movement of the tongue (e.g., tongue tie or ankyloglossia) can create gait disturbances, cause forward head posture, result in pelvic misalignment, diminish core stability, disrupt balance, and interfere with breathing [22–24]. Poor tongue placement affects how we move our jaws and engage the muscles in our throats, and thus is related to speaking [25], chewing and swallowing [26], breathing [27, 28], and sleep and sleep apnea [29]. Most optimally placed, the tongue rests against the upper palate with the tip of the tongue nestled behind the upper front teeth. In this position, there is a wholesome ripple effect through the entire lingual chain, enhancing posture, head alignment, gait, core stability, movement pattern, and respiration. Table 2.2 defines stability as a dynamic, not static, assemble and response to these many influences.

Table 2.2 Stability: Dynamic, not static

- Endurance, steadiness, firmness, and sturdiness
- Ability to reregulate after disturbance
- Resilience and resistance to sudden force, load, or disturbance
- Ability to adapt and regain postural equilibrium with mobility and ongoing micro-adjustments
- Ability to support joints during movement
- Defined by ease, not by tension
- Defined by optimally functional breathing

2.4.2 Understanding Bracing, Collapsing, and Resilience

We can enhance the quality of breathing by making note of the dynamic aspects of stability and allowing it with consciousness. Spinal stability, not outer shape, defines healthy postural alignment and natural breathing. To maximize healthy spinal range of motion and dynamism, muscles need to be relaxed, yet toned (which is not the same as not working or not contracting), *except under load*, especially shear. Ideal posture and embodiments are defined by stable ease; unfavorable postures or embodiments of shapes are defined by tension, bracing, pain, even fear—or their polar opposite, by slackness, disengagement, collapse, even terror [15, 30–32]. Interoceptive awareness is a key aspect of finding most advantageous alignment and stable mobility or dynamic stability. To bear load, muscles need to contract around the joints that move, which, in turn, limits the range of motion in these areas of the body and makes a healthy trade-off. "When under stress, stiffen; when enhancing movement, unload" [8] (p. 9). In other words, it is important not to trade range of motion for risk of joint injury.

Unfortunately, modern postural yoga often emphasizes flexibility and large ranges of motion (including *deep* breaths), instead of promoting stability and healthful alignment, posture, and breath [33–35]. Integrated holistic approaches, on the other hand, stress stability and a healthful, conscious range of motion, adapted to the factors of influence at hand. Integrated holistic positioning and movement are supportive for the body and optimal for breathing. Postural health and freedom of breath that reflect dynamic stability or the lack thereof are closely linked to the concepts of bracing, collapsing, or resilience. Understanding these patterns is helpful in designing physical breathwork preparations that increase health and resilience.

Recognizing Collapsing or Buckling

The postures and movements of individuals who are collapsing or buckling are on the disengaged end of the spectrum, perhaps unintegrated and lethargic. They are characterized by sagging, slackness, a lack of engagement, and underefforting in body or energy, often accompanied by a limited mental presence and emotions of despair, helplessness, depression, or giving up. Buckling may show up as collapsed resignation or crumpling into a position, rather than resilient and engaged yielding. There is neither much effort, nor true ease. Engagement and presence are minimal, and lines of energy seem collapsed or nonexistent.

Collapse can arise from excessive grounding or it may signal confusing relaxation with laxity or nonattachment with giving up. It often represents a *lack of stability* and engagement in key musculature, leading to unprotected, loose joints and shapes or movements that lack vigor and strength at the core. Collapse may reflect a *lack of expansiveness*, purpose, or direction—showing up as the haphazard or half-hearted embodiment of a position or movement.

Collapse may be a sign of lack of integration, disconnection from the body, apathy, or resignation. Anatomically and energetically, collapse is often accompanied by a deeply tucked pelvis (rolled posteriorly) with a rounded upper spine (arching forward) and head rolled up and back, with the throat hyperextended in front and the neck compressed in the back. This may look like severe slouching, where all effort in the body has evaporated, and there is no joyful sense of ease. Back musculature is lengthened, and chest musculature is shortened, pulling the chest and head forward while creating a rounded back. This anatomical embodiment of withdrawal or disheartenment can result in hyperkyphosis. This alignment of pelvis, rib basket, and head misaligns the spine and narrows the lower chest cavity, *interfering with free and natural breath flow*. It results in shortened psoas and hamstring muscles (interfering with the natural relationship of these muscles with one another), leading to hip and low back pain. Since shortened psoas muscles are a hallmark of a self-protective stance, this alignment can be linked to chronic sympathetic arousal that can lead to burnout, but in this context is reflective of excessive parasympathetic activation that has resulted in collapse and disengagement.

Recognizing Contracting or Bracing

Contracting, on the other hand, is marked by gripping, tension, and over-efforting, as well as physical, emotional, and mental rigidity or constriction. It can manifest as a fight against or an active and stressful retreat from the present moment's demands, rather than a yielding to current demands. There may be an aspect of stubbornness and overcontrol in bracing that reflects a mindset of needing to be on alert, over-prepared, or simply overly ambitious. Self-judgment and a chronic, pervasive sense of tension may emanate from the individual who contracts into such tightness. An overabundance of effort, untampered by the sweetness of ease or delight, sucks the joy out of life. The individual errs on the side of effort, with ease being minimal to absent; attachment to outcomes overrides the joy and delight of engaging in movement. Lines of energy are forced, lacking a sense of freedom or excitement. Everything looks like work; there is little to no play or joy.

Contraction can arise from *excessive grounding* in the sense of trying too hard to find support or connection. Bracing may signal confusing intensity with tension, commitment with obsession, and persistence with perseveration. However, excessive grounding is not always part of this type of gripping. More often, bracing signals an *excessive attempt at creating stability or safety* to the point of rigidity, forcing, clenching, or overcontrol. Contraction may include a *lack of expansiveness*, purpose, or direction—all force is directed inward or toward gaining a sense of control (often for self-protection). Inner tension and overcontrol inhibit the joy and embrace of lightness that comes from expansiveness.

Bracing may be a sign of gripping and overcontrolling, forcing or muscling into positions or movements in a way that creates tension rather than resilience. Anatomically and energetically, bracing is often accompanied by a slightly tucked pelvis (rolled slightly posteriorly but close to neutral) with a lifted chest (rolled posteriorly), a head that is rolled up and back (with a hyperextended throat and compressed neck), and excessively depressed and retracted shoulder blades. At times, the belly is sucked in with an overreliance for stability on rectus abdominus and an under-reliance on the more resilient transverse abdominis.

This alignment may look like a good posture, but upon closer inspection, the body is held with excessive effort and tension; ease and joy are absent. Back musculature is shortened, compressing the spine in the low back and neck, muscles are tense around joints, and chest musculature is lengthened, pulling the chest upward so the low ribs jut out. This anatomical embodiment of over-engagement and over-control can result in chronic muscle tension. Further, as noted above, posterior alignment of the pelvis results in shortened psoas and hamstring muscles, leading to hip and low back pain and interference with free diaphragmatic movement that impedes natural breathing. It leads to a braced core (rather than a resilient or strong core) that does not yield to load but is overefforting and overengaged. Bracing is largely due to over-engagement of the rectus abdominis in pelvic tucking and disabling of the transverse abdominis. Overall, the anatomic alignment that accompanies bracing interferes with spinal health, impedes natural breathing, and activates the sympathetic nervous system.

Recognizing Resilience or Yielding

Resilience or yielding means moving in a way that is well-balanced in body, energy, mind, action, and relationship. There is neither observable over- nor under-controlling; neither reactivity nor resignation. There is neither laxity nor excessive effort or tension. The individual is responsive to necessary aspects of position or movement, finding strength or engagement where it is needed and softness or gentleness where it is indicated. The balance of effort and ease is visible in all actions; engagement and interest emerge without striving for a particular outcome. There is a combination of grounding, expansion, and stability in just the right proportions, reflecting the middle way between effort and ease, between engagement and release.

Clear lines of energy and flow are visible in the body, along with pliability and suppleness in mind and emotions. All layers of self are present in the practice, with (self-)compassion, (self-)care, appreciative joy, and equanimity. There is evidence of awareness, attention, and mindfulness, and the individual has access to neuroception, interoception, proprioception, and exteroception (see Table 2.3 for definitions, based on Brems [36]. The window of tolerance is optimal and wide, with an accompanying experience of agency and self-empowerment embedded in compassion and lovingkindness.

Resilience arises from *stable and responsive grounding* that connects the individual to an unwavering commitment to be present, engaged, and involved. It signals a *coherent sense of stability and integration* in key musculature, breath and energy, and mind and emotion. This stability is buoyant, resilient, steady, and adaptable. Resilience reflects *purposeful expansiveness*—a joyful embrace of lightness, a sense of humor, self-acceptance, and nonattachment to an outcome, accompanied by clarity of purpose, direction, and meaning.

Resilience combines effort and ease; accesses grounding, expansion, and stability; and combines all aspects of being human into a holistic presence. Anatomically and energetically, resilience is accompanied by a slightly tilted pelvis (rolled slightly

Table 2.3 Brief review of the four 'ceptions [36]

Neuroception	Unconscious and spontaneous evaluation of the current level of safety that results in a felt sense of safety, danger, or life threat, followed by a commensurate nervous system response that activates either the ventral vagal complex (safety), the sympathetic nervous system (danger), or the dorsal vagal complex (life threat); the ability to read internal physiological reactions, along with exteroceptive inputs, translate them into an assessment of our sense of safety, and react to them quickly and efficiently to mitigate possible dangers or threats to life or safety; all of this happens outside of conscious awareness or control, being based in the pre- or subconscious and *not* mediated by conscious cognition
Interoception	Capacity to attune to, receive, process, and integrate internal signals about the internal physical, affective, and energetic state of the body, including the capacity to sense the physiological state of the body from within via sensations arising from various physiological systems of the body, including but not limited to the respiratory (e.g., breathing rhythms), cardiac (e.g., pulse or heart rate), gastrointestinal (e.g., butterflies in the stomach), thermoregulatory (e.g., temperature) and nociceptive systems (e.g., pain and discomfort)
Proprioception	Capability to grasp the body's movement, force, and speed (with which our body is moving), alignment, and positioning in space based on stimuli that arise from within the body itself, including stimuli that are received through the senses; proprioception is mediated by the cerebellum and brainstem resulting in ongoing (often unconscious) adjustments of the body in response to proprioceptive signals from receptors in muscles, tendons, and skin
Exteroception	Attunement and responsivity to stimuli originating outside the body, to perceive and take in stimulation from the outside world through the exteroceptors of the five senses of sight (i.e., photoreceptors), hearing (i.e., mechanoreceptors), touch, smell, and taste, as well as outer temperature, pressure, pain stimuli; conscious and mindful perception of these outer stimuli can then be integrated with stimuli arising from inside the body (i.e., interoception) and help inform neuroception of safety, danger, or life threat

anteriorly [~5°], but close to neutral) that allows for natural resilient spinal alignment along the vertical axis. The spine is elongated and open; it is flexible and responsive. Bones are aligned naturally in such a way as to minimize tension in muscle and connective tissue. The pelvis moves as a single unit and serves as the foundation for spinal movement and stability in all types of movements—whether sitting, bending, walking, standing, or rotating. The rib basket is slightly anterior with low ribs drawing toward the anterior superior iliac, without shortening the front body. The head, too, is slightly anterior and rests well balanced on top of the spine at the atlas, the topmost vertebra. This anatomical embodiment of resilience, of rolling with the punches, adapting and responding, supports spinal health, connective tissue cohesiveness, and muscular integrity and responsiveness. It frees the breath to move naturally and wisely through resilient and dynamic movement in the diaphragm and low rib basket. Psoas and hamstring muscles are relaxed, elastic, and supportive of an upright position. They coordinate effectively (with each other, core muscles, and diaphragm) to create balance. The core musculature is engaged but not tense, biased toward the use of deep rather than superficial abdominal muscles. Resilience integrates and embodies strength and mobility; it combines and expresses both effort and ease.

> **Resilience**
> *Physical, mental, emotional, and vital resilience, flexibility, and conditioning result in greater health and more efficient breathing. They support healthful lung functioning and enhanced lung capacity.*
> *Research indicates that lung capacity (size of the lungs) and lung function combined are excellent predictors of longevity. Even individuals with lung transplants who received larger-sized donor lungs lived longer than individuals with lung transplants using smaller-sized donor lungs* [37].

2.5 The Importance of Optimal Natural Diaphragmatic Breathing

As explained above, breathing requires coordinated movement of the diaphragm and accessory muscles. Movements of the diaphragm are primary to all breathing actions and are quite complex. They not only facilitate breathing but also contribute to core and spinal stabilization, heart activity, and organ stabilization [7, 8]. Sadly, for many people, breathing is no longer primarily diaphragmatic but relies increasingly on accessory and other muscles, with some individuals' diaphragms (especially those with chronic pain or sacroiliac dysfunction) operating far outside its actual optimal range of motion [38, 39]. This makes breathing implicitly (unconsciously) stressful, places excess strain on the heart, and reduces support for the spine inherent in diaphragmatic breathing. In other words, although all breathing involves the diaphragm, not all types of breath use the diaphragm optimally. Thus, cuing natural *diaphragmatic* breathing is valuable even if it seems slightly redundant to do so.

2.5.1 Essential Functions of Natural Diaphragmatic Breathing

To cue diaphragmatic breathing, it is helpful to have a clear sense of its various essential functions. The following summary emphasizes the *biomechanical implications* of diaphragmatic breathing. Functions related to breath *physiology* are recapitulated and augmented in the context of biochemistry in Chap. 3.

Respiratory Functions
Reliance on the diaphragm for respiration has many positive effects on breathing. For example, it slows the breath cycle, draws air deeply into the lungs, which optimizes gas exchange (including optimizing ventilation, perfusion, and O_2 uptake into

red blood cells), and prevents possible and reduces extant chemosensitivity to CO_2. It increases lung volume and optimizes tidal volume and efficiency in each breath cycle as well as decreasing dead space, which enhances lung volume. Through elastic recoil of the diaphragm during exhalation (essentially releasing diaphragmatic contraction), it facilitates full and efficient exhalation.

Postural and Alignment Functions

The movement of the diaphragm during breathing generates intra-abdominal pressure that promotes postural support, spinal alignment, and axial stability. This process has many advantages, including increased core stability and a healthfully aligned spine, neck, and head. Diaphragmatic breathing conveys several postural benefits. For example, the diaphragm is an essential part of the deep front line (a muscular chain in the anterior inner body) and, as such, contributes significantly to healthy posture and spinal alignment during breathing. The movement of the diaphragm recruits the pelvic floor and abdominal muscles during exhalation, which serves to keep these muscles toned and strong (although not rigid or hypertonic). This also supports healthy posture (which, in turn, brings ease to the breath).

Diaphragmatic breathing, through promoting alignment, helps dilate the throat during sleep, increasing the size of the airway and decreasing the occurrence of sleep apnea and (possibly) snoring. It helps move the low ribcage during breathing, strengthening the intercostals, and facilitating expansion on inhalation and strong natural recoil of the ribs during exhalation. These actions create resilience in the rib cage. This is especially helpful as we age, as aging can create stiffening in the intercostals and stuckness of the ribs in the "inhalation" position, interfering with exhalation and leading to adverse gas exchange at the alveolar and tissue level. Additionally, it helps create awareness of breathing into the side and back body, not just the abdomen. The breath thus remains efficient and resilient in many different body positions, including while prone or supine.

Physiological Functions

The movement of the diaphragm massages the heart, which, in turn, leads to increased heart rate variability, lower blood pressure, and more efficient circulation. The use of the diaphragm as the primary driver of respiration improves many other physiological functions, including, but not limited to, visceral function, lymph drainage, optimized cortisol levels, healthful cognitive function, and preservation of functional movement.

Nervous System Functions

Diaphragmatic breathing has positive effects on the nervous system, including enhanced vagal tone, increased respiratory vagus nerve stimulation via slower exhalation, calming effects on the mind, support for emotional regulation, and increased capacity to access physical and mental relaxation. It contributes to decreased pain perception and reduced pain sensitivity, and increased heart rate variability.

Fun Fact from Modern Science ...

Circulation of blood is supported by the pressure in the chest created by diaphragmatic breathing (called the thoracic pump).

Each quiet diaphragmatic inhalation creates negative pressure in the chest that draws air into the lungs and blood into the heart. It activates the sympathetic nervous system, increases heart rate, increases venous blood flow, and decreases arterial blood flow. It increases abdominal pressure and decreases thoracic pressure. Each diaphragmatic exhalation supports the forceful expelling of blood from the heart into the body and lungs. It activates the parasympathetic nervous system, decreases heart rate, decreases venous blood flow, and increases arterial blood flow. It decreases abdominal pressure and increases thoracic pressure.

The pressure differential in the chest that supports the circulation of blood is largely due to the movement of the diaphragm downward with the inhalation and upward with the exhalation, an up-and-down movement that occurs on average almost 50,000 per day and contributes to approximately 2000 gallons of blood being moved through the body per day. If the diaphragm is underutilized for breathing, the up-and-down movement is not as profound as it should be, often being only approximately 10% of its actual possible range of motion. This lack of diaphragmatic support of the breath and movement of blood results in the heart having to work harder and faster (i.e., increase heart rate and strength of the heartbeat) [40].

2.5.2   Advantages of Natural Diaphragmatic Breathing

When the breath cycle is initiated and primarily driven by the diaphragm (with support from intercostals as needed), the positive functions of diaphragmatic, as opposed to thoracic, breathing are easily realized. If the breath is observed to move high into the chest (thoracic or even paradoxical breath), especially if it moves all the way up to the clavicles, most benefits are obviated. Table 2.4 juxtaposes the impacts of natural diaphragmatic versus thoracic breathing. Thoracic breathing is commonly observed in individuals who are highly stressed, anxious, and even panicked. The chest is not meant to be the location where our daily, ordinary breath flows. Breathing high into the chest is available to support breath during extreme exertion, especially in fight-or-flight situations, or is visible as a startle response. Optimal breathing favors the diaphragm and moves breath into the belly and low rib basket. Abdominal breathing is not compared in this chart because it has very specific relaxation and calming functions and is not typically encountered in day-to-day habitual breathing. All challenges listed for thoracic breathing apply equally or more so to paradoxical breathing (which, in essence, is an extreme form of thoracic breathing).

Table 2.4 Impacts of diaphragmatic versus thoracic breathing

Natural diaphragmatic breathing	Thoracic breathing
• Generates intra-abdominal pressure that provides postural support (core stability, aligned spine, neck, and head) and spinal/axial stability	• Does not adequately recruit the diaphragm and accessory abdominal and pelvic floor muscles, which contributes to poor posture and spinal instability
• The diaphragm is part of the deep front line, another supporter of posture and spinal alignment	• Creates hypertonicity in back and neck muscles, leading to poor posture and anterior neck carriage
• Recruits the pelvic floor and abdominal muscles during the exhalation which serves to keep these muscles toned and strong (although not rigid or hypertonic), and this is associated with optimal posture	• Chest breathing is emergency breathing and appropriately kicks in to support (not replace) diaphragmatic breathing during heavy lifting, extreme exertion, or distress (such as needing to yell for help)
• Elastic recoil of diaphragm facilitates full, efficient exhalation	• Speeds up respiration and can cause hypocapnia as well as CO_2 sensitivity
• Slows respiration	• Inefficient because it uses up more oxygen because of greater muscle engagement of muscles that are not meant to be regular breathing muscles but are recruited in a state of emergency (pectorals, upper trapezoids, scalenes, levator scapulae)
• Draws air deep into the lungs which optimizes gas exchange (ventilation perfusion; O_2 uptake)	• Tightens the jaws
• Reduces chemosensitivity to CO_2	• Chronically lifts the clavicles
• Increases tidal volume and efficiency	• Creates tension in the neck and shoulders
• Decreases dead space, which enhance lung volume	• Makes the low ribs jut forward
• Improves functional movement	• Creates tension in the low back
• Improves visceral function and lymph drainage	• Triggers a sympathetic nervous system response and chronic state of arousal
• Lowers cortisol and enhances cognitive function	• Creates sympathetic hypervigilance and may lead to dorsal collapse
• Massages the heart and leads to better heart rate variability, blood pressure, and circulation	Related breath:
• Enhances vagal tone and facilitates respiratory vagus nerve stimulation via slower exhalation	• Paradoxical breathing is a traumatic breath that engages the chest breathing muscles and reverses the movement of the diaphragm up on the inhalation and down on the exhalation—Imagine being severely startled and notice how your breath reacts
• Calms the mind and regulates emotion	
• Induces relaxation	
• Changes pain perception; reduces pain sensitivity	
Related breath:	
• Abdominal breathing can seem like diaphragmatic breathing (in that the chest does not move), but it lacks the muscle tone and engagement of the pelvic floor and abs (especially TA and obliques); it does not create as much intra-abdominal pressure, is less stabilizing, and has fewer benefits (although it can be refreshing during deep supine relaxation)	

2.6   Importance of Nasal Breathing

Bridging now from the biomechanics of breathing toward biochemistry of breathing, a discussion of nasal breathing is indicated. Nasal breathing has many relationships with the biomechanics of breath, yet in a manner that often has direct impact on the breath's biochemistry. The following discussion emphasizes biomechanics. Chapter 3 addresses these concepts from a biochemical perspective.

The importance of breathing through the nose, as opposed to the mouth, cannot be overstated. Nasal breathing is essential for optimal respiration (increasing efficiency); health, wellness, and disease prevention; oral health and dental health alignment; posture and spinal alignment; protection of the airways from dehydration and inflammation; healthful and sound sleep; optimal oxygen uptake at the tissue level; and much more. Nasal breathing hydrates, moisturizes, pressurizes, and filters the air as it travels into the body and takes advantage of moist and warm air as it exits through the nose. Nasal breathing serves as a threat detection system because only the nose can smell. When we take in air through the mouth, there is no warning of odor that may signal potential harm. The nose, on the other hand, is highly sensitive to smell and wired to facilitate a survival response if necessary. This response can range from a reflexive breath hold (to prevent inhaling noxious air), to preparing for eating (when smelling something delicious and nourishing), to soothing the nervous system (when detecting a calming or familiar scent), to raising nervous system alarms that set of a flight-or-fight response to escape harm. Nasal breathing is correlated with better exercise capacity and better sports performance; for men, it is related to enhanced sexual performance [41, 42].

The mouth, on the other hand, is not a useful anatomical structure for the functions performed by the nose. In fact, mouth breathing has many disadvantages and can be a significant factor in disease, fatigue, poor health, and compromised mental and emotional well-being. Several recent findings are listed in Table 2.5. This listing is by no means complete but provides compelling arguments for nasal breathing, especially in children, followed by elderly people (for whom poor brain oxygenation secondary to oral breathing can contribute to memory impairment).

Table 2.5   Disadvantages of oral breathing

- Nasal obstruction [43].
- Negative changes in airway morphology, including decreased pharyngeal airway space [44, 45].
- Less efficient respiration and oxygen desaturation [46].
- Interference with sleep, snoring, sleep apnea; fatigue, waking up tired and restless [47].
- Reduced cognitive functioning and impaired memory [48, 49].
- Changes oral bacterial flora pH level, with concomitantly increased risk for gum disease; bad breath, dry mouth (xerostomia), and hoarseness [50, 51].
- Poor posture, moving the head forward of the shoulders into anterior head carriage [52, 53].
- Changes in facial structure development during childhood and adolescence [54].
- Poor positioning of the temporomandibular joint, leading to jaw pain, grinding, and malocclusion [45].
- Dental malocclusion and poorer dental health (e.g., cavities) [43, 55].

Nevertheless, the mouth does come in handy when nasal breathing is made impossible, perhaps due to severe colds or allergic reactions.

Fun Facts from Modern Science—Influences on the Airways
The health, size, and functionality of the airways, especially the upper airway dilator muscles, is dependent on many habits and actions that support the strength and resilience of these structures. Unhealthy airways (e.g., collapsed palate and back of the throat) reduce the volume and ease of airflow, contribute to sleep apnea, and reduce the efficiency of the breath.

Several important influences on airway health include, but are not limited to the following:

- Mouth breathing interferes with the health and resilience of the upper airway dilator muscles, contributes to a tight palate (as well as crooked teeth and challenges to dental health), and can cause a collapsed airway—the tongue rests on the floor of the mouth (rather than on the roof of the mouths as happens in nasal breathing) and obstructs airflow as well as causing long-term atrophy of the airway dilator muscles.
- Hard, forceful breaths create too much turbulence in the nose, excessive demand on the airways, and bronchial constriction.
- Eating only soft, processed food leads to an under-development of the palate, narrow mouth, crooked teeth, and collapsed airways that impair airflow through the oral cavity—chewing hard and/or tough foods is essential to strengthening the mastication muscles and this, in turn, helps open and keep open the airways [37].

Understanding the functions of the nose is key to understanding the importance of nasal breathing. As will become evident from the review that follows, it is crucially important to use the nose, not the mouth, for breathing. The mouth is used for eating, talking, tasting, and drinking. It is simply an emergency backup system for the nose when the breath cannot travel in or out of the nostrils.

2.6.1   Essential Respiratory and Related Functions and Advantages of Nose Breathing

Warming Function
Air, body, and nostrils become or stay warmer if the breath travels in and out through the nose rather than the mouth [56]. McKeown [41] reports that "air entering the nose at 42.8 °F/36 °C will be warmed to 86 °F/30 °C by the time it touches the back of the throat, and a cozy 93 °F/37 °C—body temperature—upon reaching its final destination, the lungs." Breathing through the nose helps us maintain a warmer body temperature overall, as there is less heat loss from distributing cold air through the

airways and into the lungs. Since the breath remains at body temperature during its journey through the body, when it exits through the nose, it rewarms the nostrils, keeping them warm and ready for the next chilly inhalation. Air exiting through the mouth deprives the nasal cavity of this advantage.

Moistening and Decongesting Function

The nasal passages humidify air as it travels into the nose, ensuring that air conveyed into the airways is moist and not drying to the tissues through which it travels. In fact, by the time air that travels in through the nose reaches the pharynx, its humidity is 95%. Increased humidity of the inhalation retains moisture in the entire airway and the body overall—moisture that helps protect airways against dehydration, inflammation, and congestion. Mouth breathing, on the other hand, has a dehydrating effect. Airway dryness has negative effects on speech and throat wellness. Mouth breathers tend to have hoarseness and more strained speech. Moisture loss due to mouth breathing acidifies the mouth, which can lead to dental cavities and compromised gum health, as well as bad breath. Breathing out through the mouth creates significantly more loss of moisture and leads to congestion in the nasal cavity, even if it is only the exhalation that leaves through the mouth (an unhelpful suggestion often heard in sports, yoga, and even relaxation exercises). When the exhalation travels out through the nasal passages, exhaled air remoistens nasal passages, keeping them ready and healthy for the next inhalation.

Cleansing Function

Cilia in the nostrils begin the cleansing process by filtering and trapping larger particles before the inhalation moves further into the airways. The mouth has no filtering process for inhaled air. Breathing out through the nostrils expels trapped particles. Without exhalation, nostrils cannot cleanse themselves—another potential source of congestion. Turbinates (a tiny network of bone, blood vessels, and soft tissue) create turbulence during inhalation that traps particles and infectious agents in the mucosa from which they can be removed. Mucous membranes along the airways continue to trap, filter, and clear away particles, toxins, germs, and infectious agents, including bacteria, possibly even viruses. Additional purification, in fact sterilization, occurs via circulating lysozymes, antibodies, and nitric oxide in the mucosa. This powerful antiseptic is not available to the same degree if air travels through the mouth.

Pressurizing and Efficiency Function

The small tunnel that is the nose (compared to the large tunnel that is the mouth) and its turbinates leads to less airflow and creates significantly more resistance to the air streaming in than does the mouth. The effect is a slowing of breath and strengthening and tightening of throat tissues. The latter helps prevent snoring and sleep apnea.

Slower nasal breathing creates more efficient O_2 uptake (at least a 10–20% enhancement over inhaling orally) because it provides more time for optimal perfusion of blood in the lungs and gas exchange at the alveoli. This maintains more optimal CO_2 levels (necessary for O_2 release into the tissues) and maintains a balanced body pH. Slower breathing, as naturally occurs with nasal breathing, creates healthy breathing rhythms that support relaxation, enhance physical performance, and increase aerobic capacity.

Pressurization resulting from nasal breathing supports stronger diaphragmatic action and prevents chest breathing. Nasal breathing also decreases the amount of air in the airway's "dead space" (less air outside the alveoli where gas exchange occurs), increasing efficiency in how much air is needed for adequate gas exchange.

Resistance and pressurization during nasal exhalation help maintain lung volume (leaving a greater residual volume of air in the lungs), which supports keeping breath light and easy (much as it is easier to reinflate a partially filled balloon than a completely empty balloon). Breathing out orally expels more air, reducing lung volume, which, in turn, means that more air needs to travel in with the next breath, making breathing more difficult and less efficient.

Nitric Oxide Release Function

Breathing through the nose and maxillary sinuses releases nitric oxide into inhaled air before it travels deeper into the airways [57, 58]. Mouth breathing does not release nitric oxide into inhaled air. Thus, simply breathing nasally, instead of orally, results in significantly more oxygen being absorbed into the blood when the same amount of air arrives in the alveoli. Nitric oxide levels are greatly enhanced with slow nasal exhalation and breath suspension at the end of the exhalation. The next nasal inhalation then distributes the produced NO into the lower airways and lungs [58]. The importance of nitric oxide cannot be overstated and is a larger focus in Chap. 3. A few key advantages of increased nitric oxide levels include, but are not limited to:

- Increased vasodilation (relaxation or widening of blood vessels—not a small thing, considering that the body has approximately 100,000 miles of blood vessels)
- Reduced inflammation in the airways
- Enhanced bronchial smooth muscle tone
- Better perfusion of blood (with less pooling of blood at the bottom of the lungs; a beautiful descriptive diagram of this is provided in McKeown [41] (p. 117)
- Enhanced oxygen uptake into the blood at the alveolar level and into the cells at the tissue level [59].
- Inhibited bacterial growth (especially staphylococcus), perhaps even a defense against viruses (including SARS-CoV-2) and airborne fungi [60].

Smelling Function

The nose's olfactory segment houses smell receptors that allow for the assessment of airborne risks based on detected smells. The interpretation in the brain of detected smells can then alter behavior, in general, and breathing-related behaviors, in particular. In other words, respiration patterns can be changed via powerful (survival) reflexes that are based on the types of risks detected in the air during nasal breathing. For example, certain smells may raise alarms that lead to breath retention or flight to escape threatening smells; other scents may soothe the nervous system, inviting a sense of relaxation or bringing forth positive memories. Finally, some smells prepare our physiology for food or eating, initiating the processes necessary for digestion (e.g., salivation). Breathing through the nose takes full advantage of creating food flavors. Flavor is a combination of sensations in the olfactory bulb and tongue. A congested nose diminishes the flavor of food.

Postural and Alignment Functions

Nasal breathing results in the engagement of muscles, especially those involved in posture, breathing, and coordination and balance during walking. For example, nasal breathing results in a healthier alignment of the head and neck, whereas oral breathing tends to move the head forward of the shoulders, leading to the anterior head carriage. Breathing through the nose shifts breath deeply into the abdomen, away from chest breathing. Diaphragmatic recruitment is more natural in nasal breathing than in mouth breathing, contributing to better posture.

Nasal breathing favors tongue placement at the roof of the mouth where it supports dental health, a wider palate, healthy facial and jaw development, and better sleep (with less snoring and apnea). Pressing the tongue to the hard palate strengthens the upper airway dilator muscles. In oral breathing, the tongue rests on the floor of the mouth and tends to drop to the lower jaw. This can lead to poor facial development. Thus, nasal breathing promotes and supports dental alignment and facial development, especially in children, for whom it:

Creates a wider facial structure with a U-shaped mandible and maxilla that easily accommodates all teeth supporting dental alignment; V-shapes from mouth breathing result in dental crowding

Creates a wide palate that provides ample space for clear airflow from both nostrils; narrow palates from oral breathing often pinch, restrict, or reduce the size of one nostril and are related to deviated septa

Results in a strong, well-aligned jaw; mouth breathing is related to a significantly set-back mandible

Fossil Records Reveal That, Over the Centuries, Many Things Have Changed About Human Faces

Ancient humans, when compared to modern humans, had:

- Larger face
- Strong and prominent jaws
- Straighter and stronger teeth
- Larger mouth with a wide U-shaped palate
- Larger nasal structure

These morphological changes can be attributed to several habits and practices that have changed "thanks to" civilization [37]:

- Mouth breathing
- Bottle feeding as opposed to natural nursing, which creates a larger and stronger airway because of the added effort needed to extract nourishment
- Soft and processed food that has led to less chewing, especially less vigorous chewing

When breath enters and exits the body through the mouth, many healthful functions are absent or impeded, resulting in serious health and mental health consequences. Table 2.6 juxtaposes the impacts of nasal versus mouth breathing. No wonder almost all animals breathe exclusively through the nose; no wonder humans are born breathing immediately through the nose. In fact, most babies breathe through the nose naturally and exclusively for many months. Breathing through the mouth during the early developmental period can be particularly devastating, as it may result in a change in how the face develops. Mouth breathing in children may lead to the development of a high and narrow palate, a V-shaped (rather than the more auspicious U-shaped) jaw, a set-back mandible, poor dental health with dental crowding and dental cavities, and labored breathing [61, 62]. Dentists may be particularly helpful in identifying mouth breathing in children because they can be direct observers of oral and dental changes as well as lack of appropriate jaw and facial development.

Table 2.6 Summary of the impacts of nasal versus mouth breathing

Nasal breathing	Mouth breathing
• Decongests the nose and leads to healthier breathing rhythms, exercise performance, and aerobic capacity	• Creates more nasal congestion, even if only the exhalation is through the mouth; often leads to a vicious cycle of mouth breathing
• Warms the air on the inhalation	• Has less of a warming effect, instead cold air is inhaled
• Moistens/humidifies the air on the inhalation; remoistens the nasal passage in the exhalation;	• Less moistening effect; dehydrates the oral cavity (e.g., dry mouth upon waking) and the body; dry mouth can have negative effects on dental health, hoarseness, and strained voices
• Retains moisture in the body; supports throat wellness and easeful speech	• No cleansing of the air takes place, increasing toxic exposure
• Cleanses the air via mucus and cilia that remove particles on the inhalation	• If foreign particles reach the alveoli due to mouth breathing, it takes the body 60–120 days to remove them
• If foreign particles enter the airway via the nose, it takes 15 min to remove them	• No antibodies or turbinates are available to remove infectious or toxic agents in the air
• Purifies (sterilizes) air via circulating antibodies (acting as the first defense of the immune system), nitric oxide, and hydraulics in the turbinates (see below)	• No nitric oxide is released to inhibit bacterial growth
• The small tunnel that is the nose and its turbinates pressurize/boost the inhalation's air flow which results in more efficient O_2 uptake, better perfusion, and stronger diaphragmatic action	• No turbinates to pressurize or cleanse the air.
• Nasal resistance (again—Small tunnel) expands the length of the exhalation (slows respiratory rate)—Creates healthier breathing rhythms, relaxation responses, and less dead space in the lungs	• The bigger tunnel of the mouth lacks the ability to pressurize the inhalation or provide resistance to the exhalation
• Turbinates create turbulence in the air that traps particles and infectious agents in the mucosa from where they can be removed	• Decreases the efficiency of oxygen uptake, perfusion, and diaphragmatic action
	• Creates more dead space which can lead to hypoxia
	• Increases respiratory rate, possibly contributing to hyperventilation and hypocapnia
	• Hypocapnia, in turn, is correlated with anxiety, panic, chronic pain, and cognitive challenges (low concentration, impaired memory)
• The maxillary sinuses release nitric oxide into the inhaled air; nitric oxide facilitates vasodilation (relaxation of blood vessels) and oxygen uptake; and inhibits bacterial growth (especially staphylococcus)	• The maxillary sinuses are bypassed and thus no nitric oxide is released; this leads to a stuffier nose and sets up a vicious cycle of mouth breathing
	• Hypocapnia further adds to nasal congestion

Nasal breathing	Mouth breathing
• Smell is a powerful (survival) reflex that can alter respiration patterns based on what is detected—Can raise an alarm, soothe, prepare for eating, or stop the breath	• No smell detection—No warning system • Less enjoyment of the full flavor of food
• Supports dental and gum health • Supports proper posture, and healthy head and neck alignment • Supports balanced gait	• Leads to more dental cavities and gum disease • Jaw has to move forward to facilitate mouth breathing, leading to anterior head carriage, neck strain, and hypertonic traps, scalenes, and pecs
• Tongue placement at the roof of the mouth supports dental alignment and is correlated with a wider palate and healthy facial and jaw development • Pressing the tongue to the hard palate is correlated with stronger upper airway dilator muscles, which promotes sleep due to less obstructive sleep apnea, less snoring • Healthier muscle tone in the back of the throat keeps the airway open and, during sleep, prevents snoring and sleep apnea	• Flaccid, weakened tongue may contribute to facial deformity, malocclusion, and poor jaw development, especially in children • Tongue resting at the bottom of the mouth is correlated with a narrower palate and weaker upper airway dilation, contributing to obstructive sleep apnea and snoring • Less muscle tone in and less air pressure against the soft tissue in the back of the throat leads to sleep apnea and snoring

2.7   Where We Go from Here

Nasal breathing is not only a crucial biomechanical issue but also a key aspect of breath biochemistry, as hopefully has become clear from the summary advantages of nasal breathing over mouth breathing. Modern science can explain the biochemistry of what ancient traditions practiced to preserve the subtle energy of the life force. Thus, the biochemistry of breathing is the focus of Chap. 3, as attention turns to energy and vitality produced by breath, the key to the vital layer of self, *pranamaya kosha*.

> *Everything you see has its roots in the unseen world. The forces change yet the essence remains the same.*—Rumi

References

1. Pendolino AL, Lund VJ, Nardello E, Ottaviano G. The nasal cycle: a comprehensive review. Rhinology. 2018;1(1):67–76. https://doi.org/10.4193/RHINOL/18.021.
2. Coulter D. Anatomy of hatha yoga. Body and Breath; 2001.
3. Feng H, Zhang P, Wang X. Presbyphagia: dysphagia in the elderly. World J Clin Cases. 2023;11(11):2363–73. https://doi.org/10.12998/wjcc.v11.i11.2363.
4. Stephen MJ. Breath taking. Grove/Atlantic; 2021.
5. Han MK. Breathing lessons: a doctor's guide to lung health. Norton; 2022.
6. Clark B. Your body, your yoga. Wild Strawberry Productions; 2016.
7. Lasater JH. Yoga myths.. Shambhala; 2020.
8. Clark B. Your spine, your yoga: developing stability and mobility for your spine. Wild Strawberry Productions; 2018.
9. Rothenberg R. Restoring prana: a therapeutic guide to pranayama and healing through the breath for yoga therapists, teachers, and healthcare practitioners. Singing Dragon; 2020.
10. Bordoni B, Zanier E. Anatomic connections of the diaphragm: influence of respiration on the body system. J Multidiscip Healthc. 2013;6:281–91.
11. Porges S. The polyvagal theory: neurophysiological of emotions, attachment, communication, and self-regulation. Norton; 2011.
12. Myers TW. Anatomy trains. 4th ed. Elsevier; 2022.
13. Hodges PW, Cresswell AG, Daggfeldt K, Thorstensson A. In vivo measurement of the effect of intra-abdominal pressure on the human spine. J Biomech. 2001;34(3):347–53. https://doi.org/10.1016/S0021-9290(00)00206-2.
14. Hodges PW, Gandevia SC. Activation of the human diaphragm during a repetitive postural task. J Physiol. 2000;522(1):165–75. https://doi.org/10.1111/j.1469-7793.2000.t01-1-00165.xm.
15. Porter K. Natural posture for pain-free living. Inner Traditions International; 2013.
16. Russo L, Giustino V, Toscano RE, et al. Can tongue position and cervical ROM affect postural oscillations? A pilot and preliminary study. J Hum Sport Exerc. 2020;15(3):840–7. https://doi.org/10.14198/jhse.2020.15.proc3.35.
17. Haughey JP, Fine P. Effects of the lower jaw position on athletic performance of elite athletes. BMJ Open Sport Exerc Med. 2020;6(1):e000886. https://doi.org/10.1136/bmjsem-2020-000886.
18. Alghadir AH, Zafar H, Iqbal ZA. Effect of tongue position on postural stability during quiet standing in healthy young males. Somatosens Mot Res. 2015;32(3):183–6. https://doi.org/10.3109/08990220.2015.1043120.

19. Bordoni B, Morabito B, Mitrano R, Simonelli M, Toccafondi A. The anatomical relationships of the tongue with the body system. Curēus. 2018;10(12):e3695. https://doi.org/10.7759/cureus.3695.
20. Cheng S, Butler JE, Gandevia SC, Bilston LE. Movement of the tongue during normal breathing in awake healthy humans. J Physiol. 2008;586(17):4283–94. https://doi.org/10.1113/jphysiol.2008.156430.
21. Paris-Alemany A, Proy-Acosta A, Adraos-Juárez D, Suso-Martí L, La Touche R, Chamorro-Sánchez J. Influence of the craniocervical posture on tongue strength and endurance. Dysphagia. 2021;36(2):293–302. https://doi.org/10.1007/s00455-020-10136-9.
22. Arena M, Micarelli A, Guzzo F, et al. Outcomes of tongue-tie release by means of tongue and frenulum assessment tools: a scoping review on non-infants. Acta Otorhinolaryngol Ital. 2022;42(6):492–501. https://doi.org/10.14639/0392-100X-N2211.
23. Saccomanno S, Pirino A, Bianco G, Paskay LC, Mastrapasqua R, Scoppa F. Does a short lingual frenulum affect body posture? Assessment of posture in the sagittal plane before and after laser frenulotomy: a pilot study. J Biol Regul Homeost Agents. 2021;35(3 Suppl. 1):185–95. https://doi.org/10.23812/21-3suppl-21.
24. Scoppa F, Pirino A. Is there a relationship between body posture and tongue posture? Glossopostural syndrome between myth and reality. Acta Medica Mediterranea. 2019;35:1897–907. https://doi.org/10.19193/0393-6384_2019_4_296.
25. Ito T, Caillet J, Perrier P. Stability in postural tongue control: response to transient mechanical perturbations. Paper presented at: Neuroscience 2018 - Annual Meeting of the Society for Neuroscience.
26. Shimizu A, Maeda K, Nagami S, et al. Low tongue strength is associated with oral and cough-related abnormalities in older inpatients. Nutrition. 2021;83:111062. https://doi.org/10.1016/j.nut.2020.111062.
27. Shieh W, Wang C, Cheng HK, Imbang TI. Noninvasive measurement of tongue pressure and its correlation with swallowing and respiration. Sensors. 2021;21(8):2603. https://doi.org/10.3390/s21082603.
28. Sokoloff A, Burkholder T. Tongue structure and function. In: McLoon LK, Andrade F, editors. Craniofacial muscles: a new framework for understanding the effector side of craniofacial muscle control. Springer; 2012. p. 207–27.
29. Jugé L, Knapman FL, Burke PGR, et al. Regional respiratory movement of the tongue is coordinated during wakefulness and is larger in severe obstructive sleep apnoea. J Physiol. 2020;598(3):581–97. https://doi.org/10.1113/JP278769.
30. Farhi D. Yoga mind, body & spirit: a return to wholeness. Owl Books; 2011.
31. Mitchell J. Yoga biomechanics. Handspring; 2019.
32. Schiffmann E. Yoga: the spirit and practice of moving into stillness. Gallery Books; 2013.
33. Brems C, Justice L, Sulenes K, et al. Improving access to yoga: barriers to and motivators for practice among health professions students. Adv Mind Body Med. 2015;29(3):6–13. https://www.ncbi.nlm.nih.gov/pubmed/26026151
34. Freeman H, Vladagina N, Razmjou E, Brems C. Yoga in print media: missing the heart of the practice. Int J Yoga. 2017;10(3):160–6. https://doi.org/10.4103/ijoy.IJOY_1_17.
35. Razmjou E, Freeman H, Vladagina N, Freitas J, Brems C. Popular media images of yoga: limiting perceived access to a beneficial practice. Media Psychol Rev. 2017;11:2. http://mprcenter.org/review/popular-media-images-of-yoga-limiting-perceived-access-to-a-beneficial-practice/
36. Brems C. Yoga as a mind-body practice. In: Uribarri J, Vassalotti JA, editors. Nutrition, fitness, and mindfulness: an evidence-based guide for clinicians. Springer Nature; 2020. p. 137–55.
37. Nestor J. Breath: the new science of a lost art. Riverhead Books; 2020.
38. Kolar P, Sulc J, Kyncl M, et al. Postural function of the diaphragm in persons with and without chronic low back pain. J Orthop Sports Phys Ther. 2012;42(4):352–62. https://doi.org/10.2519/jospt.2012.3830.

39. O'Sullivan PB, Beales DJ, Beetham JA, et al. Altered motor control strategies in subjects with sacroiliac joint pain during the active straight-leg-raise test. Spine. 2002;27(1):E1–8. https://doi.org/10.1097/00007632-200201010-00015.

40. Elliott S. Diaphragm mediates action of autonomic and enteric nervous systems. BMED Report. https://www.bmedreport.com/archives/8309. Updated 2010.

41. McKeown P. The breathing cure. Humanix; 2021.

42. McKeown P. Oxygen advantage: the simple, scientifically proven breathing techniques for a healthier, slimmer, faster, and fitter you. William Morrow; 2015.

43. Achmad H, Ansar AW. Mouth breathing in pediatric population: a literature review. Ann Rom Soc Cell Biol. 2021;25(6):4431–55. https://search.proquest.com/docview/2596972859

44. Thribhuvanan L, Saravanakumar MS. Influence of mode of breathing on pharyngeal airway space and dento facial parameters in children: a short clinical study. Bull Natl Res Cent. 2022;46(1):1–7. https://doi.org/10.1186/s42269-022-00802-3.

45. Hu Z, Sun H, Wu Y, et al. Mouth breathing impairs the development of temporomandibular joint at a very early stage. Oral Dis. 2020;26(7):1502–12. https://doi.org/10.1111/odi.13377.

46. Hsu Y, Lan M, Huang Y, Kao M, Lan M. Association between breathing route, oxygen desaturation, and upper airway morphology. Laryngoscope. 2021;131(2):E659–64. https://doi.org/10.1002/lary.28774.

47. Blumer S, Eli I, Kaminsky-Kurtz S, Shreiber-Fridman Y, Dolev E, Emodi-Perlman A. Sleep-related breathing disorders in children—red flags in pediatric care. J Clin Med. 2022;11(19):5570. https://doi.org/10.3390/jcm11195570.

48. Jung J, Kang C. Investigation on the effect of oral breathing on cognitive activity using functional brain imaging. Healthcare. 2021;9(6):645. https://doi.org/10.3390/healthcare9060645.

49. Lee K, Park C, Lee Y, Kim H, Kang C. EEG signals during mouth breathing in a working memory task. Int J Neurosci. 2020;130(5):425–34. https://doi.org/10.1080/00207454.2019.1667787.

50. Al-Casey M, Al-Awadi RN. Oral health status, salivary physical properties and salivary Mutans Streptococci among a group of mouth breathing patients in comparison to nose breathing. J Bagh Coll Dent. 2013;25(Special):152–9. https://doi.org/10.12816/0015133.

51. Choi JE, Waddell JN, Lyons KM, Kieser JA. Intraoral pH and temperature during sleep with and without mouth breathing. J Oral Rehabil. 2016;43(5):356–63. https://doi.org/10.1111/joor.12372.

52. Krakauer LH, Guilherme A. Relationship between mouth breathing and postural alterations of children: a descriptive analysis. Int J Orofac Myol. 2000;26(1):13–23. https://doi.org/10.52010/ijom.2000.26.1.2.

53. Okuro RT, Morcillo AM, Ribeiro MÂGO, Sakano E, Conti PBM, Ribeiro JD. Mouth breathing and forward head posture: effects on respiratory biomechanics and exercise capacity in children. J Bras Pneumol. 2011;37(4):471–9. https://doi.org/10.1590/S1806-37132011000400009.

54. Nosetti L, Zaffanello M, Bernardi D, di Valserra F, et al. Exploring the intricate links between adenotonsillar hypertrophy, mouth breathing, and craniofacial development in children with sleep-disordered breathing: unraveling the vicious cycle. Children. 2023;10(8):1426. https://doi.org/10.3390/children10081426.

55. Davidovich E, Hevroni A, Gadassi LT, Spierer-Weil A, Yitschaky O, Polak D. Dental, oral pH, orthodontic and salivary values in children with obstructive sleep apnea. Clin Oral Invest. 2022;26(3):2503–11. https://doi.org/10.1007/s00784-021-04218-7.

56. Recinto C, Efthemeou T, Boffelli PT, Navalta JW. Effects of nasal or oral breathing on anaerobic power output and metabolic responses. Int J Exerc Sci. 2017;10(4):506–14. https://www.ncbi.nlm.nih.gov/pubmed/28674596

57. Lundberg JON. Nitric oxide and the paranasal sinuses. Anat Rec. 2008;291(11):1479–84. https://doi.org/10.1002/ar.20782.

58. Lundberg JON, Weitzberg E. Nasal nitric oxide in man. Thorax. 1999;54(10):947–52. https://doi.org/10.1136/thx.54.10.947.

59. Antosova M, Mokra D, Pepucha L, et al. Physiology of nitric oxide in the respiratory system. Physiol Res. 2017;66(Suppl 2):S159–72. https://doi.org/10.33549/physiolres.933673.
60. Martel J, Ko Y, Young JD, Ojcius DM. Could nasal nitric oxide help to mitigate the severity of COVID-19? Microbes Infect. 2020;22(4–5):168–71. https://doi.org/10.1016/j.micinf.2020.05.002.
61. Trabalon M, Schaal B. It takes a mouth to eat and a nose to breathe: abnormal oral respiration affects neonates' oral competence and systemic adaptation. Int J Pediatr. 2012;2012:1–10. https://doi.org/10.1155/2012/207605.
62. Zhao Z, Zheng L, Huang X, Li C, Liu J, Hu Y. Effects of mouth breathing on facial skeletal development in children: a systematic review and meta-analysis. BMC Oral Health. 2021;21(1):108. https://doi.org/10.1186/s12903-021-01458-7.

Understanding the Physiology of Breath and Breathing

3

> *Just as we have an optimal quantity of water and food to consume each day, we also have an optimal quantity of air to breathe. And just as eating too much can be damaging to our health, so can overbreathing.*
>
> *Patrick McKeown*

3.1 Overview: The Life-Giving Vitality of Breath

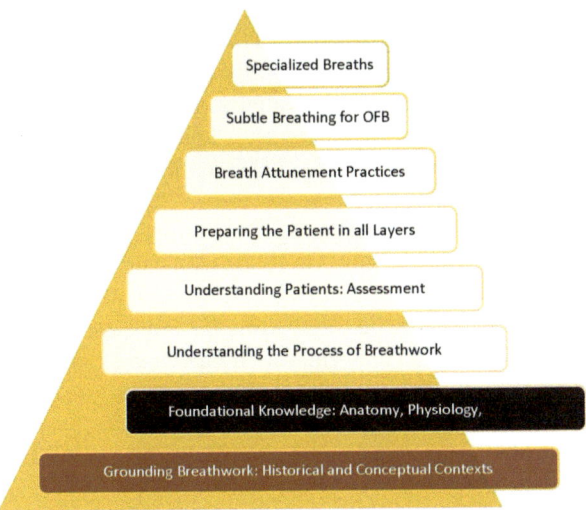

Specialized Breaths

Subtle Breathing for OFB

Breath Attunement Practices

Preparing the Patient in all Layers

Understanding Patients: Assessment

Understanding the Process of Breathwork

Foundational Knowledge: Anatomy, Physiology,

Grounding Breathwork: Historical and Conceptual Contexts

Breath is the vital energy that enlivens our body. Without breath, there is no human consciousness, no living body, no conversion of food into energy, no flow of vital energy, no thoughts, no emotions. Breath enlivens our physical being; from the moment we draw our first inhalation when we are born to the moment we let go of our last exhalation when we die. Breath is energy; breath is vitality; breath is life. It is an essential aspect of all our layers of self and infuses the entirety of our consciousness. It is the link between body and mind. The ancient yogis speak of *Prana* as the vital air or energies. This notion of *Prana* can inform our understanding of breath and breathing in tangible and subtle ways. Breath and life force are reflected in our vital layer of self, our *pranamaya kosha* (in Sanskrit). We need the air around us and the physiological processes of breathing within us to animate our body and to interact with our mind. The structures of the respiratory tract are not usable and the biomechanics of breathing are not possible unless they are enlivened by the vitality of the physiological and biochemical (autonomic) processes that steer and direct the process.

As noted previously, our physical and vital experiences (i.e., *annamaya* and *pranamaya koshas*) engage in a beautiful collaboration that gives us life. When the mind, with its many thoughts and emotions, enters this dance, it can have profound impacts on both movement and breath. In this chapter, we will explore how *prana* and physiology move breath and life force through our being, focusing on the *biochemistry* of breath and breathing. There is no doubt that ancient yogis—despite not being able to measure gases such as oxygen and carbon dioxide—had a keen understanding that subtle energies involved in breathing that either facilitated vitality and health or countered it. Ancient yoga sources (e.g., *Hatha Yoga Pradipika*), as opposed to many common modern "yoga" practices, emphasize breathing patterns and practices that optimize breath biochemistry, such as subtle breathing, tailored breath retention and suspension, or four-part breathing. Such sources also offer practices that create temporary stress or dysregulation of the breath and nervous system (which they conceived of as the *mind*) to increase resilience and recovery (to be discussed in Chaps. 10 and 11), essentially offering breathing practices of hormesis. Such practices are only then indicated when the individual already has established healthful and optimal breathing that is biomechanically and biochemically healthful, nurturing, and sound.

This chapter moves beyond breathing as a biomechanical process of the diaphragm moving downward and upward, or the turbinates in the nose channeling air into the lungs. The mechanical processes, as important as they are to healthful breathing, are only one part of the very complex equation that is respiration. The biochemical processes are as important as biomechanics, and so are a variety of psychological and mental factors related to rhythm, texture, rate, and volume of breath, to be explored in Chap. 4. Respiration, biochemically speaking, happens at multiple levels, including external, internal, cellular, and mitochondrial. Of interest to the clinician, breathing coach, or *pranayama* teacher are the external and internal levels as these are under some conscious control, with external more so than internal. The exchange of gases at the alveolar level is the process known as *external respiration*; the exchange of gases at the tissue level is the process called *internal respiration*. It is not often that we hear yoga teachers or breathing coaches talk about these two distinct aspects of breathing, and yet they are crucial to understanding healthful breathing that supports balanced biochemistry, lasting vitality, a resilient nervous system, and a composed and stable mind.

3.2 Physiology of Respiration

3.2.1 Overview of External and Internal Respiration

The primary functions of *external respiration* are related to the diffusion of gases at the junction between the alveoli and capillaries of the circulatory system that enwrap each alveolus. External respiration is concerned with:

- Steady supply of oxygen (O_2) from the atmosphere to the lungs (via the complex journey through the airways into the alveoli—explored in Chap. 2)
- Diffusion of oxygen into the capillaries at the alveolar level
- Removal of excess carbon dioxide (CO_2) via diffusion from the capillaries into the alveoli and then into the air via the reverse of the journey taken by O_2
- Protection of the airways and lungs from inhaled pathogens (via complex biomechanical processes described previously)

The primary functions of *internal respiration* are related to the diffusion of gases from the blood into bodily tissues at all levels of the body, including muscle tissue, brain, heart, organs, connective tissues, and so on. As such, internal respiration is concerned with:

- Transport of oxygen in the blood through the systemic arterial system (attached to hemoglobin in red blood cells) to the tissues,
- Transport of oxygen from red blood cells into cellular tissues,
- Diffusion of CO_2 from tissues into the blood and its transport back to the alveoli through the veinous system, and
- Regulation of body pH (via adjustments of CO_2 levels in the blood and/or via the kidneys).

Oxygen is needed by every single cell in the body to produce energy that runs all physiological processes. The transformation of oxygen into energy involves complex methods that result in the creation of carbon dioxide, water, and adenosine triphosphate (ATP), our personal energy source. It is the extraction of energy from O_2 that results in the production of CO_2. It has thus been tempting (and common practice, especially in yoga cuing) to consider CO_2 as nothing more than a waste product. However, nothing could be further from the truth. CO_2 serves vital bodily functions, including regulating pH (our acid-alkaline balance), triggering the respiratory reflex as more air is needed to continue respiration, releasing oxygen into tissues, dilating smooth muscles, supporting relaxation, and more. To recap, internal respiration involves the uptake of oxygen molecules into tissues to support energy production in the mitochondria of all cells. It involves the release of accumulating carbon dioxide molecules into the blood. Closing the loop with external respiration, from the blood, CO_2 diffuses into the alveoli, while O_2 diffuses from the alveoli into the blood. CO_2 is then transported out of the body via the airways.

Oxygen
Oxygen, and thus breathing, is more essential to energy production in our bodies than food, or eating. In fact, it has been argued that oxygen should be defined as an essential nutrient, despite the fact that its optimal entry into the body is through the nose, not the mouth. Oxygen is fundamental to the transformation of macronutrients (fat, protein, carbohydrates) into energy and micronutrients. It is also related to hormones that either stimulate appetite or signal us to stop eating [1].

The process of involuntary breathing is tied directly to *broad* levels of oxygen in the blood and, much more importantly, to carefully calibrated and *narrow* levels of concentration of carbon dioxide, as well as CO_2's effect on body pH level. Gas exchange at the alveoli and capillaries (O_2 into the blood; CO_2 into the alveoli) and at the tissues and capillaries (CO_2 into the blood; O_2 into the tissues) relies on: (1) the tendency of *fluids to move from high concentration to low concentration,* and (2) of *gases to move from high pressure to low pressure.* In scientific language, the flow of blood (a fluid) in the capillaries at the alveoli is called perfusion; it is strongly affected by the diameter and health of involved blood vessels. The movement of air (gases) into and out of the lungs is called ventilation; it is strongly affected by the diameter of the airways (bronchioles, for the most part). Ventilation (presence of air in the lungs) and perfusion (adequate flow of blood into the alveoli via pulmonary capillaries) need to be balanced for breath to nourish tissues optimally. Following is an exploration of the biochemistry of this process.

3.2.2   Understanding Basics of Partial Pressures and Gas Exchange

Breathing is strongly tied to physical laws related to how gases move and exert pressure on the surfaces they contact. This notion was already explored in the context of air moving through the lungs based on changing pressure gradients inside the lungs, caused by diaphragmatic movement. When muscular movement changes the chest cavity's volume, it automatically inversely changes pressure within the lungs (Boyle's law). When it comes to the cellular level (i.e., transport and exchange of oxygen and carbon dioxide), things get even more interesting.

The pressure of our atmosphere (the air) is the sum of all gases contained within that air. The pressure of our planet's atmosphere (calibrated to sea level—so things are slightly but meaningfully different at high altitudes; we will ignore that for now) is 760 mmHg (*millimeters* of mercury [*Hg*] *pressure*). There are many gases contained in the air, each gas contributing a portion to overall air pressure. This is called partial pressure and is the most common reference seen when gas pressures are reported. Each gas, in a mixture of gases, has its own partial pressure. In our atmosphere, at sea level, nitrogen contributes the greatest portion of pressure, specifically 78.6% or 597.4 mmHg. Oxygen contributes 21% to the total composition of air or 158.8 mmHg; water vapor is next at 0.04% or 3 mmHg; followed by carbon dioxide at 0.0004% or 0.3 mmHg. The rest is contributed by a variety of gases for a total atmospheric pressure at sea level of 760 mmHg.

3.2.3 Partial Pressures and Gas Exchange in External Respiration

Why are the physics of gas exchange important to breathing? It helps to remember that differences in partial pressures in different physical structures support the diffusion of gases from one structure to the other. Partial pressures determine where a gas will move because gases (of the same kind) equalize their pressure in regions that are connected (in the case of breathing: in the lungs overall, their connection via the airway to the air outside the body). The larger the difference in pressure of a particular gas in one region, the faster the movement of gas from the high-pressure to the low-pressure region. Following, this process is applied to the body for diffusion of oxygen and carbon dioxide at the alveoli during external respiration.

Oxygen Diffusion During External Respiration
Because of Boyle's law, the partial pressure of oxygen in alveolar air is approximately 104 mmHg (on average, across exhalations and inhalation). This partial pressure of oxygen differs significantly from that in the venous blood, which is 40 mmHg. Thus, oxygen diffuses from high-pressure alveoli to low-pressure pulmonary venous blood, creating a partial pressure of oxygen of 104 mmHg in newly oxygenated blood. If there is an insufficient pressure gradient between partial pressures of oxygen in the alveoli and the blood (as might happen at high altitudes or due to certain lung pathologies that restrict airflow into the alveoli), diffusion of oxygen into the blood becomes less efficient. Generally, in healthy lungs, partial pressure of oxygen at the junction between alveoli and capillaries is high enough to expose hemoglobin in red blood cells to sufficient oxygen that a transfer of O_2 to the blood, red blood cells, and hemoglobin happens easily. Each hemoglobin molecule (a combination of the protein globulin and a nonprotein heme portion) can carry four O_2 molecules (there are about 250,000 hemoglobin molecules in each red blood cell).

When blood first arrives from tissues at the alveoli, its hemoglobin molecules are completely deoxygenated, which means they have a very low affinity for O_2. This requires a higher partial pressure of O_2 outside of the hemoglobin molecule to bind oxygen (which is fortunately what we have at the junction between venous capillaries and alveoli). Interestingly, however, once the first O_2 molecule has attached to hemoglobin, the next three attachments happen more easily (in the presence of less partial pressure of O_2). Once hemoglobin is oxygenated, its affinity for O_2 is strong (i.e., it strongly binds with O_2). Thus, blood stays oxygenated until the right conditions support the release of O_2 from hemoglobin and into the tissues. This will become important to understand when exploring internal respiration, that is, the release of O_2 from hemoglobin into tissues.

Carbon Dioxide Diffusion During External Respiration

Carbon dioxide diffusion is a bit more complicated, in part because the level of CO_2 in blood has several life-sustaining functions. Most importantly, it is related to body alkalinity or acidity (the body's pH level has a very narrow range before it has deleterious effects on the body which, if severe, can be life-threatening) and to the release of O_2 molecules from hemoglobin, so that it may be released into the tissues (part of the process of internal respiration). Biomechanically, the optimal presence of CO_2 dilates the airways and blood vessels. But, back to CO_2 diffusion as a physiological process of respiration in the context of partial pressure and gas exchange: Carbon dioxide is taken up into the blood from the tissues (as a byproduct of metabolism) and dealt with in two ways. First, it is carried through the body for calibration of the body's pH level. Second, the rest of CO_2 (the portion not needed in the body; i.e., *excess CO_2*) is transported to the capillaries surrounding the alveoli. From here, excess CO_2 diffuses into the alveoli to be released into the airway and carried out of the body. This diffusion depends on partial pressures in the involved gases and regions. The partial pressure of CO_2 in venous capillaries (at the alveoli) is 46–48 mmHg. The partial pressure of CO_2 inside the alveoli is 40 mmHg—a pressure gradient that is much smaller than that for oxygen. Yet, CO_2 has a much easier time diffusing through tissues than oxygen (about 20 times faster) and can easily travel from blood into alveoli despite this relatively small pressure gradient. Once enough CO_2 has diffused into the alveoli to equalize the pressure between the alveoli and blood, the (now also *oxygenated*) blood will have a partial pressure of CO_2 of 40 mmHg.

The arterial partial pressure of CO_2 must remain at approximately 40 mmHg to make sure enough CO_2 is in the bloodstream to maintain proper blood pH levels for optimal health and even survival. To maintain this constancy of arterial partial pressure of CO_2, alveolar partial pressure of CO_2 also has to be at 40 mmHg (remember that atmospheric pressure of CO_2 is only 0.3 mmHg!). Thus, if alveolar partial pressure of CO_2 decreases, so does arterial CO_2 pressure, resulting in dysregulation of blood pH. *This happens if too much CO_2 is expelled.* In other words, over-breathing results in alveolar hypocapnia and can have significantly negative consequences for health. Unfortunately, over-breathing is very common and the source of much suffering; it thus can become the starting point for useful breathing interventions that can restore health by changing the rate and volume of breathing (as will be explored in detail below). A summary of external respiration is shown in Table 3.1.

Table 3.1 Tabular summary of external respiration

External respiration or pulmonary gas exchange	
CO_2 is unloaded from the blood into the alveoli	
O_2 is loaded into the blood from the alveoli	
What occurs when blood arrives at the alveoli	*What occurs when blood leaves the alveoli*
• *Deoxyhemoglobin* arrives—No or a single O_2 attached to the hemoglobin molecule • Hemoglobin is bound to lots of CO_2 (to about 20% of the CO_2 in the blood) and protons (positively charged) → hemoglobin is in the deoxygenated state and hangs on to CO_2 • Additional CO_2 exists in other forms; these too can diffuse to the alveoli • Deoxyhemoglobin has a low affinity for oxygen (i.e., does not easily take it up).	• *Oxyhemoglobin* departs—All hemoglobin molecules are loaded with oxygen • Hemoglobin begins to bind to oxygen; this allows carbon dioxide to leave the red blood cells (the first O_2 molecule has trouble binding; each subsequent O_2 is more easily loaded onto hemoglobin) → hemoglobin is in the oxygenated state and hangs on to O_2 • Oxyhemoglobin has a high affinity for oxygen (i.e., hangs on to it) and a low affinity for CO_2

• Partial pressure of CO_2 in the alveoli = 40 mmHg
• Partial pressure of CO_2 in the blood = 45 mmHg
  → small pressure gradient
  OK as CO_2 easily diffuses (20 * easier than O_2)
• Partial pressure of O_2 in the alveoli = 104 mmHg.
• Partial pressure of O_2 in the blood = 40 mmHg.
  → large pressure gradient
  Helpful as O_2 does not diffuse as easily as CO_2
	• Partial pressure of CO_2 in the alveoli = 40 mmHg
	• Partial pressure of CO_2 in the blood = 40 mmHg
	  → no pressure gradient
	
	• Partial pressure of O_2 in the alveoli = 104 mmHg.
	• Partial pressure of O_2 in the blood = 104 mmHg.
	  → no pressure gradient
	  Transport of O_2 in the blood to the tissue

• *Haldane effect* is relevant—O_2 is needed to release CO_2 from hemoglobin when red blood cells arrive at the alveoli; this requires a high O_2 pressure gradient—Luckily, in health, we have this; however, conditions that result in low partial pressures of oxygen in the alveoli (e.g., high altitude, poor ventilation due to various pathologies) present a problem	• *Bohr effect* is relevant—CO_2 is needed to unload O_2 from hemoglobin and into the tissues; this requires adequate partial pressure of CO_2 in the blood (at least >37 mmHg)—In health and with optimal functional breathing, we have this; however, chronic hyperventilation leading to hypocapnia presents a problem

3.2.4   Partial Pressures and Gas Exchange in Internal Respiration

Gas exchange also, and very importantly, happens beyond the alveoli at the tissue level. Oxygen molecules have to be delivered into cells all over the body and carbon dioxide molecules have to be picked up from tissues to be either redistributed to support the body's pH balance (the bulk of absorbed CO_2) or exhaled (a small proportion). For transport of both oxygen and carbon dioxide, the respective gas has to diffuse into the bloodstream and then into red blood cells (also called erythrocytes). An exploration follows describing how this process happens, specific to all gases involved.

Oxygen's Story During Internal Respiration

When oxygen is released into capillaries at the alveoli, it begins its journey throughout the body. As noted above, to be carried along in blood, oxygen molecules have to enter red blood cells. Red blood cells are slightly donut-shaped and produced in bone marrow. They live for about 3 months and are continuously replenished. Once O_2 has entered red blood cells, it attaches to resident hemoglobin molecules, important proteins abundant in each red blood cell (as long as there is sufficient iron). Each hemoglobin molecule can bind four oxygen molecules, becoming *oxyhemoglobin*. It will hang on to these O_2 molecules to deliver them where they are needed and will then release O_2 molecules for diffusion into tissue. To increase the oxygen-carrying capacity of blood, we need more red blood cells (we cannot increase the amount of O_2 carried by any one individual erythrocyte). Exercise can help increase the number of red blood cells and the amount of hemoglobin available; iron-rich food can also be helpful (although excess iron has its own set of potentially serious problems). As the number of red blood cells increases in the blood, so does the capacity to carry oxygen to tissues.

Release of oxygen from hemoglobin molecules (related to the degree of affinity between O_2 and hemoglobin) is regulated by several important conditions: pH level, *partial pressure of carbon dioxide*, carbon monoxide, and internal warmth (e.g., increased body temperature from exercise). If the partial pressure of CO_2 falls below 40 mmHg, blood pH will increase in red blood cells and surrounding tissue. As pH rises out of its ideal zone toward greater alkalinity, the bond (or affinity) between hemoglobin and O_2 strengthens. In other words, *hemoglobin hangs onto O_2, rather than releasing it into tissues where it is needed*. The presence of carbon monoxide competes with the binding of O_2 to hemoglobin, creating carboxyhemoglobin. If carbon monoxide is present on even one of the four sites on the hemoglobin molecule, even if the other sites are filled with O_2, oxygen will not be (easily) released into the tissue. Arterial partial pressure of oxygen will be normal (a pulse oximeter registers normal because it cannot differentiate between carboxyhemoglobin and oxyhemoglobin), but O_2 affinity is so high in hemoglobin, that *tissues become hypoxic* because O_2 is not released to diffuse into tissues.

Our physiology is primed to maintain a high level of oxygen saturation in the bloodstream, namely, approximately 98%. Oxygen saturation, then, refers to the ratio of oxygen that is bound to hemoglobin as compared to how much oxygen *could* be carried by hemoglobin. The higher the saturation, the larger the percentage of hemoglobin that is loaded with oxygen molecules. Oxygen saturation level stays stable even during short to moderate breath holds, during diving, and other breath-challenging activities. It needs to drop to almost 50% before O_2 detectors trigger an inhalation and/or increase in breathing rates. *The primary trigger for natural breathing thus is not oxygen; it is carbon dioxide.*

The challenge is that if hemoglobin does not release O_2 into the tissue, our blood may be well-saturated with oxygen, but our tissues are starving. O_2 is tightly bound to hemoglobin when pH is alkaline, partial pressure of CO_2 is low, our bodies are so cold that transfer of oxygen to the cells is impaired, or carbon monoxide levels are high. The *Bohr effect*, named after Christian Bohr [2] who identified this failsafe of constant oxygen saturation levels in the blood, refers to the reality that CO_2 plays a major role in the strength of the bond between hemoglobin and oxygen. *In the presence of insufficient partial pressure of CO_2* (below 40 mmHg), the commensurate increase in pH, and the strengthened bond between O_2 and hemoglobin, *diffusion into the cells of the tissues where oxygen is needed is impaired.*

The relationships between these factors can be captured via the oxygen dissociation curve, which plots oxygen saturation against the partial pressure of CO_2, showing the fraction of hemoglobin that is occupied by O_2 [3]. If this curve shifts to the right from normal (lower fraction of hemoglobin is occupied), the curve shows that hemoglobin has decreased affinity with O_2, releasing it into the surrounding tissues more readily. A shift to the left from normal (larger proportion of hemoglobin is occupied), on the other hand, shows increased affinity, meaning that hemoglobin is hanging onto the O_2 that is bound to it. Partial pressures of carbon dioxide, pH, temperature, carbon monoxide, and other factors affect whether affinity between oxygen and hemoglobin rises or drops, that is, whether the oxygen dissociation curve moves to the right or left. A right shift supports tissue oxygenation; a left shift impairs it. Figure 3.1 and Table 3.2 provide more detail.

To make the take-home message very clear: low levels of CO_2 and/or high levels of blood pH (alkaline) result in oxygen deprivation of bodily tissues, including brain tissue; vasoconstriction; and out-of-balance pH levels (even in the presence of high O_2 saturation). Warmth can help release more oxygen (e.g., exercise can support O_2 release into tissues). However, *maintaining optimal blood CO_2 levels is literally the*

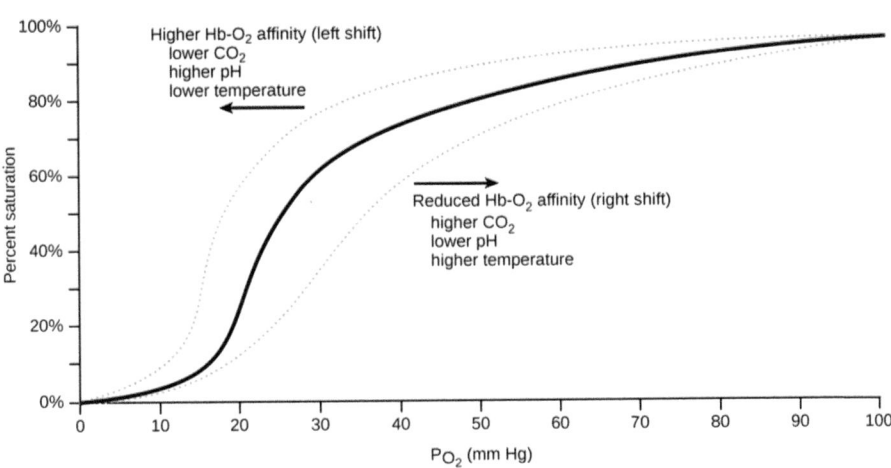

Fig. 3.1 Oxygen dissociation curve. (Data source: OpenStax Biology, licensed under CC BY 4.0; retrieved from https://openstax.org/books/biology/pages/39-4-transport-of-gases-in-human-bodily-fluids)

Table 3.2 Effects of left versus right shift in the oxygen dissociation curve

Left shift—increased Hg Affinity = poorer tissue oxygenation	Right shift—decreased Hg Affinity = better tissue oxygenation
• Increased pH (alkalinity) • Decreased partial pressure of carbon dioxide (e.g., from hyperventilation or over-breathing) • Colder temperatures (e.g., from very cold weather/climate) • Lack of exercise (lower metabolic rate of the muscles) • Presence of carbon monoxide • High altitude	• Decreased pH (acidic) • Increased partial pressure of carbon dioxide (e.g., from healthful natural breathing—Soft, light, diaphragmatic, nasal) • Warmer temperatures (e.g., from exercise or warm weather/climate) • Adequate amounts of exercise (increased metabolic rate of muscles) • No significant presence of carbon monoxide • Sea level

key to health and well-being. This is accomplished by maintaining healthful breathing patterns—the primary focus of the integrated holistic breathing practices that are the focus of this book.

> **Great YouTube Resources About External and Internal Respiration by Ninja Nerd**
> https://www.youtube.com/watch?v=yUtngVm93-c = External Respiration: Ventilation Perfusion Coupling
> https://www.youtube.com/watch?v=Wn_f23qus1k&list=PLTF9h-T1TcJjdJppplKVsgPWNQ_beElaG&index=11 = External Respiration: Thickness & Surface Area of Respiratory Membrane
> https://www.youtube.com/watch?v=YGGG_gKi0m8 = External Respiration: Partial Pressures & Solubilities
> https://youtu.be/Lo6kRuC0ruU = Internal Respiration
> https://www.youtube.com/watch?v=bhJarMGNFw4 = Oxygen-Hemoglobin Dissociation Curve

Carbon Dioxide's Story During Internal Respiration

Although often described as a waste gas, CO_2 is much more than that. While it *is* a byproduct of metabolism (fueling its label as waste), CO_2 has many essential bodily functions. In proper proportions, it supports oxygen release into tissues, nitric oxide release, pH level regulation, vasodilation, and more. If CO_2 levels are not ideal, there are significant negative health effects, as described below. Following is an exploration of CO_2 in our bodies.

CO_2 is produced in tissues during metabolism. It then is released from tissues into the blood to serve its various functions. Once released from tissues into the blood, the bulk (about 90%) of absorbed carbon dioxide diffuses into red blood cells. Here, carbon dioxide combines with water and forms carbonic acid, which then breaks down into hydrogen and bicarbonate ions. The increase in hydrogen that results from this process lowers the pH level in red blood cells (pH is the partial pressure of hydrogen; pH = 7 is neutral; pH < 7 is acidic; pH > 7 is alkaline). Bicarbonate atoms diffuse into blood plasma where they create lactic acid. In other words, the amount of CO_2 in the red blood cells helps determine the amount of hydrogen and bicarbonate present in red blood cells and blood plasma, contributing to the regulation of blood pH. The relationship between carbon dioxide, pH, and bicarbonate concentration is captured in the Henderson-Hasselbach equation: pH = [HCO3] ÷ PCO_2 (where PCO_2 refers to the partial pressure of carbon dioxide, which is regulated by breathing; HCO3 refers to the concentration of bicarbonate, which is regulated by the kidneys).

Although it is not necessary to remember this equation, its implications are meaningful. Most importantly, this equation suggests that *breathing is a crucial aspect of moment-to-moment acid-alkaline regulation in the body and hence a mediator of health and well-being*. The amount of hydrogen (pH) affects the strength of the bond between O_2 and hemoglobin and ultimately the release (or lack of release) of oxygen into the tissues. Decreased CO_2 leads to increased pH which leads to decreased release of oxygen (as described in Oxygen's Story above). When too much CO_2 is off-loaded (exhaled) via over-breathing, too much bicarbonate and not enough hydrogen atoms are the result. Blood becomes too alkaline and action is needed to make adjustments to prevent respiratory alkalosis. When this happens acutely (occasionally or situationally), it is no problem; the body's chemistry is set up for situational recalibration. Optimal CO_2 levels are so important to health and well-being that the profound effects of variations of CO_2 away from optimal (either too high or too low) are explored in more detail below.

Nitric Oxide's Story in Internal Respiration
An important function of healthful levels of CO_2 includes the release of nitric oxide, a powerful vasodilator we met in Chap. 2's biomechanics section (as nitric oxide is released in the nose during exhalation and breath holds after exhalation). Increased CO_2 and reduced pH stimulate the release of nitric oxide. Through vasodilation, nitric oxide causes vessels to widen, increasing blood volume and arterial blood flow which, in turn, increases oxygen and glucose supply to the cells. Hypocapnic conditions (low partial pressure of CO_2) diminish the release of nitric oxide; that is, when CO_2 levels drop (e.g., from over-breathing), less nitric oxide is released. Less nitric oxide leads to vasoconstriction and increases the likelihood of blood clotting (because of its effect on blood platelets). Nitric oxide is also a signaling molecule with effects on almost all physiological systems. It affects vasoregulation, homeostasis, neurotransmission, immune defense, respiration, and more—see the following *Fun Facts from Science*. It helps reverse arterial plaque and reduce cholesterol. It can enhance ciliary movement in the airways and, during nasal breathing,

sterilizes inhaled air. In other words, nitric oxide is helpful to human health and wellbeing and its levels can be profoundly affected by healthful breathing, biochemically and biomechanically. Diet, too, can affect nitric oxide production, with some whole foods having a particularly beneficial effect, especially leafy green vegetables (e.g., arugula) and some root vegetables (e.g., beets). A summary of all aspects of internal respiration is offered in Table 3.3.

Table 3.3 Tabular summary of internal respiration

Internal respiration or tissue-level gas exchange	
O_2 is unloaded from the blood into the alveoli	
CO_2 is loaded from the alveoli into the blood	
What occurs when the blood arrives at the tissues	*What occurs when the blood leaves the tissues*
• *Oxyhemoglobin* arrives—All hemoglobin molecules are loaded with oxygen	• *Deoxyhemoglobin* departs—No or a single O_2 attached to the hemoglobin molecule
• Oxyhemoglobin has a high affinity for oxygen (i.e., hangs on to it) and a low affinity for CO_2	• Deoxyhemoglobin has a low affinity for oxygen (i.e., does not easily take it up)
• Adequate levels of partial pressure of CO_2 in the blood and a large pressure gradient of O_2 in the blood versus the tissues is necessary for O_2 to unload to the tissues	• Pressure gradient of O_2 in tissues and blood are the same and hemoglobin is saturated with CO_2—This carbaminohemoglobin means the red blood cells are deoxygenated
• Partial pressure of CO_2 in the tissues = 45 mmHg	• Partial pressure of CO_2 in the tissues = 45 mmHg
• Partial pressure of CO_2 in the blood = 40 mmHg → small pressure gradient OK as CO_2 easily diffuses (20 * easier than O_2)	• Partial pressure of CO_2 in the blood = 45 mmHg → no pressure gradient Transport of CO_2 in the blood to alveoli
• Partial pressure of O_2 in the tissues = 40 mmHg	• Partial pressure of O_2 in the tissues = 40 mmHg
• Partial pressure of O_2 in the blood = 104 mmHg → large pressure gradient Helps O_2 diffuse from the blood to the tissue	• Partial pressure of O_2 in the blood = 40 mmHg → no pressure gradient
• *Bohr effect* is relevant—CO_2 is needed to unload O_2 from hemoglobin and into the tissues; this requires adequate partial pressure of CO_2 in the blood (at least >37 mmHg)—In health and with optimal functional breathing, we have this; however, chronic hyperventilation leading to hypocapnia presents a problem → too little O_2 will move into the tissues	• *Haldane effect* is relevant—O_2 is needed to release CO_2 from hemoglobin when red blood cells arrive at the alveoli; this requires a high O_2 pressure gradient—Luckily, in health, we have this; however, conditions that result in low partial pressures of oxygen in the alveoli (e.g., high altitude, poor ventilation due to various pathologies) present a problem

Fun Facts from Modern Science …

Nitric oxide, increased by optimal natural breathing and optimal levels of carbon dioxide in the blood, has documented health benefits [4–6].

Several studies have demonstrated that nitric oxide, the very chemical that is released thanks to nasal breathing and balanced CO_2, has a variety of health benefits. Specifically, nitric oxide may:

- enhance vasodilation and bronchodilation
- lower blood pressure
- have antimicrobial effects (bacteria, viruses, and fungi)
- decrease muscle soreness and increase glucose transport to skeletal muscle
- enhance athletic performance and endurance
- help manage Type 2 diabetes (via its relationship with insulin and blood glucose levels)

3.3   Biochemistry of Breathing

Given the importance of CO_2 to O_2 release into tissues (internal respiration) and to maintaining ideal pH levels in the body, it is no surprise that CO_2 levels are the primary physiological triggers for breathing, not O_2 levels (which, as noted above, are amazingly constant absent disease or strong exertion). In other words, the urge to breathe and the basis for oxygen/carbon dioxide exchange generally comes not from a need for O_2, but rather due to too much or too little CO_2. CO_2 is of particular importance as it is a crucial contributor to blood pH (which has to be maintained in a very narrow range of 7.35–7.45; the average normal is 7.365).

3.3.1   Triggers for Breathing

The slightest change in CO_2 level triggers adjustments in the actions of the muscles of respiration to regain proper balance of CO_2 and O_2 and, relatedly body pH (which is regulated primarily by CO_2 and secondarily via regulation of bicarbonate by the kidneys). When the medulla receives a bodily signal about high CO_2 levels in the blood, it triggers contraction in the diaphragm (i.e., inhalation) via the phrenic nerve. O_2 affects breathing only if its blood levels have become dangerously low (e.g., via extreme exertion or hypoventilation, often due to disease, such as COVID-19 infection), which is relatively rare as blood oxygen saturation tends to be stable, regardless of breathing rhythm.

In good health, the respiratory system flexibly and easefully adjusts CO_2 and O_2 levels (maintaining healthy blood pH) simply by altering breath rate and volume. For example, when we increase the rate or volume of breathing during vigorous exercise, we take in more O_2 and expel more CO_2, recruiting accessory and ancillary muscles in the chest and neck to facilitate greater blood flow and air intake. This increase in respiration results in changes in blood pH out of the ideal range. The body, under these circumstances, immediately addresses this shift in pH via the autonomic nervous system (as non-optimal pH level can be life-threatening). Greater deviations from the ideal balance point of CO_2 and pH result in a signal to the cerebral cortex that there is impending danger and we become consciously alarmed and motivated to change our actions.

All action involved in involuntary breathing is monitored and regulated by the medulla oblongata and pons, the respiratory center at the base of the brainstem, in response to sensory feedback from the body. Feedback (traveling via the phrenic nerve) includes signals from chemoreceptors about blood carbon dioxide levels, stretch receptors in smooth muscles of the airway, baroreceptors regarding blood pressure, and baroreceptors regulating stroke volume of the heart.

Specifically:

- Chemoreceptors sense blood pH levels, as well as concentrations of carbon dioxide and oxygen. They send signals to the medulla oblongata which, in turn, signals the diaphragm to adjust breathing rhythms accordingly. When partial pressure of CO_2 rises above an acceptable level (most typically 40 mmHg), the medulla triggers a diaphragmatic breath to remove excess CO_2 from the blood. When the partial pressure of CO_2 drops below the optimal range of 35 mmHg, the medulla sends signals to the body to slow down the breathing rate.
- Signals are sent to the pons, where breath texture is monitored. The pons receives this feedback and signals needed adjustments to create optimal smoothness of airflow.
- Stretch receptors signal excessive stretch in smooth muscles of the airways to the medulla oblongata during inhalation. This information about stretch in the lungs results in an exhalation via inhibitory signals to the diaphragm and external intercostal muscles. This feedback loop, called the Hering-Breuer reflex, prevents hyperinflation of the lungs.
- Baroreceptors in arteries and large veins signal the amount of pressure against the walls of these blood vessels. In response, the medulla oblongata facilitates changes in cardiac output and arterial tension.
- Baroreceptors in the heart provide feedback to the medulla via the vagus nerve. Sensations noted in the heart are linked to pressure against the heart based on the amount of air in the lungs. This feedback results in a speeding up and intensifying of the heart's stroke volume with the inhalation (signaling sympathetic arousal); conversely, it results in slowing down and lessening of the stroke volume with the exhalation (signaling a parasympathetic shift). It is this cycling in heart rate and stroke volume that is called respiratory sinus arrhythmia, which is difficult to measure. However, its proxy measure of heart rate variability is easily measured, even with smartwatches.

We can affect the actions of the medulla oblongata and pons by overriding brainstem reflexes via control from the cortex; this reality informs the teaching of *pranayama*. However, if CO_2 levels get too high or too low (e.g., due to illness), the autonomic nervous system reclaims control from the prefrontal cortex and forces an inhalation. Chronic hyperventilation resets the medulla to become less tolerant of CO_2 concentrations that are actually normal. In fact, just 24 hours of overbreathing can reset the medulla's chemosensitivity to a new trigger level for PCO_2. Change in the medulla's sensitivity to blood CO_2 levels leads to excessive or premature air hunger and a vicious cycle of over-breathing. Resetting this nervous system sensitivity is difficult and yet key to healthful breathing in daily life as well as during breathing practices; it may be accomplished via the slow-paced breathing strategies offered in Chap. 9. Changes in chemosensitivity are made visible in unhealthful breathing patterns, such as hyperventilation or over-breathing, and require careful assessment and ongoing reassessment of breathing. Thus, breath observation and (re)assessment are important foci in the *application* of breathing practices offered in Chaps. 8 and 9.

3.3.2 Understanding the Crucial Relationship of CO_2 and Breathing

Many factors, including stress and other lifestyle factors associated with modern life, can lead to chronic hyperventilation and, commensurately, chronically low CO_2 blood levels. Even minor over-breathing, if chronic, may lead to low concentrations of CO_2 (hypocapnia), making breathing less efficient and more resource-demanding than necessary. Fast (short), shallow breaths (e.g., during chest breathing, especially while stressed or in pain) mean that the bulk of breath does not reach the lungs "depths" (i.e., the alveoli where gas exchange takes place) but stays in the airways and is reexpelled before much gas exchange can occur (i.e., before sufficient O_2 moves into and before much CO_2 is released from the blood). Slow and light breaths, facilitated by the diaphragm [7, 8], and breathed nasally [9] reach the lungs' depths and are more efficient in terms of the percentage of O_2 extracted from any given breath. To be explored in Chap. 4, the ideal number of breaths per minute is 5.5–8. This is in stark contrast to the average number of breaths most adults take per minute, which is 12–20. We have become a stressed *"culture of overbreathers"* [10] (p. 86).

Acute excess release of CO_2 (acute over-breathing) is dealt with by the body via breath rhythm adjustments [11]. The medulla slows the breath rate to allow CO_2 to re-rise in the blood. However, with chronic over-breathing, bicarbonate ions keep accumulating and pH becomes increasingly alkaline. Such respiratory alkalosis can become life-threatening; thus, the body has a fail-safe system via the kidneys. With ongoing dysregulated breathing, the kidneys step in to regulate body pH as reregulation via breath rhythm is no longer possible. This fail-safe literally saves our lives; pH is restored. However, although it regulates pH and bicarbonate, this process does not regulate CO_2. In other words, while the threat to life has been removed by rebalancing pH, carbon dioxide concentration in the blood remains low; this is called hypocapnia.

Chronic hypocapnia or low levels of CO_2 (below 35–37 mmHg), over time, bias the medulla's perception of the need to breathe, giving us air hunger (strong need to breathe) at CO_2 levels that are *not actually dangerously high*. The set point for CO_2 is lowered and chemosensitivity is such that a breath is triggered at levels of CO_2 that are lower than ideal for natural breathing. In fact, some claim that we have become a culture that is CO_2 intolerant, that we experience air hunger in the presence of normal levels of $_{CO2}$, having adapted to chronic hypocapnia [10, 12]. Our medullae, in other words, have become hypersensitive to CO_2. We no longer have the ability to maintain an optimal CO_2 level, so crucial for the uptake of O_2 into the tissues. Through this mechanism, chronic hyperventilation keeps us at the brink of disease.

If this is the case, it is helpful to use breathing exercises that increase CO_2 concentrations as well as CO_2 tolerance, such as breath holds at the end of the exhalation or slow, light, diaphragmatic breathing (if that sounds like *pranayama*, that is so, because it is). Such practices can return our organism to optimal CO_2 levels, which has many health and mental health benefits. Before we discuss this, we need to explore the impacts of optimal, chronically low, and chronically high levels of CO_2 in the blood.

Benefits of Optimal CO_2 Levels in the Blood

Optimal levels of CO_2, approximately 40 mmHg, dilate blood vessels, facilitate the release of oxygen molecules into tissues, and help produce energy (ATP) more efficiently [13]. Since CO_2 is a catalyst for hemoglobin to release oxygen into tissues (Bohr effect), the optimal presence of CO_2 supports the release of O_2 from red blood cells and proper oxygen saturation of blood and tissues. CO_2 facilitates a sense of ease, mental clarity, and emotional peacefulness because energy is available through optimal gas exchange in the lungs (external respiration) and tissues (internal respiration). It invites an autonomic nervous system state that signals that it is okay to relax, rest, and restore, because smooth muscles are openly relaxed, blood flow is easeful, and breath is calm. Benefits arising from optimal CO_2 levels *and* healthful CO_2 sensitivity (partial pressure of CO_2 between 35 and 45 mmHg, accompanied by optimal oxygen saturation) are summarized in Table 3.4.

Clearly, balanced CO_2 and optimal CO_2 tolerance (optimal chemosensitivity of the medulla) are wonderful goals to strive for in daily breathing and *pranayama* practices (through which we increase ranges of tolerance, cultivate subtle energetics, and attain optimal breath health).

Consequences of Chronically Low CO_2 Blood Levels

If CO_2 concentration drops *too low* (*hypocapnic*; partial pressure of $CO_2 < 35$ mmHg) blood becomes alkaline. To recap quickly, acute or chronic hyperventilation leads to low levels of CO_2. During lower levels of partial pressure of CO_2 in the blood, the bond of O_2 to hemoglobin strengthens, and there is less release of O_2 from the blood, leading to less tissue oxygenation. Hyperventilation can be acute due to blowing off too much CO_2 too fast, causing acutely low CO_2 blood levels (as occurs during a panic attack, after exertion, or due to asthma [14]; or chronic with habitual overbreathing that has reset our medulla's CO_2 setpoint (e.g., due to chronic perceptions of stress, food sensitivities, or other lifestyle factors). Occasional acute episodes of

Table 3.4 Benefits arising from optimal CO_2 levels *and* healthful CO_2 sensitivity

Nervous system benefits
- Accurate chemoreception
- Stimulation of the vagus nerve leading to decreased heart rate and application of vagal brake on sympathetic nervous system activation
- Enhanced heart rate variability and respiratory sinus arrhythmia
- Reduction in and prevention of inflammation (acetylcholine, released by the vagus nerve when stimulated, reduces pro-inflammatory cytokines)

Physiological benefits
- Healthy pH level in the blood—Necessary for many aspects of physiological functioning, repair, and regeneration of tissue
- Increased concentration of nitric oxide
- Enhanced vasodilation of smooth muscle
- Improved circulation

Respiratory benefits
- Improved bronchodilation
- Enhanced breathing rhythms
- Easeful slow breathing
- Normalized ventilation
- Reduced breathlessness

Emotional and mental benefits
- Calming of the mind
- Emotional peacefulness and wellbeing
- Enhanced mental clarity

hyperventilation are on a situational basis either by the autonomic nervous system or additional external aids, such as breathing into a paper bag (to bring more CO_2 back into the body as the air expelled into the bag is higher in CO_2 concentration that outside air) or into one's hands cupped over nose and mouth (preferable to the paper bag as this has the desired effect on CO_2 while still providing adequate levels of oxygen in inhaled air).

Chronic excess in ventilation of CO_2 (chronic hyperventilation) can be caused by unhealthful breathing. Constant chest breathing and/or chronic sympathetic arousal due to perceived stress are often involved in chronic hypocapnia. Relatedly, chronic anxiety often involves breathing patterns that lead to chronic hypocapnia [15, 16]. This is one reason why treatment of anxiety disorders ideally includes breath intervention to increase CO_2 tolerance and decondition the anxious feeling associated with low CO_2 levels (as well as the muscle tension that is associated with hypertension and other types of dysregulated breathing [14]. Living or spending an extended period at a high altitude can lead to hypocapnia, as can prolonged fever. Due to the thermoregulation function of breath, high body temperature (e.g., fever, heat stroke) tends to increase the rate of respiration. Heat also can interfere with the attachment of O_2 molecules to hemoglobin in the blood—another reason why we have to breathe harder in extreme heat or when overheating due to vigorous exercise.

If hyperventilation becomes chronic, it can lead to CO_2 hypersensitivity in the medulla, which triggers air hunger even at normal CO_2 concentration. This air hunger then leads to the strong desire to breathe more, creating more hyperventilation and, thus, starting a vicious cycle of over-breathing. This vicious cycle can have grave consequences for physical and mental health and well-being. A few

Table 3.5 Challenges associated with chronic hypocapnia

- Chronic sympathetic arousal
  - Readies us for SNS-based activity (fight, flight, action of any sort)
  - Leads to more over-breathing if no such activity takes place (which it often does not as we are glued to our chairs/offices)
  - Perpetuates the unhealthy breathing cycle and physical and emotional dysregulation
  - Increases anxiety, irritability, and emotional reactivity
- Bronchoconstriction
- Muscle spasms, muscle pain, and stiffness, even weakness, due to excessive lactic acid, electrolyte imbalance, and/or under-oxygenation of tissues
- Numbness or tingling, especially in fingers, toes, and around the mouth
- Increased vasoconstriction
  - Non-cardiac chest pain migraines
  - Hypertension and cardiovascular disease
- Constriction of the carotid artery, with increased risk for cerebral hypoxia (decreased oxygen to the brain)
  - Anxiety, panic
  - Brain fog, lack of concentration, and compromised memory and problem-solving
  - Dizziness, lightheadedness, fainting
  - Confusion, disorientation
  - Headaches that can feel like tension headaches or even like migraines
- Insomnia and generally poor sleep, including greater risk for sleep apnea
- Gastrointestinal disturbances such as irritable bowel, cramping, or bloating
- Low vitality and metabolic disturbance
  - Fatigue and weakness
  - Compromised endurance
  - Low threshold for exercise and poor stamina during exercise

challenges associated with hypocapnia (= partial pressure of $CO_2 < 35$ mmHg, typically accompanied by good oxygen saturation) are shown in Table 3.5, which is by no means all-inclusive.

Consequences of Chronically High CO_2 Blood Levels

Under-breathing is much less common than over-breathing. It is most typically associated with specific disease conditions that create breathing challenges, involving insufficient expelling of air. This leads to chronically high blood levels of CO_2, called hypercapnia (partial pressure of $CO_2 > 45$ mmHg). Hypercapnia results from not expelling enough air, either due to acute or chronic under-breathing or incomplete exhalation. Acute episodes of hypoventilation are easily managed by our physiology. The body is prepared for short breath holds such as occur during swimming or diving, for example. Chronic under-ventilation of CO_2 is more likely associated with chronic physical illness, anatomical changes due to aging or lack of movement (e.g., a chronically hyperinflated rib basket), or due to a conditioned and deeply ingrained nervous systems style of physiological collapse in the face of life threat (dorsal vagal state [17]). Physical conditions correlated with hypercapnia include—but are not limited to—smoking (and related downstream illness, including chronic obstructive pulmonary disease [COPD]), asthma, sleep apnea, and, in more recent history, COVID-19. Even age-related stiffening of the ribcage that interferes with proper exhalation can result in this chronic condition. If CO_2 concentration rises too high, the blood becomes too acidic, which can become life-threatening. Hypercapnia is a less common physiological pathology than low CO_2 levels (the latter being mediated by more common human factors, such as stress and incorrect breathing). Although high CO_2 leads to vasodilation, we cannot reap the benefit of widening arteries because blood O_2 levels are indeed low, leading to an undersupply of oxygen to tissues and brain. Not surprisingly, too much CO_2 on a chronic basis can have significant health consequences that can then layer on top of already compromised health conditions that caused inadequate exhalation to begin with. Challenges associated with chronic hypercapnia (partial pressure of $CO_2 > 45$ mmhg, typically accompanied by low oxygen saturation) are summarized in Table 3.6.

Comparison of Various Blood CO_2 Levels

Table 3.7 compares and contrasts various CO_2 levels and their impacts on health, respiration, nervous system, immunity, and more. This comparison is offered as

Table 3.6 Challenges associated with chronic hypercapnia	• Irregular respiratory rates, bradypnea, and possibly tachycardia • Low tidal volume and poor gas exchange in the alveoli • Less resilience and more reactivity emotionally and mentally • Dizziness, drowsiness, trouble concentrating, memory problems • Confusion, disorientation (even seizures) • Cardiac arrhythmia • Tremors, spasms • Fatigue, sluggishness, sleepiness • Headaches • Flushed skin • Sleep disturbance • Anxiety, panic, agitation

Table 3.7 Biochemistry of breathing: Impacts of various CO_2 levels

Balanced CO_2 and CO_2 tolerance	Hypocapnia (low CO_2)	Hypercapnia (high CO_2) (see note)
• Functional breathing balances CO_2 • CO_2 is a catalyst for hemoglobin to release oxygen into tissues (Bohr effect) • Facilitates accurate chemoreception • Increases concentration of nitric oxide • Enhances vasodilation of smooth muscle	• Acute or chronic hyperventilation leads to low levels of CO_2 • Stronger bond of O_2 to hemoglobin, resulting in less oxygenation of tissues • If chronic, leads to CO_2 sensitivity in the medulla, which triggers air hunger even at a normal CO_2 concentration	• Insufficient expelling of air leads to high levels of CO_2 • Most typically caused by illness or disease— Respiratory failure, smoking, asthma, COPD, neurological impairment • High CO_2 leads to vasodilation; however, O_2 levels in the blood are low and there is undersupply of oxygen to tissues and the brain

(continued)

Table 3.7 (continued)

Balanced CO_2 and CO_2 tolerance	Hypocapnia (low CO_2)	Hypercapnia (high CO_2) (see note)
• Regulates breathing rhythms • Facilitates slow breathing • Normalizes ventilation • Reduces breathlessness	• Leads to air hunger or a strong desire to breathe more • Leads to hyperventilation and a vicious cycle of over-breathing	• Leads to irregular respiratory rates, bradypnea, and possibly tachycardia • Leads to low tidal volume + poor gas exchange in alveoli • Could be linked to dorsal vagal collapse, resulting in reduced respiratory drive, which can cause hypoxemia
• Stimulates the vagus nerve, which decreases heart rate. • Increases heart rate variability. • Improves circulation. • Reduces inflammation (acetylcholine, released by the vagus nerve when stimulated, reduces pro-inflammatory cytokines)	• Creates chronic sympathetic arousal, which readies us for SNS-based activity (fight, flight, action of any sort) and leads to more over-breathing if no such activity takes place (which it often does not as we are glued to our chairs/offices)	
• Supports a healthy pH level in the blood which is necessary for many aspects of physiological functioning, repair, and regeneration • Calms the mind • Creates emotional peacefulness • Supports mental clarity	• Increases alkalinity in the blood, which can be life-threatening. • Causes vasoconstriction and cerebral hypoxia • Reduced oxygen to the brain often results in greater anxiety, brain fog, lack of concentration, poor memory	• Acidity in the blood as CO_2 diffuses into the red blood cells as carbonic acid, can be life-threatening • Less resilience and more reactivity emotionally and mentally
• All systems are go	• Muscle spasms and pain due to excessive lactic acid and under-oxygenation • Migraine-like headaches • Fatigue, breathlessness • Insomnia • Dizziness, lightheadedness, fainting • Non-cardiac chest pain • Inflammation • Low vitality and low threshold for exercise	• Dizziness, drowsiness, trouble concentrating, memory problems • Confusion, disorientation • Cardiac arrhythmia • Tremors, spasms • Fatigue, sluggishness, sleepiness • Headaches • Flushed skin • Sleep disturbance • Anxiety, panic, agitation

Note: The label "hypercapnia" is at times used in the yoga literature to indicate increased CO_2 tolerance. In those contexts, the reference is to increasing the ability to move out of chronic hypocapnia and CO_2 sensitivity, in essence rebalancing CO_2 to a more natural level. In this table, hypercapnia is described in its pathological state motivation to find optimal breathing patterns that support efficient gas exchange and biomechanics. Fortunately, breath is not only under autonomic control but *can be altered by conscious choices* via the prefrontal cortex. This ability to remediate breathing patterns to improve biochemistry, biomechanics, and breath rhythms is the story to be told in later chapters.

3.4   The Importance of Understanding Influences on Breath Biochemistry

Many processes contribute to dysregulating breathing and commensurate changes in breath biochemistry, such as changes in CO_2 chemosensitivity of the medulla. Some are the result of certain physical or environmental influences. Many are linked to modern lifestyles and behaviors and their effects on breathing and CO_2 levels. Others are related to existing mental health or physical health conditions and habits that can have a bi-directional relationship with breathing, breath chemistry, and chemosensitivity. Existing breathing patterns, rhythms, and habits, including breath biomechanics also play a role, as can deliberate breathing exercises. It helps to understand these influences as a means of having multiple avenues for intervention and guidance about which types of breathing practices to choose for a given individual.

3.4.1   Possible Physical Factors That May Affect Breath Biochemistry (and Biomechanics)

Hypocapnia, or low blood levels of CO_2, can occur due to various physical factors [18, 19]. Breathing guides need to be careful not to step outside of their scope of practice when it comes to possible physical considerations of contributors to disordered breathing. Referral to, and collaboration with, qualified healthcare providers are crucial if physical or mental health factors appear implicated. For example, breathing instructors need to understand the following connections:

- Lung diseases such as chronic obstructive pulmonary disease (COPD), asthma, pneumonia, and pulmonary embolisms can lead to increased ventilation and hypocapnia due to impaired gas exchange in the lungs.
- Elevated body temperature, including but not limited to fever, can increase respiratory rate and lead to hypocapnia.
- Mechanical ventilation in intensive care settings obviously affects breath mechanics and can disrupt breath chemistry, if ventilator settings are not properly adjusted.
- Pathologies affecting the brainstem or central nervous system, such as brain injury, stroke, or encephalitis, can disrupt respiratory control mechanisms and lead to altered brain chemistry.

- In severe cases of sepsis or systemic infection, metabolic acidosis can stimulate increased ventilation, resulting in hypocapnia.
- Hepatic encephalopathy, a complication of liver failure, can lead to respiratory alkalosis and hypocapnia due to alterations in acid-base balance in the body.
- Salicylates-containing medications or herbal preparations (e.g., aspirin; willow bark), can stimulate the respiratory center in the brain, leading to hyperventilation and hypocapnia.
- Certain medications, such as stimulants, bronchodilators, and some anesthetics, can increase respiratory rate and cause hypocapnia as a side effect.

3.4.2   Lifestyle Factors That May Affect the Biochemistry (and Biomechanics) of the Breath

A listing of lifestyle patterns that affect breath physiology and chemistry follows. This listing is offered to raise awareness about the variety of factors that can affect how auspiciously we breathe—and hence how healthy we feel. Given their importance to breathwork applications, these factors are touched on again in later chapters when we explore retraining breath through breath awareness, optimal functional breathing, and complex breathing strategies. For example, it helps to understand the lifestyle effects on breath and breathing:

- Stress, especially of the low-grade chronic variety, that we encounter in modern life
- Lack of exercise and movement, in general, especially as related to our sedentary lifestyles that frequently involve hours of being in one position without moving much at all, regardless of whether this means standing (e.g., at a cash register) or sitting (e.g., at a desk)
- Poor posture—not just when seated but also while walking, exercising, running, or standing, and its reverberations into our rib basket, chest, neck and shoulders, and head carriage
- Over-eating, mindless (unconscious or habitual) eating and snacking, eating foods to which we have a sensitivity, and/or eating processed and unnatural foods, especially those that acidify the body
- Food sensitivities, especially if there is a lack of awareness of the sensitivity and the sensitive foods are not avoided
- Alcohol consumption
- Frequent talking, such as in professions like teaching, public speaking, sales, and so on that require lots of talking for much of the workday
- Mouth and chest breathing (as opposed to nasal and diaphragmatic breathing) during rest, sleep, and activity

- The belief that it is necessary to take deep or complete breaths during exercise or to induce a sense of relaxation (e.g., mistaking a big sighing exhalation as a "cleansing breath") [20].
- Overly heated homes with rare experiences of feeling cool, especially overly heated conditions during sleep
- Lack of moderation in almost any activity or lifestyle habit—mistaking more for better, striving for perfection, or, at the opposite end of the spectrum, not caring enough, lacking initiative

Modern Life—A Perfect Storm for Hypocapnia

To recap, optimal levels of carbon dioxide are necessary for the release of oxygen into the tissues and are crucial to healthful pH levels in the blood and body. Our body has careful fail-safe systems to calibrate pH and CO_2 via breath rates and the kidneys. These systems work perfectly if needed situationally. They break down when needed chronically.

Modern life, unfortunately, sets up chronic conditions that tend to result in CO_2 levels that are too low. We are chronically hypocapnic and hyperventilating. Why is this?

One possible and common scenario is as follows:

Our modern lives require us to sit a lot, to be relatively inactive. Physical *inactivity results in less CO_2 being produced* by our tissues. Additionally, we are exposed to *chronically high levels of stress*. This IV drip of stress throughout the day, as James Nestor puts it, tends to make us overbreathe. Overbreathing in effect means that we are blowing off more CO_2 than is healthful.

If we combine those two factors—first, inactivity which produces too little carbon dioxide to begin with, and second, high stress and hyperventilation which blows off too much CO_2—we have a prescription for disaster. We become increasingly hypocapnic. Our kidneys have to kick in as a failsafe to recalibrate the pH level in our blood and tissues. The pH crisis is resolved but CO_2 stays low—our medulla is confused by these disparate signals. If this happens occasionally, it is no big deal. The body recalibrates. If this happens chronically, *the medulla resets itself for lower carbon dioxide levels in the blood. Being reset for a "new normal" of low CO_2, the medulla begins to trigger breathing at partial pressures of carbon dioxide below 35 mmHg.* This premature initiating of a new breath continues the vicious cycle of hyperventilation and leads to poor oxygenation of our tissues—including our brains.

As Patrick McKeown put it (in a workshop in December 2022), *"we run on the inside and we sit on the outside."* From this typical Western lifestyle, we reap poor health.

One possible and very simple solution: breathe less, move more.

3.4.3 Physical and Mental Health Conditions Correlated with Breath Chemistry

A variety of physical and mental health conditions are correlated with hyperventilation and a (probably) partial listing follows. The direction of the relationship between the condition and dysfunctional breathing varies. For some of these conditions, it is unclear whether the condition causes over-breathing or if over-breathing (at least partly) causes the condition (e.g., asthma, anxiety [16]). For others, it is most likely that breath dysfunction may cause a condition (e.g., erectile dysfunction), often via moderating or mediating influence or factor. For others, the condition may cause unhealthful breathing patterns (e.g., emphysema). However, regardless of the relationship's direction, it appears that working with breath can help enhance breath chemistry and ameliorate the related physical health conditions (e.g., asthma [21] and sleep apnea) [22]. Similarly, evidence is accumulating that depression and anxiety disorders can be significantly ameliorated by returning to natural, functional breathing (even if they may have served to create the dysfunctional breathing at its onset [23–25].

Conditions correlated with dysregulated breathing and breath chemistry include asthma, exercise-induced asthma, insomnia, sleep apnea, snoring, erectile dysfunction, depression, anxiety, attention deficit disorder, and panic disorder.

Stress and Breath

When we are stressed, our breath rate increases—we breathe faster and sigh more often. We tend to breathe through the mouth (rather than the nose) and into our chest (rather than diaphragmatically). Our breath becomes noticeable: it is louder, choppier, and involves more body movement, such as a heaving chest. This type of breathing sets off a vicious cycle. Once we breathe in this way, our vagus nerve relays signals to the brainstem that something is amiss and the brain initiates a sympathetic nervous system response. This adds further validity to our perception of stress.

Chronic stress, and commensurate over-breathing and vascular constriction, can lead to physical and mental health challenges, including anxiety, panic, elevated blood pressure, cardiovascular disease, and more. This is particularly true if we do not have something to balance us out—such as exercise, healthful food, breaks for chilling out and socializing, or practices that relax and release the overstimulation of our nervous system. Chronic stress keeps our physiology prepared for danger, which is a risky and resource-depleting way of existing in the world [17]. Much of this can be ameliorated by reducing stress; even more by reducing our rate and volume of breathing [26–28].

3.4.4   Yogic Breath Control and Western Breathing Exercises

As we will explore in detail in Chap. 4, rhythms of breath interact profoundly with its biochemistry. The same is true for breath biomechanics as shown in Chap. 2 (especially the sections on nasal versus mouth and chest versus diaphragmatic breathing). With regard to anatomy, the most profound influence on breath biochemistry arises from diaphragmatic versus chest breathing and from nasal versus mouth breathing. For example, thoracic breathing tends to speed up respiration and can cause both hypocapnia and, over time, CO_2 hypersensitivity in the medulla. Thoracic breathing also results in less efficient use of oxygen, as well as increased use of oxygen by increasing exertion in muscles not typically necessary for breathing. Similarly, mouth (as opposed to nasal) breathing increases respiratory rate, possibly contributing to hyperventilation and hypocapnia. It also bypasses the maxillary sinuses and thus does not result in the release of nitric oxide.

Breathing Practices of Hormesis

Some breathing practices, both based on yoga (e.g., *kapalabhati*) and Western exercises [29] use hyperventilation and/or long breath holds that can result in hypocapnia, blood alkalinity, and hypoxia. Given these impacts, these breathing exercises can lead to chronic disruption of healthful breathing and breath biochemistry if *misunderstood as recommended daily* or as typical breathing practices. Instead, it is important to view these practices as exercises in hormesis—exercises that stress the body to promote vigorous and healthy stress responses that lead to adaptation and serve as a means of inoculating the organism against stressors.

Such practices can be adaptive and healthful [30], if used with caution. In other words, challenging breathing practices do not have to be shunned. It is, however, important to understand their intention and specific applications. They are used with caution and by breathers who

- have already mastered the art of breathing healthfully;
- understand what they are creating biochemically, biomechanically, and with regard to nervous system (dys)regulation; and
- are in good health, especially free of cardiovascular disease, respiratory illness (e.g., asthma), brain pathologies, and mental health disorders (such as panic disorders, anxiety, PTSD, and more).

Using *pranayama* or Western breathing practices that encourage over-breathing and strong breath holds can create great imbalances in the breath, physiology, musculoskeletal function, and nervous system of students and clients [20]— something neither students or clients nor teachers or clinicians are always fully aware of. Lowered CO_2 level and increase in blood pH can lead to a variety of side effects [31, 32]. For example, practitioners have reported a "claw hand" effect with such breathing, where hands clench, sometimes for very extended periods. Such reports are sometimes made with little recognition that this is a signal that breathwork may not be optimally matched to the client [33]. Other students have reported little recognition of the nervous system impacts of such breathing, which can be sympathetically arousing, creating even more stress in an already chronically stressed organism. Significant hypoxia can have harmful effects, including on the brain due to inadequate oxygen supplies to all tissue [34].

3.5   Where We Go from Here

The good news about the causes and correlates of disrupted breathing patterns and less-than-optimal biochemical signaling is that we can return our body to health by cultivating healthful breathing and embracing health behavior changes that support ongoing respiratory health. We can use our capacity to exert executive control (via our prefrontal cortex) over our behavior and breathing rhythms. To apply conscious control over breathing, we need to understand how chemosensitivity in the medulla develops biochemically and how these changes affect breathing. This understanding helps provide motivation to engage in important health behavior changes that support resilient breathing. Breathing changes that support healthy biochemistry and biomechanics are an important focus of Chaps. 8 and 9. For now, we will turn to exploring various rhythms of breath as well as the breath's relationship to the nervous system states. Based on the science about these aspects of breath and breathing, Chap. 4 provides a definition of coherent and resilient breathing that allows for adaptive responses to life circumstances to maintain breathing rhythms that serve our human anatomy, physiology, and psychology.

If you are quiet enough, you will hear the flow of the universe. You will feel its rhythm. Go with this flow. Happiness lies ahead.—The Buddha

References

1. Trayhurn P. Oxygen—a critical, but overlooked, nutrient. Front Nutr. 2019;6:10. https://doi.org/10.3389/fnut.2019.00010.
2. Bohr C, Hasselbalch K, Krogh A. Über einen in biologischer Beziehung wichtigen Einfluss, den die Kohlensäurespannung des Blutes auf dessen Sauerstoffbindung übt. Skandinavisches Archiv Für Physiologie. 1904;16(2):402–12. https://doi.org/10.1111/j.1748-1716.1904.tb01382.x.
3. Patel S, Jose A, Mohiuddin SS. Physiology, oxygen transport and carbon dioxide dissociation curve. StatPearls Publishing; 2022. https://www.ncbi.nlm.nih.gov/books/NBK539815/
4. Besco R, Sureda A, Tur J, Pons A. The effect of nitric-oxide-related supplements on human performance. Sports Med. 2017;42:99–117. https://doi.org/10.2165/11596860-000000000-00000.
5. Gamboa A, Shibao C, Diedrich A, et al. Contribution of endothelial nitric oxide to blood pressure in humans. Hypertension. 2007;49(1):170–7. https://doi.org/10.1161/01.HYP.0000252425.06216.26.
6. Sansbury BE, Hill BG. Regulation of obesity and insulin resistance by nitric oxide. Free Radic Biol Med. 2014;73:383–99. https://doi.org/10.1016/j.freeradbiomed.2014.05.016.

7. Bradley H, Esformes J. Breathing pattern disorders and functional movement. Int J Sports Phys Ther. 2014;9(1):28–39. https://www.ncbi.nlm.nih.gov/pubmed/24567853

8. Russo MA, Santarelli DM, O'Rourke D. The physiological effects of slow breathing in the healthy human. Breathe. 2017;13(4):298–309. https://doi.org/10.1183/20734735.009817.

9. Trevisan ME, Boufleur J, Soares JC, Haygert CJP, Ries LGK, Corrêa ECR. Diaphragmatic amplitude and accessory inspiratory muscle activity in nasal and mouth-breathing adults: a cross-sectional study. J Electromyogr Kinesiol. 2015;25(3):463–8. https://doi.org/10.1016/j.jelekin.2015.03.006.

10. Nestor J. Breath: the new science of a lost art. Riverhead Books; 2020.

11. Litchfield PM. Good breathing, bad breathing. https://www.breatheon.com/media/docs/Peter-Litchfield-on-goodbad-breathing-CapnoTrainer8.pdf. Updated 2006.

12. McKeown P. The breathing cure. Humanix; 2021.

13. Gilbert C, Chaitow L, Bradley D. Recognizing and treating breathing disorders. 2nd ed. Elsevier Health Sciences; 2013.

14. Ritz T, Meuret AE, Bhaskara L, Petersen S. Respiratory muscle tension as symptom generator in individuals with high anxiety sensitivity. Psychosom Med. 2013;75(2):187–95. https://doi.org/10.1097/PSY.0b013e31827d1072.

15. Leyro TM, Versella MV, Yang M, Brinkman HR, Hoyt DL, Lehrer P. Respiratory therapy for the treatment of anxiety: meta-analytic review and regression. Clin Psychol Rev. 2021;84:101980. https://doi.org/10.1016/j.cpr.2021.101980.

16. Lehrer PM, Woolfolk RL. Principles and practice of stress management. 4th ed. Guilford Press; 2021.

17. Porges S. The pocket guide to the polyvagal theory: the transformative power of feeling safe. Norton; 2017.

18. Palmer BF, Clegg DJ. Respiratory acidosis and respiratory alkalosis: Core curriculum 2023. Am J Kidney Dis. 2023;82(3):347–59. https://doi.org/10.1053/j.ajkd.2023.02.004.

19. Curley G, Laffey JG, Kavanagh BP. Bench-to-bedside review: carbon dioxide. Crit Care. 2010;14(2):220. https://doi.org/10.1186/cc8926.

20. Gilbert C. Better chemistry through breathing: the story of carbon dioxide and how it can go wrong. Biofeedback. 2005;33(3):100–4. https://search.proquest.com/docview/208148631

21. Burgess J, Ekanayake B, Lowe A, Dunt D, Thien F, Dharmage SC. Systematic review of the effectiveness of breathing retraining in asthma management. Expert Rev Respir Med. 2011;5(6):789–807. https://doi.org/10.1586/ers.11.69.

22. Kimura A, Chiba S, Capasso R, et al. Phase of nasal cycle during sleep tends to be associated with sleep stage. Laryngoscope. 2013;123(8):2050–5. https://doi.org/10.1002/lary.23986.

23. Annapoorna S, Wale GR. The effect of Anulom Vilom pranayama on levels of depression in geriatric population in selected areas of Hutti, Raichur District, Karnataka. Asian Pac J Nurs. 2019;6(2):87–90. https://mcmed.us/downloads/02201987-90.pdf

24. Kumar N, Pradhan B. Immediate role of two yoga-based breathing technique on state anxiety in patients suffering from anxiety disorder: a self as control pilot study. Int J Yoga Philos Psychol Parapsychol. 2017;5(1):18. https://doi.org/10.4103/ijny.ijoyppp_9_16.

25. Marshall RS, Basilakos A, Williams T, Love-Myers K. Exploring the benefits of unilateral nostril breathing practice post-stroke: attention, language, spatial abilities, depression, and anxiety. J Altern Complement Med. 2014;20(3):185–94. https://doi.org/10.1089/acm.2013.0019.

26. Kalaivani S, Kumari MJ, Pal GK. Effect of alternate nostril breathing exercise on blood pressure, heart rate, and rate pressure product among patients with hypertension in JIPMER, Puducherry. J Educ Health Promot. 2019;8(1):145. https://doi.org/10.4103/jehp.jehp_32_19.

27. Raghuraj P, Telles S. Immediate effect of specific nostril manipulating yoga breathing practices on autonomic and respiratory variables. Appl Psychophysiol Biofeedback. 2008;33(2):65–75. https://doi.org/10.1007/s10484-008-9055-0.

28. Saravanan L, Anu S, Vairapraveena R, Rajalakshmi G. Impact of alternate nostril breathing exercises on vascular parameters in hypertensive patients - an interventional study. Natl J Physiol Pharm Pharmacol. 2019;9(3):210–4. https://doi.org/10.5455/njppp.2019.9.1237308012019.

29. Hof W. The Wim Hof method: activate your full human potential. Sounds True; 2020.

30. Ji LL, Dickman JR, Kang C, Koenig R. Exercise-induced hormesis may help healthy aging. Dose Response. 2010;8(1):73–9. https://doi.org/10.2203/dose-response.09-048.Ji.
31. Kasperk C. Hypercalcemic crisis and hypocalcemic tetany. Internist. 2017;58(10):1029–36. https://doi.org/10.1007/s00108-017-0311-3.
32. Macefield G, Burke D. Paraesthesiae and tetany induced by voluntary hyperventilation: increased excitability of human cutaneous and motor axons. Brain. 1991;114(1):527–40. https://doi.org/10.1093/brain/114.1.527.
33. King JC, Rosen SD, Nixon PG. Failure of perception of hypocapnia: physiological and clinical implications. J R Soc Med. 1990;83(12):765–7. https://doi.org/10.1177/014107689008301205.
34. Curley G, Kavanagh BP, Laffey JG. Hypocapnia and the injured brain: evidence for harm. Crit Care Med. 2011;39(1):229–30. https://doi.org/10.1097/CCM.0b013e3181ffe3c7.

Understanding the Psychology of Breath and Breathing

4

> *When the breath is unsteady, all is unsteady; when the breath is still; all is still. Control the breath carefully. Inhalation gives strength and a controlled body; retention gives steadiness of mind and longevity; exhalation purifies body and spirit.*

> *Goraksasathakam (eleventh century)*

4.1 Overview: Vital and Psychological Aspects of Breath and Breathing

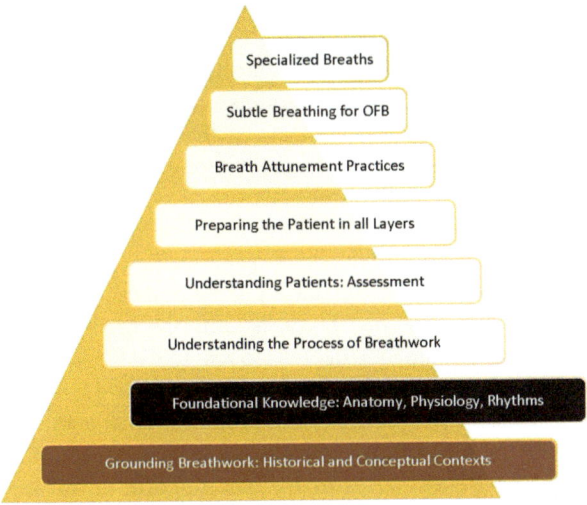

In a vital and rhythmic manner, breath links all experiences in body, vitality, and mind. Biomechanics (involving anatomy and the collaborative, interconnected nature and movement of physical structures) and biochemistry of breathing (involving vital physiology and pulsation of life) interact and interdepend in a profound manner. The biochemistry and biomechanics of breathing, while largely under autonomic nervous system control, are further profoundly affected by the mind, emotions, and psyche. Lifestyle factors, such as food choices, movement, alcohol, stress exposure, and stress perception, accompany environmental factors, such as temperature, altitude, and cleanliness of air, to shape breathing in a variety of ways. Conscious breath control can be claimed (to a degree) when we understand that what we do and how we breathe can alter our biology, anatomy, and physiology of respiration. *Manomaya* and *vijnanamaya koshas*, our layers of conscious and wisely compassionate decision-making, discernment, and behavioral and relational choices, can enter into the breathing equation by becoming vehicles for breath awareness and attention, as well as for lifestyle and health behavior changes that allow us to rediscover physical, mental, and emotional well-being. This chapter explores the rhythms, textures, sounds, and psychological features of breath and breathing. It explores how the autonomic nervous system and breath interact and how breath provides a portal into emotional, mental, and psychological self-regulation and is an important strategy for health promotion. It ends with a clear definition of resilient and coherent breathing, paving the way for the practical application of the science of breathing to the art of therapeutic breathwork.

4.2   Rhythms of Breath and Breathing

Breath awareness is central to understanding the rhythms and subtle vibrations of breathing. It is the starting point and remains a central practice even for advanced breathing practices. Breath awareness is a practice of attunement that hones interoceptive and proprioceptive skills. It is a practice that helps us become familiar with neuroception and recognize autonomic states or energetic ways of being and coping in the world. As such, gaining breath awareness is essential to the development of deeper self-awareness and self-understanding, as well as the capacity to self-regulate all aspects of human functioning, including healing the breath. In turn, healing the breath can help heal the mind and body; healing the breath leads to greater resilience, enhanced co-regulation, and decreased reactivity. Central to breath awareness is the understanding of various breath dimensions that can become the focus of attunement. This awareness eventually is recruited to change breathing rhythms and patterns to become more healthful and supportive of desirable breath biomechanics and biochemistry. Awareness helps us become mindful of default nervous system states, opening our hearts and minds to new possibilities and perspectives. Following is an exploration of science-based rhythms and qualitative characteristics of breath and breathing as well as nervous system-based understandings of self-expression and their relationship to breath, breathing, and therapeutic breathwork.

4.2.1 Understanding Breath Cadence

Breath biomechanics and biochemistry interact profoundly with breath cadence, as represented by rate, volume, and timing, as well as being directly affected by breath characteristics such as texture, sound, location, and resting pauses. Understanding breathing characteristics is a direct link to breath-informed clinical practice and teaching, in that considerations of breath cadence and related factors are how we can optimally cue and instruct breathwork. In reviewing various breath characteristics, it helps to remember that these breath features interact. Although they are discussed separately, in real life, they are completely interrelated; indeed, they may interdepend and correlate in particular habitual, even diagnostic, ways.

Respiratory Rates or Breaths Per Minute

When googling or reading scientific papers about human breath rates, it is typically asserted that the average adult, at least in the Western world, takes approximately 12–20 breaths per minute (BPM), with a statistical mean *spontaneous respiratory rate* for adults of 14 bpm, and a daily total of approximately 20,160 breaths [1]. Interestingly, this average respiration rate (RR) *does not represent the optimally healthy rate of breathing*. That rate, as we are beginning to learn, is much lower [2–4]. The optimal respiratory rate at rest is 5.5–8 BPM—much lower than the reported average [5]. The implication is clear—most of us take more BPM than is ideal for health and well-being. As noted previously, such overbreathing presents many challenges. Conversely, slower, lighter, nasal, and diaphragmatic breathing (of up to 10 BPMs with a light volume of approximately 5–6 L/min) has many benefits, as shown in Table 4.1.

Breath Rates

Interestingly, ancient chants and mantra practices in Buddhism, Hinduism, and yoga use rhythms that are equal to approximately 5.5 BPM. Prayer techniques of indigenous cultures in the Americas, Japan, Africa, and Hawaii also induce this particular breath rhythm.

When investigated with modern methods, this slow breathing rhythm, whether implemented based on the original practices (such as the Buddhist mantra, yogic breath practices, or the Latin version of the Christian rosary) or "newly" developed strategies (e.g., coherent or resonant breathing), has significant benefits. It increases blood flow; increases heart rate variability; reduces blood pressure; and coordinates the heart, lungs, and nervous system so they function in coherence with one another. It also supports easier respiration at high altitudes (think Tibetan Buddhists) [6, 27–31].

Table 4.1 Benefits of slow-paced, nasal, diaphragmatic breathing

- Enhanced autonomic nervous system functioning with greater access to rest and repair [6–8].
- Positive effects via stimulation of somatosensory afferent fibers of the vagus nerve [9].
- Enhanced mental and emotional well-being [10, 11].
- Deeper and more frequent sense of calm [12, 13].
- Decreased perceptions of stress and increased sense of relaxation [14–16].
- Decreases in anxiety and panic [17–19].
- Enhanced cardiovascular functioning (including increased heart rate variability, lowered blood pressure, and enhanced vasodilation [5, 11, 20].
- Enhanced pulmonary function (e.g., reduced chemosensitivity to carbon dioxide; enhanced oxygen saturation during exercise; efficient ventilation [6, 21].
- Increased exercise tolerance and athletic performance [22].
- Carefully calibrated CO_2 levels leading to more efficient respiration [22, 23].
- Enhanced executive function and emotional regulation [24, 25].
- Profound coherence through which all systems in our body and mind work together at peak efficiency and in balance with one another [26].

Fast breathing or overbreathing, which is "average" or "normal" breathing in the sense that it is typical of many adults (and often encouraged in yoga classes), has many downsides. It is more likely to activate the sympathetic branch of the autonomic nervous system, has unfortunate effects on physiology, and often brings with it emotional challenges of depression, anxiety, and even panic, along with reduced stress resilience and increased stress perception [32, 33]. Chronic fast breathing has become a Western standard as our lives unfold in ways that contribute to increased respiratory rates. Stress, poor food choices, inadequate sleep, lack of exercise, the belief that *deep* breathing is important, talking a lot, and excessively warm temperatures in homes (especially during sleep) contribute to chronic overbreathing. If we eat a food to which we are sensitive or that is highly processed, we can feel this. We can do our own experiments and measure BPM before we eat something that we know in our hearts is not good for us; we can remeasure after we have eaten. Almost inevitably, the breath rate has increased. Of course, if we always eat unhealthfully, we may already be overbreathing chronically before we eat, and there is no pre-post difference (because we start with too many BPM to begin with).

Average and above-average respiratory rates correlate strongly with reduced CO_2 levels and the commensurate challenges of hypocapnia explored in Chap. 3, such as vasoconstriction, lightheadedness, panic, fatigue, poor concentration, irritability, and more. Unnecessarily high breath rates also correlate with decreased (external) respiratory efficiency. Faster breathing means less absorption of O_2 at the alveolar level because air moves too quickly through the airways and lungs to facilitate an optimal rate of gas exchange. Air often does not even reach the lower alveoli (and the lower part of the lungs then contains stale air). In fact, at 20 BPM, only 50% of oxygen in inhaled air is used at the alveoli; this increases to 75%, with a reduction to 12 BPM, and 85% at 8 BPM. In other words, the faster we breathe, the less oxygen is actually extracted from the same amount of inhaled air [2].

Respiratory Volumes and Capacities

In addition to being curious about how many breaths we breathe per minute, we also need to become aware of the amount of air we take in and release with each breath, as well as our potential volume capacity. *Average tidal volume* (TV or Vt) is the amount of breath moved in one breath cycle; it equals approximately 500 mL for adults (mL = milliliter; approximately ½ a quart of air). Tidal volume, as explored below, can be combined with respiratory rate to define how much breath moves in and out in the span of 1 minute. This combination of respiratory rate * respiratory volume is called *minute volume* or *minute ventilation* (MV). Before we explore the complexity of respiratory rate and volume interactions, a few other volume- and capacity-related terms need to be defined [34]. This information is summarized in Table 4.2.

Inspiratory reserve volume (IRV) is the additional air that can be breathed in after an average inhalation. If the tidal volume of an in-breath was the typical TV (500 mL of air), IRV on average can be about 2500–2800 mL (another 2½ quarts of air; to visualize this, imagine the volume of 2½ quarts of water). In other words, more breath can be taken in at any time (as needed) than during normal daily breathing. We rely on this capacity to inspire more air when the need arises, for example, during hard exercise. We also do this deliberately in some breathing practices, such as when we add more inhalations after having already inhaled before we exhale (e.g., breath of joy).

Expiratory reserve volume (ERV) is additional air that can be breathed out after an average exhalation. If the average exhalation is 500 mL, ERV is an additional 1000 mL (approximately). Breathing out the reserve volume of expiration is something we do when we sigh, for example. We also might breathe out additional air during exercise such as swimming or diving. At times, we do this deliberately in yogic breathing, when we add more exhalations after having already exhaled (e.g., viloma).

Even after we have removed extra exhalation, which represents the expiratory reserve volume, some residual air remains in the lungs, which is called *functional residual capacity* (FRC) . This air is important to keep the lungs from collapsing (remember the balloon example in the biomechanics section—residual air helps us reinflate the lungs more easily than if we had to start from nothing). To summarize, FRC (also called *residual volume*; RV) is the volume that remains after a "complete" exhalation. The residual volume is approximately 1500 mL.

IRV, ERV, and RV are understood in the context of average total lung capacity, or the total volume of air the lungs can hold at any moment. The average *total lung capacity* (TLC) is approximately 6000 mL (figures vary across sources, reflecting significant individual variation based on bioindividual and environmental factors). From TLC, we can calculate three additional interesting *vital capacities*:

- Average *vital lung capacity* (VC) is the amount of air one is able to move in one breath. This total can be expressed as follows: VC = TV + IRV + ERV. It averages approximately 4500 mL (again, figures vary—some sources give a reference range of approximately 3400–4800 mL).
- *Inspiratory capacity* is the maximum capacity an individual is able to inhale in any single inhalation. This capacity can be expressed as follows: IC = TV + IRV
- *Expiratory capacity* is the maximum capacity an individual is able to exhale in a given exhalation. This can be expressed as follows: EC = TV + ERV

Table 4.2 Summary of respiratory volumes and capacities

Type of volume or capacity	Abbreviation	Definition
Average tidal volume	TV or Vt	Amount of breath moved in one breath cycle
Minute volume or minute ventilation	MV	How much breath moves in and out in the span of 1 minute
Inspiratory reserve volume	IRV	Additional air that can be breathed in after an average inhalation
Expiratory reserve volume	ERV	Additional air that can be breathed out after an average exhalation
Functional residual capacity or residual volume	FRC or RV	Volume that remains after a "complete" exhalation
Total lung capacity	TLC	The total volume of air the lungs can hold at any moment
Vital lung capacity	VC	Amount of air one is able to move in one breath
Inspiratory capacity	IC	Maximum capacity an individual is able to inhale in any single inhalation
Expiratory capacity	EC	Maximum capacity an individual is able to exhale in a given exhalation

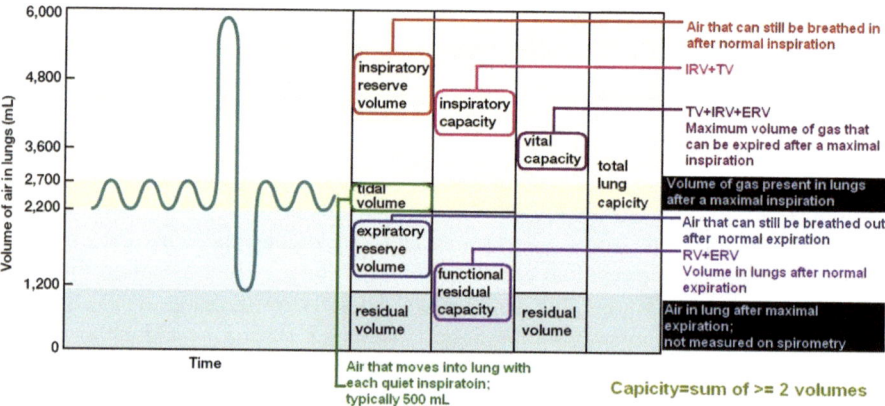

Fig. 4.1 Lung capacities and respiratory volumes. (Data Source: https://commons.wikimedia.org/wiki/File:Respiration_physiology.JPG; Creative Commons Attribution 3.0)

Figure 4.1 provides a visual display of these aspects of lung capacity and respiratory volumes. It provides estimates of *averages* for each value. However, it is important to realize that no two sets of lungs are the same. Capacities and volumes vary widely from person to person. They are strongly influenced by lifestyle factors, possibly by genetics, certainly by illness or diseases, possibly by physical changes in anatomy (e.g., due to rib baskets stiffening with age), and definitely by situational variables (e.g., exercise, air quality, even restrictive clothing).

Cadence: Respiratory Rate and Tidal Volume Combined

Breath rhythms are a combination of respiratory rate (BPM) and respiratory volume (tidal volume or amount of air moved in one breath cycle). These two aspects combine to create *minute ventilation* (MV; aka minute volume), which is the amount of breath moved in 1 minute; it *can* be expressed as MV = TV*RR (we will make this formula slightly more complex in a moment). Average minute ventilation for Western adults is approximately 4–7 L (4000–7000 mL), based on approximately 12 BPM at approximately 500 mL/breath (12*500 mL = 6000 mL). An individual during a panic attack may move as much as 20 L of air/min; individuals with asthma have been shown to average 13 (± 2) L of air [35]; and those with sleep apnea 15 (± 2) L of air [36]. These examples begin to hint at an important fact: moving more air is not healthier. In fact, moving more air tends to be correlated with disease and is more inefficient than slower, lighter breathing.

As the formula for MV shows, the amount of air moved in a single breath can vary widely based on two different factors (that can change individually or in combination): how *fast* and how *voluminously* we breathe. It is not enough to cue or count BPM; we know little about a person's breathing merely based on how often they inhale and exhale/min. We also need to know how much air (how much tidal volume) they move with each breath, and vice versa. A few mathematical examples in Table 4.3 clarify the relationship between respiratory rate and tidal volume that results in a particular minute volume.

Now for the additional complexity. The respiratory rate has a greater impact on *alveolar* minute volume than on tidal volume. What does this mean? The speed at which we breathe affects how much air reaches the alveoli and is involved in the actual process of external respiration (diffusion of O_2 into capillaries at the alveolar level). Two people may move the same amount of minute volume (see Average Breathers A to C in the above table). However, an individual with a higher respiratory rate (more BPM) will have less alveolar minute volume (air available for gas

Table 4.3 Examples of minute volume as constituted by respiratory rate and tidal volume

Sample breathers	Respiratory rate	Tidal volume	Resulting minute volume
Average breather A	15 bpm	400 mL	6000 mL
Average breather B	12 bpm	500 mL	6000 mL
Average breather C	10 bpm	600 mL	6000 mL
Fast breather	20 bpm	500 mL	10,000 mL
Deep breather	12 bpm	1200 mL	14,400 mL
Fast deep breather	20 bpm	1200 mL	24,000 mL
Slow breather	6 bpm	500 mL	3000 mL
Light breather	12 bpm	300 mL	3600 mL
Slow light breather	6 bpm	300 mL	1800 mL

exchange) than the individual with a slower respiratory rate. In the above table, Average Breather C has the largest alveolar minute volume; that is, this person has more air involved in gas exchange than Average Breathers A or B. As a result, Average Breather C has better respiratory efficiency.

Why is this happening? The answer takes us back to breath anatomy. The upper airway is a respiratory dead space; no alveoli here means no gas exchange. During every breath, approximately 150 mL of inhaled air is in this dead space (designated as DV = dead volume). This means that if we inhale 500 mL of air, only 350 mL becomes available at the alveoli during that breath cycle. In other words, for each breath/min, we need to subtract 150 mL from the overall tidal volume to obtain the more important *alveolar tidal volume*. Clearly, the more times per minute we breathe, the more often we have to subtract 150 mL from minute ventilation [30].

Table 4.4 shows three breathing patterns, all with a tidal volume of 500 mL. The efficiency loss (EL) column shows that the amount of air that reaches the alveoli is greatly reduced with faster breathing patterns. The individual breathing 15 times a minute loses 2250 mL (15 * 150 mL) of air each minute; the individual breathing 12 times per minute loses 1800 mL/min; and the person breathing 10 times loses 1500 mL/min. A greater percentage of air is "lost" with faster breathing than with slower breathing at the same tidal volume. That is, increased efficiency reveals that with slower breathing, less air must be moved to absorb the same amount of oxygen into the blood at the level of the alveoli.

We can exert conscious control over respiratory rate; we can slow down or speed up the breathing cycle, as well as change the length and ratio of inhalations to exhalations. We can also consciously affect tidal volume, either by increasing or decreasing inspiratory or expiratory volume moved with each breath and, thus, changing tidal volume and total vital lung capacity (over time). Effects of either rate or volume or both in combination can be described as follows:

- Lengthening the breath slows the respiratory rate
- Shortening the breath speeds up the respiratory rate
- Deepening the breath increases tidal volume
- Making the breath shallower decreases tidal volume
- Breathing at 4 to 6 to 10 gentle BPM has positive effects on heart rate variability and is a common respiratory rate during mindful *pranayama*

Table 4.4 Complexity about the three breathers

Sample breathers	Respiratory rate	Tidal volume	Resulting minute volume	Minute volume at the alveoli	Efficiency loss (EL)*
Formula			MV = RR * TV	aMV = RR * (TV-150)	EL = MV - aMV
Breather X	15 bpm	500 mL	15 * 500 = 7500 mL	15 * (500–150) = 5250 mL	2250 mL
Breather Y	12 bpm	500 mL	12 * 500 = 6000 mL	12 * (500–150) = 4200 mL	1800 mL
Breather Z	10 bpm	500 mL	10 * 500 = 5000 mL	10 * (500–150) = 3500 mL	1500 mL

* It is a loss of 150 ml of usable air per breath and thus increases as number of breath per minute increase

Combinations of Respiratory Rate and Tidal Volume Leading to Hyperventilation

Hyperventilation can result from increased respiratory rate and/or increased tidal volume. This may happen because of too many BPM without a reduced volume or because of too much volume with each breath without a reduced rate. As discussed in the biochemistry section, hyperventilation is one possible reason for hypocapnia. Hyperventilation results in increased oxygen saturation (in blood instead of tissues) and reduced levels of carbon dioxide in alveoli, arterial blood, and venous blood. The harder and faster we breathe, the less oxygen is delivered to the tissues because less CO_2 is present to support the release of O_2 from red blood cells' hemoglobin (Bohr effect). Reduced CO_2 increases blood pH; high blood pH, in turn, further constricts blood vessels, especially small arteries and arterioles, reducing blood flow to the spinal cord and brain, *no matter how well oxygenated the blood.* Vasoconstriction due to hyperventilation occurs immediately throughout the body (affecting the approximately 50,000 miles of blood vessels), including in the brain. Decreased levels of arterial CO_2 can result in lightheadedness, panic, fatigue, poor concentration, irritability, and even fainting. It may induce panic, which will worsen hyperventilation because the individual will try to bring even more breath into the body as they feel as though they are suffocating.

If an individual has an acute episode of hyperventilation, it can help to have them breathe into a paper bag or their own hands cupped over their nose and mouth (this is obviously not a long-term solution). The excess carbon dioxide expelled due to hyperventilation is breathed back in, returning CO_2 levels to normal, ending vasoconstriction and feelings of panic. Hyperventilating and then holding the breath can cause a person to pass out. This has implications for breathing exercises. For example, the yogic practice of *bastrika* (strong, forced inhalations and exhalations) can cause hyperventilation—we do not want to follow up such breath with breath retention. With practice (of *pranayama* or acclimating to high altitude), cerebral circulation can adapt to and increase tolerance of lower CO_2 blood levels without arterial constriction. This allows more oxygen to migrate into the brain and spinal cord, increasing alertness and well-being. All of this requires a carefully sequenced practice that spans many sessions and weeks.

Table 4.5 lists the challenges associated with hyperventilation syndrome. This list is based on a somewhat dated (yet still relevant) textbook by Timmons and Ley [32] and *The Breathing Cure* by McKeown [2], with additions from Tavel [37]. A review of this listing explains why respiratory values have also been identified as crucial pieces of data in medical settings to help identify certain pathologies or disorders (e.g., cardiac or respiratory illness) [38].

Combinations of Respiratory Rate and Tidal Volume Leading to Hypoventilation

Hypoventilation can occur due to decreased respiratory rate and/or tidal volume. It can result from too few resting-state BPM (e.g., fewer than eight breaths) without

Table 4.5   Symptoms of hyperventilation syndrome

Cardiovascular
- Palpitations
- Arrhythmias
- Tachycardia
- Angina
- Capillary vasoconstriction
- Cold extremities

Respiratory
- Shortness of breath, breathlessness, air hunger
- Irritable cough, wheezing
- Air hunger
- Inability to breathe deeply
- Sighing, yawning
- Sniffling
- Panting or breathlessness while speaking
- Hoarse, creaky, or breathy voice
- Dry and inflamed upper airways
- Exercise-induced asthma

Psychological
- Tension
- Anxiety, phobias, panic
- Feeling unreal, dissociation
- Nightmares

Gastrointestinal
- Difficulty swallowing
- Air swallowing
- Globus (lump in throat)
- Dry mouth and throat
- Gastric reflux
- Flatulence
- Belching, burping.
- Bloating

Neurological
- Dizziness
- Instability
- Feeling faint
- Headaches
- Paresthesia (numbness, deadness, tingling)

Muscular
- Stiffness
- Cramping
- Weakness
- Pain, especially neck and shoulders
- Soreness after exercise
- Poor exercise tolerance

Immunological
- Allergies
- Food sensitivities

Autonomic
- Emotional reactivity
- Decreased vagal tone
- Chronic sympathetic nervous system arousal
- Inability to relax

General
- Exhaustion
- Poor concentration
- Impaired memory
- Decreased performance
- Poor sleep, restless sleep
- Sleep apnea, snoring
- Blocked nose and dry mouth upon awakening
- Emotional sweating

increased volume. As noted above, hypoventilation is generally not encountered and is typically caused by toxins or a chronic disease state. Hypoventilation with too little volume with each breath, without increased rate, is also generally caused by diseases, including COPD, asthma, sleep apnea, airway edema, and similar conditions. Hypoventilation results in reduced levels of oxygen and increased levels of carbon dioxide in the alveoli, arterial blood, and venous blood. Increased levels of CO_2 (i.e., hypercapnia) in arterial blood dilate small arteries and arterioles, increasing blood flow to the spinal cord and brain. However, O_2 saturation in the blood is low. This undersupply of oxygen leads to a sense of being smothered, a warning that the brain and spinal cord are not receiving sufficient oxygen. In healthy people, this is remedied with a few deep breaths. If it is temporary, hypercapnia can lead to acute symptoms of respiratory acidosis, such as headache, confusion, anxiety, or drowsiness. If chronic (e.g., due to COPD), it can be asymptomatic but in time may lead to memory challenges, sleep disturbances, myotonic jerks, gait disturbance, tremor, and more.

The Solution: Slow Subtle Breathing

Balanced breathing that results in optimal blood and tissue levels of CO_2 and O_2 is neither too fast nor too slow, and is neither too deep nor too shallow. Ideally, breathing is slow and subtle, nasal and diaphragmatic, moving approximately 6000 mL of air via fewer than 8–10 BPM. Interestingly, the concept of slow and subtle breathing is nothing new. It is the essence of a central aphorism about *pranayama* in the *Yoga Sutras of Patanjali*. According to Sutra 2.49, *pranayama* is about slowing and braking the force of energy (while biomechanically depending on a perfected meditation posture). Through subtlety and slowness, *pranayama* invites the expansion of awareness that stabilizes the mind, offering tranquility and resilience. Slow subtle breathing, according to many interpretations of this sutra, is the very foundation of *pranayama*. This is an often overlooked fact of yoga, especially in the Western world. Yogic breathing in daily life is subtle and soft, not hard and deep. In other words, traditional yoga is about practices that *preserve* energy, not about practices of awesome feats that take our breath away. Subtle, slow breathing is covered in detail in Chap. 9. It will be referred to as optimal functional breathing and is the underpinning of breathing practices promoted for teachers, clinicians, and students. For now, we turn to other breath characteristics important to healthful breathing and breath awareness.

Sutra 2.49
Once posture has been perfected, the slowing or braking of the force behind and of unregulated movement of inhalation and exhalation is called breath control and expansion of prana.

tasmin sati shvasa prashvsayoh gati vichchhedah pranayamah

4.2.2 Breath Texture and Sound

Breath texture provides information about physical health, energetic state and vitality, emotional well-being, and mental state. It is autonomically controlled by the pons (of the brain stem) but can be affected by conscious breathing, focused on smooth breaths that flow easily and freely. Breath texture is often correlated with breath sounds. Uneven breath textures tend to bring with them noisy breathing, from wheezing to panting to gasping. The link between texture and sound is not a given; the two can vary and change independently of one another. It is useful to examine both separately and in conjunction.

Breath texture is best understood by reviewing descriptors used to refer to smoothness versus roughness of breathing. Smoothness may define breath as

Table 4.6 Breath textures and possible related sounds

Characteristics of breath smoothness:	Characteristics of breath roughness:
• Buttery, silky, soft, smooth, even, velvety, unfluctuating, consistent, stable, steady, honeyed, pleasant	• Jerky, hesitant, choppy, pausing, ragged, with hitches or glitches, with hiccups, staccato, spasming, halting
• Feathery, downy, relaxed, light, bright, weightless, easeful, peaceful, easy, calm, effortless, flowing	• Heavy, tense, strained, harsh, disturbed, full of friction, worried, heavy, hefty, troubled, distressed, gagged
• Gentle, quiet, silent, light, calm, mild, tender, inaudible, noiseless, tranquil, serene, pleasant	• Hoarse, noisy, loud, breezy, wheezy, husky, huffy, throaty, croaky
• Free, unencumbered, clear, empty, unblocked, free-moving, released, clean, fluid, unbroken, graceful, fluent	• Restricted, sticky, stuffy, constricted, tight, limited, bound up, clogged, restrained, congested, choked, blocked, obstructed
• Comfortable, cool, warm, content, relaxed, carefree, unlabored, easeful	• Uneasy, uncomfortable, cold, hot, slippery, overcontrolled, laboring, struggling

buttery, easeful, free-flowing, or peaceful. Roughness may be described as choppy, staccato, harsh, or strained. Table 4.6 offers alternatives to provide variety for cuing and assessment.

Breath sounds arise from turbulence caused by inhalation and exhalation and can come from the lungs, airways, nose, or mouth. Breath sounds vary in pitch, loudness, and coarseness. They might be continuous or discrete (yet repetitive). Some breath-related sounds may only occur intermittently. Examples (and descriptors) of breathing sounds include, but certainly are not limited to, sounds such as sighing, sniffling, sputtering, choking, heaving a sigh, gasping, snorting, snuffling, breathing out noisily, groaning, yawning, panting, sounding winded or breathless, rasping, whistling, or similar audible breathing-related sounds. Other breathing-related sounds that may provide hints about respiratory health are sounds such as clearing the throat, coughing, hoarseness, breathy speech, and speech interrupted by breath sounds.

Breath sounds may be made deliberately by the breather, especially in the context of yoga classes, such as in ujjayi or bhramari breathing, during which the breather deliberately constricts portions of the upper airway. Breathing sounds may be habitual, such as among yogis who have brought ujjayi breathing into their daily lives on the (mistaken) assumption that this is useful. Breath sounds may be situational, such as panting or gasping sounds of labored breathing during or after strenuous exercise. Some breath noises sound more like a blowing or a rustling. Breathing through the nose engenders different sounds than breathing through the mouth. Many people, especially in Western yoga classes, think that it is typical to hear the breath. This is not the case; natural breathing, generally speaking, is quiet and mostly inaudible. Thus, the main sound to hope and look for in one's own and that of students' or clients' breathing is the sound of silence.

Medically, there are four classes of breath sounds. Often, these are perceived with the use of a stethoscope; sometimes, however, they are clearly audible. *Crackles* are small rattling, clicking, popping, snapping, or bubbling sounds heard mostly during inhalation. They can be associated with fluid in the alveoli. *Rhonchi* are a little bit like the low-pitched sound of light snoring, but the person is awake. They are usually coupled with a rough breath texture and may be associated with phlegm in the bronchi. *Stridor* is a harsh-sounding, vibrating breath sound heard generally during inhalation, sometimes indicative of an obstruction in the back of the throat or trachea. *Wheezing* is a high-pitched sound heard during exhalation and may be associated with a narrowed airway (such as in asthma).

Breath texture and sound may signal anatomical obstructions (as might happen due to a very large tongue or a tongue that chronically rests at the bottom of the mouth; due to foreign objects or infection; or fluid in the lungs) or any other blockage of the airway (such as swelling or inflammation from an allergen) that impairs smooth and quiet flow of breath. A high and narrow palate can impair nasal breathing because it may pinch or reduce the size of a nostril. Sinus congestion can result in wheezy or labored breath textures and sounds.

Texture and sound can also reflect mental or emotional states; unease and reactivity may become notable to oneself and others as disrupted flow of breath, not so much in terms of volume or depth but in terms of how roughly, smoothly, or noisily breath moves through the body. Texture and sound can reflect the mind's emotional state and are helpful ways to explore mental preoccupations (*vrittis* in yoga's Sanskrit language), emotional reactivities (*kleshas*) , and mind states. A disrupted mind state may result in choppy or disrupted breath that lacks smooth and easy flow. It may contribute to breath that is loud, labored, or variable in sound. Breath texture and sound are best accessed through mindful attention to breath and interoceptive awareness of how the breath feels as it flows into and out. Just as fingertips can become increasingly sensitive to surface textures with practice (e.g., think about learning to read in braille), interoceptive awareness of breath textures and sounds can be honed through practice and mindful attention. Offering clients the above descriptors can help them become more sensitively attuned to breath texture and sound across time and more aware of what different textures and sounds may communicate.

If breath sounds persist (despite efforts to let go of them) or are coupled with breathlessness, difficulty breathing, or strong recruitment of accessory breathing muscles in the chest and neck, referral for diagnosis by a credentialled healthcare provider may be needed to rule out obstructions, inflammation, infection, fluid, or other possible causes.

4.2.3 Breath Location and Space

Another breath characteristic that communicates a tremendous amount of information about the state of body, vitality, and mind (including thoughts and emotions) is related to bodily locations where breath is perceived or felt most easily or tangibly. Breath can be traced through attending to movement in the nostrils, throat, abdomen, lower ribcage, side body, upper ribcage, clavicle region, and back body. As noted in Chap. 2, the diaphragm is ingeniously constructed to allow breath to mold itself to the shape of the surrounding body, to posture and movement. Anything other than that would mean that during much of our day, the breath would become constricted or inefficient. Instead, the body's wisdom is such that the lungs move with the expansion and contraction of the rib basket, perfectly molding themselves to the inner shape of the thoracic cavity. The diaphragm can move in different ways—either contracting and moving downward or contracting and moving the lower ribs outward and upward. It is supported by a range of accessory muscles that can help move the diaphragm out of the way upon inhalation (making space for the lungs to expand) and help the diaphragm relax and recoil back into its resting position upon exhalation (reducing the size of the thoracic cavity to support efficient expulsion of air). Thus, depending on position or motion, we feel the breath in different places in the body.

Table 4.7 shows the possible locations and space parameters that can be attended to, to note where the breath is most tangible at any given moment. Not all these places are equal in terms of the utility of muscular action depending on the position. For example, feeling breath high in the chest and clavicles during rest is not desirable, as it suggests hyperventilation (for any number of reasons). It is important to be clear why we are exploring regions of the body—*it is not to suggest that we _should_ feel the breath there* (a common misunderstanding). Rather, it is to *notice* where the breath is palpable, for better or worse. We can also compare side-to-side differences in breathing to explore whether breath travels through the body symmetrically or asymmetrically. Perhaps one side of the rib basket moves appropriately, whereas the other side hardly moves at all. Maybe we breathe easily into the front body, but when it is necessary to breathe into the back body (e.g., while lying prone), we struggle to catch our breath. Perhaps when we twist to one side, our breath stays smooth and efficient; when we rotate to the other side, perhaps the texture changes and breath becomes labored or noisy.

Breath location, and how space is inhabited by breath, can be accessed consciously through mindfulness, proprioception, and interoception. Neuroception can play a role as well, becoming notable as a perception of threat versus danger versus safety—all reactions that affect breathing and breath via the autonomic nervous system and polyvagal system. Just as form and movement can help increase sensitivity to the body's experience in the here and now, sensitizing to perceptions of ease, unease, disease, healthfulness, and more in the physical body, interoceptive

Table 4.7 Exploration of breath in location and space

Body location in which to explore the breath	Distribution of breath within the body space
• Nose and mouth	• Front versus back body
• Throat and neck	• Right side versus left side
• Abdomen	• Upper chest versus abdominal region
• Lower rib basket and midriff	• Central body versus peripheral body
• Middle rib basket and/or mid-torso	• Symmetrical versus asymmetrical
• Mid torso and upper ribcage	• Flowing versus stagnant
• Upper ribcage and clavicles	• Outward versus inward
• Back body and side body	• Upward versus downward

awareness of how the breath inhabits space and where it is most habitually located is honed through breathing practice. This attunement provides important feedback about nervous system states and mental or emotional fluctuations.

4.2.4   Breath Phases

Another notable exploration revolves around the fact that each breath cycle has four phases:

- inhalation
- pause or rest at the top of breath
- exhalation, and
- pause or rest at the bottom of breath

Biochemically, the brief hiatus after inhalation facilitates perfusion of O_2 from the alveoli into the blood and CO_2 from the blood into the alveoli (external respiration); biomechanically, it maintains postural stability via air in the lungs and intraabdominal pressure due to the diaphragm's downward contraction. Biochemically, the brief hiatus after exhalation facilitates enhanced oxygenation of tissues, including brain tissue, and uptake of CO_2 into the blood (internal respiration); biomechanically, it maintains postural stability via intraabdominal pressure arising from contractions in abdominal (and possibly pelvic floor) muscles. Psychologically, the rests at the top and bottom provide a brief pause for the mind—a gap in our constant sense of arousal, thinking, and doing; a space for discernment. Along with the exhalation, as the *Yoga Sutras of Patanjali* tell us, pauses still the mind's many fluctuations, worries, preoccupations, and distractions.

Sutra 1.34
The mind is also calmed by regulating the breath, particularly attending to exhalation and the natural stilling of breath that comes from such practice.

prachchhardana vidharanabhyam va pranayama

In essence, four-part breathing brings together the psychology (including rhythm or cadence), biochemistry, and biomechanics discussed thus far. Inhalation, retention at the top, exhalation, and suspension at the bottom increase awareness of physiological processes that occur during breathing and their relationship to the autonomic nervous system. Four-part breathing is a portal into facilitating intentional, conscious, and functional breathing and provides a clear way to communicate the advantages of functional breathing as well as the disadvantages of dysfunctional breathing. It has important implications for mindfulness and meditative awareness, in that it creates gaps in our *doing*-oriented nature, inviting us into simply *being*, at least for a moment. Four-part breathing is nothing new or modern; in fact, it is the very essence of yogic breathing, as reflected in an important aphorism in the *Yoga Sutras of Patanjali*.

Sutra 2.50

Pranayama has three aspects of **external or outward flow (exhalation)**, *inter-**nal or inward flow (inhalation)**, and the third, which is the absence of both during the transition between them, and is known as* **retention or suspension**.

These are regulated by place, time, and number, with breath becoming slow and subtle.

bahya abhyantara **stambha** *vrittih desha kala sankhyabhih paridrishtah dirgha sukshmah*

Four-part breathing is an acknowledgment that yogic breathing is not about breathing hard or deep or with long breath-holds, although this is often cued in modern Western yoga classes. Instead, yogic breathing, as the sutra clarifies, is about setting the breath free to allow it to unfold its essence with a slow and subtle rhythm; a cadence that honors the yogic principle of preserving energy through moderation in all we do. Retention refers to the pause at the top of the inhalation (breath has been drawn in and is retained for a moment); suspension refers to the pause at the bottom of the exhalation (breath has been released outward, and all action is suspended for a moment). It is important to note that Sutra 2.50 uses the Sanskrit word "*stambha*," which denotes a subtle and natural pause, not an intentional or strong holding of the breath. *Stambha* is the transition period between the active phases of the breath when no action is necessary either to inhale or exhale. *Intentional* lengthening of these transition periods is called *kumbhaka* in Sanskrit and is an entirely different, more advanced, *pranayama* practice of using breath-holds for particular purposes in body (biomechanically), breath and energy (biochemically), and mind or psyche (psychologically). *Kumbhaka* practices are more typically practices of hormesis; *stambha* practices are practices of cultivating optimal functional breathing. Many Western yoga teachers are unaware of this crucial difference.

Also notable about Sutra 2.50 is the recognition—more than 2000 years ago—that *place* (where in the body we feel the breath), *time* (how long each breath takes to complete itself), and *number* (how many times we breathe in a particular span of time) determine the quality and healthfulness of breathing. This is a deep acknowledgment of the characteristics of breath we have explored in this section from the perspective of modern science, including rate and volume of breath (as well as their combination as minute volume); posture, location, and body space; and breath phases. Modern science is catching up to these ancient wisdoms (see Table 4.8). As yoga practitioners, clinicians, and teachers, we need to be conscientious about acknowledging the deep history of breathing subtly and lightly, with a rhythmic cadence and healthful alignment [39]. We need to resist the temptation to view *pranayama* from the perspective of Western postural yoga, which has often led to harsh, regimented, rapid, and deep (voluminous) breathing, a regimen *not* in line with intentions of ancient practices (which emphasize subtlety and transcendence of breath), nor in accordance with research about wholesome breathing in daily life [4].

Table 4.8 Ancient wisdom and scientific principles of four-part breathing

Aspect of breath	Biochemistry	Biomechanics
Inhalation	Sympathetic shift as vagal brake lifts lightly; energy lifts; nitric oxide increases; air moves into the alveoli; cleansing and purification of *air*	The diaphragm contracts into the abdomen and low ribs lift; intra-abdominal pressure supports posture and spinal stability; decreasing pressure in the lungs invites air flow in
Retention after inhalation	Facilitates O_2 diffusion from lungs to blood	Postural stability is maintained by diaphragmatic action; inhaled air is retained in the lungs
Exhalation	Respiratory vagus nerve stimulation; parasympathetic shift; air moves out of the lungs; remoisturizing and cleansing of *airway*	The diaphragm relaxes upward; pressure in intrathoracic pressure increases and invites air to flow out; core muscles may lightly engage and create stability
Suspension after exhalation	Arterial CO_2 increases and facilitates O_2 release into tissues, resulting in enhanced oxygenation of tissues, brain, etc.	Core engagement continues to support postural stability; residual volume of air is retained in the lungs

4.3   Breathing and the Autonomic Nervous System

The act of breathing involves deep interactions with the human nervous system, in part because it stimulates the vagus nerve, which is central to the autonomic nervous system. Breath has a powerful function as a portal (granted, one of many) that provides conscious access to nervous system regulation. Simply by breathing, we can create access to a state of restoration and well-being versus a state of distress and agitation. Through optimal breath and specific breathing practices, we can affect our state of well-being, stress, resilience, and functioning. In turn, autonomic resilience translates into greater physical and mental health, groundedness, and enhanced functioning of cardiovascular, respiratory, immune, endocrine, and respiratory systems.

4.3.1   Brief Overview of the Human Nervous System

The human nervous system has several collaborating and interdependent, integrated components. The central processing unit, so to speak, is the *central nervous system*, consisting of the brain and spinal cord. The CNS receives sensory signals from the body, processes and integrates sensory information, and sends out motor signals. It supports consciousness in that it is responsible for processing inputs from all senses; for forming thoughts and emotions, desires and aversions, discernment and decision-making; and more [40–42]. It has crucial coordinating functions that keep our body humming smoothly, including coordination of movement; breathing, heart rate, and blood pressure; all organ functions; endocrine, neurotransmitter, and immune responses; body temperature, hunger, thirst, and pain reception; and much more.

The spinal cord is the conduit for information between the body (via signals collected from the peripheral nervous system; see below) and the central nervous system. It also mediates important musculoskeletal reflexes that are crucial to rapid responsiveness to ensure survival, health, and well-being.

The central nervous system collaborates and interdepends with the *peripheral nervous system* (PNS). The PNS is a communication center that connects the entire body to the CNS, constantly exchanging information between the body and CNS [43, 44]. The PNS consists of all nerves that branch off the brain (i.e., cranial nerves) and spinal cord (i.e., spinal nerves). It relays sensory and motor signals to and from all parts of the body, connecting them to the CNS. Some nerves in the PNS are dedicated to relaying motor signals from the brain to the body (motor or efferent nerves); others relay sensory information from body to brain (sensory of afferent nerves); and some have a mixed function, being able to relay sensory data to the brain as well as returning motor commands to the body (mixed nerves with efferent and afferent fibers).

The peripheral nervous system has two parts, depending on how, with whom, or what it communicates. Involuntary reactions are steered by the *autonomic nervous system*. Voluntary actions, such as moving into an asana or taking an extra-deep breath, are steered by the *somatic nervous system*. Of particular interest in the context of breathwork is the breath's profound relationship with the autonomic nervous system (ANS). The ANS has two branches of interest in this context, the sympathetic and parasympathetic nervous system (a third branch being the enteric nervous system, not covered here). All aspects of the ANS are linked by their role in ensuring the organism's survival. As survival depends on the seamless and healthful functioning of all organ systems, all are under ANS control. This is great news since we would not want to be in charge of consciously keeping our hearts beating, lungs breathing, or liver and kidneys clearing toxins.

4.3.2   Branches of the Autonomic Nervous System

The two branches of the ANS work together to help humans achieve allostasis and homeostasis—the capacity to *adapt* to changing environmental demands in a sufficiently adaptive manner (allostasis) and to *return* to a state of balance (homeostasis). The sympathetic nervous system typically takes over when fast reactions are needed for the organism's safety (i.e., physical survival), mobilizing the organism into action and initiating a *"fight-or-flight"* reaction. The parasympathetic nervous system comes into play when fight-or-flight mobilization is not needed (or, as we will explore below, is no longer sufficient). This allows the organism to lower its defenses, regain a state of calm, and return to the business of being a thriving organism, prepared to *"rest and restore,"* to heal and rejuvenate, and to connect and stay safe.

Vagus Nerve

The primary nerve that transmits and organizes signals within the ANS is the vagus nerve (i.e., the tenth cranial nerve). It innervates all major organs, the only cranial nerve that reaches (or wanders) this far into the body (other cranial nerves being mostly focused on the neck, head, and face). The vagus nerve functions outside of conscious control to surveil and regulate bodily functions, such as breathing, heart rate, and arousal. It is a mixed nerve with afferent and efferent fibers, with afferent fibers dominating [45]. In fact, 80% of information conveyed by the vagus nerve is sensory information from the body to the brain. The vagus nerve mediates nervous system responses and is responsible for activating the parasympathetic nervous system response by inhibiting (via the vagal brake) the sympathetic nervous system response [46].

The vagus nerve is the primary conduit for communication about internal states and exteroceptive inputs as perceived through various sensory systems to the brain. It relays physical, mental, and environmental sensory input (from the bottom of the brain) via the anterior cingulate cortex and insula to the prefrontal cortex (to the top). It integrates emotion, cognition, and conscious deliberation about sensory input from the top to the bottom, creating integration across brain structures that allows for the collaboration of top-down and bottom-up pathways. It connects to and interacts with the enteric nervous system, relaying bottom-up signals and top-down responses to optimize functions in the digestive system, along with all systems affected by neurotransmitters created and resident in the enteric nervous system. It promotes the achievement of top-down bottom-up integration, which, in turn, helps the organism gain access to the ventral vagal space, inviting a sense of calm, integration, and resilience. It enables us to engage with others positively through verbal and nonverbal communication.

Recent research on the vagus nerve [46–48] has expanded the understanding of the ANS's parasympathetic branch, becoming more complex, *less reciprocal* (or mutually exclusive), and *more interactive and integrated* with the SNS. Specifically, the vagus nerve has been shown to have *two distinct branches* that surveil and regulate the parasympathetic nervous system, resulting in two profoundly different ways to cool down (or put the brakes on) the sympathetic nervous system response of mobilization (i.e., fight-or-flight) or to help us exist and stay safe in the world. The two separate and distinct, yet interactive and integrated, branches are called the dorsal vagal (DVC) and ventral vagal (VVC) complexes. Although both responses originate within the parasympathetic nervous system (PSNS), they mediate intensely different responses to stimuli or inputs arising through inner visceral and outer environmental sensations. This recognition has innumerable clinical applications and implications and significant implications for breath and breathing [46, 48–53].

The *ventral branch* of the vagus nerve responds to perceptions of safety and results in prosocial behavior. Through increased neural complexity first noted phylogenetically in mammals, the ventral branch of the vagus nerve evolved a *social engagement system* [48]. It is linked to sensory nerves above the diaphragm and, as such, is associated with the heart and hypothalamus-pituitary-adrenal (HPA) axis. The social engagement system facilitates prosocial behavior, verbal and nonverbal communication, and adaptive emotional responses to occurrences around and inside the organism. In humans, this profound social connection and embeddedness, coupled with complex reasoning ability and multifaceted brain power, likely paved the way for the development of human culture, language, technology, politics—and, less advantageously, the human assertion of power over other creatures and the planet.

The *dorsal branch* of the vagus nerve responds to perceptions of extreme danger, in fact, life threats, and results in immobilization (e.g., playing dead, fainting, dissociating, or shutting down behaviorally and/or emotionally). This branch of the vagus nerve is very ancient and can be seen very readily in the behaviors of reptiles who are under life threat. It is linked to sensory nerves below the diaphragm and hence is related to visceral responses.

Neuroception and Its Effects

The vagus nerve is crucial to the body's surveillance (or threat detection) system— unconscious, subcortical processes that rely on implicit memory and procedural memory to assess or appraise any and all situations, and to prepare us for an action-based response. It collects and sends (bottom-up) sensory signals from the body, endocrine release, and other internal and external signals of environmental conditions (e.g., sensory information coming from outwardly-oriented senses that provide input about what is happening around us, including others' facial expressions, gestures, voice quality, and actions). This information (collected and conveyed to the brainstem by the vagus nerve) is the foundation of *neuroception*—the ability to read internal physiological reactions, along with exteroceptive inputs, translate them into an assessment of our sense of safety and react to them quickly and efficiently to mitigate possible dangers or threats to life or safety [46, 48]. This lightning-fast appraisal occurs outside of conscious awareness or control, is based on our pre- or subconscious, and is not mediated by conscious cognition. Neuroception can be viewed as an appraisal response that is subcortical, unconscious, and non-cognitive. It comprises three stages: noticing or orienting to what is happening, preparing a reaction, and executing it [54].

Neuroception of sensory inputs from the environment and visceral inputs about internal states can result in three basic perceptions of what is happening (as well as combinations thereof; more about this later): *safety, danger,* or *life threat* (terror). Based on types of stimuli received via neuroception and their lightning-fast, unconscious interpretation as indicating either safety, danger, or threat, the autonomic nervous system activates either the sympathetic branch (danger), ventral vagal (safety), or dorsal vagal branch (life threat) of the parasympathetic nervous system. ANS activation, regardless of branch, affects, alters, and adapts all organ systems to be prepared for the most appropriate response given the neuroceptive interpretation of incoming stimuli. These effects are particularly notable in the respiratory, cardio-vascular/circulatory, endocrine, musculoskeletal, and gastrointestinal systems, as well as in voice, hearing, and metabolism. Over time, and based on repetitive experiences and conditioning, especially in early childhood, reactive patterns and defaults are developed and remain present even if the original circumstances in which they developed no longer apply. Patterns that were once adaptive and functional in response to actual outer stimuli can begin to unfold even in situations that do not reflect the original conditions and nervous system response [48, 55, 56]. Each default neural platform of safety, danger, or threat carries specific behavioral and respiratory patterns. These patterns are based on implicit somatosensory memories and procedural learning that are now applied in contexts that may or may not actually warrant these responses. The following three patterns can emerge: neuroception of safety, danger, or life threat.

1. *Neuroception of safety activates the PSNS ventral vagal complex (VVC), creating behavioral and respiratory patterns of social engagement.*

    The social engagement system ties us to one another. When we are in a ventral vagal state of safety and connection, the vagus nerve connects to physiology above the diaphragm, especially the region of our faces. We attune to one another's facial cues, nonverbal communication, tone of voice, expressiveness of the eyes, and meaning of gestures. We attune to human voices and tune out auditory ranges of lower sounds. When we are in a ventral vagal state, we are in a state of co-regulation—our natural habitat. We are evolved to be embedded in an interpersonal matrix, a connected web of life. Infants need parenting, community, and embeddedness. Only when they have internalized a sense of trust and safety can human children move out and explore their world increasingly freely—with periods of rapprochement to reconnect and refill their tank of human connection [50, 57].

    Neuroception of safety results in physiological restoration and recovery, emotional processing and interoception, mental and emotional (self-)regulation, and prosocial behavior (including socially engaging voices and facial expressions, and relaxed posture). Breath is soft, smooth, and gentle; heart rate and blood pressure are calm and within typical limits for the individual; digestion is chugging along; endocrine hormones for social engagement are released (e.g., oxytocin); fascial muscles relax; the voice is melodic and has the prosody of relaxation; and hearing is optimally attuned to human voices. We relax into contact with other human beings, ready for conversation, connection, interaction, collaboration, even playfulness and shared joy.

    The ventral vagal state is our natural, resilient way of being in the world. It is our coping state that allows us to create relationships and stay connected. When we are in a ventral vagal space, we are open-hearted, ready to communicate, nondefensive, and emotionally balanced [58]. We are ready to be in relationships and to give and receive love, kindness, and compassion. We can engage in easy conversation, relax in the presence of others, and enjoy our connection to our community. We are ready to play and have fun. We sense our connectedness, our interdependence.

    When we are in a ventral vagal space, the vagus nerve puts the brakes on the sympathetic nervous system, communicating that we are safe with no need to increase heart rate, increase respiration, or prepare skeletal muscles for fight or flight [16, 59]. The vagal brake on the SNS leads to optimal opportunities for developing and maintaining health, cultivating resilience, facilitating growth, supporting restoration and regeneration, and sustaining healing. A ventral vagal state is associated with slow diaphragmatic breathing, smooth breath rhythms with little to no sound, balanced inhalations and exhalations, and nasal breathing. These breathing rhythms support the sense of calmness, relaxation, safety, and social engagement that is so distinctive of the ventral vagal state. However, because life has challenges and ups and downs, none of us stays in a ventral vagal state forever. We move to other states as needed when environments or relationships become challenging. If all goes well, we return to a ventral vagal sense of social connection and safety when the crisis has resolved.

2. *Neuroception of danger releases the vagal brake on the SNS, creating specific behavioral and respiratory patterns of sympathetic arousal.*

   In the presence of perceived danger, we move out of the ventral vagal state of social engagement, and the sympathetic nervous system activates, mobilizing a fight-or-flight response to increase the likelihood of survival. In other words, if arousal increases due to an increased perception of danger or challenge, our VVC response may transform—the vagal brake loosens its grip on the SNS. Playfulness may become more aggressive, dance may turn into preparation for a show of strength and fierceness, and collaboration may turn into competition. We shift our focus of attunement; our attention turns to different aspects of our experience—away from faces and eyes, and away from hearing human voices. We move into auditory hypersensitivity for sound ranges of potential danger (such as the low growl of a tiger) and away from being able to hear human voices [50, 57].

   The release of the vagal brake on the SNS results in increased muscle tone, redirection of blood flow from the periphery to the core, inhibition of the gastrointestinal system, dilation of the bronchi, and increased respiration and heart rate (among other physiological responses) to prepare the organism for a vigorous, proactive survival response. Breath and heart rate increase, skeletal muscles tense in readiness for action, digestion is turned down or off, stress hormones are released (e.g., cortisol), and the voice becomes hard and threatening or insistent and alarming (to relay the perception of stress to others in our group), and hearing shifts to optimize the reception of extremely high and low sounds of threat (shifting away from optimal perception of human voices).

   When we are in an *acute sympathetic* state, we see the world as dangerous and are more likely to interpret the actions of others as aggressive or threatening. Given this perspective, we are preparing to fight and defend ourselves, our loved ones, and our tribe. If we cannot defend successfully, we are ready to flee our dangerous circumstances. We lose social connections beyond our tribe and lose the willingness to negotiate or talk with those to whom we do not feel we belong. We are less interested in communicating to resolve conflict; we are ready to pounce and defend instead. We are in survival mode and care more about our own and our tribe's survival than the well-being of others who are seen as potential threats or dangers. This reactivity sets up a vicious cycle of potential interpersonal disconnection, even violence. We threaten, express rage and anger, we

defend and fight; we scream, and stop listening; we become physically threatening or aggressive—all actions that serve to bring others into their own sympathetic nervous system response as well.

When we are in a *chronic state of hyperarousal* (as many of us are due to
ongoing chronic stress or perception of stress), over time, physical and emotional health becomes compromised. Because we cannot seem to return to the
ventral vagal space, blood pressure may remain chronically high; digestion may
start to fail, and gut flora might suffer; we may always be on alert or prone to
anxiety and excessive worry; we might resort to drugs or alcohol to try to calm
our nerves; and we ready for action and self-defense. In time, our adrenals may
wear out, and we lose energy and start to feel worn out and unable to cope [57].
We want to muster our resources to stay in the fight, but we cannot do it any-
more. We burn out; we lose our resilience—our ability to bounce back.

Chronic sympathetic arousal is associated with shallow or rapid breathing,
typically into the chest via the recruitment of accessory breathing muscles. Oral
breathing is more likely, further disrupting primary diaphragmatic recruitment.
Breath patterns tend to be erratic with an imbalance between inhalation and
exhalation, disrupted breath texture, and noise breathing. Respiratory rate may
be chronically increased, leading to hyperventilation and chronic hypocapnia,
changing the medulla's CO_2 sensitivity. Respiratory muscles are hypertonic and
further heighten the perception of danger and the need for preparedness to fight
or flee. Only if the threat or danger is neutralized (by whatever means, including
having received help from someone) can we return to a ventral vagal state, put
the (vagal) brake on SNS reactivity, and return to a neutral and socially connected state.

3. *Neuroception of life threat activates the PSNS dorsal vagal complex (DVC), creating behavioral and respiratory patterns of immobilization.*

   The sense of terror instilled by neuroception of life threats results in the following: shutting down, freezing, or playing dead; decreased muscle tone and
   cardiac output; reflexive defecation and urination; and other physiological
   responses that reduce life functions to the least amount needed for survival. This
   nervous system state represents a profound departure from our natural human
   evolution as co-regulators [50, 57, 60]. In an extreme dorsal vagal state, we disconnect from co-regulation, from one of the most basic traits of what it means to
   be human (or a mammal). It is much harder to reemerge from dorsal vagal collapse or immobilization than from sympathetic arousal. It is important to remember that we do not consciously choose the nervous system state that is activated
   in response to neuroception. Neuroception is unconscious and noncognitive,
   rooted in implicit memory; the same is true for our response—it is a *reaction*,
   deeply rooted in procedural memory. Moving into a dorsal vagal state is as much
   (or even more so) a survival or self-protective mechanism as is the movement
   into a sympathetic state. Evolution has clearly demonstrated the effectiveness of
   dorsal vagal collapse and immobilization for self-preservation.

   If a perceived danger cannot be resolved (via fight or flight or social engagement) and turns into a perceived threat to our lives or psychological integrity,

and we see no solution for escape or potential for supportive and helpful others, we become overwhelmed, feel alone, and shut down—physically, energetically, mentally, emotionally, and relationally.

When we are in an *acute dorsal vagal* space, we perceive the world as distant and others as removed, emotionally unavailable, unhelpful, and not supportive of our very (physical, affective, mental, or emotional) existence. Given this (unconscious, subcortical, noncognitive) perspective, we shut down—we are no longer able to or interested in communicating; we have given up on defending ourselves. We have become physically or emotionally immobilized or numb; we cannot muster any resources other than withdrawing, even playing dead (literally or figuratively) to try to save ourselves [48, 49, 57].

When we have experienced significant or complex trauma, we may move into a faulty neuroception of life threat when there is none. From this neural platform, we begin to live in a *chronic dorsal vagal* state. Because we cannot return to the ventral vagal space of human connection and trust, we develop emotional difficulties and a myriad of physical challenges, even illness. Emotional distress takes us out of supportive relationships. We expect to be re-traumatized and hurt. We may develop pains and aches that keep us inactive and disengaged from life; we may lose the drive to create a better life; we might give up on ever feeling connected again. We may move through life in a depressed and defeated way. We may become suicidal.

Physical challenges arise related to the shutdown of physiological processes and negatively affect the immune system, digestion, cardiovascular health, respiration, and even sleep hygiene [57]. A chronic dorsal vagal state is associated with disrupted and irregular breathing rhythms and patterns, along with decreased respiratory rates as the body tries to conserve resources. Breath becomes shallow and constricted, accompanied by a sense of tightness or tension in the chest. Minimal movement of the diaphragm and oral breathing contribute to the freezing response, heightening the helpless sense of stagnation, heaviness, and immobilization. Excessive pauses may be noted in breathing; in fact, breath may be marked by breath holds that exacerbate the state of extreme fear or expectation of life threats.

Only if the threat to life or psychological integrity is neutralized (by whatever means, including having received help from someone or having been able to mount an escape after all) can we return to a ventral vagal state, reconnect to others, and return to a state of wellness and ability to heal and recover. More often than not, escape from dorsal vagal collapse occurs through sympathetic arousal (as opposed to movement into social connection). We regain the capacity to fight; from there, if successful, we might move back into social connection.

The Value of Dorsal Vagal Collapse

Observation of animals clarifies the value of dorsal vagal immobilization and collapse. This nervous system state has a clear survival value—even if this is not as self-evident as the survival and self-protective value of a sympathetic fight-or-flight response. Table 4.9 shows a few reasons from animal behavior that support the

Table 4.9 The value of dorsal vagal collapse or immobilization

- Lack of motion signals lack of danger. Animals who sense danger (to themselves or their offspring) are more likely to attack than animals who simply sense the presence of another being. Immobilization is a way to become completely non-threatening to others. Aggressors may lose interest in an immobilized being, thus allowing this being to escape aggression. In Alaska, during encounters with wild animals with babies (whether a moose with calves or bears with cubs) in tow, the best response is to freeze into immobility; to make no sound, barely to breathe. This immobilization (which has a bit of SNS activation mixed in) serves to keep everyone safe
- Most predatory animals are less likely to eat the carcass of an animal that is already dead as their instinct warns them away from possibly spoiled and dangerous food. Animals in dorsal vagal collapse appear dead—Hence, they have a greater likelihood of not being eaten. In Alaska, where any backcountry hiking invites encounters with predators stronger than humans, hikers are given the advice to play dead in encounters with aggressive grizzly bears
- Dorsal collapse results in the release of chemicals that reduce pain perception, slow down time, decrease heart and breath rate, and stop emotional or affective reactivity and arousal. This protects the potential victim from pain and extreme fright
- Sympathetic arousal is heavily resource-demanding and draining; dorsal collapse preserves human functioning at the most basic level of physical survival. It helps the potential victim optimally conserve physiological resources should a moment arise when flight or fight becomes a possibility. Prolonged SNS arousal would be an energetic threat to our system; a profound and destructive (catabolic) drain on our resources. Dorsal collapse preserves our life energy

evolutionary utility of moving into a dorsal vagal state (partially based on [55]). In the animal world, a being who survives the threat from which it protected itself via dorsal vagal collapse, will reemerge from this state via behaviors that mimic (or actually call upon) actions of sympathetic arousal. They shake, play out imaginary fights, and engage in a chase with other animals. In other words, they always discharge the energy that was constrained in dorsal collapse. In humans, this healing reaction to a state of DVC is often absent. It is constrained by cultural expectations, ongoing terror or fear, or other variables that preclude this evolutionary successful resolution of the dorsal vagal response. It is the lack of resolution of the DVC that can lead to longer-term symptoms in response to this nervous system response.

4.3.3 Types of Nervous System Responses

Ventral vagal, sympathetic, and dorsal vagal (i.e., polyvagal) responses can manifest in their pure form; however, perhaps more commonly, they interact. The branches of the ANS are not mutually exclusive; rather, they are balanced with one another, allowing for smooth transitions from one to the other and allowing for a mixture of polyvagal states. To understand this, it is important to remember that the autonomic nervous system overall is not simply a system of defense—it is *a system of allostasis and homeostasis*. It is a system that evolved to maintain health, restore functioning after disruption, facilitate growth and regeneration, and support well-being. Mounting a sympathetic nervous system response in a defensive state is therefore different from mounting a sympathetic nervous system response in a socially engaged state. Similarly, collapsing into a withdrawn and distant dorsal vagal state in a moment of self-protection against life threats is not the same as moving toward dorsal vagal quietude and inhibition of movement while also remaining socially engaged.

There are pure states of sympathetic nervous system arousal—these serve defensive or self-protective functions—and mixed states of SNS arousal that occur in the context of social engagement. Mixed SNS/VVC states are what we enter into during competitive sports, vigorous (especially movement-based) play, and moments of interpersonal assertiveness. There are pure states of dorsal vagal complex arousal—serving a last-ditch self-protective function—and mixed states of dorsal withdrawal and quietude in the context of social engagement. Mixed DVC/VVC states are what we enter during moments of physical stillness of intimacy (e.g., nursing a baby, cuddling with a loved one) or in moments of deep relaxation, such as in meditation or contemplative yoga practices. There are even mixed states of SNS/DVC. This mixture of nervous system states can serve as a final attempt at creating safety or as a way of releasing from dorsal vagal collapse and returning outward. A summary of the three pure states (VVC, SNS, DVC) and several mixed states is shown in Table 4.10. An excellent summary of the pure and mixed polyvagal states by the German psychologist Mathias Thimm is available at https://www.youtube.com/watch?v=CM7GNeX42tc.

Table 4.10 Many polyvagal states: Our physiology of safety

Neural platform	Description	Summary label
• Pure VVC → Perception of safety	• Live in a socially engaged parasympathetic nervous system; relaxed, engaging, and restorative (myelinated) ventral vagal space	• *Social engagement*
• (VVC + SNS) → Perception of the need for safe and interpersonally engaged action with mobilization in the service of personal or collective growth, health, competition, and play	• Sympathetic arousal that is slightly downregulated and accompanied by the desire or need for social engagement; assertiveness (as opposed to aggressiveness) that leaves open a door for collaboration	• *Preparedness, play* (especially play involving physical movement)
• (SNS + VVC) → Perception of the need for safe and interpersonally engaged action with mobilization in the service of assertive (as opposed to aggressive) self-defense, self-protection, or defense and protection of loved ones or one's community	• This state of self-assertion leaves open a door for collaboration and negotiation; emotions stay regulated and manageable; opportunities remain for finding peaceful solutions and social reconnection outside of the tribe	• *Assertiveness*

(continued)

Table 4.10 (continued)

Neural platform	Description	Summary label
• Pure SNS → perception of danger	• Prepared for danger, live in a near-constant state of sympathetic arousal, isolation, and physiological overload or breakdown; mobilized SNS state of fight or flight	• *Mobilization*
• (SNS + DVC) → perception of the need to survive by ceasing mobilization and collapsing into immobilization in service of survival in the face of being overcome	• Collapse into a dorsal state with echoes or traces of the urge to fight or flee; an inadvertent effort to ensure physical and psychological survival	• *Freeze, submit*
• (DVC + SNS) → Perception of the need to survive by increasing mobilization in service of bringing physical, energetic, mental, emotional, and social engagement functions back on line	• Active effort to rally resources of the SNS to reemerge from dorsal collapse	• *Rallying, hope*
• Pure DVC → Perception of life threat; parasympathetic NS is at an extreme state of withdrawal, surrender, and hopelessness	• Develop a habitual pattern of shrinking back from life, withdrawing, disengaging—Even dissociating—From human experiences and relationships	• *Immobilization*
• (DVC + VVC) → Perception of the need for safe immobilization without significant active interpersonal engagement in the service of rejuvenation (e.g., healing from an injury, supporting growth or immunity, regeneration of physical or energetic resources)	• Dorsal state of calm and of letting go, a state of deep relaxation or surrender as might be experienced in yoga or meditation, a state of concentrated mind with physical immobilization; this nervous system state may be accessed in a solitary or communal setting	• *Relaxation, trance*
• (VVC + DVC) → Perception of the need for safe, trusting and interpersonally engaged immobilization in the service of prosocial activities	• Dorsal state of surrender or relinquishment of control and effort, accompanied by strong human connection and engagement	• *Intimacy, shared stillness* (e.g., childbirth, nursing, sadness, collapse in laughter)

Table prepared with gratitude to Stephen Porges as experienced in workshop environments

4.3.4   Shifting Neuroception and Autonomic Reactivity

As noted above, moving into a sympathetic nervous system (SNS) response, dorsal vagal collapse and withdrawal (DVC), or ventral vagal social engagement and collaboration (VVC) is not intentional—it reflects implicit memory-based reactivity and elicits overpowering behavioral, respiratory, and relational patterns. It is an unconscious, noncognitive reaction driven by neuroception based profoundly on our physiology. Neuroception is *not* the same process as perception. Perception includes cognitive awareness and transforms (i.e., slows) reactivity into responsiveness. *Neuroception occurs before perception. It is neither conscious nor cognitive; it is subcortical.* The result of neuroception (i.e., movement into SNS, DVC, VVC, or mixed states) is outside of conscious control and is not mediated by cognitive contemplation. Changes in neuroception and subsequent reactivity rely on changes in perceptions and interpretations of physiological bottom-up signals. This requires a shift in physiology and a shift toward gaining access to and consciously using cognitive resources available to us via the prefrontal cortex.

Neuroception and the Prefrontal Cortex
While neuroception is reactive, it nevertheless utilizes the *resources* of the prefrontal cortex to keep us alive [52]. However, despite this connection to the cortex, neuroception invokes reactivity, not responsiveness in a contemplated or discerning manner, because it taps into implicit, not explicit, memory. However, neuroception *is* linked to the cortex and influenced by our lifetime of experiences and subsequent predictions and expectations about the world. Each event of neuroception is registered by the nervous system and prefrontal cortex. This learning, however unconscious or implicit, influences future reactions to similar circumstances. The cortex makes ongoing predictions about how life will unfold. This tendency influences neuroception. This reciprocal relationship is a true interaction of bottom-up sensory experience and top-down behavioral control.

The fact that neuroception is shaped by relationships and experiences within our biopsychosociocultural context helps us understand our unconscious or implicit adjustments to life events, especially events that felt dangerous or threatening. Lifetime experiences of trauma leave particularly deep grooves and profound traces in our physiology and anatomy that shape neuroception as well as predictions and expectations that emerge from our prefrontal cortex [56, 57]. Trauma attunes the body to become increasingly conservative—moving ever faster into self-protective states of SNS arousal or dorsal vagal detachment or collapse. In other words, traumatic experiences of violations of trust, especially as experienced in significant relationships, wire themselves deeply into our nervous system and our physiology. They embed themselves into our energy and tissues; they guide predictions and expectations and affect emotional reactivity. Violations of trust, especially in attachment relationships, trigger self-protection (i.e., SNS or DVC) because there is no experience of safe co-regulation, a necessary ingredient for social engagement. When relationship partners prove to be untrustworthy (especially if the expectation was otherwise), self-protective instincts take over. The more often or profoundly trust is violated, the deeper the grooves embed themselves in our nervous system and layers of consciousness. Habitual ways of responding to the world become increasingly powerful (even overwhelming) and pattern-locked. Reactions to the outer world become increasingly habit-driven, reactive, and symptomatic; they come from a profoundly altered physiological (neuroceptive) place of scanning for danger and threat; of expecting the worst to happen yet again [49, 60].

Porges [48], and before him, Levine [55], postulated that trauma-based reactivity results from a lack of access to successful resolution in moments of great challenge (because of the absence of inner self-regulation due to vulnerability or the absence of outer co-regulation due to violation of trust). Sympathetic states and dorsal vagal states have resolution phases if they are allowed to unfold naturally. This can be seen in a dog who has chased a rabbit—when the chase is over, the dog either had success and got the rabbit, which resolves the chase. If the dog is out-maneuvered, the dog will shake off the tension that was created by the sympathetic arousal and action. In the modern world, humans are often in situations that do not allow them to resolve a dorsal vagal or sympathetic state to allow the nervous system to get closure. Instead, contextual demand may force us to stay in a state of tension or collapse, a lack of re-regulation that can lead to potentially permanent physiological (and commensurate affective and vital) changes. For example, if we are in an altercation with our boss and move into sympathetic arousal, context forces us to stay calm on the outside, even though we are fighting on the inside. This mismatch in physiology and possible action needs to be resolved. If we are lucky, we can let off steam after work during a fast run or a soccer match. If not, the traces of sympathetic tension may embed themselves permanently in our tissues and may lead to chronic nervous system up-regulation. In other words, unresolved dorsal or sympathetic states can leave traces in our physiology and anatomy, leading to permanent physical changes that will affect how we take in the world and respond to it. Badenoch [57] traces these changes in all parts of the body, from how our eyes focus, how our ears attune to selective ranges of vibration, to how our skin responds to touch, and to how we breathe.

Neuroception and the Inner Physiological States

Neuroception is not only in a two-way relationship with the prefrontal cortex. It is also affected by inner physical states that are *not related to current* outer events or situations that require our response. Specifically, neuroception can be mediated by inner sensations of pain, especially chronic pain, irritable bowel syndrome, stomach distress as caused by *H. pylori*, and other physical conditions (e.g., Ehlers-Stanos syndrome). It is strongly correlated with breath and breathing; therefore, breathing patterns that are not aligned with a ventral vagal state can contribute to signaling of danger or threat even if neither is present. Engaging the VVC through specific PVT-informed strategies, such as rhythmic, slow, balanced, smooth, and quiet breathing, can transcend the impact of physical states to help our physiology recognize that there is safety despite inner sensations or signals of pain or discomfort that might otherwise mean the opposite (i.e., be interpreted by our nervous system as dangerous).

4.4   Polyvagal States, Breathwork, and a Return to Resilience

Clearly, challenges to wellness arise. Chronic, complex, or perhaps traumatic life experiences in our given biopsychosociocultural context (especially during early childhood); chronic or acute physical illness; and other experiences, such as accidents or unexpected events, can condition our nervous system to default to neural platforms of defense (self-protection) instead of safety. We become likely to see the world as dangerous or threatening and either mobilize (SNS reactivity) or shut down (DVC disengagement or collapse) at the expense of interpersonal connection. Through experience, we develop patterns of responses ("pattern locks" in science; *samskaras* in Sanskrit) that are driven by habit and conditioning, rather than being based on what is actually happening in a given moment. Some of us have life experiences that help us become more likely to perceive safety (living more commonly in a relaxed, engaging, and restorative ventral vagal space); some of us grow up or learn to expect danger (living in a near-constant state of sympathetic arousal, isolation, and physiological overload or breakdown); and a few of us come to expect life threats or trauma and develop a habitual pattern of shrinking back from life, withdrawing—even dissociating—from human experiences. The influence of biopsychosociocultural context on our affinity for a particular neural platform is clear.

Resilience refers to operating from a neural platform of expecting safety, social connection, and interpersonal reciprocity. It is the ability to move smoothly and integratively between the three pure autonomic nervous system states (via mixed states), especially between social engagement and mobilization responses, as needed to secure survival and well-being. Most commonly, we need to be able to put on the brakes and connect with others (moving into a ventral vagal state). At times, we need to be able to mobilize and put resources toward responding rapidly and vigorously on our own behalf (activating our sympathetic nervous system response). At times, we need to surrender and preserve life energy purely for survival (moving into a dorsal vagal state). Breath can become a powerful mediator of adaptive shifts in nervous system responses.

4.4.1   Neural Platforms and Yogic Notions of the Basic Qualities of Human Nature

The polyvagal notion of neural platforms (SNS, VVC, and DVC) aligns well with the yogic concept of the *gunas* or fundamental qualities or expressions of nature [51]. In ancient yoga psychology, three expressions of nature are inherent in us, articulated most commonly in combination with one another: *sattva* (wholesomeness and clarity), *rajas* (motion, enthusiasm, and activation), and *tamas* (groundedness, quietude, and inertia).

Sattva refers to wholeness, holism, or wholesomeness, as well as resilience or clarity (the literal translation is "goodness"). It is a way of being in the world that allows us to connect to others, feel safe, be in a state of trust, and cope with resilience and stamina. It involves a state of harmony, balanced responsiveness, resilient arousal, and healthful engagement with the world. The *sattvic* individual is neither too fast nor too slow to respond to a situation, is discerned without being discriminating or judgmental, seeks careful awareness when making decisions, and exudes a sense of equanimity and peacefulness. *Sattva* aligns well with a ventral vagal neural platform.

Rajas refers to a state of strong energy and activation; it can bring with it enthusiasm or hyperactivity. Generally speaking, it is associated with readiness for action, especially in the service of self-protection and readiness. *Rajas* is useful because it ignites passion and enthusiasm, encouraging us to engage vigorously with the world. It may show up at work, in play, and in sports. Individuals who have a default *guna* that is rajasic are passionate, goal-oriented, and always ready to take charge of a situation. They can be enthusiastic and can quickly come up with new ideas. Their minds are sharp and always active. *Rajas* aligns well with a sympathetic neural platform.

Tamas refers to a state of lethargy, inertia, or exhaustion that may bring with it bluntness in emotional responsiveness, withdrawal, and a stance of distrustfulness toward the world and others. However, *tamas* can also be a grounding force that allows us to settle into the moment with solidity when it invites us to rest and restore with clarity and intention. People who are *tamasic* tend to be solid and deliberate, with little perceived need for change or action. They are reliable and can be counted on for their presence and stability. They tend to be committed to their way of life with little motivation to rock their boat. *Tamas* aligns well with a dorsal vagal neural platform.

Many of us in the Western world pivot between the extremes of *rajas* and *tamas*, rather than finding a resiliently settled and balanced state in *sattva* or engaging with *rajas* and *tamas* in a contextually-indicated way. We over-engage, over-breathe, and over-activate at work, in sports, in hobbies and in relationships—or we collapse into exhaustion, lethargy, and dullness, feeling tired and worn out. Ideally, we find balance in *sattva*—in a state of clarity and openness that allows us to be in the world in an engaged and balanced way, with a rhythmic and resilient breath pattern, finding a bit of *rajasic* energy to get up and get going when we need to and releasing into a bit of rest, stability, and solidity when we need to recover and ground. The yogic concept of the *gunas* provides an alternative language to use with clients and students—perhaps a less balanced way of introducing the idea of neural platforms, default nervous system styles, and emotional and mental reactivities or pattern-locks. In the context of yoga-based breathwork, using the terms *sattva*, *rajas*, and *tamas* may be more familiar and resonant for clients than the science-based language of polyvagal theory. Basic strategies and cuing, however, remain consistent regardless of the chosen approach.

4.4.2   Basic Strategies for Self-Regulation and Nervous System Re-Training

While we cannot intentionally change neuroception, we can become familiar with our state of arousal and affect breath and energy, and mental and emotional reactivity. We can learn to become aware of our reactions and to read our own signals when we have slipped into SNS (*rajas*), VVC (*sattva*), or DVC (*tamas*). With increased awareness, we become more knowledgeable about our physiology and what it signals about our nervous system adjustment or basic human self-expression. We can begin to read our own as well as others' nervous system state or *guna*—a primary goal of breath attunement exercises. Once we recognize physical, affective, arousal, cognitive, emotional, behavioral, and relational patterns, we can begin to retrain our nervous system. The process of retraining our nervous system and physiology starts with sensing our body, energy (i.e., breath), and affect, along with accessing strategies that engage our ventral vagal complex. Once we can recognize our sense of arousal and affect based on awareness of body, breath (vitality), and mind and emotions, we can begin to *choose* strategies for creating changes in our default nervous system state, mental and physical habit patterns, and emotional reactivity.

Strategies for Returning to Social Engagement

Regulated and attentive breathing is one of the primary ways in which we can affect our nervous system, moving into a ventral vagal or *sattvic* state of being [7, 11]. Chapters 8 and 9 provide ample evidence for this assertion. Beyond breathwork, many yogic and psychological strategies invite co-regulation and support the return to social engagement.

Here are a few examples:

- Simply letting people talk something out can be helpful—especially if they can talk without being interrupted until their arousal rebalances and their affect neutralizes. Lending an ear to someone can be healing.
- Sensing the body can help us begin to become familiar with how the body feels in different situations and how it may reflect habitual activation or shrinking from the world. Attunement to our felt sense—our experience of body, breath, energy, and affect as a whole—can help us begin to notice when our nervous system is dysregulating and when we move into pattern-locked reactivity. Such awareness is a first step in encountering our symptomatic adjustment to experience and its transformation.
- Acoustic stimulation that is received by the nervous system as safe and sound can help re-regulate our nervous system into neuroception of safety (e.g., the Safe and Sound Acoustic Protocol developed by Porges [52]).
- Movement, ranging from simply fidgeting for a moment, or shaking or tapping, to a formal practice like asana, taking a run or going for a walk can shift our nervous system state
- Taking a break from a difficult conversation can help to gain distance from the emotional reactivity of the interaction.
- Getting a drink of water can invite us to reset or gain emotional distance during a challenging moment that seems unsafe to threatening.
- A self-compassionate moment of conscious awareness can attune us to dysregulation and shift our intention to conscious re-regulation.
- Tuning into the safety of a co-regulating relationship, whether the individual is immediately present or simply a resource in our interpersonal context that we can remember and imagine, can help us regain resilience in the moment.

Safety, especially safety in relationship, is the treatment or healing.—Stephen Porges (in workshop presentation)

Physical embodiment and movement, as well as specific ways of breathing, are extremely supportive of understanding and resetting the nervous system, returning to the organism to social engagement, and accessing ventral vagal co-regulation. All of us can access breathing practices to cultivate keener awareness of personal and others' nervous system states; *we can learn to use breath and breathing to reset.* Feeling embodied and attuned to breath during a difficult relationship or challenging situation is transformative and healing. Breathwork, as simple as taking a break to focus on long exhalations or as complex as choosing an appropriate breathing exercise (e.g., rapid expulsion of the exhalation to reactivate to prevent dorsal vagal collapse, or bumble bee breath (a calming breath with the sound of "mmm" on exhalation) to prevent dysregulation into a sympathetic state), can return us into a ventral vagal space [11, 61]. Chapters 8 and 9 focus on breathing applications, from breath observation to optimal functional breathing to more specialized breathing practices, and address how breath and breathing practices can be tailored to our nervous system state (or guna) and used to shift pattern locks to create more healthful responsiveness and resilience. Before turning to specific breathing strategies, it is helpful to take a look at how breathwork can be used in the context of recognizing and resetting pattern-locked and habitual ways of being in the world with regard to physical presence, nervous system state, vitality and affect, and thoughts, opinions, attitudes, expectations, and emotions.

4.4.3 Breathwork for Self-Regulation and Nervous System Re-Training

To tailor breathwork to the nervous system or polyvagal states, it is important to recognize which polyvagal states or gunas are our defaults and to choose breathwork that supports the most natural nervous system re-regulation and self-expression. As we become familiar with neuroception and typical (or default) nervous system reactivity via self-awareness and self-understanding, our capacity increases to self-regulate using specific breathing practices or variations that suit our needs to create change, healing, and thriving. Targeted or specific breathing practices can be used to alter autonomic states and move us toward more healthful, responsive, equanimous, and resilient energetic states as well as toward neuroception of safety and groundedness. Depending on the polyvagal state identified, different breathing practices can be chosen to create the most useful and tailored practice for a given patient.

For example, breathing practices can be tailored to enhance a greater sense of ease, calm, softening, freedom from desire or aversion, tranquility, and peace. Alternatively, breathing exercises can focus on cultivating effort, energy, courage, strength, engagement, or determination. In time, all breathwork is used to invite our innate capacity to achieve balance or coherence, in which there is ease balanced by effort or effort balanced by ease. For individuals who tend to live in sympathetic arousal, calming and grounding breathwork may be most often indicated; for students who tend toward a dorsal vagal state, energizing and expansive breathwork may be helpful. For all patients, starting with balancing and stabilizing breathing, especially using breath awareness and observation, is a great entrée into breathwork if it is not yet clear which nervous system state predominates.

Just as we offer variations to clients in a particular form (*asana*) or movement (*vinyasa*, *kriya*), variations can be offered with regard to breathing practices. Variations of the same breathwork practice can be taught in a group class by offering choices about how to engage with a particular breathing practice (e.g., giving a choice about attending more to the inhalation versus the exhalation). The same breathing practice (e.g., four-part breathing) may be adapted to patients' energetic needs via slightly different emphases or intentions in how we teach the practice. We take a quick look at such tailoring here; however, specifics related to each breathing technique are detailed in Chaps. 9, 10, and 11.

Balancing or Stabilizing Breathing Practices

Balancing breathing is functional breathing that supports the stabilization of the autonomic nervous system, anatomy (biomechanically), physiology (biochemically), breath (energetically), and mind (mentally and emotionally). As a bottom-up process of enhanced and accurate self-awareness and top-down emotional self-regulation, it focuses on balanced and stable inhalations and exhalations, gentle breath retention, balanced speed and vigor of breath, awareness of breath location (including interoceptive awareness of nasal versus mouth and diaphragmatic versus chest breathing), attention to breath texture, and clarity about the four parts of the breath—inhalation, pause at the top, exhalation, and pause at the bottom. It invites a parasympathetic shift in the nervous system to a ventral vagal way of being present; balances mood, energy, and physical arousal; provides an opportunity to explore emotional and mental reactivity; and invites social engagement, a sense of safety, and equilibrium.

Balancing or stabilizing breathing can be adjusted to be more or less active or calming, depending on the beginning state of clients' experiences and presence. However, its central feature is the cultivation of physical, energetic, affective, mental, and emotional balance. Balancing breathing is nasal, diaphragmatic, slow, and light; it is rhythmic and easeful (balancing effort and ease). It is cued with an intention to create a sense of ease, subtlety, and lightness in the student's energy while still actively engaging with the breath—either through breath awareness or breath control. Stabilizing breathing is centered in the abdomen and relies primarily on the diaphragm with regard to breath biomechanics. It is slowed to achieve a balanced breath rate of no more than 10 BPM, while maintaining breath volume at a light load without being either shallow or forced. This combination of breathing—nasal, slow, light, and diaphragmatic—stabilizes breath biochemistry, achieving CO_2 levels in an ideal range of comfort to maintain an optimal breath cadence.

Balancing or stabilizing breathing practices work well for individuals with a strong tendency toward sympathetic nervous system reactivity. Action is emphasized in cuing at the beginning, and then, calming becomes predominant toward the end of a breathwork session. Balancing or stabilizing breath is essential for patients who tend toward a dorsal vagal reactivity of shutting down in the face of challenge. Cuing emphasizes ease and calm at first, slowly adding small increments of

Table 4.11 Features of autonomically balancing or stabilizing breathing

- Smooth, balanced, stable, steady, fluid, silky, smooth, natural, steady, even, uniform, sweet, tranquil, serene, unlabored
- Moving into the abdomen and low rib basket with compassion and mindfulness
- Refreshing, rejuvenating, harmonizing, stabilizing, soothing, steadying, or revitalizing
- Balancing, stabilizing, even
- Inviting of self-agency, clarity, or resolve
- Attentive to and/or balanced between inhalations and exhalations
- Even with regard to breath texture during inhalation and exhalation
- Even with regard to lengths of inhalation and exhalation
- Stable and steady in rhythm and volume, inviting a balance between effort and ease
- Able to stimulate the vagus nerve as notable by increasing relaxation, ease, and social engagement
- Mindful of and adaptive to physical, mental, emotional, and environmental stimuli and experiences

increasing effort. Clients who tend to live in a state of resilient social engagement resonate well with all balancing and stabilizing breathing practices, and activation versus calming might be adjusted depending upon external variables (such as time of day and demand characteristics in the individual's life). Table 4.11 outlines the features of balanced or balancing breathing.

Vitalizing or Energizing Breathing Practices

Energizing breathing, as a bottom-up process of awareness and top-down process of upregulation of the nervous system to access emotional and physical balance, focuses on inhalation, intentional speed or vigor of breath, and the combination of breath and movement. It recalibrates an immobilized or collapsed nervous system, up-regulates mood, energy, and physical vitality; provides an opportunity for exploring *kleshas* and *vrittis*; and invites engagement, action, and initiative. It counteracts a *tamasic* breath that tends to be slow, ineffective, high in the chest, and through the mouth.

Energizing breathing practices are applied to activate the nervous system and shift arousal from the dorsal vagal parasympathetic to the sympathetic branch of the autonomic nervous system, with the ultimate goal of achieving a ventral vagal state. Their central feature is the cultivation of increased arousal and upregulated more pleasant affect. Energizing breathing is slightly more active, faster, diaphragmatic, and measured with regard to the volume of breath inhaled. The focus is on inhalation over exhalation and on the right nostril over the left nostril. It prefers nasal over mouth breathing.

Energizing breathing intends to create a sense of engagement and expansion in the individual's energy and nervous system. Energizing breathing can initially be activated via chest breathing but ultimately becomes centered in the abdomen and low rib basket, relying primarily on the diaphragm with regard to breath biomechanics. It initially speeds up the breath rate (perhaps even to more than 10 BPM) and/or increases breath volume. This combination of breathing—nasal, faster, more intense, diaphragmatic, and geared to the sympathetic branch of the ANS—may

Table 4.12 Features of autonomically vitalizing or energizing breathing

- Energetic, strong, robust, active, spirited, brave, decisive, lively, dynamic, determined, vigorous, resilient, buoyant
- Moving into the belly with intention, resolve, commitment, determination
- Enlivening, strengthening, invigorating, stimulating, refreshing, or revitalizing
- Creating strength, determination, fortitude, willpower, resolve, and courage
- Attentive to the inhalation and encouraging of lengthening or emphasizing the inhalation
- Easing up on the exhalation, letting the exhalation move naturally
- Intent on lengthening each breath with determination yet without creating a sense of gasping for air
- Inviting of a sturdy rhythm and volume without forcing or chest breathing
- Marked by ease being balanced by effort
- Able to invite the vagus nerve to ease the vagal brake on the sympathetic nervous system
- Mindful of and responsive to physical, mental, emotional, and environmental stimuli and experiences

initially destabilize and then restabilize the breath's biochemistry, cultivating CO_2 levels in an ideal range of comfort that helps maintain an optimal cadence of breath. Vitalizing breathwork increases vitality, energy, and alertness. It is used deliberately based on patient needs and never indiscriminately. Vitalizing breathing may be contraindicated for individuals with a history of cardiovascular disease (especially uncontrolled hypertension), stroke, or seizure disorders. It is not appropriate during pregnancy or acute illness. Table 4.12 outlines the features of vital or vitalizing breathing.

Calming or Grounding Breathing Practices

Calming breathing, as a bottom-up process of awareness and top-down process of nervous system down-regulation to access emotional and physical balance, focuses on exhalation, decreased speed or vigor of breath, and the combination of breath and resting. It recalibrates a sympathetically aroused nervous system, downregulates affective reactivity or excess, energy, and physical activation; provides opportunities to explore emotional and mental reactivity; and invites gentle curiosity, calming, and relaxation. It counteracts a sympathetically driven breath that tends to be fast, panting, high in the chest, and through the mouth. It can be used targetedly for a specific purpose, such as helping with inducing sleep.

Calming breathing practices are applied with the intention of (re)grounding the nervous system and shifting arousal from the sympathetic to the parasympathetic branch of the autonomic nervous system. Their central feature is the cultivation of reducing arousal and downregulating affective reactivity and unpleasantness. Calming breathing is nasal, slow, diaphragmatic, and light—with focus on exhalation over inhalation and on the left nostril over the right nostril.

Calming breathing intends to create a sense of ease and relaxation in practitioners' energy and nervous systems. It is centered in the abdomen and low rib basket and relies primarily on the diaphragm to breathe. It is slowed *across time* to achieve a balanced breath rate of fewer than 10 BPM while maintaining breath volume at a light load without being shallow. The combination of breathing nasally, slowly,

Table 4.13 Features of autonomically calming or grounding breathing

- Soft, calm, calming, sweet, gentle, tender, light, easeful, loving, feathery, compassionate, kind
- Moving the breath into the abdomen with minimal engagement of accessory muscles
- Soften, light, relaxing, easeful
- Inviting of ease, peace, lightness, comfort, and effortlessness
- Actively inviting an emphasis on the exhalation and gently inviting a lengthening of the exhalations
- Easing up on inhalations, letting inhalations move naturally
- Marked by slow, long breathing without creating a sense of gasping for air
- Inviting of increasingly slow rhythms and decreased volume without losing a sense of easefulness
- Marked by effort being balanced by ease
- Able to invite the vagus nerve to engage a strong vagal brake, tamping down activity in the sympathetic nervous system
- Mindful of and responsive to physical, mental, emotional, and environmental stimuli and experiences

lightly, diaphragmatically, and in a manner that stimulates the parasympathetic branch of the ANS stabilizes the breath's biochemistry. It can reset the medulla's sensitivity to CO_2, thus creating CO_2 levels in an ideal range of comfort to maintain an optimal cadence of breath.

Calming and grounding breathwork decreases exertion and effort, invites restful and relaxed states, and soothes the mind and emotions. Although it is likely safe for the majority of patients, it is still used deliberately based on patient needs. Calming breathing may be contraindicated for individuals with certain mental health concerns, such as depression or suicidality; it is contraindicated for acute panic states. It may not be appropriate during pregnancy or acute illness. Table 4.13 outlines the features of calm or calming breathing.

4.5   Resilient and Coherent Breathing

Based on the anatomy, physiology, nervous system states, and breath rhythms and characteristics, a definition emerges for what it means to breathe resiliently. Specifically, resilient breathing is coherent—it is defined by healthy biomechanics, optimal biochemistry, auspicious cadence and characteristics (rate, volume, texture, space, and rest), and optimized energetic flow and awareness. It is a breath that supports coherence in the entire organism [61, 62], in that it creates harmony and balance and reflects the interconnectedness and interdependence of all layers of self—body; energy, arousal, and affect; mind with its range of thoughts and emotions; wisdom-based perspective-taking, compassion, and insightful discernment; and joyful recognition of interpersonal embeddedness. Resilient or coherent breathing is nasal, diaphragmatic, slow, subtle, and rhythmic; it is free of respiratory habits or pattern locks. It is captured (mostly) in the *BREATHE* acronym offered by Watkins and Wilber [62]. (p. 115): **B**reathe; **R**hythmically; **E**venly; **A**nd; **T**hrough the; **H**eart; **E**veryday.

This definition of resilient or coherent breathing is *consistent with yogic wisdom and scientific research*, both of which support a rhythmic, peaceful, balancing, and easeful breath when we are at rest; a breath that calms and heals when we are stressed; a breath that vitalizes and nourishes when we are tired; and a breath that promotes resilience and balance in our daily lives. Resilient or coherent breathing is linked propitiously to the autonomic nervous system via important somatosensory feedback from the entire body and helps us adapt to the specific demands of any given moment [13, 63, 64]. In all types of coherent breathing, the inhalation represents a link to the sympathetic nervous system, as does the right nostril (increasing, for example, our heart rate). The exhalation represents a link to the parasympathetic nervous system [65], as does the left nostril (decreasing, for example, our heart rate).

Resilient breathing can take many forms, depending on the circumstances in which we find ourselves. In the context of a restful, easy, relaxed, ventral vagal or sattvic presence, coherent breath is in its most natural state, a state we can refer to as *optimally functional breath*. Such natural breathing is also known as *eupnea* or *quiet breathing*; it is favorably (not excessively) slow, gentle, and light. Eupnea facilitates a calm mind state, balances emotions, provides clarity of thought, and fosters mindful presence. In states of deep calm (e.g., meditation, concentration), intimacy (e.g., during nursing a baby, quiet togetherness), or restfulness (e.g., yoga nidra, relaxation exercises) breath may become resiliently slowed, calm, smooth, and subtle. If taken to an extreme, such slowing of the breath can turn into *hypopnea*, a breath rhythm that is slowed so much and moves so little volume that there is a drop in capillary oxygen saturation (i.e., O_2 levels in the blood are too low as not enough breath is taken in). Hypopnea may be related to dorsal vagal collapse, as the organism shuts down all systems to preserve as much energy or vitality as possible. Care needs to be taken in teaching resilient breathing not to reduce breath to a level that is so subtle or slow that it is a life threat or reaches the dimensions of hypopnea. Nevertheless, it is important to be able to apply strategies of calming breathing that reduce the volume and speed of breath, creating smooth, subtle rhythms of breathing that trigger the parasympathetic nervous system to engage the vagal brake.

In situations of high demand, stress, strenuous activity, or fight-flight activation, resilient breath can become appropriately fast, forceful, or voluminous to prepare the organism for action and to support exertion in the service of well-being or survival. Such activated breathing can, however, become dysregulating for body, mind, and emotions if it occurs in a context that does not truly require significant sympathetic nervous system arousal. As noted previously, many humans in the modern world have an overly activated breath (i.e., chronically hyperventilate) because of chronic sympathetic arousal in stressful contexts that do not allow for the physical discharge of excess breath. Such forceful and rapid breathing is also called *hyperpnea*, signaling by its label (*hyper* = too much) that it involves more vigorous and additional muscular effort than quiet breathing, and than necessary in daily life. In the final analysis, strong and deep breathing is not typically the most helpful approach to routine breathwork, as more students and clients than not may already be in a chronic state of overbreathing. Nevertheless, it is useful to be aware of and apply vitalizing breathwork strategically for students or clients whose breath is indeed too shallow, slowed, collapsed, restricted, or tentative.

Calming or grounding and activating or vitalizing breathing were briefly introduced above. Chapter 10 (under Variations Based on Polyvagal States) elaborate on these types of strategies, offering instructions and cuing from the perspective of creating accessible, person-centered, resilient breathing. This approach emphasizes tailoring breathwork to clients' presentation, applying activating variations and cuing in the presence of chronically restricted or overly subtle or subdued breath, and grounding or calming breathing in the presence of chronic overbreathing.

Generally speaking, when in doubt, more patients are likely to benefit from breathwork focused on slow and light over fast and deep (i.e., voluminous) breathing, especially in daily life, during rest and sleep, and even during light to moderate exercise. A detailed definition of optimal functional breathing (OFB) follows; detailed instructions for helping patients cultivate OFB are offered in Chap. 8.

4.5.1   Defining Optimal Functional Breathing

Drawing on breath anatomy, breath physiology, and breath characteristics, a definition of optimal functional breathing has emerged that can guide intervention (whether on a yoga mat, in a breathwork session, or in clinical practice) as well as daily breathing during rest, sleep, motion, and (light) exertion. OFB is marked by several traits that are present regardless of circumstances and that can be cultivated with ongoing breathing practices. Specifically, OFB can best be described via the following traits:

- *Nasal*: silent breathing in and out through the nose at all times (including at night and during exertion; mouth breathing in emergencies only)
- *Biasing the diaphragm*: breathing is diaphragmatic in the sense that the primary movements notable are abdominal and low rib basket movements; upper chest, shoulder, and neck muscles stay relaxed and passive (unless purposefully or intentionally engaged)
- *Slow*: 5.5–10 BPM
- *Light, silent, and subtle*: inhalation is neither shallow nor forced but rather tailored to move just the right amount of air given respiratory rate, leading to a normal volume of 5–6 L of breath/min; exhalation is easeful and quiet
- *Rhythmic*: breath oscillates with a soft texture and rhythm that is neither rigid nor too relaxed—there is a balance of ease and effort; resting pauses at the top and bottom of breath may be notable, but their length is adapted to the individual; there is no gasping or grasping

4.5.2   Virtuous Cycle of Optimal Functional Breathing

Optimal functional breathing creates a virtuous cycle of harmonious breathing (shown in Fig. 4.2). Calm, subtle, and light breaths have a peaceful rhythm that soothes the nervous system. A long, smooth, and slow diaphragmatic breath stimulates the vagus nerve and results in signals to inhibit overbreathing and unnecessary arousal. The medulla downregulates the breath's speed, and the pons keeps its texture smooth and gentle. This slower rate of breathing invites the possibility of recalibrating the medulla's hypersensitivity to carbon dioxide, inviting a virtuous, self-perpetuating cycle of healthful, coherent, and resilient breathing. These changes decrease minute ventilation and result in efficient use of air that is being moved through the respiratory system. Fewer breaths are taken per minute without losing optimal gas exchange in the tissues or alveoli. The breath is so gentle that we feel a soft pause at the bottom of the breath to invite the new inhalation at just the right moment. Over time, we find a set-point in the medulla for a balanced breathing rhythm that meets our ongoing and situational needs and optimizes physiology and biochemistry.

This flow of breath is akin to the four-part breath that is described in Patanjali's Sutra 2.50. It involves inhalation, rest (however subtle) at the top of the inhalation, exhalation, and rest at the bottom of the exhalation. It is naturally adapted to situational demands and free to vary in pacing, time, texture, sound, and body location as needed. It is unencumbered by habits or pattern locks that force a particular way of breathing or using energy across all circumstances. Four-part breathing, natural breathing, is adaptable and wise.

Optimal functional breathing that relies on a four-part breath occurs during breathwork and in daily life. Whether we teach optimal functioning breathing to clients or students on a yoga mat or practice *pranayama* at home, we try to create a practice environment and context that offers maximum opportunity for safety and open-heartedness; is carefully prepared to create an intentional practice that incorporates all *koshas* and limbs; honors our context, connections, and relationships; creates optimal access to and experience of the practice; and supports the unfolding of joy, wellness, and happiness.

Fig. 4.2 Virtuous cycle of optimal functional breathing

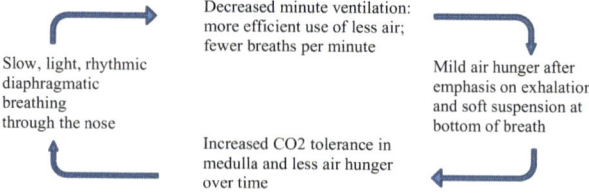

Slow, light, rhythmic diaphragmatic breathing through the nose

Decreased minute ventilation: more efficient use of less air; fewer breaths per minute

Increased CO2 tolerance in medulla and less air hunger over time

Mild air hunger after emphasis on exhalation and soft suspension at bottom of breath

Table 4.14 Impact of slow, light, rhythmic breathing

- Enhanced autonomic nervous system functioning with greater access to ventral vagal complex
- Enhanced Well-being and a greater sense of calm
- Decreased perceptions of stress
- Decreases in anxiety and panic
- Enhanced cardiovascular and pulmonary functioning, including increased heart rate variability, lowered blood pressure, enhanced vasodilation, and greater lung efficiency
- Increased exercise tolerance and athletic performance
- Carefully calibrated CO_2 levels leading to efficient respiration
- Creates coherence, with all systems working at peak efficiency in balance with one another

4.5.3   Summary of Impacts of Optimal Functional Breathing

Resilient and coherent breathing optimizes all physiological systems, including respiratory, cardiovascular, immune, endocrine, and digestive systems. It invites autonomic balance with a bias toward a ventral vagal parasympathetic state with preparedness for activation of the sympathetic nervous system as needed. It maintains optimal O_2 and CO_2 levels in the blood and, as such, maintains the body's pH balance and optimal tissue oxygenation, energy production, and cellular function, including in all organs, tissues, and the brain. It supports the movement of lymph, healthy dilation of smooth muscle, maintenance of healthful posture and spinal stability, and emotional balance. Such breathing is the *pranayama* of the yoga sutras; it is the coherent breath of modern science [11, 13, 24, 25, 61].

Optimal functional breathing supports a calm state of mind, resilient emotionality, and well-functioning cognition with good concentration and memory. It is subtle and light; it stills the fluctuations of mind and emotions [58]. It invites us into quietude necessary for inner practices of yoga or practices focused on mental health and well-being, such as guarding of the senses (*pratyahara*), deep concentration and single-pointed focus (*dharana*), and cultivation of awareness in meditation (*dhyana*) during practice and in daily life. Table 4.14 summarizes the positive effects or impacts of optimal functional breathing in a format that can be used with clients or students, inviting motivation for disciplined commitment to ongoing breathwork for health and thriving.

4.6   Where We Go from Here

Optimal functional breathing stimulates the respiratory vagus nerve in a manner that decreases default mode network (DMN) activity and increases communication between the DMN and the executive control network, increasing cognitive control and enhancing the capacity for behavioral inhibition [24, 51, 66]. Not surprisingly, breathwork that moves us toward harmonious, balanced, and individually tailored breathing has been shown in the research literature to enhance heart rate variability [61, 62] and resilience and to reduce sympathetic and dorsal reactivity [13, 30]. From this perspective, the breath functions as a bridge between mind and body and allows us to explore and reregulate personal energy level, quality of affect, degree of arousal, and auspicious behavioral patterns [61, 62, 67].

Understanding these linkages was the final scientific puzzle piece to put in place in preparation for the practice and teaching of breathwork. With a broad understanding of resilient and coherent breathing as grounded in anatomy, physiology, breath characteristics, and breath's relationship with the autonomic nervous system, *we are now ready to transition from exploring the ancient wisdom and modern science of breathwork to its application in clinical practice*—whether in healthcare, mental healthcare, or therapeutic yoga settings.

In the dance of polyvagal theory, breathing becomes the choreographer,
   orchestrating the interplay between safety and threat, connection and disconnection.—
Stephen Porges

References

1. Tortora GJ, Derrickson BH. Principles of anatomy and physiology. 16th ed. Wiley; 2023.
2. McKeown P. The breathing cure. Humanix; 2021.
3. Nestor J. Breath: the new science of a lost art. Riverhead Books; 2020.
4. Rothenberg R. Restoring prana: a therapeutic guide to pranayama and healing through the breath for yoga therapists, teachers, and healthcare practitioners. Singing Dragon; 2020.
5. Lehrer PM, Gevirtz R. Heart rate variability biofeedback: how and why does it work? Front Psychol. 2014;5:756. https://doi.org/10.3389/fpsyg.2014.00756.
6. Bernardi L, Gabutti A, Porta C, Spicuzza L. Slow breathing reduces chemoreflex response to hypoxia and hypercapnia, and increases baroreflex sensitivity. J Hypertens. 2001;19(12):2221–9. https://doi.org/10.1097/00004872-200112000-00016.
7. Gerritsen R, Band G. Breath of life: the respiratory vagal stimulation model of contemplative activity. Front Neurosci. 2018;12:1–25. https://doi.org/10.3389/fnhum.2018.00397.
8. Mather M, Thayer JF. How heart rate variability affects emotion regulation brain networks. Curr Opin Behav Sci. 2018;19:98–104. https://doi.org/10.1016/j.cobeha.2017.12.017.
9. Noble DJ, Hochman S. Hypothesis: pulmonary afferent activity patterns during slow, deep breathing contribute to the neural induction of physiological relaxation. Front Physiol. 2019;10:1176. https://doi.org/10.3389/fphys.2019.01176.
10. Lehrer PM, Woolfolk RL. Principles and practice of stress management. 4th ed. Guilford Press; 2021.
11. Shao R, Man ISC, Lee TMC. The effect of slow-paced breathing on cardiovascular and emotion functions: a meta-analysis and systematic review. Mindfulness. 2024;15(1):1–18. https://doi.org/10.1007/s12671-023-02294-2.
12. Van Diest I, Verstappen K, Aubert AE, Widjaja D, Vansteenwegen D, Vlemincx E. Inhalation/exhalation ratio modulates the effect of slow breathing on heart rate variability and relaxation. Appl Psychophysiol Biofeedback. 2014;39:171–80. https://doi.org/10.1007/s10484-014-9253-x.
13. Zaccaro A, Piarulli A, Laurino M, et al. How breath-control can change your life: a systematic review on psycho-physiological correlates of slow breathing. Front Hum Neurosci. 2018;12:353. https://doi.org/10.3389/fnhum.2018.00353.

14. Laborde S, Hosang T, Mosley E, Dosseville F. Influence of a 30-day slow-paced breathing intervention compared to social media use on subjective sleep quality and cardiac vagal activity. J Clin Med. 2019;8(2):193. https://doi.org/10.3390/jcm8020193.

15. Malhotra V, Hulke SM, Bharshankar R, Chouhan S, Ravi N, Patrick KP. Effect of slow and deep breathing on brain waves in regular yoga practitioners. Mymensingh Med J. 2021;30(4):1163–7. https://search.proquest.com/docview/2579089112

16. You M, Laborde S, Ackermann S, Borges U, Dosseville F, Mosley E. Influence of respiratory frequency of slow-paced breathing on vagally-mediated heart rate variability. Appl Psychophysiol Biofeedback. 2024;49(1):133–43. https://doi.org/10.1007/s10484-023-09605-2.

17. Meuret AE, Ritz T, Wilhelm FH, Roth WT, Rosenfield D. Hypoventilation therapy alleviates panic by repeated induction of dyspnea. Biol Psychiatry Cogn Neurosci Neuroimaging. 2018;3(6):539–45. https://doi.org/10.1016/j.bpsc.2018.01.010.

18. Meuret AE, Rosenfield D, Hofmann SG, Suvak MK, Roth WT. Changes in respiration mediate changes in fear of bodily sensations in panic disorder. J Psychiatr Res. 2009;43(6):634–41. https://doi.org/10.1016/j.jpsychires.2008.08.003.

19. Paul M, Garg K. The effect of heart rate variability biofeedback on performance psychology of basketball players. Appl Psychophysiol Biofeedback. 2012;37(2):131–44. https://doi.org/10.1007/s10484-012-9185-2.

20. Shaffer F, Meehan ZM, Zerr CL. A critical review of ultra-short-term heart rate variability norms research. Front Neurosci. 2020;14:594880. https://doi.org/10.3389/fnins.2020.594880.

21. Bilo G, Revera M, Bussotti M, et al. Effects of slow deep breathing at high altitude on oxygen saturation, pulmonary and systemic hemodynamics. PLoS One. 2012;7(11):e49074. https://doi.org/10.1371/journal.pone.0049074.

22. Borges U, Lobinger B, Javelle F, Watson M, Mosley E, Laborde S. Using slow-paced breathing to foster endurance, well-being, and sleep quality in athletes during the COVID-19 pandemic. Front Psychol. 2021;12:1–8. https://doi.org/10.3389/fpsyg.2021.624655.

23. Spicuzza L, Gabutti A, Porta C, Montano N, Bernardi L. Yoga and chemoreflex response to hypoxia and hypercapnia. Lancet. 2000;356(9240):1495–6. https://doi.org/10.1016/S0140-6736(00)02881-6.

24. Laborde S, Allen MS, Göhring N, Dosseville F. The effect of slow-paced breathing on stress management in adolescents with intellectual disability. J Intellect Disabil Res. 2017;61(6):560–7. https://doi.org/10.1111/jir.12350.

25. Laborde S, Allen MS, Borges U, et al. The influence of slow-paced breathing on executive function. J Psychophysiol. 2022;36(1):13–27. https://doi.org/10.1027/0269-8803/a000279.

26. Brown RP, Gerbarg PL. Non-drug treatments for ADHD: new options for kids, adults, and clinicians. Norton; 2012.

27. Critchley HD, Nicotra A, Chiesa PA, et al. Slow breathing and hypoxic challenge: cardiorespiratory consequences and their central neural substrates. PLoS One. 2015;10(5):e0127082. https://doi.org/10.1371/journal.pone.0127082.

28. Lin IM, Tai LY, Fan SY. Breathing at a rate of 5.5 breaths per minute with equal inhalation-to-exhalation ratio increases heart rate variability. Int J Psychophysiol. 2014;91:206–11. https://doi.org/10.1016/j.ijpsycho.2013.12.006.

29. Mason H, Vandoni M, deBarbieri G, Codrons E, Ugargol V, Bernardi L. Cardiovascular and respiratory effect of yogic slow breathing in the yoga beginner: what is the best approach? Evid Based Complement Alternat Med. 2013;2013:743504. https://doi.org/10.1155/2013/743504.

30. Russo MA, Santarelli DM, O'Rourke D. The physiological effects of slow breathing in the healthy human. Breathe. 2017;13(4):298–309. https://doi.org/10.1183/20734735.009817.

31. Srinivasan T. Entrainment and coherence in biology. Int J Yoga. 2015;8(1):1–2. https://doi.org/10.4103/0973-6131.146040.

32. Timmons BH, Ley R. Behavioral and psychological approaches to breathing disorders. Springer; 1994.

33. Ley R. Panic attacks during relaxation and relaxation-induced anxiety: a hyperventilation interpretation. J Behav Ther Exp Psychiatry. 1988;19(4):253–9. https://doi.org/10.1016/0005-7916(88)90054-7.

34. Chambers D, Huang C, Matthews G. Basic physiology for anaesthetists. Cambridge University Press; 2019.
35. Chalupa DC, Morrow PE, Oberdörster G, Utell MJ, Frampton MW. Ultrafine particle deposition in subjects with asthma. Environ Health Perspect. 2004;112(8):879–82. https://doi.org/10.1289/ehp.6851.
36. Radwan L, Maszczyk Z, Koziej M, et al. Respiratory responses to chemical stimulation in patients with obstructive sleep apnoea. Monaldi Arch Chest Dis. 2000;55(2):96–100. https://www.ncbi.nlm.nih.gov/pubmed/10949866
37. Tavel ME. Hyperventilation syndrome: a diagnosis usually unrecognized. Intern Med Prim Healthc. 2017;2(1):1–4. https://doi.org/10.24966/IMPH-2493/100006.
38. Scott JB, Kaur R. Monitoring breathing frequency, pattern, and effort. Respir Care. 2020;65(6):793–806. https://doi.org/10.4187/respcare.07439.
39. Sterios P. Gravity and grace. Sounds True; 2019.
40. Cozolino LJ. The neuroscience of psychotherapy. 3rd ed. Norton; 2017.
41. Damasio AR. Self comes to mind: constructing the conscious brain. Vintage; 2012.
42. Siegel DJ. Aware. Penguin; 2018.
43. Scaer R. 8 Keys to brain-body balance. Norton; 2012.
44. Ratey JJ. A user's guide to the brain: perception, attention, and the four theaters of the brain. Pantheon; 2001.
45. Prescott SL, Liberles SD. Internal senses of the vagus nerve. Neuron. 2022;110(4):579–99. https://doi.org/10.1016/j.neuron.2021.12.020.
46. Porges S. The polyvagal theory: neurophysiological of emotions, attachment, communication, and self-regulation. Norton; 2011.
47. Porges SW. The polyvagal theory: new insights into adaptive reactions of the autonomic nervous system. Cleve Clin J Med. 2009;76(Suppl 2):S86–90. https://doi.org/10.3949/ccjm.76.s2.17.
48. Porges S. The pocket guide to the polyvagal theory: the transformative power of feeling safe. Norton; 2017.
49. Dana D. The polyvagal theory in therapy: engaging the rhythm of regulation. Norton; 2018.
50. Dana D, Porges S. Clinical applications of the polyvagal theory: the emergence of polyvagal-informed therapies. Norton; 2018.
51. Sullivan MB, Erb M, Schmalzl L, Moonaz S, Taylor JN, Porges S. Yoga therapy and polyvagal theory: the convergence of traditional wisdom and contemporary neuroscience for self-regulation and resilience. Front Hum Neurosci. 2018;12:67–82. https://doi.org/10.3389/fnhum.2018.00067.
52. Porges SW. Polyvagal theory: a science of safety. Front Integr Neurosci. 2022;16:871227. https://doi.org/10.3389/fnint.2022.871227.
53. Rosenberg S. Accessing the healing power of the vagus nerve. North Atlantic Books; 2017.
54. Payne P, Crane-Godreau MA. The preparatory set: a novel approach to understanding stress, trauma, and the bodymind therapies. Front Hum Neurosci. 2015;9:178.
55. Levine P. Waking the Tiger: healing trauma. North Atlantic Books; 1997.
56. van der Kolk B. The body keeps the score. Penguin; 2014.
57. Badenoch B. The heart of trauma: healing the embodied brain in the context of relationship. Norton; 2018.
58. You M, Laborde S, Zammit N, et al. Emotional intelligence training: influence of a brief slow-paced breathing exercise on psychophysiological variables linked to emotion regulation. Int J Environ Res Public Health. 2021;18(12):6630. https://doi.org/10.3390/ijerph18126630.
59. You M, Laborde S, Zammit N, Iskra M, Borges U, Dosseville F. Single slow-paced breathing session at six cycles per minute: investigation of dose-response relationship on cardiac vagal activity. Int J Environ Res Public Health. 2021;18(23):12478. https://doi.org/10.3390/ijerph182312478.
60. Schwartz A. Applied polyvagal theory in yoga: therapeutic practices for emotional health. Norton; 2024.

61. Sevoz-Couche C, Laborde S. Heart rate variability and slow-paced breathing: when coherence meets resonance. Neurosci Biobehav Rev. 2022;135:104576. https://doi.org/10.1016/j.neubiorev.2022.104576.

62. Watkins A, Wilber K. Wicked and wise: how to solve the world's toughest problems. Urbane; 2015.

63. Hsu S, Tseng C, Hsieh C, Hsieh C. Slow-paced inspiration regularizes alpha phase dynamics in the human brain. J Neurophysiol. 2020;123(1):289–99. https://doi.org/10.1152/jn.00624.2019.

64. Sakakibara M, Hayano J. Effect of slowed respiration on cardiac parasympathetic response to threat. Psychosom Med. 1996;58(1):32–7. https://doi.org/10.1097/00006842-199601000-00006.

65. Birdee G, Nelson K, Wallston K, et al. Slow breathing for reducing stress: the effect of extending exhale. Complement Ther Med. 2023;73:102937. https://doi.org/10.1016/j.ctim.2023.102937.

66. Vukojević B, Vater C, Laborde S. The role of resonance frequency in slow-paced breathing: systematic review. Curr Issues Sport Sci. 2024;9(2):80. https://doi.org/10.36950/2024.2ciss080.

67. Bhagat V, Simbak N, Husain R, Mat KC. A brief literature review retraining amygdala to substitute its irrational conditioned fear and anxiety responses with new learning experiences. Res J Pharm Technol. 2020;13(8):3987. https://doi.org/10.5958/0974-360X.2020.00705.2.

Part III

Clinical Applications of Breathwork

Setting the Stage for Breathwork

5

Some students are in a hurry to begin 'real' pranayama. They go right to the later stages without first laying a quality foundation, and their practice often suffers. First find out <u>what is</u>.
This is also part of the answer to the question <u>Who am I</u>?

Richard Rosen in The Yoga of Breath: A Step-by-Step Guide to Pranayama

5.1 Overview: Understanding Integrated Holistic Breathwork

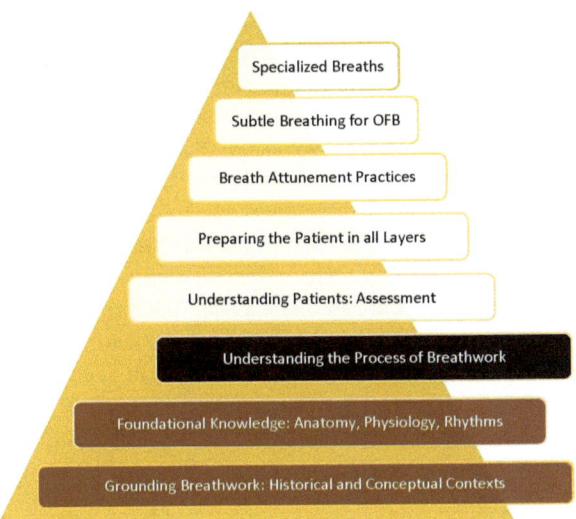

Integrating yogic wisdom with the science of biomechanics, biochemistry, and psychology of breathing, this chapter begins with the application of these foundational understandings to the clinical practice and teaching of integrated holistic breathwork. Although it may not be possible to remember all the little details, it is helpful to understand and put into action the central messages of breath anatomy and physiology, psychological and mental aspects of breath rhythms and cadence, and intricacies related to autonomic nervous system platforms. In applying the science of breathing to the art of breathwork, this chapter highlights how some of the teachings about breathing in the context of Western or modern postural yoga do not always support optimal, natural, and functional breathing in daily life. Simply copying what we have learned in yoga classes or using what we have read in popular books about breathing may not serve our clients and students clinically. We begin to realize that breathwork needs to be adapted to each individual—that one size does *not* fit all.

This is not to imply that yogic breathing encountered in yoga classes is not useful—it can be. However, many yoga and Western breathing practices (e.g., bellow's breath, skull-shining breath, breath holding, and ujjayi) have specific purposes and are not meant as daily or continuous breathing practices. Although many teachers ask students to use ocean-sounding breathing (*ujjayi*) *throughout* a yoga class, now that we understand breath biomechanics and biochemistry, is this meaningful instruction? Natural breathing is meant to be silent and soft, unlabored, and free. We may hear teachers ask students to box breathe, that is, equal length of inhalation and exhalation and retention at the top and suspension at the bottom of the breath. Given our understanding of breath biomechanics and biochemistry, do we now understand that this may be a difficult practice for many practitioners? In fact, is such a breathing technique perhaps a practice that goes well beyond healthful, accessible, and appropriate breathing for many people? Teachers instruct students to engage in breath-holds after skull-shining (repetitive forceful exhalations and passive inhalations). Do we now understand that this technique may result in dizziness and discomfort for some?

As breathing guides or coaches, we need an integrated holistic framework for *what* we are practicing and teaching and how to take the skills and practices that we cultivate on the mat or in the office into daily life. Integrated holistic practice requires intention, clarity of purpose, and open hearts and minds. Integration and wholism (introduced in Chap. 1) are not new ideas; they honor the wisdom of ancient and modern yoga psychology. The Yoga Sutras of Patanjali, the Hatha Yoga Pradipika, and other classic yogic and Buddhist texts are clear that breathwork is *situated in a greater context* of safety, commitment, and physical preparation; breathwork is, after all, only one of many integrated practices. To have a holistic and integrated practice, we bring sensitivity to nonviolence, truthfulness, moderation, and purpose to the practice in each and every moment. We set up an environment that honors ethical principles to create maximum opportunity for well-being within available circumstances and parameters. We create intention and explicit motivation and purpose that honors interconnection, creates meaning, and encourages commitment to serve a greater good. We strive to understand how our bodies function and move, and how their functions, shapes, and movements interact with breath. We link breath to the experience of thoughts and emotions and become increasingly aware of profound interconnections between body, mind, heart, behavior, and relationships. This chapter explores how to set the context or stage for integrated holistic breathwork.

5.2   Integrated Holistic Breathwork Principles

It is important for yoga teachers or clinicians to understand that they are not simply teaching students or clients how to engage in a particular breathing practice. Instead, they are teaching their patients how to become wise practitioners who can make informed and knowledgeable personal choices about breath and breathing, on the mat, in the office, and in daily life. Optimally accessible breathwork (whether in the context of a yoga class or in healthcare) includes not only instruction about how to breathe in certain systematic ways, but also education about the biomechanics, biochemistry, and psychology of optimal functional breathing. Careful breathing instructors empower practitioners to listen to feedback from their bodies and to respect this information with truthfulness and nonviolence. Cultivating self-awareness, including interoception and neuroception, teaches patients to tailor self-care and healthcare practices in general, breathing practices in particular, and daytime (at rest, during stress, during exertion) and nighttime breathing most importantly. Thus, breathing guides (whether teachers or clinicians) *explicitly* hold in mind and, over time, teach clients how to choose and adapt breathwork to individual needs and how to transition these practices from the office into wholesome functional breathing in daily life. The basic principles of integrated holistic yoga (introduced in Chap. 1) are very helpful in this regard and merit a review of their application to breathwork.

5.2.1   Intentionality in Breathwork

Intentionality occurs on two levels. The teacher or clinician has clarity about the intention and purpose of each session as well as across time. The student or client develops intentionality in each session and purpose or meaning for breathing practice across time. Intentionality is grounded in the individual needs of students and is based on careful assessment and self-reflection. As such, assessment explores the type of suffering with which clients are presenting, as well as possible proximal and distal causes. Once the client and clinician understand what the presenting concerns are and how they may arise in context and relationships, goals can be set to guide the intention of breathwork in the long term. It is then up to the teacher to create a plan across time that slowly and deliberately moves the client toward the breathing goals that were developed. In addition to having clarity for breathwork across time, the clinician also responsibly develops a sequence for each session that slowly and intentionally guides the work toward these goals. All planning, across time and within each session, is grounded in sound pedagogy to result in sequences that are tailored to the client, ensuring meaningful, beneficial, accessible, and healthful work. Patients are also invited in each session to stay aligned with their defined goals and to set a deliberate intention. They are encouraged to let session-based intentions be grounded in personal needs and resources, as well as in the overall goals for therapeutic breathwork across time.

5.2.2   Beneficence in Breathwork

A universal principle in healthcare is *"first, do no harm"* (*primum non nocere* in Latin; often mistakenly attributed to Hippocrates). This principle reminds us that in all interventions with students, clients, or patients, the most important guideline for working together is not to inflict unnecessary harm or suffering. Framed as a more positive foundational principle, healthcare providers choose interventions that reflect beneficence—the commitment to creating well-being, nurturance, support, encouragement, and healing—and to prioritize the interest of each individual patient. In the context of breathwork, this means that clinicians maintain safety and reduce the potential for harm to clients by attending to the following:

- Developing wholesome and shared goals for breathwork based on careful assessment and understanding of the student
- Honoring affiliative and ethical variables in the client-clinician relationship
- Assuring safety, security, and accessibility in the healthcare or practice environment
- Creating the most wholesome way of sequencing breathwork across time and within sessions
- Tailoring breathwork to the physical and energetic presentation of the patient
- Supporting clients' anatomy and physiology of breath in optimally functional ways
- Honoring patients' nervous system states and subtle energies in the choice of breathwork
- Inviting autonomy, agency, nonstressful effort, and meaning in offered breathing practices
- Refining practices continuously, based on new information from the student
- Integrating new information from modern science as it emerges in the research literature
- Maintaining clarity of intention and purpose throughout

Beneficence in breathwork reflects clinicians' and teachers' understanding of optimal functional breathing, careful sequencing that is grounded in careful assessment and goal-setting, and ongoing reassessment and refinement of offered practices. Beneficence also means that breathing instructors commit to helping students and clients develop a knowledge base about breath and breathing that they can use to generalize practices offered on the mat or in the office into daily life. This means that clinicians help clients understand how to listen to body, breath, and mind feedback (through enhancing neuroception, interoception, and proprioception) consistently to make wholesome choices about their personal breathing practices in class and at home.

5.2.3 Accessibility in Breathwork

Accessibility has many facets and manifestations. This summary is by no means complete and simply serves as a motivation for each clinician to reflect on how to invite clients into the practice in the most intentional, beneficial, holistic, integrated, tailored, appropriate, caring, compassionate, joyful, and thoughtful manner. Accessibility ensures that clinicians choose breathing practices and variations appropriate for students' state of health, nervous system, state of mind, and in-the-moment needs. As is true for all aspects of anatomy and physiology, breathing is subject to tremendous individual variations as well as environmental or external factors. Anatomy (e.g., number of ribs, degree of thoracic kyphosis), physiology (e.g., hypersensitivity to carbon dioxide), psychology (e.g., polyvagal state), air quality, air temperature, type of movement, and many other variables affect breathing and, in turn, are affected by the breath. These individual and environmental factors require that breathwork (similar to movement practices) be adapted to individual clients and their specific breathing patterns, contexts, and needs.

Accessibility includes the offering of appropriate props, such as blankets, bolsters, blocks, and more. However, it does not end there. Accessibility honors all layers of self and the biopsychosociocultural context of each patient. Accessibility is reflected in the environment in which the breathwork takes place (whether in a yoga or medical space) that may signal or fail to convey inclusivity and openness, equity and social justice, beneficence and compassion, professionalism and ethical commitment. Accessibility is reflected in language and cuing—via connotations of inclusivity versus exclusivity, authority versus autonomy, directiveness versus agency, compassion versus judgment, criticism versus open-minded exploration, and so much more. Clearly, whole books could be and, in fact, have been written about creating accessibility across a range of human dimensions. As breathing guides, we must educate ourselves about how to make practices optimally beneficial and accessible by taking advantage of the wonderful resources that already exist [1–6].

5.2.4 Wholism in Breathwork

Challenges in breath and breathing can reverberate into all tangible layers of experience (see Chap. 1 for a review)—body, energy and vitality (affect and arousal), mind and emotions, actions and relationships, with downstream effects on intentions, thoughts, actions, relationships, and communal ways of being. It is helpful, as we name clients' presenting concerns or students' intentions for seeking breathing practices, to note which layers of experience are affected. This is true even if clients seemingly voice issues only in one way of experiencing themselves. Our layers of being (body, breath, mind, heart, community) are interdependent and co-arising; they are a holistic and dynamic system of mutuality. Challenges or well-being in any particular layer reverberate into all others. For example, if clients present with a physical complaint (such as asthma, bronchitis, allergies), this physical challenge most likely has repercussions for their vitality, may preoccupy their thoughts, may challenge them emotionally, and could even profoundly affect their behaviors, relationships, and communities. Regardless of the presenting concern, good clinicians always listen to the effect and ripples into all *koshas* or layers.

Once challenges have been identified in all layers of experience, it is helpful to understand what is contributing to and maintaining identified suffering. Presenting concerns are always grounded in a greater context that can be explored comprehensively via four factors of influence—biological, psychological, social-sociological, and cultural-familial—combined, abbreviated as *biopsychosociocultural* [7, 8]. These factors of influence affect clients' approaches to life, perceptions of self, medical histories, and their greater collective grounding in cultural, familial, and social matrices that shape their way of being in the world and in relationships. For example, contexts and relational webs provide the backdrop for our development and influence how we live and relate. They shape affects, energies, mind states, beliefs, attitudes, and stories that contribute to suffering in general and self-created suffering in particular. This process starts not simply at birth but even before we are born as we accumulate experiences in utero that arrive through our senses and the physiology shared with our mothers. At the earliest point in development, we develop a nervous system style that reflects whether we entered the world in a context of safety, danger, or even (perceived) life threat. As noted in Chap. 4, yoga refers to our basic nature or temperament (*gunas* in Sanskrit). Modern neuroscience defines our basic styles of reacting and relating, best captured by the nervous system states elucidated by polyvagal theory [9]. Basic nervous system states or gunas contribute to health or suffering depending on how they develop and emerge in daily life. Understanding context and nervous system style helps shape interventions and guides clinicians or teachers toward more tailored breathwork.

To summarize the main point—wholism, via attention to the *koshas* and biopsychosociocultural context, ensures that breathwork is tailored to the specific needs and larger contexts of each client. It leads to not applying a one-size-fits-all approach to breathwork. Offering tailored and individualized intervention differentiates therapeutic breathwork from simply offering *techniques*.

5.2.5   Integration in Breathwork

Given the reality that wholism explores presenting concerns and their etiology in the context of patients' *koshas* and life circumstances, it is no surprise that interventions have to be carefully tailored and draw on more than one strategy or tool to effect change. The very definition of integration is that we never simply offer a single tool—instead, we offer many possible ways of improving symptoms and lives. The remainder of this book assumes that this is the approach teachers and clinicians take when they begin to integrate breathwork into their extant toolbox—they use breathing and breath interventions in combination with other approaches to help their clients. Breathwork is integrated into a greater treatment plan that is comprehensive and wraps around the client in a meaningful, intentional, beneficial, and accessible manner. Breathwork minimally is grounded in the other limbs of yoga, always based on ethical practices, life commitments that create purpose and meaning, physical practices that address symptoms and promote physically healthful applications of breathing practices, and inner practices that explore mental, emotional, behavioral, and relational aspects of why clients or patients seek healthcare or why students choose yoga and breathwork to enhance their well-being.

5.3   Creating a Physically and Psychologically Safe Environment for Breathwork

Successful teaching and therapeutics, especially in the context of integrated holistic therapeutic breathwork, depend on the creation of a psychological holding space or environment that conveys beneficence, in the form of compassion, kindheartedness, and appropriate ethical boundaries; accessibility, equity, and inclusion; and goal-directedness, intentionality, and purpose. It is an environment that offers clarity about procedures and rules, boundaries and priorities, the management of group dynamics, respect for each student, and insight into individual versus group needs in the teaching environment. A supportive and therapeutic environment honors the ethical guidelines of relevant healthcare and yoga professionals, as well as provides clarity about motivation, discipline, and commitment. The environment needs to express attunement to client needs as related to their layers of experience (or *koshas*). It is an environment that creates a deliberate and committed atmosphere of consent. Such an environment is created via attention to the physical and psychological safety of all clients and clinicians.

5.3.1   Creating Optimal Opportunities for Physical Safety

Opportunities for physical safety arise from environments and relationships with healthcare providers that create structures and logistics that provide consistency, predictability, respect, and clear safety-based boundaries and policies. Consistency, predictability, and safety in an environment can be created via the following features and behaviors embraced by all clinicians and staff who interact with patients:

- *Language*—have a way of using language and prosody that is predictable
- *Lighting levels*—maintain a consistent pattern that is adjusted to the time of day, availability of windows, etc.

- *Noise and sound*—have a predictable pattern of noise level and management in the clinical space (e.g., use of white noise machines if indicated); have predictability about the use of music and tolerance of noise by patients (e.g., how the environment handles chatter, excessively loud breathing, snoring during savasana)
- *Environmental features that convey thoughtfulness and signal safety*
  - Maximize and optimize the degree of privacy and confidentiality
  - Ensure the availability of emergency exits
  - Make conscious decisions about how to deal with windows and/or window coverings
- *Safe and supportive containment in the room*
  - Select accessible and comfortable floor coverings
  - Have appropriate props (e.g., blankets, pillows, bolsters, blocks) available for use with disclosure about how hygiene for props is attended to
  - Minimize clutter and maximize the ease with which the space can be navigated
  - Choose wisely how to use or not use mirrors
  - For groups, select an appropriate group size for the available space
- *Assistants/helpers, and substitute teachers/clinicians*—make sure there is consistency in how clinicians use helpers and choose substitutes (e.g., when on vacation or sick leave); clarify that the clinician is the one who holds responsibility for the behavior of staff or assistants
- *Routines and rituals*—commit to a flow or sequence that has predictability and creates an opportunity for patients to feel a sense of safety
- *Culture of consent*—stay committed to ongoing consent procedures regarding patient freedom to choose variations, policies related to touch, and level of directiveness
- *Time management*—start and end breathwork sessions on time; provide a clock that faces the clinician; for group sessions, have rules about late arrival and/or early departure; have clarity about time after class to respond to and deal with students' or clients' questions, reflections, and concerns

5.3.2   Creating Optimal Opportunities for Psychological Safety

Opportunities for psychological safety arise from physically safe environments, as described above, as well as from psychological variables in the environment that convey respect, compassion, inclusivity, equity, and commitment to advocacy and empowerment. Additionally, and perhaps most importantly, psychological safety arises in the context of empowering and respectful relationships between care providers and clients.

Environmental Psychological Safety Cues
Environments that optimize the perception of safety in patients or students promote positive relationship development between clinicians and clients by expressing awareness of and not abusing power dynamics in the healthcare or yoga context.

Table 5.1 Commitments necessary for psychologically safe environments

- Maintaining boundaries with patients
- Staying responsive and trying not to be reactive toward clients
- Remaining defenseless and open-hearted, especially vis-à-vis input, comments, or feedback from clients
- Holding space for the relationship and remembering that breathwork is about students' needs
- Listening and helping patients feel seen, heard, and understood
- Minimizing interruptions (not being distracted by phones or electronic media)
- Engaging in common courtesy and rules of etiquette
- Ensuring privacy and confidentiality, including understanding limits and boundaries of information exchange with other staff members regarding clients seen for breathwork
- Making referrals and engaging in interprofessional collaboration as needed, with appropriate consent and release of information from clients
- Addressing rules related to contact between client and clinician outside of the breathwork context
- Debriefing and consulting as needed, especially after challenging clinical situations with a patient

They express explicit respect for each student by promoting a culture of listening attentively and respectfully to patients, respecting and honoring their points of view, beliefs, and culture. Staff and clinicians are expected to speak truthfully, politely, and directly to clients and to strive for the most compassionate and kind ways of providing information, including performance feedback, to patients and one another.

Psychologically safe environments also promote patient (self-)empowerment, autonomy, and agency. One way in which patient autonomy is supported is via clarity about touch/no-touch, use of props, selection of mat location in class or seat in a session, and clients' self-rule about variations and adaptations. In group settings, such environments are clear about how they balance individual client needs and desires with group needs. Finally, psychologically safe environments do what they can to reduce the perceived power of the clinician over the patient, such as making discerning language choices, adjusting choices and pacing for intervention, and making thoughtful choices about cuing and assisting. Psychologically attentive systems prioritize patient needs ahead of clinician needs (unless patient behavior is offensive, unethical, or dangerous) by ensuring clinicians, staff, supporters, and assistants are committed to assuring a patient-centered approach to care (see Table 5.1).

Personal Traits of a Breathwork Clinician or Teacher to Support Psychological Safety

In addition to being properly trained and working within their proper scope of practice, breathing instructors develop an awareness of personality traits, biases, and preferences they bring to their clinical practice and have clear intentions and approaches to relationships with clients. These capacities are supported by clinicians' disciplined commitment to ethical clinical practice and disciplined personal practice (in a yoga context, to Limbs 1 and 2), as well as deep mindfulness, personal inner or contemplative practice, and (self-)compassion (as promoted by yoga's

Limbs 5, 6, and 7). The presence or absence of these qualities can greatly enhance or detract from the teachings and have a strong impact on the clinician-client relationship.

Personal insight into strengths, weaknesses, and biases is crucial. Breathing instructors can lead students only as far as they themselves have progressed in their practice. Clinicians who have become self-aware of their own development know how they function and interact most typically and habitually. The most successful breathwork instructors have attained the capacity to be deeply compassionate, wise, and insightful. They embody equanimity, curiosity, non-judgmentalism, gratitude, and a desire to be of service. They are also keenly aware of their personal qualities—attunement that is essential to truthful, safe, and committed teaching. Being self-aware can make the difference between ethical and successful work versus work that is unsafe for clients.

Auspicious personal qualities and practices (described in Table 5.2) create meaningful client-clinician relationships and environments that are psychologically and physically arranged to optimize cues and opportunities for safety. They support practice accessibility through a deep appreciation for patients' empowerment, self-agency, and resilience. While several personal and interpersonal qualities are summarized below, this listing is not meant to be all-inclusive. Many other qualities and

Table 5.2 Essential traits of a breathwork instructor

Cultural skillfulness and sensitivity
- Deep understanding of the biopsychosociocultural context and its impact on development and developmental opportunities; relationships and power structures; experiences and opportunities in the world; exposure to trauma, racial and other bias, and oppression
- Deep understanding of the biopsychosociocultural model and its impact on systems and the perpetuation of white supremacy, as well as systemic and institutionalized racism
- Awareness of the impact and manifestation of personal biases, prejudice, and privilege
- Understanding and embracing differences with a strong commitment to diversity, equity, and inclusion
- Knowledge, awareness, and skills of cultural differences and diversity, lived and applied with sensitivity and humility
- Open-mindedness about values, behaviors, and approaches to life
- Restraint from imposing personal values, standards, or beliefs
- Openness about personal characteristics of diversity, such as gender identity, race, culture, religion, age, levels of ability, socioeconomic factors, educational opportunities, and more
- Non-offensive, nonsexist, non-ageist, and nonracist language
- Ability to discern the intention *and* impact of actions, speech, and even thought
- Ability to apologize and make amends for microaggressions or missteps—Along with non-defensiveness and humility
- Willingness to have challenging conversations with others—Clients, peers, supervisors, the general public—When bias, oppression, and other diversity and equity issues emerge
- Willingness to seek cultural consultation
- If White, active solidarity and advocacy that elevates Black, indigenous, and people of color, shrinks back from speaking for groups with different diversity characteristics than one's own, and active commitment to expose, counter, and repair systems of white supremacy

(continued)

Table 5.2   (continued)

Interpersonally relevant traits for relationship-building
- Being interpersonally attuned via empathy, kindness, compassion, and mindful awareness of personal impact on clients, peers, and assistants
- Being interpersonally perceptive with the ability to listen attentively and fully, read nonverbal communication, and be respectful
- Being able to joyfully celebrate patients' successes
- Embodying and demonstrating calmness, groundedness, and equanimity in general and especially under pressure and during challenge
- Reducing interpersonal power differentials to communicate clearly that clients are in charge of their bodies, are invited to exercise self-agency, have the power to say "no," and have the power to make choices they deem ideal for themselves
- Respect patients' points of view, beliefs, and culture
- Listen attentively and respectfully
- Speak truthfully, politely, and directly to clients

Clinical preparedness
- Have a clear plan for the session:
  - Establish a clear intention for the session
  - Develop a defined plan with the flexibility to modify it as needed given how the client presents
  - Feel centered and ready to teach
  - Stay mindful of self and breath
  - Be mentally and physically ready to teach and interact with patients
  - Be prepared to assert etiquette and boundary guidelines
- Be mentally, emotionally, energetically, and physically prepared to ensure personal capacity to:
  - Be fully present
  - Respond to the demands of each moment
  - Remain emotionally centered and mentally balanced
  - Feel able to offer an environment and context that invites safety, promotes collaboration, and supports engagement and mutuality
- Be knowledgeable about and prepared for the type and level of breathwork being taught with a capacity to:
  - Use modifications and variations in each session based on client presentations
  - Adapt breathwork to meet clients where they are in the moment
  - Change a breathing lesson plan based on unexpected circumstances (such as historical events, student presentations, teacher challenges, and more)
  - Shift gears with regard to how breathwork is cued or taught based on new information that emerges about a patient
- Be skillful in addressing and honoring individual needs of patients:
  - Strive to accommodate diverse learning styles in communicating
  - Be self-aware and discerning about the tone of voice (e.g., non-commanding, clearly audible, warm, inviting, modulated to present-moment occurrences)
  - Be self-aware and discerning about choice of language (e.g., gender-sensitive, trauma-sensitive, invitational, respectful of individual choices)
  - Do not allow personal beliefs and values to adversely influence the relationship with clients
  - Do not impose personal beliefs on students

(continued)

Table 5.2 (continued)

Personal preparedness
- Remain mindful of and attuned to self and others
- Maintain equanimity (i.e., optimize capacity to stay in a ventral vagal space) in times of challenge, stress, or crisis through teacher preparedness
- Have an emotional safety plan for distressed students as well as for the clinician once the session is over
- Maintain awareness of and effectively resolve transference and countertransference
- Stay attuned to clients, especially the level of arousal as related to polyvagal states
- Be able to help clients re-regulate if a crisis occurs in a breathing session and become attuned to their capacity to do so
- Stay attentionally connected to patients as much as possible—Note their physical and energetic resources and responses
- Stay responsible for the conduct of staff, assistants, helpers, or supporters and have clarity about their role with the clinician and the clients

biopsychosociocultural influences affect clinician-patient relationships. Ongoing mindfulness, vigilance, and humility are essential to being an open-hearted and open-minded breathwork guide.

From the contextual understanding of the five principles of integrated holistic practice (i.e., intentionality, beneficence, accessibility, wholism, and integration) and environmental and relational considerations, we can begin to shape person-centered and tailored work with each individual client. This shaping relies on a clear understanding of our clients and their biopsychosociocultural context, their specific reason for seeking support with breath and breathing, the goals and intentions that emerge from this understanding, and the specific plan for intervention. We now turn to a comprehensive paradigm of conceptualization that serves as the foundation for the application of breathwork.

5.4   Conceptualization in Integrated Holistic Breathwork

Conceptualization for each client in the context of integrated holistic breathwork relies on a comprehensive paradigm for conceptualizing clients' presentations and needs [7, 8], rooted in Ayurvedic and Buddhist ways of understanding health, *panchamaya kosha* model of the yoga tradition (first described in the *Taittiriya Upanishad*), modern healthcare, and integral psychology broadly (re)interpreted [10, 11]. Four steps or components form the basis of the conceptualization model and are overviewed in Table 5.3 in modern and ancient terminology. In Buddhism, the four steps parallel the four noble truths (cf., *catvāri āryasatyāni* [12, 13]; in Ayurveda, they derive from the systems model of the body (cf., *vyuha* model; sutra 3.28 in the *Yoga Sutras of Patanjali*). True to its ancient origins and modern understanding, the conceptualization model is developmental in nature and premised on the fact that humans evolve and change throughout their lifespan within a web of relationships that supports, nourishes, or hinders health and thriving.

Table 5.3 Four-step/four-component model for client conceptualization

Medical terminology	Ancient wisdom terminologies[a]	Translation of Sanskrit terminology	Breathwork terminology
Diagnosis	Dukkha	Unsatisfactoriness, suffering, pain, stress, dysfunction	Defining presenting concerns, challenges, or symptoms
	Heya (2.16)	That which is to be discarded	
Etiology	Samudaya	Cause, arising, coming into existence, roots of suffering	Identifying primary and secondary (or proximal and distal) causes (or roots) of suffering
	Hetu (4.11)	That which causes false impressions of identity	
Prognosis and goal setting	Nirodha	Cessation, releasing, removal, letting go, quieting	Kindling hope and planning the goals for and path of transformation
	Hana (2.25)	That which is to be removed	
Treatment or intervention	Marga	Path, steps, strategies, practice, discipline	Embarking on the healing path, engaging in ongoing assessment of the patient, and refinement of the intervention
	Upaya/Hanopaya (2.26)	The means for removal of suffering	

Note: Based on Brems [8]
[a]The first term refers to the Buddhist conceptualization; the second derives from Ayurvedic practice (with reference to the relevant sutra in the Yoga Sutras of Patanjali; although these sutras do not really speak to therapy but to spiritual practice)

This framework deeply acknowledges that we need to understand—for each patient—why we are engaging in breathwork, what we hope to accomplish, why we choose to offer certain practices over others, and what mechanisms we employ to create change that leads to enhanced coping, healing, and thriving. The model encourages us to apply the science covered in Chaps. 2, 3, and 4, by realizing that change mechanisms that are inherent in breathwork (while arising from ancient wisdom) can be expressed in terms of modern science. Specifically, the primary change mechanisms that result in healing and thriving through breathwork are as follows:

- *Enhancement of biomechanics* (teaching nasal and diaphragmatic breathing, attending to posture, teaching tongue placement, and more)
- *Enhancement of biochemistry* (teaching about internal and external respiration, CO_2 sensitivity, oxygenation of blood versus tissues, and more)
- *Enhancement of breath rhythms* (enhancing breath cadence, rate and volume, texture and sound, breath phases, and more)
- *Facilitation of awareness of bottom-up processes* (enhancing neuroception, interoception, proprioception, and exteroception)

- *Facilitation of self-regulation* via *engagement of a top-down process* (providing psychoeducation and encouraging motivation, discerning choices, and informed decision-making)
- *Stimulation of the vagus nerve* that enhances the vagal brake; increases vagal tone, heart rate variability, and resilience, and reduces sympathetic and dorsal reactivity (via diaphragmatic breathing, social connection, and co-regulation)

By going through the four-step process of diagnosis, etiology, prognosis and commensurate goal-setting, and intervention planning, we, as clinicians, can discern which types of breathwork approaches are most likely to result in changes that are needed for each patient based on the specific symptoms and contexts they bring to us as healthcare providers or yoga professionals.

5.4.1   Step 1—Diagnosis: Defining Presenting Concerns

The first step (*dukkha* or *heya*) represents the start of any healing journey and invites us to attune open-heartedly and open-mindedly to the reality that humans experience various forms of challenges (or suffering), problems, stress, pressure, struggle, sorrow, discontent, or friction. To embark on a healing path via breathwork, it is important to understand and define the challenges (or suffering) with which clients present. In healthcare, this process results in a diagnosis. In breathwork or other therapeutic contexts (including yoga therapy or therapeutic yoga), *defining the presenting concern or challenge* may be appropriate terminology, as clients may seek breathing practices for wellness, prevention, or resilience—not necessarily for a specific medical or mental health diagnosis (although the latter may be present and have triggered referral for breathwork).

Challenges can occur in any or all of the koshas—body, energy (affect, vitality, arousal), mind, emotions, and all downstream aspects of our lives, such as actions, relationships, and ways of being in the community. We are human; hence, by definition, we are prone to physical and mental or emotional illness, injury, disease, aging, and—yes, death. Due to having a human brain, we tend to compound painful or challenging experiences with thoughts of aversion, craving and clinging, confusion, and fears for our lives, identity, or survival. We meet our challenges with minds that can become agitated and disorganized, distracted and inattentive, tired and hopeless. Our emotions can take us from the deepest lows of depression, despair, and shame, to the depths of anxiety or panic, to the out-of-control feelings of anger or rage, to a sense of hurt, grief, or betrayal. When physical, mental, or emotional challenge or pain reaches significant dimensions of suffering, it may begin to interfere with daily functioning, relationships, resilience, and the ability to cope. These human experiences of challenge, dissatisfaction, discomfort, and pain are captured by the word *dukkha*, which has no clear or definitive single translation into English.

Dukkha is always captured in our breathing. Breath is directly linked to mind and body and intimately interwoven with the nervous system, as elucidated in Chaps. 2, 3, and 4. Thus, even in the context of breathwork, recognizing and defining the presence of challenge, pain, or sorrow (as well as their varied manifestations in day-to-day life, relationships, body, mind, and energy) as suffering in the sense of *dukkha* is the first step in the process toward healing and thriving. It is important to remember that the word *dukkha* is meant to describe human unease, unsatisfactoriness, and discomfort as applicable to all tangible layers of self or consciousness. As such, suffering as defined by the word *dukkha* does not have a single translation in English. Pain may mostly refer to *dukkha* manifested in the body; sorrow and distress may reference *dukkha* in the mind; struggle or pressure may best describe *dukkha* in our vital layer of being. Strained breathing rhythms, overbreathing, gasping or dysregulated breath texture, reverse breathing, and any other forms of "disordered" breathing are all signs and symptoms of pain, distress, or struggle. Breath is a profoundly helpful feedback mechanism about the disturbance of the organism and, as such, a wonderful portal into healing. Assessment of breathing and all related aspects of functioning is an important and integral aspect of this first step in working with patients. This topic deserves great attention and is covered in Chap. 6.

5.4.2 Step 2—Etiology: Understanding Causes and Conditions

Once extant pain and unsatisfactoriness, as expressed in breathing challenges and related aspects of functioning, have been identified and defined, the second step toward healing and thriving via more wholesome breathing begins. This next step is to understand the factors that contribute to and maintain identified suffering (i.e., proximal and distal causes; *samudaya* or *hetu*). The exploration of a client's presenting concerns is always grounded in a greater context that considers many potential influences on breath, health, and thriving. This context is explored most comprehensively via four factors of influence, namely, biological, psychological, social-sociological, and cultural-familial, abbreviated as *biopsychosociocultural* [7, 14]. These factors of influence affect clients' approaches to life; perceptions of self, medical and mental health histories; and their greater collective grounding in cultural, familial, and social matrices that shaped their way of being in the world and in relationships—even the way they breathe. Suffering, pain, friction, stress, sorrow, diagnoses, discontent, or challenges develop in our patients' biopsychosociocultural context and interpersonal matrix. Our context and embeddedness in the community influence development, life trajectory, and health as well as the unfolding of our koshas. This biopsychosociocultural developmental context, however, is often buried in implicit memories and unconscious affective, emotional, mental, and relational patterns and habits.

The biopsychosociocultural paradigm invites breathing guides to gain an in-depth understanding of clients' webs of relationships and connections. The roots of presenting concerns (and all life experiences, of course) are always relational and contextual. Thus, it is crucial to understand biopsychosociocultural contexts that have had and continue to have a bearing on clients, development, experience, and way of breathing. Relationships and biopsychosociocultural contexts are ever-emerging, always changing, and in flux—adding complexity, ambiguity,

BIO		PSYCHO
Biological Influences	**Intersection of Bio-Psycho**	**Psychological Influences**
o genetics		o temperament
o physical disabilities		o personality
o developmental issues	**Behavioral Health**	o self-identity
o health issues	o nutritional choices	o resilience and coping
o accidents and injuries	o exercise	o affect and emotion
o nutritional status	o sleep hygiene	o cognitive style
o sleep quality	o hydration	o learning styles
o medications	o addiction	o intellectual capacity
o medical family history	o time in nature	o executive functioning

	Public Health	**Familial Health**	
Intersection of Socio-Bio	o access to healthcare	o family dynamics	**Intersection of Psycho-Cultural**
	o access to health education	o family structure	
	o access to insurance	o family process	
	o food insecurity and quality	o family communication	
	o air and noise pollution	o family competence	
	o access to nature	o family affect	
	o environmental safety	o family values and myths	

o affordable, safe housing	o oppression or bias	o group memberships
o neighborhood safety	o discrimination	o values, ethics, and morals
o educational access/quality	o microaggression	o prejudice, stereotypes
o educational opportunity	o intergenerational trauma	o choices and options
o employment, career, work	o privilege, supremacy	o religion and spirituality
o socioeconomic equity	o gentrification	o language, speech, symbols
o political systems		o historical trauma
o social support networks	**Sociocultural Health**	o customs, rituals, standards
o legal structures/equity		o dress, style, appearance
o crime exposure/definition		o expectations and openness
	Intersection of	
Social and Societal Influences	**Socio-Cultural**	**Cultural Influences**
SOCIO		**CULTURAL**

Fig. 5.1 Biopsychosociocultural influences on well-being and development

uncertainty, and volatility to our understanding of clients. However, this ever-evolving context or matrix also represents hope—the fact that the biopsychosociocultural context can change directly signals that change is also possible in the individual. Healing and thriving rely on the fluidity of context and influences. Understanding our patients' and our own context allows us to change it or to emphasize and draw on different aspects of it. It invites us to find new communities, new relationships, and new ways of co-regulating and living. The Fig. 5.1 details the four biopsychosociocultural factors individually as well as their cross-sections. It is important to understand that the figure is simply offered for ease of communication. In actuality, these factors coexist, influence each other, co-arise, and interact deeply and profoundly—they are connected.

The four factors and their intersections/interrelationships provide clinicians with a roadmap for exploring clients' contexts for breathwork—both in the sense of understanding their current symptoms and devising healing plans. Information from clients' biopsychosociocultural contexts guides clinicians toward a deeper understanding of the developmental level (or primary kosha) and factors that contribute to clients' presentation and trajectory. With this information, clients can be understood in the context of habitual neurological platforms (based on polyvagal theory:

perceptions of life as safe, dangerous, or threatening), affective predispositions (inclined toward attachment, aversion, ego, fear, or confusion), and mental preoccupations (e.g., with the past, future, relationships, circumstances), and more. They help determine the distal and proximal causes of the presenting concerns and provide a context for exploring how to set individualized and tailored goals with each individual client. Once presenting concerns and biopsychosociocultural etiologies (as shapers of neural platforms, affective and arousal patterns, habitual thoughts and emotions, and behavioral and relational pattern locks or habits) have been explored, the determination of possible goals and outcomes for breathwork becomes possible.

5.4.3 Step 3—Prognosis and Goal-Setting: Kindling Hope and Setting Goals

Together, client and breathing guides use their insights about presenting concerns and possible underlying or contributing causes and conditions identified in Steps 1 and 2 to develop a roadmap for change, including the determination of possible outcomes and the establishment of hope and motivation. As Buddhism, yoga, and science reassure us, while there will always be pain and challenges in a human being's life, suffering can end and transform. This transformation can be facilitated in the context of many different healthcare and allied healthcare professions, including breathwork and therapeutic yoga. Each of these modalities differs; it is important for patients and healthcare providers to be clear and hopeful about progress that is possible and to define desired aims or goals in a manner tailored to each individual patient. In medicine or mental health, this process of discernment may be referred to as prognosis and goal-setting. In yoga classes, this understanding between student and teacher may be best referred to as clarity for the aims of the shared class; for breathwork and therapeutic yoga, this understanding may include specific health, mental health, behavioral health, or lifestyle-related goals.

Relying on assessment data (see Chap. 6) collected for Steps 1 and 2, Step 3 helps care providers understand how forces and contexts in clients' lives predispose them to suffering, what experience may have precipitated breathing challenges, and what factors serve to perpetuate unhelpful and unhealthful ways of breathing, and influences may serve to protect respiratory well-being and health, getting in the way of resilience and equanimity. A definition of these four factors of influence is provided in Table 5.4. These factors interact with one another and with influences that can further mediate or moderate experiences, perceptions, and sufferings of the individual and his or her collective.

Different clients have differing needs, experience unique life circumstances, are embedded in particular webs of relationships, exist in idiosyncratic biopsychosociocultural contexts, define different goals, and desire specific outcomes. Understanding how these various factors combine and function to predispose the patient to difficulties, how they may have triggered current symptoms or the decision to seek help with breathing, how they perpetuate detrimental breathing or behavioral patterns, and how they may be useful in becoming protective for the patient is crucial to

Table 5.4 Four Ps—predisposing, precipitating, perpetuating, and protective factors

Factor	Definition	Breathing-related examples
Predisposing factors	Factors present chronically or for an extended period that increases the likelihood an individual may experience the world in a particular manner, may develop a specific personal style, may have a certain way of relating to others, may experience suffering, or may develop certain symptoms	*Biological*: chronic respiratory disease, food sensitivities, environmental allergies *Psychological*: emotional difficulties, underdeveloped coping capacity, lack of self-compassion, pessimistic mental set *Social/sociological*: racial discrimination, oppression, poverty, food insecurity, stressful work environment *Cultural/familial*: complex trauma, beliefs about breathing, stigma about seeking help *Environmental*: exposure to toxins, lack of clean air
Precipitating factors	Factors that trigger acute suffering *or* impel the individual to take an action (including seeking help); these factors arise acutely, suddenly, unexpectedly, or intermittently—they are triggers that exceed current coping resources	*Biological*: sudden illness (e.g., COVID-19), exposure to a respiratory toxin, accident or injury, rape *Psychological*: unexpected event or stressor that exceeds coping resources, unexpected threat to self-identity or self-confidence *Social/sociological*: sudden job loss, unexpected lawsuit, incident of discrimination *Cultural/familial*: sudden family move, unexpected parental divorce, sudden loss of faith, a profound encounter of prejudice *Environmental*: earthquake, natural disaster, outbreak of war
Perpetuating factors	Factors that maintain challenges or positive traits—manifesting as vicious or virtuous cycles; patterns that often started because they helped the client cope with a difficult situation (i.e., once served a self-protective purpose) but have now become reactive and less functional	*Biological*: poor eating habits, non-avoidance of known allergens, high-risk behaviors leading to frequent injury *Psychological*: affective reactivity, negative attitude about behavior change, rigid mental sets, unwillingness to change *Social/sociological*: uninterested in education, staying in a destructive employment situation, rejecting social supports *Cultural/familial*: choosing a perpetual caretaker role, engaging in destructive behaviors toward others, embracing prejudice *Environmental*: never seeking out nature
Protective factors	Factors that bolster the individual against stress, contributing to resilience and coping capacity; strengths clients can bring to bear on their suffering; available resources and supports (often overlooked)	*Biological*: healthful lifestyle, well-nourished, generally healthy respiratory system, strong muscles, good sleep hygiene *Psychological*: positive attitude, history of resilient coping, self-efficacy, motivation for change *Social/sociological*: sound employment, strong educational resources, health insurance *Cultural/familial*: strong community, supportive family, life purpose, no stigma related to seeking help *Environmental*: access to nature, clean air, and environment

completing Step 3. Specifically, for each client, we explore which changes could enhance their breathing and general functioning. We consider their unique presentation and circumstances and the influences that created and perpetuated them. We share our insight gently and with discernment with the patient to collaborate on creating hope and motivation for change, drawing on existing strengths and resources. Once areas of possible respiratory change, healing, and thriving are identified, goals and objectives are defined that move clients toward transformation and away from suffering. By working together, clinicians and patients use this understanding to identify realistic goals for joint breathwork, as well as to address goals that may require referral to or collaboration with other types of healthcare providers. The goals for the joint work naturally define the healing path that is deemed most patient-centered.

5.4.4 Step 4—Intervention: Embarking to the Healing Path

After goals for breathwork have been determined based on shared clarity about presenting concerns, contributing influences, and desired goals, the plan for creating respiratory thriving or healing is implemented. Healing pathways toward wholesome breathing are hardly ever straight—they can be adapted and blended based on developments and evolutions that emerge as breathwork progresses. Yet, pathways offer a direction that decreases the possibility that breathwork proceeds without a roadmap or a clear intention.

Ancient traditions and modern science of breathwork (as a part of the eight limbs of yoga) provide a toolbox and strategies for building respiratory resilience and thriving. These strategies address all layers of experience. They honor and address the causes of identified breathing challenges. They move clients toward the goals enumerated for their breathwork. Choosing optimal breathing and related strategies results in an action plan that is tailored to individual needs and utilizes a full array of strategies—not simply breathwork in isolation. As noted, the path will likely include appropriate referrals and collaborations with other healthcare professionals to ensure that breathing instructors remain within their professional scope of practice and code of ethics, especially if there are breathing challenges whose causes are rooted in physical or psychological illness.

Breathwork from the integrated holistic perspective does not simply include breathing practices per se. It may include movement and postural intervention; it may draw on contemplative practices and mindfulness to work with one's mind and emotions to transcend unhelpful thought patterns and transform beliefs, attitudes, and opinions. In fact, how clients breathe and move is even informed by their ethical (such as truthfulness and non-harming), compassionate (such as gratitude and non-judgment), and lifestyle-based (such as harmful or salutary behaviors and communities) relationships with their body, vitality, and mind. Breathwork also explores and works with how patients engage with all of these practices to express their greater purposes with discipline and commitment. How various interventions are combined and developed is an important part of the individualization of person-centered and adaptive breathwork. It brings to bear the power of the four-step conceptualization model by offering clients an integrated holistic breathing practice that feels authentic and meaningful, honors the complexity of their experiences and context, and is embedded in an interpersonally therapeutic context of deep caring, comprehensive understanding, and compassionate intention. The implementation of the healing path is carefully sequenced and developed honoring each patient's needs. Fortunately, there are a few principles that can help us develop the best possible path for and with each client—principles for *sequencing* the therapeutics we offer to our patients.

5.5   Sequencing of Integrated Holistic Breathwork

The four-step model foreshadows that breathing practices do not unfold randomly, but are constructed and implemented with great care and discernment—tailored and individual to each person who breathes. Understanding *why* we or our clients breathe *how* we or they breathe matters; it makes a difference in how breath shows up biomechanically, biochemically, psychologically, emotionally, and mentally. It affects us on the macrolevel in terms of overall health and well-being, including the capacity to maintain a sense of safety and to stay connected in relationships. It affects us on the microlevel, including breath efficiency, optimization of gas exchange, and production of energy. Breathwork is rooted in science and ancient wisdom about how to breathe, when to alter the breath, and why to breathe in different ways to meet specific situation demands or to reach particular goals or intentions. The structure of breathwork is an art firmly grounded in science. As outlined above, breathwork honors integrated holistic principles and creates an individualized framework for each student or client that honors their context, needs, and layers of self. Basic structures for how to sequence breathwork across time and within each session are extremely useful. These structures are integrated with other approaches, including movement practices, meditation, lifestyle changes and commitments, medical care, occupational therapy, physical therapy, and mental health treatment.

   To create optimally sequenced structures, it helps to recall a few important points about breathwork. Some breathing practices free the breath to create access to the natural flow of breath that results in optimally functional patterns for daily life. These practices help us become aware of our breathing so that we may develop a default or spontaneous breathing pattern that serves our biomechanics, biochemistry, psychology, and cognition. Once awareness has been achieved, attention can begin to shift to altering the breath as needed. A great start is the exploration of how patients may develop breathing rhythms that are aligned with optimal functional daily breathing. Once clients know how to begin to regulate their breath, without constraining or overefforting, more demanding breathing practices can be introduced that are tailored to students' specific needs and challenges. Once tailored practices have begun to help clients reshape their breathing, they may be ready (although this is not necessary) for breathing practices that are deliberately stressful to create enhanced resilience.

Stressful breathing practices create challenging breathing patterns for short periods to increase resilience and awareness of the highly variable impacts of the breath on anatomy, physiology, autonomic nervous system responses, mind, emotions, and psychology. They challenge us to realize that our nervous system can dysregulate with certain types of breathing and help us notice that, as long as we consciously breathe in ways that allow for recovery, our nervous system can also naturally re-regulate themselves after a stressful event. They are designed to help us understand our breathing better so that we can remain resilient under stress. They are practices of hormesis. Not every client needs or benefits from these practices although they have become quite common in certain circles. Careful sequencing of breathing practices considers the needs of each individual in offering intentional and holistic practices that are non-harming, truthful, necessary, compassionate, beneficial, and appropriate to context and circumstances.

What Is Hormesis?
Our bodies have the amazing capacity to bounce back from exposures to exertion, fasting, stress, toxins, extreme temperature, and even short bouts of oxygen deprivation with extra resilience, compensating for and even improving on the temporary challenge or damage that was caused by such exposure. Vaccines are a great example of medical hormesis: minute exposure to a potentially harmful virus results in the body's creation of antibodies to provide resilience against future exposure. Daily life examples include cold showers that create temporary challenges to body temperature to increase cardiovascular health and immune functioning; intermittent fasting to stimulate the use of fat and protein reserves, ultimately increasing longevity, cognitive function, and cellular health; or strength training that results in minor tears in muscle tissue that lead to stronger, more resilient muscles.

Forceful breathing, breath holds, and other challenging breathing practices operate on the same principle of stressing the body to invite a self-protective response that results in improved health. Through forceful breathing or strong breath holds, we stress the nervous system and challenge the lungs to operate outside of their typical parameters. We can then observe our nervous system reregulate and gain better autonomic control of our breathing, such as resetting CO_2 sensitivity in the medulla or breaking the conditioned stimulus-response cycles between increased breath rate and panic or even asthma attacks.

5.5.1   Sequencing of Breathwork Across Time

Breathing practices can be offered as a way to help clients and students become specialists or experts of their own breath across time. They enable clients to become discerning about how to breathe and how to adjust the breath for an auspicious way of being in their bodies, relationships, and communities. Breathwork ideally proceeds through several stages across time (i.e., multiple sessions) based on proper preparations, assessments, and motivations (assessment and motivation are covered in Chap. 6). This progression slowly moves us or our clients through breathing practices in a manner that makes ample space for new learning, unlearning, and relearning—neither going too fast nor too slow in changing breathing. This progression allows for collaboration between teachers and students to build increasingly tailored breathing practices as students develop increasing interoception, proprioception, exteroception, and neuroception to have a better sense of what does and does not serve the body, energy, mind, psyche, emotions, and relationships. Thinking of breathwork as unfolding deliberately and thoughtfully across time increases the likelihood of clients' success, sustained motivation, self-determination, personal agency, and empowerment. Commensurately, it decreases the risk of harm being done in any of the layers of experience.

The model of sequencing across time summarized in the table below does not necessarily unfold exactly in this manner for each student. As explored in Chap. 6, assessment and motivation help guide students and clinicians to the most appropriate starting point in the sequence. For example, clients who have had long-standing self-awareness (e.g., meditation) practices may be ready to jump directly into exploring optimal functional breathing. Others who have been engaging in stressful breathing practices may need to be guided back to basic awareness. The sequencing framework is useful for group classes in which individualization is more difficult. It offers a sequence that is accessible to most, if not all, clients or students—everyone can start again at the beginning. Breath awareness is useful even for experienced students, inviting everyone to participate in each practice with a beginner's mind. In individualized work, it is possible to be more selective and discerning. However, even in an individual context, especially if there is still some uncertainty and a need for more assessment, this sequencing is unlikely to cause harm. Table 5.5 provides an overview of the carefully sequenced, progressive approach, each step of which is explored in detail in the applied breathwork chapters that follow.

5.5.2   Sequencing of Breathwork Within Single Sessions

Just as it is important to understand that breathing practices unfold with intention and purpose across time (i.e., across sessions), it is crucial to note that each breathing session optimally unfolds in a predictable flow. Consistent sequencing within any given session creates predictability for clients and contributes to the sense of safety and holding environment created in the client-clinician or student-teacher relationship. While many possible ways to sequence consistently exist, one approach is offered here. Individual breathing instructors may differ in how they create predictability, and not all may follow the offered outline exactly. The main takeaway is

Table 5.5 Overview of wholesome breathwork sequencing across time

Breathing practices can be presented as a way to help clients become experts of their own breath, able to begin to use discernment about how to breathe and how to adjust the breath for an optimal way of being in their body, mind, relationships, and world. Over time, as clients move from being beginners to more advanced breathers, breathwork ideally proceeds through the following progression:

Preliminary steps
- Assessment—knowing from whence we start
- Psychoeducation—knowing the reasons for what we do
- Preparation in all koshas—feeling wholeheartedly motivated to engage with the practice

Breath attunement on the mat/in the office and in daily life
- Development of breath observation skills: learning to read breath patterns and nature
- Development of breath awareness: learning to read nervous system signals and subtle energies

Cultivation of healthy daily breathing
- Optimal functional breathing—slowly, lightly, quietly, nasally, and diaphragmatically
- Avoidance of stress apnea (including email apnea—the tendency to hold the breath while emailing)—noticing when our breath stops and when overbreathing starts while under challenge and using more wholesome breathing strategies
- Attention to nighttime breathing patterns—learn how we breathe while asleep
- Avoidance of sleep problems—using strategies for improved night-time breathing, including the consideration of mouth taping to support nasal breath and to prevent or heal sleep apnea

Basic breathing exercises
- Practice of targeted breathing strategies to develop resilient and coherent breathing via exercises with intention and clarity, including:
- Subtle breathing
- Breathing with mindfulness of the phases of the breath
- Alternate nostril breathing

Advanced and tailored breathing exercises
- Application of breathing exercises tailored to specific intentions and needs:
- Breathing with sound
- Breathing with force

All breathing practices are offered with a multitude of variations; those consistently encouraged include:
- Coordination of breath with movement, emphasizing the union of breath and movement during practice and in daily life for wholesome functional breathing
- Tailoring of breathwork for calming, energizing, or balancing, inviting optimal autonomic nervous system function based on client needs to encourage breath coherence and resilience
- Applications of breathwork in daily life, providing hints and tips about how to use specific breathing practices to support ventral vagal resilience and coherence off the mat

to create a consistent, intentional, and predictable framework that creates a structure and relationship of safety for clinicians and clients and for teachers and students.

In the offered within-session sequencing model, each breathing session begins with a ritual that reminds clients of the safety that has been created in the environment and relationship with the clinician. Each session consciously (re)invites motivation or purpose in the form of deliberate intention-setting at the outset of practice.

The clinician arrives with an intention; the client is invited to set an intention. Once contextual safety has been (re)created and motivation is present, the work moves into physical and mental preparation. Asanas and movements are offered in specifically designed ways that prepare practitioners for breathing practices to come. That said, breath awareness, breath observation, and functional breathing can be great ways to *start* any intervention, especially with students or clients in the context of therapeutic healthcare (non-yoga-based) settings. Breath awareness is followed by movement that is specifically preparatory for the tailored breathing practices to be offered (e.g., alternate nostril breathing or equal breathing) and that engages optimal functional breathing during physical exertion and preparation. Physical practices include movements to create rib basket resilience, core recruitment to support breathing, openness of chest musculature, and attunement to the rhythmic relationship between body and energy.

Once physically prepared, the session can move students into specific breathing practices. Cuing of breathing overall and specific breathing practices honor breath anatomy, physiology, and nervous system impacts, along with addressing subtle energy experiences from yoga or other contemplative traditions. The session can end with contemplation and resting in silence to integrate experiences, absorb new learning, and invite conscious reflection and introspection, creating the opportunity to realize and dedicate the personal and collective merit that arose from the practice.

The process of integrating breathing into a greater practice context is key throughout any session. It is important to remember that even when we begin to discuss each individual breathing practice separately (Chaps. 8 and 9), they are rarely taught in isolation. They are most effectively and beneficially taught, practiced, and explored, embedded in the greater context and sequencing offered by a skilled breathwork clinician. Proper sequencing integrates motivation and intention, attention to all eight limbs of yoga (or equivalent), and the development of an arc that reflects the integrative nature and purpose of a complete breathwork session. Integration of diverse practices and greater purpose results in a class of balance, beauty, and joy. In demonstrating, observing, and assisting, clinicians pay attention to these principles—embodying them in demonstrations, searching for them in observation, giving feedback about them in response to observation, and using them to assist, vary, modify, and (yes, even) correct themselves and their clients.

Thoughtful within-session sequencing creates an arc that moves toward a specific (or multiple) breathing practice(s), allowing the sequence to provide meaning and purpose in all layers of experience. Such an integrated, sequenced class may unfold via the steps shown in Table 5.6 that follow.

Table 5.6 Careful sequencing of an individual breathwork session

1. Opening centering and/or conditioned stimulus for mindfulness (e.g., verbal welcome, opening bell, shared breath)
2. Opening comments
   - Setting the stage if new students are present
   - Introduce props that may be needed
3. Presentation of the motivation or intention for the class
   - Grounded in an explicit aspect of yoga philosophy, yoga psychology, and/or science
   - Carried through the rest of the class—explicitly and/or implicitly
   - If a multi-class sequence, refer back and tie to prior sessions
4. Centering practice
   - Coming into the moment and space
   - Connecting to all koshas
5. Intention setting for the students (sankalpa)
6. Breath attunement practice
   - Inviting observation, attention, or awareness
7. Preparatory form and movement practice
   - Warm-up for the body
   - Preparatory asana and movement for the specifically-chosen *pranayama*, such as:
     - Removing nasal obstruction
     - Tongue strengthening
     - Recruiting the core
     - Resilience in the rib basket
     - Releasing neck and shoulders
8. Specific *pranayama* practice(s)
   - Breath preparation as needed
   - Introducing a specific breathing practice with clear instructions and demonstrations
   - Practicing the specific breathing practice(s)
   - Debrief, refine, and repeat as often as needed and possible
9. Reflective practices
   - Resting/relaxation posture
   - Guided meditation or concentration
   - Touch on body, breath, mind, intuition, bliss
   - Silence (length determined by perceived needs and risks presented by students)
   - Intentional reentry (e.g., return to senses, return to koshas, transition to a seat)
10. Closing comments
    - Tie back to the class and personal motivation or intention
    - Link breathing practice on the mat to breathing in daily life and/or
    - Integrated positive new learning or experience
    - Invite dedication of merit
11. Expression of gratitude

5.6   Where We Go from Here

The exploration of the principles of integrated holistic breathwork, the model for conceptualizing how breath develops and can be healed, and the commitment to discerning sequencing and environmental preparation has readied us for the pragmatic aspects of working with students and clients (or for devising personal self-care practices). The comprehensive understanding of breathwork suggests that the next in the process is assessment. Assessment is crucial to all steps: in Step 1, to defining the breathing-related challenges; in Step 2, to discerning etiological factors; in Step 3, to developing realistic and tailored goals for the work; and in Step 4, to assessing the success of the implementation of breathwork in the context of integrated holistic healthcare, mental healthcare, and/or therapeutic yoga settings. Assessment is necessary to understand the kinds of challenges patients bring along, how their suffering came about, how to set goals and choose interventions; and how to introduce breathwork in a tailored and carefully sequenced manner. Assessment guides the way into the specifics of whether to develop intervention plans around change mechanisms related to breath anatomy, physiology, psychology, or (as in most cases) a carefully sequenced integration of all, leading to tailored and patient-centered approaches to breathwork.

> *No matter what we eat, how much we exercise,*
> *how resilient our genes are, how skinny or young or wise we are –*
> *none of it will matter unless we're breathing correctly.*—James Nestor in Breath

References

1. Bondy D. Yoga for everyone: 50 poses for every type of body. Dorling Kindersley; 2019.
2. Heyman J. The teacher's guide to accessible yoga. Rainbow Mind; 2024.
3. Heyman J. Yoga revolution: building a practice of courage and compassion. Shambhala; 2021.
4. Johnson MC. We heal together: rituals and practices for building community and connection. Shambhala; 2023.
5. Johnson MC. Skill in action: radicalizing your yoga practice to create a just world. Shambhala; 2021.
6. Stanley J. Every body yoga. Workman; 2017.
7. Brems C, Rasmussen CH. A comprehensive guide to child psychotherapy and counseling. 4th ed. Waveland; 2019.
8. Brems C. Yoga for mental health: cultivating emotional resilience and mental fortitude. Self-published; 2024.
9. Porges S. The pocket guide to the polyvagal theory: the transformative power of feeling safe. Norton; 2017.
10. Wilber K. Integral psychology. Shambhala; 2000.
11. Wilber K. Integral meditation: mindfulness as a path to grow up, wake up, and show up in your life. Shambhala; 2016.
12. Mingyur Rinpoche Y, Swanson E. Joyful wisdom. Three Rivers Press; 2009.
13. Boccio FJ. Mindfulness yoga: the awakened union of breath, body, and mind. Wisdom Publications; 1993.
14. Brems C. Refinement of a multi-dimensional data collection tool for assessment, treatment planning, and outcomes tracking. Paper presented at: Symposium on Yoga Therapy and Yoga Research; 2019 June; Newport Beach, CA.

Motivation and Assessment for Breathwork

6

Maybe you are searching among the branches for what only appears at the roots.

Rumi

6.1   Overview: Clarifying the Importance of Breathwork

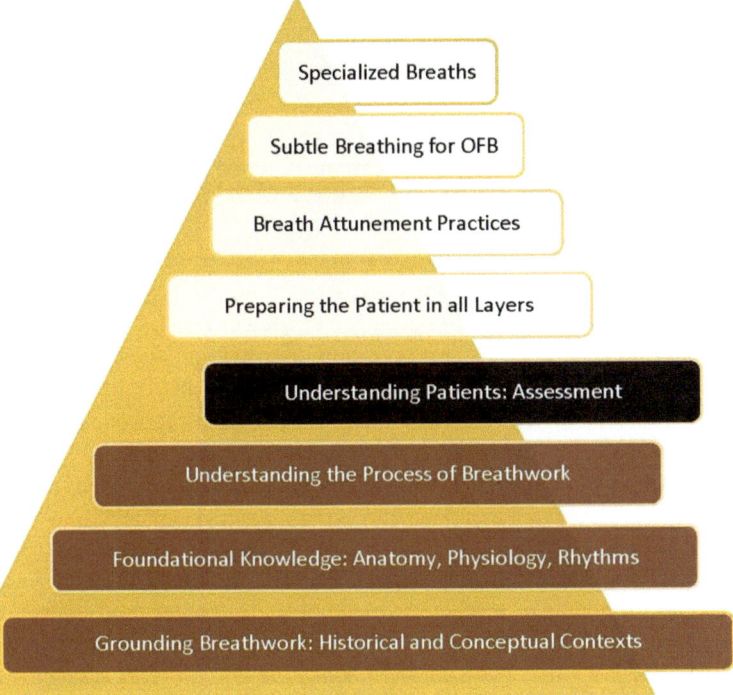

Specialized Breaths

Subtle Breathing for OFB

Breath Attunement Practices

Preparing the Patient in all Layers

Understanding Patients: Assessment

Understanding the Process of Breathwork

Foundational Knowledge: Anatomy, Physiology, Rhythms

Grounding Breathwork: Historical and Conceptual Contexts

C. Brems, *Therapeutic Breathwork*,
https://doi.org/10.1007/978-3-031-66683-4_6

When clients seek out breathwork, they typically present a specific concern that has motivated them to seek assistance. When the acuity of symptoms is high, motivation to start breathwork may peak. However, regardless of acuity of symptoms, it is helpful to address motivation and set goals with patients at the outset of breathwork to help them appreciate possible gains from breathwork that may reach beyond resolution of initial symptoms that prompted them to seek help. Thus, it is helpful to review possible benefits of breathing healthfully with patients and to work collaboratively with them to create intentional goals for taking offered breathing and supportive practices beyond the clinical (or yoga) context into daily life. Motivation is greatly supported by an understanding of how breath and related physical and psychological factors manifest. Thus, breathwork is well served by a careful assessment with clients that can help them begin to appreciate how their breath functions currently and what kind of changes, enhancements, and optimizations may be possible with disciplined practice.

This chapter lays the foundation for enhancing and clarifying motivations—essentially greatly supporting the goal setting that happens as part of conceptualizing breathwork (as outlined in Chap. 5). This chapter offers a thorough framework for assessment (to facilitate Steps 1 and 2 in the conceptualization process), necessary to clarify the etiology of symptoms and challenges, to set realistic goals for breathwork, and to commit to a path toward resilient and coherent breathing via a specific individualized plan for intervention (Step 4 in the conceptual model). Careful assessment defines the path toward healing and thriving, guiding clinicians toward appropriate strategies that address the specific biomechanical, biochemical, psychological, and nervous system-related symptoms and etiologies presented by the patient.

6.2   Psychoeducation to Increase Motivation to Change

Modern science, practice of yoga, and many wisdom traditions provide ample evidence that insightful, tailored, and clear goal setting leads to purposeful action—initially on our own behalf, but ultimately for the greater good. Discipline, introspection, and commitment to a greater purpose help us create a cohesive change-embracing motivational set that inspires our life plans (or goals) and trajectories and moves us toward greater awareness, compassion, insight, and capable action. Drawing on modern science, we can integrate the yogic work of discipline, introspection, and creation of purpose with the modern clinical approach of motivational interviewing [1].

Motivational interviewing is a method of supporting clients, students, or ourselves in finding inner, self-inspired reasons for wanting to embark on a journey into healing. As clinicians or teachers, we do not impose outer motivations or standards for students or clients, but instead help guide them to an introspective and self-directed awareness that leads to the *intrinsic desire to create changes* that support the amelioration of suffering in all layers of consciousness—often starting one small goal or step at a time. Teachers or clinicians serve as sounding boards or empathic others who provide information to increase knowledge and ask honest questions to invite self-inquiry (or *svadhyaya* in Sanskrit). The most successful clinicians, including the most effective breathing instructors, refrain from giving advice or commands, instead offering information, options, variations, and choices; they offer opportunities for students to listen inward to become self-directive while feeling heard and acknowledged.

Relationships between teachers and students collaborating on breathwork are therefore *client-centered*, that is, clients' needs and resources are primary and direct the pedagogy, cues, and encouragements used by clinicians to help students enter the healing path with commitment and open-heartedness. Teachers express genuine caring for students and clearly prioritize students' perspectives, experiences, and values. In other words, teachers or clinicians encourage clients to find their own path to healing and toward a personal *raison d'etre*. Teachers have and likely radiate their own values, ethics, convictions, and commitments; however, they do not impose these views, perspectives, practices, or experiences on students. Instead, we remember that each human being has a unique biopsychosociocultural context and therefore has highly idiosyncratic experiences, needs, and solutions for their challenges.

That said, helping students develop motivation to embark on a healing path means encouraging change and transformation—by definition. As teachers, we invite students to develop a committed practice and set of goals that can relieve suffering and invite healing. This process requires discipline (*tapas* in Sanskrit) and clarity (*saucha* in Sanskrit). Students seek healthcare, yoga, and breathwork for a reason; teachers or clinicians help them develop commitment, engagement, and contentment (*santosha*) to persevere. In motivational interviewing, encouragement of clients by clinicians is framed as *directiveness without imposing specific goals, choices, or practices*. The power of choice lies with our clients; we make offerings of knowledge and curiosity and empower them to decide. An important aspect of students' self-inquiry (or *svadhyaya*) is finding a teacher and the thirst for new learning via readings, based on scientific and wisdom resources. It is a legitimate role of teachers to share knowledge and wisdom and to share principles, practices, and science about breathing. Once information has been shared, it is up to students or clients to resolve any ambivalence about making changes, to make the most affirming treatment and lifestyle choices, and to be discerning in intention, thought, speech, and action.

Achieving motivational goals together means that student and teacher, client and clinician, are in a caring relationship with one another. This relationship is grounded in trust, respect, compassion, caring, and kindness (all the traits that were outlined as crucial to wholesome breathwork in Chap. 5). It is a relationship of open and honest communication that invites clients into their own experience and into an honest relationship with their own bodies, affects and vitality, thoughts and emotions, actions, and relationships. The *relationship and communication between care providers and clients* are such that they invite clients to ponder for themselves (within a relational context of profound compassion and support) how they are suffering and the causes and consequences of this suffering; what they might want to change based on how they come to understand the causes of their suffering; why there is cause for hope and optimism that change and transformation of suffering are possible; and what may be their therapeutic intentions and goals.

As discussed in detail in Chap. 5, these four aspects of communication (recognizing suffering, its roots, and its effects; attuning to advantages of creating change; kindling hope and confidence; setting goals and committing to behavior change via a path toward healing) are ancient yogic and modern clinical practices at their very heart. They are *central definitions of change talk in motivational interviewing*, grounded in a strong evidence base. They are central lifestyle commitments in the yogic limb of disciplined practices called *niyamas*. Table 6.1 explores the alignment of motivational interviewing and yogic wisdom.

Clearly, it is in the spirit of yoga overall, and breathwork in particular, to help students and clients develop motivation. How providers speak to clients can be crucial to the development of a positive and healing relationship and creation of an environment that invites a sense of safety, respect, and accessibility. Teachers invite students to explore their suffering (without overwhelming them), to access their desire to create healing and transformation, to develop hope about change and a different way of being in life and relationships, and to set specific goals for a healing path. As practitioners, we have to do this for ourselves, perhaps based on reading and learning in ways other than with a teacher. Either way, the process necessitates *knowing why* we want to try to heal ourselves, how appropriate goals may be defined, and what types of breathing practices will be useful.

Motivation and direction thus arise from knowledge—from realizing that there are legitimate reasons for creating change. Knowledge about optimal functional breathing leads to motivation to do something, to choose the practice, to make changes to the breath, and to transform how we live in our bodies and move our energy. With regard to *creating knowledge* that guides our commitment to breathwork, we create motivation through learning the anatomy and biomechanics; physiology and biochemistry; functions of the nervous system; and rhythms, patterns, and subtle energies of breath. We learn about the importance of nasal breathing and the functions of the nose versus the mouth. We learn about the importance of diaphragmatic breathing and the functions of the diaphragm in collaboration with other muscles and tissues. We begin to recognize symptoms of dysfunctional breathing and consequences of overbreathing (e.g., blood vessel constriction, decreased O_2 exchange at the tissue level, poor health and resilience, anxiety). We understand advantages of optimal functional breathing and its positive downstream effects on health. Armed with information, we - and our clients - can make choices about how and if we want to explore and commit to breathwork practices on the mat and in daily life.

Table 6.2 summarizes essential motivating facts that can support a committed breathing practice. Many more scientific findings that can fuel motivation to change how we breathe were offered in Chaps. 2, 3, and 4 about the science of breathing. It is helpful to share this scientific content and yogic wisdom with clients and students *as motivational resources*. Ongoing study of newly emerging breathing-related science is important as knowledge continuously evolves, changes, and adapts to new circumstances and realities.

Table 6.1 Motivational interviewing and yogic discipline

Change talk in motivational interviewing	Alignment with yogic disciplines in breathwork
• Recognizing disadvantages of the status quo and of causes and conditions for current behaviors, beliefs, ways of being in the world, that lead to challenges	• Exploring the disadvantages of current breath patterns via self-reflection and self-inquiry (*svadhyaya*), grounded in contentment and balance (*santosha*)
• Appreciating advantages of change, by envisioning what could be different; exploring what shifts are possible, desirable, and important	• Diving into breath self-assessment with an open-heart and the recognition that help from teachers and teachings may be supportive (*svadhyaya*)
• Developing optimism about changes, sensing into the possibilities of what is possible to create a more healthful and satisfying life (e.g., breath)	• Lighting a fire of hope (*tapas*) for a new way of breathing, that is different and clears space for a less conflictual relationship with our breath (*saucha*)
• Becoming clear about new intentions, goals, and purpose committing to the intention to change outlining a path [1]	• Setting breathing goals—Step by step—To move toward better breath and overall health with commitment and purpose (*ishvara pranidhana*)

6.3 Assessment and Self-Awareness to Increase Motivation to Change

Despite its importance, abstract knowledge is hardly ever sufficient. Motivation and commitment to a healing path also depend on self-awareness—on the recognition that current behaviors or actions may or may not align optimally with healthful living. We need to assess honestly and openly who we are, how we function, and what we can aspire to. Self-awareness is key for clinicians and clients. There needs to be a shared understanding of symptoms, etiologies, goals, and commensurate strategies to created change. Change is tailored to patient needs and plots a clear course toward better health and well-being—including toward increasingly optimal, coherent, and functional breathing. Thus, in addition to enhancing knowledge, it draws students, clients, and ourselves into *assessment to create awareness* of current breath and breathing challenges as well as possible goals related to how breathing might evolve auspiciously. With knowledge *and* awareness, commitment to change and an ongoing practice path become truly meaningful, intentional, and sustainable.

The assessment (or, in the case of a first session, the intake) process can be a formal interview with a client or student (or a self-check-in) to make a conscious assessment of breathing characteristics, respiratory health, and breathing-related challenges. Alternatively, and perhaps depending on context, assessment can consist of self-administered questionnaires that collect relevant information from students, clients, or ourselves for the purpose of drawing attention to important and relevant behaviors and experiences related to breathing and goal setting. It is beyond this book to describe a complete clinical intake or assessment process; our interest here is specific to assessment of breath and breathing. In that context, assessment focuses on several issues, all related to the science presented in Chaps. 2, 3, and 4, that is,

Table 6.2 Motivating facts about optimal functional breathing

• Enhanced well-being and greater sense of calm and equanimity	• Greater overall health
• Decreased perceptions of stress	• Enhanced sleep and ability to rest and restore
• Decreases in anxiety and panic	• Carefully calibrated CO_2 levels leading to efficient respiration
• Enhanced autonomic nervous system functioning with greater access to adaptive cycling between sympathetic and parasympathetic arousal	• Enhanced cardiovascular and pulmonary functioning—e.g., increased heart rate variability, lowered blood pressure, enhanced vasodilation, greater lung efficiency
• Enhanced preparedness to deal with challenge and ability to move into rest, restoration, regeneration, and growth	• Increased exercise tolerance and athletic performance
• Increased brain plasticity, supporting new learning, habits, resilience, and adaptability	• Increased coherence, with all systems working at peak efficiency and in balance with one another

Simply put,
optimal breathing means:
We breathe more healthfully
We feel more resilient and hopeful
We deal with challenges more effectively
We think more rationally and remember more fully
We heal more rapidly and restore more completely
We interact more compassionately and patiently
We exercise more joyfully and effectively
We sleep and rest more soundly
We age more gracefully
We live better

related to anatomy, physiology, rate and rhythm, and characteristics such as texture, sound, location, and resting breaks. To capture all dimensions of breath and breathing, assessment looks at the following dimensions (the science for all of which is provided in Chaps. 2, 3, and 4):

- *Breath anatomy* (i.e., nasal versus oral, diaphragmatic versus chest; posture- and movement-related aspects)
- *Breath physiology* (with focus on the controlled breath pause as a proxy for medullar CO_2 hypersensitivity)
- *Breath rhythms or cadence breath* (i.e., breath rate and volume)
- *Breath characteristics* (i.e., breath locations and spatial distribution, breath textures and sounds, and breath phases)
- *Breathing-related patterns* reflecting state of mind, emotions, and nervous system
- *Breathing-related symptoms* (e.g., apneas, obstructions, labored breathing)

Self-assessment and observation of these breathing variables can be augmented by objective *physical measurements* that may include formal measurement of controlled breath pauses, nasal obstructions, and momentary nostril dominance—all defined in detail below. Standardized questionnaires related to breathing and breathing-related well-being also exist and are referenced below. In using assessments, clinicians and teachers take care to stay within their scope of practice and seek collaborations and referrals with other healthcare professionals as needed. The assessments covered here are generally within the purview of therapeutic yoga practitioners, especially those with healthcare credentials.

Assessment of breath characteristics based on self-awareness of the breath may not be possible early in therapeutic work. It depends on patients' extant capacity for interoception, proprioception, and neuroception. For some individuals, it may take weeks of teaching breath and physical self-awareness before they can truly and in an informed manner answer the questions explored via (self-)assessment. Assessment questions are also an excellent way to monitor treatment progress and outcomes. As patients are increasingly capable of voicing their inner experiences and perceptions, they demonstrate an increase in self-awareness and sensitivity. As such, assessment is never separate from treatment; the two inform and support one another.

Because clients' self-awareness may need to develop over time, clinician observations are very helpful along the way. Care providers may understand a patient's breath rhythm before the individual does. Clinicians may be able to discern changes and progress in breathing patterns, helping clients recognize their own progress and evolution. All assessments detailed in this chapter can thus be inquired about as well as observed. All can be enhanced and supported by, and sometimes even depend on, breath attunement exercises outlined in Chap. 8.

6.3.1   Assessment of Breath Anatomy

Primary features assessed in terms of anatomy relate to differentiating nose versus mouth breathing and diaphragmatic versus chest breathing. Generally, this assessment is relatively observable by the care provider. Clients, however, may be relatively unaware of the degree to which they breathe nasally versus orally and into the chest versus the mid-torso. They may be quite surprised by what they uncover as they begin to become more self-attuned. Assessment can unfold over time with increasing self-awareness and observation, starting in the session with the clinician who can provide helpful insights about how to observe the breath in the here and now. Once clients are relatively self-aware and able to discern how they are breathing anatomically, they can be encouraged to take this self-assessment off the mat and out of the session. As they make observations in daily life, they become increasingly aware of how mouth-versus-nose and chest-versus-abdominal breathing are used in a variety of situations, including during times of rest, time of exertion, times of challenge, while alone, while with others, while exercising, and so on.

Assessment of Nasal Breathing and Nostril Dominance

Most people can quickly and easily discern oral versus nasal breathing, both in the present moment and then increasingly in daily life under a variety of circumstances. It helps to provide guidance about how to begin to make these observations—and it is best to simply ask clients to observe first and to define what needs to change (and how) at a later time. Table 6.3 provides suggestions about how to begin to direct patients' focus on nasal versus oral breathing.

If students are not sure how often they mouth-versus-nose breathe, they can place tape over their lips to prevent themselves from breathing through the mouth to notice if this creates a significant challenge in their breathing. This strategy is a technique for helping clients retrain themselves to nose breathe, and it is addressed in more detail in Chap. 8. Another self-assessment of nasal versus mouth breathing can be made with the help of a small handheld mirror or the screen of a smartphone (turned off). The task is simply to exhale onto the mirror or screen of the turned-off cell phone to obtain a moisture ring (a footprint of the breath). The way to use this assessment is to exhale onto the mirror via the mouth and to make note of the size of the moisture ring. Then, we again exhale onto the mirror, but breathe out via the nose. We can now compare the size of the moisture rings obtained via mouth versus nasal breathing to obtain a visual representation of how much more moisture is lost via the mouth than the nose.

The second way to use this assessment is to assess nostril dominance by comparing moisture rings for the two nostrils. We exhale onto the mirror via the nose again, but only via the right nostril (using a finger to block the left side of the nose). We note the circles of moisture and let the wetness dissipate (or wipe it away). Then, the process is repeated for the left nostril. We can then compare whether one nostril is more blocked than the other by comparing the size of the moisture rings. Alternatively, nostril dominance can be assessed by gently closing one nostril and taking a forceful breath in; this process is then repeated with the other nostril. It will be easy to feel and hear which nostril is more open and which is more restricted by the amount of air that flowed in easily or by the sound of the breath (the more blocked nostril will produce a higher pitch). It is important to recall there are normal variations in nostril dominance; sometimes one side is more blocked than the other. To glean specific information about possible more permanent nostril blockages or

Table 6.3   Nasal breath assessment

Do you breathe mostly through the nose or the mouth?
- Is your mouth dry more often than not?
- Do you wake up with a dry mouth?
- Do you need to drink water at night?
- Do you wake up with a sore throat?
- Does the tongue rest more at the bottom of the mouth or nestle to the roof?
- Is the tongue strong or flaccid?
- Is your mouth open a lot when you talk or laugh?

How do the above observations change, depending on:
- Activity (e.g., during rest, with gentle physical exertion, with cardiovascular workouts, during walking)
- Body position (e.g., standing, walking, sitting, lying down)

How do the above observations change, depending on:
- Mental and emotional state (e.g., when you are confused, mentally taxed, distracted, focused, stressed, sad, anxious, or angry)
- Contextual circumstances (e.g., when you are alone… with a loved one… With boss or someone who is difficult, challenging, …)

preferences, this assessment is repeated several times a day for several days. If natural variation is present, this is not a notable result. However, if one nostril always produces a smaller moisture ring than the other, a blockage may exist in that nostril. Investigating this further with a qualified healthcare professional may be indicated.

The third way this assessment can be used is as an outcomes measurement. We measure overall or nostril-specific moisture rings before starting a breathing practice. We make note of the size(s) and then move into the breathing practice. After completing a particular breathing exercise or the entire breathwork session, we remeasure to note whether the nostrils have cleared (looking for a larger moisture ring post-breathwork than pre-breathwork). We compare side-to-side differences. For example, after a practice of only right nostril breathing, we may expect to see a larger moisture circle on the right than on the left. Similarly, after nasal clearing exercises, we can expect to have larger moisture circles on both sides of the nose. Such immediate physical feedback can be very empowering and motivating to maintain breathing practices over time.

Assessment of Diaphragmatic and Other Types of Breathing

Chest versus thoracic versus abdominal breathing tends to be harder for individuals to discern and observe than nasal versus oral breathing. Guiding questions can help (see Table 6.4 for examples); however, sometimes it is necessary to devise external methods of feedback. One strategy is to place the hands in various locations on the torso to experience physical movement in this region of the body through the hands. For some clients, this may be insufficiently concrete feedback. For them, adding a resistance band, gently tied around the chest—moving it up and down in several positions—can be helpful. Patients can begin to feel the stretch of the band and gain more insight into where expansion and contraction are occurring in the rib basket. For some students, a resistance band may not be helpful, but they can begin to feel the difference by using a non-stretchy band (such as yoga strap or scarf). It is important to note that this may be contraindicated for some individuals (e.g., those with complex trauma histories, severe anxiety disorders, or asthma). It is recommended to use these strategies in the order in which they were described. Table 6.4 provides suggestions about how to inquire about diaphragmatic breathing.

Clinician observation can be very helpful in supporting patients as they try to become more attuned to how the breath moves in their torso. Clinicians have a clear understanding of different types of breath (or can review Chap. 2 for this information) and can typically draw helpful conclusions or develop clarifying inquiries from observing how patients breathe and where movement is visible in their bodies as breath travels in and out. It is particularly noteworthy how breathing patterns change under varying circumstances (see aforementioned table). Most clients present with a default pattern that appears predictably in a variety of circumstances; others evidence specific patterns when encountering specific demand characteristics. Natural variation in accessing differing breath types is expected and adaptive. If we did not need to be able to breathe into the thorax at times, the body would not have developed this capacity. As is true for most patterns—the key to dysfunction is

Table 6.4 Diaphragmatic breath assessment

Do you breathe mostly with the diaphragm or with the muscles of chest and neck?
- Which part of the torso moves when you breathe in and out?
- Do you feel more movement in the lower rib basket, middle, or up high?
- Do your clavicles move when you breathe in and out?
- Do your shoulders rise up when you breathe in?
- Do your low ribs move outward and upward when you breathe in?
- Do you tense your stomach when you breathe out?
- Do you tense your neck muscles when you breathe in?
- Does it feel like work to breathe?

How do the above observations change, depending on:
- Activity (e.g., during rest, with gentle physical exertion, with cardiovascular workouts, during walking)
- Body position (e.g., standing, walking, sitting, lying down)

How do the above observations change, depending on:
- Mental and emotional state (e.g., when you are confused, mentally taxed, distracted, focused, stressed, sad, anxious, or angry)
- Contextual circumstances (e.g., when you are alone… with a loved one… With boss or someone who is difficult, challenging, …)

generally the indiscriminate and habitual emergence of the same pattern (i.e., pattern locks or *samskara* in Sanskrit) in most, if not all, circumstances. We need to be able to reverse breathe when we jump in to a cold lake and have to let our nervous system adapt to the sudden and unexpected change in temperature. However, if we note that a client reverse-breathes habitually, concern emerges about the individual's breathing patterns, lung capacity, and breath efficiency. Similarly, thoracic breathing can be adaptive occasionally (e.g., to feel empowered). However, when it is the default breathing pattern during rest and relaxation, this may indicate imbalanced, less than optimal breathing with less efficient carbon dioxide removal and decreased oxygen at the level of the alveoli. A brief summary of indicators that breathing instructors can explore (or observe) to help clients discern various breath types is provided in Table 6.5.

Additional inquiries about how breath is related to physicality are discussed further in the context of assessing how patients experience the flow of breath. These inquiries revolve around how breath is experienced in terms of space and location. Explorations of types of breath and experience of the breath in the body overlap significantly and can help provide more clarity when considered in combination. Finally, even posture is useful for discerning breathing type. This topic is where we turn next.

Assessment of Postural Effect on Breathing

Additional aspects of breath anatomy assessment relate to posture and movement characteristics (collapsing, bracing, and resilience), which may have a significant effect on how breath travels through the body. The science of posture and movement characteristics in relation to breath anatomy was explored in Chap. 2. Following are observational strategies to illustrate this relationship in a manner that is useful to client self-awareness and clinician observation. Primary postural anatomical (self-)

Table 6.5 Indicators for discerning breathing types

Type of breath	Physical signs	Breath and emotional signs	Other notes
Thoracic breath	• Shallow or no abdominal movement • Little to no movement low in the rib basket or flared ribs • Visible movement high in the chest • Visible movement of the clavicles • Perceptible shoulder or neck tension or tightness	• Feelings of breathlessness • Feeling the urge to breathe mode • Gasping for air • Large inhalations • Rapid breathing • Feelings of anxiety • Feelings of stress or worry • Braced or collapsed posture • Flat lumbar spine	• Can be empowering in flight-or-flight situations—Noted by bracing and flared ribs • Can be constricting, especially if breath is clavicular and shallow, and posture is collapsed
Paradoxical/reverse breath	• Abdomen moves inward and upward with inhalation • Abdomen moves outward with exhalation • Enlarged rib basket on inhalation • Shallow breathing • Poor posture	If chronic, • Highly upregulated nervous system • Feelings of anxiety, panic • Confusion when encountering breathing cues • Fatigue and loss of energy • Decreased athletic performance	If non-habitual: • Accompanied by a strong startle response • Quick recovery of natural breath
Abdominal breath	• Relies only on the diaphragm, with no additional muscle recruitment • Abdominal wall moves visible outward • No movement in the low ribs • No chest movement at all	• Completely relaxed exhalation • General relaxation in body, breath, mind, and emotion • Less air exchange • Imperceptible breath	• Useful in contexts of relaxation, yoga nidra, meditation • Not natural for standing, walking, or moving
Natural diaphragmatic breath	• Visible abdominal and low rib basket movement outward and upward • Minimal upper chest and no clavicular movement • Relaxed shoulders and neck • Suppleness in muscles. • Good posture while moving and at rest	• Adaptive resilient breath rate • Nasal breathing • Smooth breath texture • Generally silent breath • Emotional resilience • Healthy breath rate, rhythm • Breath adapts to postural changes	• Resilient response to stress or challenge with good fluidity between nervous system states • Supports focus and mindfulness

observations are related to alignments of pelvis, spine, and head along the central axis of the body. Particular spinal alignment dysfunctions have specific implications for muscular movements along the spine, assembly of organs in the abdominal cavity, range of motion of the diaphragm, and movement of the rib basket. These postural changes create profound alterations in how breath can be distributed inside the body space, how the lungs and thorax can increase and decrease in size and/or volume, and how much recruitment of accessory muscles is necessary to move sufficient air. The implications for breathing are varied, with labored breathing, shortness of breath, constricted or restricted breathing, gasping for air, and other possible effects.

The following questions can help guide posture-related inquiries specific to the spine. The set of questions is followed by Table 6.6 that elaborates on the physical and breathing-related implications. In combination, the questions and table can be useful in guiding inquiries for patient self-assessments and clinician observations. Generally, breathing patterns that are linked to postural dysfunction cannot be improved via breathwork alone. They require additional support to retrain posture and spinal alignment. Breathing instructors need to be aware of their scope of practice and collaborate with other healthcare providers as necessitated by each patient's specific physical and energetic presentation.

Questions to Guide Patient Self-Assessment and Clinician Observation (*looking at the client from the side*)

1. Is the spine in its natural curves with a natural lordosis (curve) in the lumbar and cervical spine and a natural kyphosis in the thoracic spine and sacrum?
   - Is there:
     - Hyper- (too much rounding forward) or hypokyphosis (standing at attention) in the thoracic spine?
     - Hyper- (a hollow low back) or hypolordosis (slumping) in the lumbar spine?
     - Distortion in the natural curve of the cervical spine, perhaps manifesting in forward head posture or hyperlordosis in the neck?
   - Is the pelvis overly tucked (flat) or tilted (with a hollow lumbar spine) or anchored in a natural and healthy balance that has a slight anterior tilt?
   - Is the low rib basket flared or too drawn in versus able to expand outward and upward with inhalation, and inward and downward with exhalation?
   - How do any distortions that are present in individual's typical spinal alignment seem to affect the breath?

2. How is the plumb line alignment? The line should pass:
   - Through the center of the ear
   - Through the center of the shoulder
   - Through the center of the waist
   - Through the center of the hip joint
   - Slightly anterior to the knee joint
   - Slightly anterior to the ankle and heel
3. Is there bowing in the spine and pelvic region forward or backward (beyond the natural curves)? Consider the following questions or dimensions:
   - Is any bowing distributed across the whole length of the body? Or are there opposing bows forward or backward in the upper versus lower portions of the body or in other portions?
   - Is the top of the ear slightly higher than the eyebrow (as opposed to chin jutting forward moving eyes higher than ears)?
   - Is the center of gravity of the head above the shoulders? Is the head forward of the body with the neck in too little extension at the upper cervical region?
   - Is the center of gravity of the shoulders above the hips?
   - Is the pelvis tilted anteriorly or tucked posteriorly?
   - Is the sacrum at its proper 30° angle (i.e., *not* vertical)?
4. Is there bowing elsewhere in the body forward or backward? Ponder the following questions or dimensions:
   - Are the hips above the knees?
   - Are the knees above the ankles?
   - Is there hyperextension in the knees?
   - Is there excessive plantar or dorsiflexion in the ankle?

Table 6.6 Implications of problematic spinal curve patterns for the breath

Type of spinal dysfunction	Physical patterns	Impact on breath
Hyperkyphosis in thoracic spine = excessive forward curvature of the thorax with impact on the lumbar spine; likely posterior pelvic tilt (tuck)	• Shortened chest muscles (pectoralis minor, major, and fascia around them) and lax back muscles (rhomboids, mid traps) • Tight external hip rotators, weak adductors, tight hamstrings • May have back, sciatica, or disc herniations • May experience numbness, tingling, or weakness in extremities	• Restricted breath • Decreased rib basket resilience • Restricted chest expansion • Reducing lung capacity • Shortness of breath • Difficulty breathing

(continued)

Table 6.6 (continued)

Type of spinal dysfunction	Physical patterns	Impact on breath
Anterior head carriage = head is forward of shoulders; neck is likely hyperextended at C1 and C2 to keep gaze on horizon	• Tight chest muscles • Restricted blood flow and nerve impingement in cervical spine • Likely posterior tilt of pelvis • Respiratory muscle weakness • Decreased exercise tolerance	• Labored breath • Decreased lung capacity • Change in diaphragmatic function with over-recruitment of accessory muscles • Shortness of breath
Hyperlordosis in lumbar spine = lumbar spine is too concave; thorax may be too flat; likely anterior tilt of pelvis	• Sway back posture has hips pushed forward and middle thoracic goes into kyphosis • Tight hip flexors • External rotation of hip joints and legs • Respiratory muscle fatigue • Overreliance on accessory muscles of breathing	• Restricted breath due to restricted rib basket mobility • Diaphragm cannot contract effectively in inhalation • Chest/thoracic breathing or reverse breathing • Shortness of breath
Overly tucked tailbone or sacrum = sacrum is not at its proper 30° angle (excessively posterior), which results in destabilization of the spine and SI joints	• Creates excessive weight-bearing on vertebral body and discs; may compress discs • Places the weight of the organs onto the pelvic floor, which weakens pelvic floor muscles, puts pressure on bladder, uterus, and prostate and may cause malfunction (e.g., incontinence) and/or prolapse • May cause neck pain as entire spinal alignment is imbalanced	• Reduced diaphragmatic range of motion • Shallow breathing with little abdominal movement • Decreased lung ventilation and capacity • Shallow breathing • Labored breathing • Excess recruitment of accessory breathing muscles
Lack of natural curves in spine, aka flat back = no natural lordosis in lumbar spine; no natural kyphosis in thorax and sacrum; cervical spine tends to be overly lordotic at the base and overly extended at the head	• Intervertebral joints compress and weight distributes poorly • Likely shortening of hamstrings • Pelvis tilt is off—Either too posterior or anterior; more muscle power is needed to stay upright; can make sitting hard on discs • Often accompanied by excessively externally rotated feet and knees and functional loss of height • Can lead to chronic pain, tension in neck and cervical spine, pain in low back	• Reduced mobility in rib basket • Reduced lung capacity and ventilation • Diaphragm cannot contract effectively in inhalation • Over-recruitment of accessory muscles leads to chest or clavicular breathing • Shallow breathing • Labored breathing

Assessment of Impact of Movement Characteristics on Breath

Primary movement characteristics (self-)observations are related to general patterns of *collapse* versus *bracing* versus *resilience* [2–5]. As teachers, we encourage attunement to and observe collapse/resignation and contraction/tension versus resilience/yielding in clients' expression across all layers of self to learn more about physical, energetic, mental, and emotional adjustments that may facilitate resilient breath. Assessment of physical, energetic, and even mental or emotional presence hints at whether clients have a tendency (or habitual way) to give up, resign, collapse, and buckle; grip, tense, over-effort, and grind; or respond, adapt, adjust flexibly, and yield to the demands of the practice (or life, for that matter). Patterns, habits, or ruts in any layer of self can close down choices, shut down openness, impair the free flow of breath, and limit possibilities for practitioners. Habits of collapse or bracing (and lack of resilience) tend to shut down agency, disempower, and short-circuit discernment and choice—they dysregulate breathing and prevent optimal breath rhythms. Noticing tendencies and habits related to collapsing, gripping, or yielding invites clients back into the beginner's mind, to a place of unlimited possibility, a place of exploration and options. It supports self-awareness that can lead to greater agency, resilience, and self-efficacy, as well as to more resilient ways of breathing.

Following are suggestions for observing or inviting clients to self-assess these three primary patterns of movement (collapse, bracing, and resilient) in body, breath and vitality, mind and emotions, and even in actions and relationships. In assessing these patterns, it is important to remember that everyone has all of these patterns at some point in time. Of interest here is to assess whether one of these patterns predominates to the degree of crowding out others, limiting choices, and disempowering more resilient breath, action, or movement.

1. Are there consistent patterns of <u>collapse</u>, evidenced by some of the following features?
   - *In the physical layer*: under-exerting, under-efforting, inadequate presence or use of force or strength, lack of sufficient tone in the muscles
     - Slouched posture
     - Tucked (posterior) pelvis
     - Rounded spine (overly anterior rib basket)
     - Head rolled up and back—throat (front) hyperextended, neck (back) compressed
     - Back muscles are lengthened, weak, and tight
     - Chest muscles are shortened and tight
     - Psoas and short hamstrings are shortened and tight, leading to nervous system collapse
   - *In the vital or energetic layer*: burnt-out or collapsed breath and vitality; tamasic or dorsal vagal energy; lack of resilience and recovery in the breath; hypoarousal and unpleasant feeling tones
     - Shallow, restricted, or collapsed breathing
     - Weak or anxious breathing
     - Lax or lifeless energy

- Absence of engaged affect
- Withdrawn energy and affect
- *In the mind layer*: thoughts and emotions of hopelessness, confusion, and lack of focus
  - Sluggish, hopeless, and/or depressive thoughts
  - Confused, disorganized, or muddled thoughts
  - Perceptions of futility
  - Depression, despair, hopelessness
  - Fear, dread, anguish
  - Neither drawn to action/agency nor grounded in simply being
2. Are there consistent patterns of _bracing_, evidenced by some of the following features?
  - *In the physical layer*: over-efforting and over-exertion, excessive use of muscular force or strength, creation of traction, excessive tension, muscular gripping in places irrelevant to the circumstances (e.g., gripping in the jaws or tongue; grimacing)
    - Upright stance
    - Neutral to slightly tucked (posterior) pelvis
    - Lifted chest with posterior rib basket and flare in the lower ribs
    - Excessive scapular depression and retraction
    - Belly drawn in to create a braced core with overreliance on rectus and disabling of transverse abdominus
    - Shortened upper back muscles and lengthened chest muscles
    - Excess tension in muscles around joints and excessive muscular action
    - Short hamstrings and psoas leading to sympathetic nervous system arousal
  - *In the vital or energetic layer*: excessive arousal; rajasic or sympathetic nervous system energy; lack of resilience and predictability in the breath; uneven flow of breath and breath sounds
    - Hyperventilation or over-controlled breathing
    - Uneven texture of breath with hitches and glitches
    - Hyperreactive and/or hyperkinetic energy and arousal
    - Noisy, agitated breath
    - Tendency toward negative affect
  - *In the mind layer*: thoughts and emotions of agitation, distraction, or hyperfocus (at the expense of soft awareness and presence)
    - Driven thoughts with a tendency toward agitation and striving
    - Agitated and distracted thoughts and actions
    - Forceful clinging, grasping, or wanting
    - Strong emotions of anger, aversion, even hatred
    - Strong defense of self and ego
    - Forceful, even overpowering, presence in relationships
    - Driven to action over being
3. Are there consistent patterns of _resilience_, evidenced by some of the following features?
  - *In the physical layer*: softness in strength and strength in softness; stillness in movement and movement in stillness; healthy muscle tone that supports the

pose with easeful effort; finding the physical middle way that integrates effort and ease
- Upright stance
- Neutral to slightly tucked (posterior) pelvis
- *In the vital or energetic layer*: easeful breath that is adaptive to respiratory needs; breath stays regulated despite increasing or decreasing demands; balanced breath of a ventral vagal nervous system state; appropriate affective connection; balanced or easily rebalancing (i.e., adaptive and allostatic) levels of arousal
  - Optimal natural (light and subtle) breath rhythm with smooth texture, nasal, without sounds
  - Even flow of breath without hitches or glitches
  - Adaptable arousal with a wide window of tolerance
  - Balanced, sattvic ventral vagal energy, arousal, and breath
  - Pleasant affective tones
  - Capacity to easily reregulate in the presence of pleasant or unpleasant affect
- In the mind layer: clarity in thoughts, willingness to surrender habitual ways and views, inspired ways of analyzing what is happening/present, mental and emotional clarity and presence
  - Willingness to learn, unlearn, and relearn
  - Accurate appraisal of physical and emotional needs
  - Optimal interoception, proprioception, and exteroception
  - Accurate self-awareness leading to openness to change and exploration
  - Agency, initiative, and self-empowered with accurate self-appraisal
  - Openness to exploration
  - Appreciation of feedback and new ideas

Table 6.7 presents synonyms for labeling these three concepts that can be applied across all aspects of self. These synonyms can guide observation—allowing clinician to frame the concepts explored in these three categories of experience and expression. Synonyms are often very helpful to patients as they learn to recognize or self-assess (and ultimately transform) patterns of buckling, grasping, and yielding.

6.3.2 Assessment of Breath Physiology—Controlled Breath Pause

Three types of breath pauses can be measured to gain insight into breath physiology. The *comfortable* pause is a pause after exhalation until a gentle urge to inhale is perceived. The *controlled* breath pause is a pause after the exhalation that is held until there is a strong yet manageable urge to breathe (e.g., there is a sensation of involuntary movement of the diaphragm). Finally, the *maximum* pause, also known as the break point, is a pause after exhalation until the urge to breathe is so strong that inhalation essentially forces itself onto the breather [6, 7]. The comfortable pause is useful as a baseline for learning to extend the pause after exhalation, as we retrain breathing with specific breathing exercises to change the medulla's CO_2 sensitivity. We return to this notion in Chap. 9 in the context of developing optimal

Table 6.7 Synonyms for talking about collapse, contraction, and resilience

Too loose—Collapsed, buckled

• Buckling	• Limp	• Crumpled	• Having given up
• Under-efforting	• Nonresponsive	• Loose	• Re- or unmoved
• Tamasic	• Uninvolved	• Dull	• Disinterested
• Dorsal vagal	• Unintegrated	• Disconnected	• Indifferent
• Disengaged	• Indifferent	• Detached	• Apathetic
• Flaccid	• Fragmented	• Disheartened	• Slack
• Drooping	• Hopeless	• Downhearted	• Careless
• Sagging	• Withdrawn	• Lax	• Haphazard
• Removed	• Dissociated	• Self-deprecating	• Resigned
• Dispirited	• Dissociative	• Inattentive	• Passive
• Absent	• Despairing	• Listless	• Submissive

Too tight—Contracted, grasping

• Bracing	• Clenched	• Holding	• Tense
• Over-efforting	• Overly determined	• Greedy	• Insistent
• Rajasic	• Grasping	• Gripped	• Resolute
• Sympathetic	• Obsessive	• Scrunched	• Unbendable
• Over-engaged	• Forced	• Driven	• Unyielding
• Tight	• Strained	• Coerced	• Stubborn
• Reactive	• Hyper	• Constricted	• Trapped
• Overinvolved	• Overactive	• Stressed	• Restricted
• Inhibited	• Overconfident	• Overly ambitious	• Perseverative
• Overcontrolled	• Self-judging	• Squeezed	• Dogged
• Grim	• On alert	• Strongminded	• Tightly wound

Just right—Resilient, yielding

• Stable	• Calm	• Unwavering	• Pliable
• Easeful effort	• Invigorated	• Committed	• Uncomplicated
• Sattvic	• Involved	• Established	• Safe
• Ventral vagal	• Cohesive	• Secure	• Hopeful
• Engaged	• Focused	• Durable	• Self-compassionate
• Relaxed	• Attentive	• Maintainable	• Alert
• Responsive	• In the sweet spot	• Sustainable	• Serene
• Peaceful	• Integrated	• Elastic	• Buoyant
• Balanced	• Natural	• Resilient	• Free
• Grounded	• Steady	• Coherent	• Lucid
• Fully present	• With the middle way	• Nonattached to outcome	• Persistent not insistent

functional breathing. The control pause is useful in assessment—our focus here. The maximum pause is used to support nasal clearing and is a powerful practice that can be used as a preparation to pave the way for nasal breathing (covered in Chap. 7). Maximum pause has to be used with care as it can induce a sense of panic in some clients or students.

The control pause, or as we will call it here—controlled breath pause (CBP)—provides a window into breath physiology. It is a way to measure the ability to hold the breath comfortably at the end of a natural breath cycle. It is (somewhat confusingly) known as the *comfortable pause* among some yoga teachers [8], as well as the body oxygen level test (*BOLT) score* in the Oxygen Advantage System [9]. CBP provides a measure of breathlessness, functional breathing, and exercise readiness and is a proxy variable for chemosensitivity of the medulla oblongata to CO_2 levels in the blood. Actual partial pressure measurement of CO_2 is complex and requires expensive equipment (i.e., a capnometer). CBP provides highly correlated information that is easy to gather anywhere, anytime, and under any circumstance. It gives clients access to a quick and easy self-assessment of the state of health in the respiratory system (and beyond). CBP can be measured regularly and repeatedly and represents a helpful outcomes assessment for clinicians who want to help clients assess the impact of prescribed breathing practices on physiology. It can be measured immediately before, several times during, and 5–10 min after breathwork for immediate biofeedback about how that practice may have altered the breath. Notable changes in CBP can become powerful motivators to practice. It is important to remember and to remind clients that the controlled breath pause is an assessment tool, *not* a practice. Measuring the control pause does not change its length—the practice of breathwork does. CBP serves to measure baselines and progress. It can be easy, especially for perfectionists or performance-driven humans, to strive for an ideal CBP and to become slightly obsessed with results. This is not the point of this assessment. Instead, it is a means of biofeedback that provides a proxy measure for the breath's healthfulness and biochemistry.

Instructions for Controlled Breath Pause Measurement

The controlled breath pause is most reliably measured in the morning, but can be taken anytime, and is especially useful directly before and after breathwork. It can be taken repeatedly throughout the day to obtain feedback about respiratory changes over time and in response to possible activities and triggers. It is imperative to remember that there are natural variations in CBP length across the day; it is generally higher in the evening than in the morning. CBP is a useful outcomes measurement across weeks and months of breathing practice. The control pause can also be used to make decisions about types of breathwork that may or may not be indicated.

In measuring the control pause, it is important not to create significant strain or stress while holding the breath at the bottom of the exhalation. The measurement is based on mild air hunger—when the urge to breathe takes hold (e.g., via notable but not strong diaphragmatic contraction). It is a measurement of how long the breath can be held and still return to normal breathing when the breath suspension is released. If neck or abdominal muscles begin to spasm, the hold exceeded the CBP (and may have become a maximum pause). The control pause is not based on willpower or force. If there is a gasping or spasming after the breath hold is released, the hold was too long and the measurement needs to be repeated after a reasonable break for breath recovery. To measure the controlled breath pause, it is best to rest for 10 min before taking the measurement. Ideally, no heavy meal was consumed immediately before the measurement.

Once ready, the following steps are recommended:

- After the rest period, be prepared with a stopwatch
- Gently inhale nasally
- Lightly exhale nasally
- Pinch the nose shut (optional, but preferable) and simultaneously start a stopwatch
- Suspend the breath after exhalation *until the first significant sign of air hunger* (i.e., desire to inhale, perhaps signaled by a gentle diaphragmatic contraction); neither wait too long (this could become a maximum pause) nor stop too soon (this could simply be a comfortable pause)

- On the arising of air hunger, check the stopwatch to note the breath suspension duration in seconds; time registered on the stopwatch in that moment equals the length of CBP
- Now open the nose, inviting an inhalation and monitor the quality of the next inhalation:
  - If the inhalation is normal (i.e., not labored or gasping), CBP measurement is likely reliable
  - If the inhalation is a gasp, the breath suspension was too long; in this case, wait a few minutes (allowing the breath to resettle) and repeat measurement to reach a lesser level of desire to breathe

Controlled Breath Pause Interpretation

CBP assessment is a measure of CO_2 tolerance in the medulla; higher CBPs indicate greater tolerance of higher levels of CO_2 in the blood. Lower levels are indicative of CO_2 hypersensitivity, the likely consequence of chronic hyperventilation and commensurately chronic hypocapnia (low blood CO_2 levels). Generally, as control pause decreases, breath rate and volume increase. According to McKeown [10], breath-related symptoms are strong with low CBPs and ease as CBP rises, with notable improvement for every increment of 5–10 seconds. For individuals who start with a control pause of <10 s, it can take several weeks to reach a CBP of 20 s and symptom relief. Once individuals reach a CBP of 20 s, they often reach a plateau with little change for a few weeks. To reach a CBP above 30 s requires physical exercise. Interpretations of exact scores vary slightly by source; however, the following guidelines (expressed in seconds) offered by McKeown [10, 11] are useful.

- <=10 s: very low CO_2 levels with likely CO_2 hypersensitivity and commiserate dysregulated breathing patterns (hyperventilation, chest breathing)
- >10–15: low CO_2 with likely vulnerability to CO_2 hypersensitivity and the tendency to be triggered into reactivity in breathing patterns
- >15–20: healthy CO_2 levels and a stable and resilient respiratory system
- >20–30: good vitality and health with near optimal tolerance and levels of CO_2
- >30: mild to no breathlessness during exercise; excellent vitality and CO_2 tolerance

Lower CBPs are strongly correlated with faster breathing, irregular sighing, mouth breathing, upper chest breathing, and a breath that is very noticeable, either because it is highly visible (e.g., heaving chest) or audible (noisy and accompanied by gasps, yawns, coughs, throat clearing, or similar sounds). High CBPs, on the other hand, are associated with slow, regular, soft, light nasal and diaphragmatic breathing that is hardly noticeable. For those who want more detail about the larger meanings and implications of the controlled pause, Table 6.8 provides general guidelines about implications of CBP values for various breath dimensions and qualities. (based on detailed research reviews of McKeown [10, 11] and other resources). Table 6.9 translates CBP scores and their implications into recommendations related to necessary preparations, breathwork sequencing across time, and physical movement and exertion across time.

Table 6.8 Clinical Implications of Controlled Breath Pause scores

Implications for:	CBP < 10	CBP = 10–15	CBP = 15–20	CBP = 20–30	CBP > 30
CO_2 levels and chemosensitivity	Very low CO_2 levels with likely CO_2 hypersensitivity	Low CO_2 with likely vulnerability to CO_2 hypersensitivity	Healthy CO_2 levels	Near optimal tolerance and levels of CO_2	Excellent vitality and CO_2 tolerance
Breath rate	~20–25 BPM	~16–20 BPM	~14–16 BPM	~12–14 BPM	~<12 BPM
Breath volume	Higher or lower than typical	Higher than typical	Higher than typical	Typical	Light
Breath texture	Highly irregular, rough, and choppy	Irregular and not smooth	Mostly regular and smooth	Smooth and regular	Smooth, calm, and regular
Breath sound	Noisy, labored, noticeable, gasping; yawning, sighing; wheezing	Noisy and noticeable; yawning, sighing	Less noisy and less notable; some sighing	Quiet	Quiet and inaudible
Breath location	Mouth and upper chest breathing; paradoxical breath	Mouth and chest breathing	Could be any	Could be any	Most likely nasal and diaphragmatic
Natural pause post-exhale	Impossible due to extreme air hunger; breath stacking (inhalation starts before exhalation is complete)	No natural pause	Starting to be possible; ~1 s	Likely; ~1–2 s	Present; ~2–3 s
Breathlessness at rest	Moderate to severe; effortful, erratic breath	Moderate	None	None	None
Breathlessness with exercise	Severe; fighting for air	Moderate	Mild	Normal	Likely none
Common breath-related symptoms	Blocked nose, coughing, fatigue, insomnia, snoring, asthma, panic, anxiety	Blocked nose, coughing, fatigue, insomnia, snoring, asthma, anxiety—symptoms are easing	Symptoms are easing significantly	Symptoms are mostly gone but may come back with triggers	Symptoms are gone

Table 6.9 Intervention recommendations related to Controlled Breath Pause scores

Implications for:	CBP < 10	CBP = 10–15	CBP = 15–20	CBP = 20–30	CBP > 30
Primary breathwork focus	Nasal; honing proprio- and interoception; calming	Nasal, soft, and diaphragmatic; interoception, calming	Nasal, soft, quiet, light, and diaphragmatic; interoception and neuroception, calming	Any as needed	Any as desired given intention
Energetic, mental, and physical preparations for breathwork	Strong focus on centering, calming; focus on energetic and emotional prep	Continue with all calming practices at start and end; add physical and postural preparations as indicated via assessment	Continue brief opening centerings and integrated cuing for calmness; emphasize physical preparations	Continue brief opening centerings and integrated cuing for calmness; emphasize strength in physical work	Recommend ongoing self-guided relaxation and calmness practices; fine for all physical practices as appropriate
Breath attunement recommendations	Gentle breath observation practices focused on calming; no observation of pauses	Gentle breath observation for all breath dimensions, including pauses	All breath observation practices; any breath awareness practices	As needed for calming and resilience	As desired for calming and resilience
Breathwork recommendations	Introducing the idea of nasal and bumble bee breathing; teach breath recovery	Exploring nasal and bumble bee breathing; possibly add other subtle breaths; begin diaphragmatic breathing	Emphasize all subtle breathing practices for regular use, including during exertion; add 4-part breathing	Refine all practices offered to date; can add longer breath holds and more forceful practices	All practices can be offered with intentions and clarity of purpose
Breathwork cautions	No work related to breath holds or breath pauses; no forced or loud breathing; observe closely for energetic dysregulation	No breath holds; introduce the idea of breath pauses without creating them; no forced or loud breathing; observe closely for energetic dysregulation	Look for dysregulation and make sure recovery can be managed by the patients themselves as they take breathwork into daily life	Most practices can now be integrated into daily life; ensure patient understands interoceptive and neuroceptive signals and how to adjust accordingly	Consider ending collaborative work as patients continue any and all practices on their own; leave door open for check-ins
Movement recommendations	Slow gentle movement, including slow walking	Light movement with more physical practices offered; walking	Moderate exercise; more vigorous physical movement; brisk walking	Strong exercise; running; all physical movement practices can be offered as needed	All levels, including HIIT and all physical movement practices as needed

Controlled Breath Pause Cautions

CO_2 sensitivity and, thus, CBP can be affected by many lifestyles and other factors, including but not limited to trauma, high-stress environments or relationships, hormonal variations (e.g., progesterone can increase breath rate), and genetic predispositions for certain disorders with breath-related symptoms (e.g., asthma, panic disorder). Similarly, making progress with CBP based on breathwork may be slowed or facilitated by these factors, as well as by the following factors:

- Inability to handle stress resiliently
- Chronic infection, including tonsilitis and rhinitis
- Food sensitivities
- Disturbed sleep
- Ongoing mouth and chest breathing
- Chronic long-term illness (for each decade of illness, a change in CBP takes a year [11])
- Severe illness

Increasing the comfortable pause reflects the alteration of our physiology in response to our breathing practice. If CBP changes quickly it means the biochemistry is changing rapidly as well. It is possible to develop *temporary* detoxification symptoms. These symptoms typically resolve on their own, usually in a short period of time. However, according to McKeown (workshop presentation; 12.10.2022) and Ayurvedic wisdoms, it can be helpful to drink a glass of water a day with a teaspoon of saltwater to help ameliorate this reaction. It is helpful to be aware of this possibility and to debrief it with clients. However, this is best done in a way that does not suggest fragility or scare clients away from increasing the controlled breath pause. Detoxification can include the following symptoms, although they may vary significantly in number and intensity given our human bioindividuality:

- Insomnia
- Fatigue
- Headache
- Feeling like having a head cold
- Loss of appetite
- Runny nose
- Increased urine output
- Lightheadedness
- Emotional upset
- Yawning
- Metallic taste in the mouth

6.3.3   Assessment of Breath Rate and Volume

As noted previously, breath cadence is a combination of rate (number of breaths per minute) and volume (amount of breath inhaled and exhaled in each breath cycle).

Healthy cadence implies fewer than 10–12 BPM, with a moderate volume of air breathed in each cycle. Optimal functional breathing may be even slower than this, being optimized at 5.5–6 breath cycles per minute, coupled with light to moderate volume. It is important to recall that we do not make up for the slowness of the rate with increasing volume. In other words, we always consider rate and volume at the same time. Assessment of breath cadence thus rests on gaining an understanding of how many breaths our clients are breathing *and* how voluminous each breath cycle is. Minute volume is strongly correlated with breath physiology, as covered in Chap. 3. It is useful to recall that standard healthcare definitions of breath rate may *not align* with the breath rates recommended in the breathing science literature. Tachycardia (too many breaths per minute) tends to be defined as more than 20 BPM; bradycardia (too few breaths per minute) is defined as fewer than 12 breaths [12]. Clients may fit into the 12–20 BPM window and yet are hyperventilating.

Breath rate can be assessed simply by measuring how many times we breathe a complete breath per minute. To measure number of breaths, it is important to track that *full and partial* breaths are counted. A full breath includes an inhalation and an exhalation. If the count starts with an inhalation and ends with an exhalation, this will yield total number of breaths per minute. However, if the count starts with an inhalation and ends with an inhalation, the last count is only half a breath. Does it matter terribly if we are exact about 10 versus 10.5 breaths? Probably not. However, if we are also assessing changes in breath rate over time, even a half breath's worth of change may make a difference, if only psychologically, in that it signals improvement. Additionally, it is important to accurately measure the breath rate for *a full minute*. Common (time-saving) practices, such as counting for only 15 s and then multiplying that rate by 4, have been shown to overestimate the number of breaths per minute [13]. To recall, breath rate varies with inhalation and exhalation. If we count for only 15 s, we may capture two inhalations and one exhalation, or two exhalations and one inhalation. Hence, such estimations are not as reliable as a full-minute count.

The following instructions might be helpful for <u>counting</u> breaths:
- Take a few moments to tune into your breath, become familiar with sensing your breath to be able to count how often it moves through you in a given time period.
- To count the breath, you might count the number of inhalations [*explain this further as needed*], OR the number of exhalations [*explain this further as needed*], OR the number of times you feel your abdomen rise or fall [*explain this further as needed*]. *Perhaps take a practice run before the actual count.*
- Once you have a clear sense of your inhalations and exhalations and your breath seems to flow naturally, let me know and we can begin the count.
- Once you can reliably locate or identify a breath cycle (i.e., the beginning and end of an inhalation as well as an exhalation), I will start a timer that is set for 1 min.
- Count the number of breaths while the timer is running for the full minute (*no short-cuts*). When I say STOP, use the current or most recent count (*make sure clients do not add or drop a count*)

The following instructions might be helpful for <u>determining</u> breath rate:
Note the reported count and determine breath rate as follows:
- If you counted by using the rising and falling of the abdomen, the total count is your rate of breaths per minute.
- If you counted inhalations and you started on an inhalation and ended on an exhalation, your total count is your breath rate; if you started on an inhalation and ended on an inhalation, your breath rate = total count − 0.5 (e.g., if you counted inhalations and also ended on an inhalation and your count was 8, your breath rate equals 7.5 because one of the breath cycles was not complete)
- If you counted exhalations and you started on an exhalation and ended on an exhalation, your total count is your breath rate; if you started on an exhalation and ended on an exhalation, your breath rate = total count − 0.5 (e.g., if you counted exhalations and also ended on an exhalation and your count was 10, your breath rate equals 9.5 because one of the breath cycles was not complete)

Breath volume can be objectively assessed but generally not in a yoga or breathwork context, as it requires equipment that is not typically available. Formal assessment is beyond the scope of this chapter (although if the equipment is available and the clinician knows how to use it correctly, by all means, it can be used). However, as breathwork guides, we can use proxy measures for volume by subjectively evaluating via observation or client self-assessment the amount of breath that is traveling in and out with each complete breath cycle. We can try to categorize the breath at the two extremes (not at all voluminous versus very voluminous) with descriptors such as light, shallow, minimized, limited, restricted, paltry on the non-voluminous end and descriptors such as full, deep, massive, heavy, expansive, maximized, at the more voluminous end. Average breath volume is approximately 500 mL. A very voluminous (deep, expansive) breath might move 1000 mL of air or more; a very non-voluminous (light or shallow) breath may move as little as 200 mL.

For assessment (and eventually breathing practice) purposes, we can plot breath rate and volume graphically, an exercise that can be very helpful for client and clinician to begin grasping the nature of a patient's breath (as well as ultimately the unfolding of particulars of the various breathing exercises). To create a visual breath representation, volume (how much air is breathed in or out with each breath cycle) can be plotted on the vertical/left (Y-axis or ordinate) of the graph; rate (number of full breaths per minute) can be plotted on the horizontal/bottom (X-axis or abscissa) (Fig. 6.1). The resulting line or wave is a map or metaphor for breath or breathing practices. A few examples can explain this process of creating a visual of our breath. The anchors for the Y-axis are shown in mL in the examples. However, the graph could also be created with descriptive anchors such as those offered earlier (perhaps ranging from shallow to light to average to deep to expansive, for which client and clinician can create these anchors or definitions collaboratively).

Breathing graphs can be a powerful way of assessing and demonstrating breath physiology. They can be used to show various forms of excessive or insufficient breathing and to discuss their implications and possible consequences. They can be

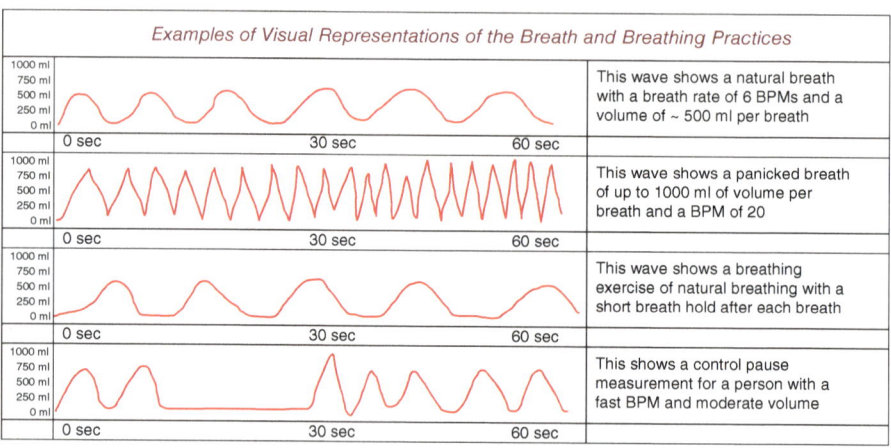

Fig. 6.1 Visual representations of various types of breath and breathing practices

used to demonstrate likelihood of hyperventilation, hypoventilation, and the likely results with regard to oxygen uptake in the tissues and carbon dioxide levels in the blood. This information can be harnessed to begin linking certain breathing cadences to certain symptoms of less-than-optimal breath physiologies. For example, the second wave in the aforementioned graph can be used to demonstrate the reciprocal relationship between breath cadence and emotional state. A breath of high rate and high volume can induce panic; alternatively, panic can create hyperventilation. This same wave may also be used to see what happens in asthma and why calming the breath may actually serve to prevent or rescue a client from an asthma attack.

6.3.4   Assessment of Breath Locations and Spatial Distribution

Related to breath anatomy, and yet moving beyond it, is assessment that focuses on areas where students can discern the unfolding of breath in their body and the way in which breath distributes itself in patients' physical beings. This assessment moves beyond anatomy in that it may start with concrete physical sensation of breath in the body, but also includes more subtle vibrations of breath and vitality in clients' beings. This assessment can thus even include an exploration of yoga's *prana vayus* or the subtle energies or winds of the breath (covered in detail in Chap. 8). Subtle aspects of breath and breathing may not be accessible to students right away. Thus, this dimension of breath assessment, more so than any other, may require breath awareness work and tends to develop over time (hence, its coverage in Chap. 8).

Often assessment of breath locations begins by attuning to where breath is felt in the body while seated—quite similar to how breath anatomy assessment unfolds. The breath can be consciously traced through various locations, including the nose, throat, abdomen, low rib basket, and chest. Then, assessment explores how breath distributes itself in the body—symmetrically; flowingly; to the front, back, or sides; and so on. We help clients create increasingly subtle awareness of locations and distribution of the breath in a tangible way while the body is at rest and then at increasing levels of exertion or action. This can start with breath assessment on the yoga mat, at rest, or during a gentle restorative *asana* practice. From there, assessment can continue during more vigorous movement, such as in stronger *asana*, flow, or *kriya*. Once clarity emerges about breath areas and distribution in all various situations, we assess how location and space of breathing change in clients' bodies as they alter their position, shape, and movement. We help students begin to recognize how their body expands in many directions and that breath and vitality can become palpable in various physical locations, even those not directly anatomically or physiologically connected to the breath (such as feeling the vibration of breath in the toes or feeling pulsation of breath in every cell in the body).

Finally, assessment of area and distribution can be moved off the mat and into daily waking hours to notice how and when breath travels through the nose or mouth, via the diaphragm or high into the chest—differentiating these data for different times of day, types of activities, or physical, emotional, or mental demands. It helps to understand variation of breath locations in context, such as during moments of calm and rest, moments of exercise or exertion, moments of difficulty or challenge, moments of anger or conflict, and moments of fear and worry. If possible, it also helps to learn how the breath manifests anatomically during sleep. Table 6.10 provides suggestions for inquiry and observation.

Table 6.10 Examples of breath location assessment

Where in the body can the breath be felt tangibly (e.g., via *movement, energy, temperature*):
- Nose or mouth
- Low, mid, or upper throat
- Low, mid, or upper abdomen
- Low, mid, or high rib basket
- Low, mid, or high chest
- Clavicles or neck muscles
- Low, mid, or upper back body
- Side body
- Which parts of the body move or pulse the most?
- Do you consciously direct the breath to certain body areas? Why?

How does the breath distribute itself in the body:
- Front versus back body
- Evenly on both sides or more to one side than the other
- Into the abdomen or the chest; where in the chest
- Symmetrically or asymmetrically
- Outward or inward
- Upward or downward
- Into the center (e.g., abdomen, chest) or periphery (e.g., hands, feet) of the body
- Is there a difference in quality of the breath depending on distribution (e.g., more or less subtle, pulsing, or vibrating)

How do the above observations change, depending on:
- Activity (e.g., during rest, with gentle physical exertion, with cardiovascular workouts, *during* walking)
- Body position (e.g., standing, walking, sitting, lying down, folded—Such as in child's pose)

How do the above observations change, depending on:
- Mental and emotional state (e.g., when you are confused, mentally taxed, distracted, focused, stressed, sad, anxious, or angry)
- Contextual circumstances (e.g., when you are alone… with a loved one... With boss or someone who is difficult, challenging, …)

As awareness increases about breath distribution, so does awareness of subtle breath energies. Clients begin to feel energy, vibration, or pulsation of breath and vitality in places not directly connected to the breath, such as in the toes or fingertips, third eye, pit of the stomach, or other locations in or just beyond the body. Students may begin to feel breath as the pulsation of aliveness, energy beyond breath in a heartbeat, or in the expansion of compassion for themselves or others. Location and distributions in which patients notice breath, energy, vitality, and lifeforce can become increasingly subtle and meaningful and provide feedback about fluctuations in the mind and experiences of emotions and affects. It is through this more subtle aspect of breathwork that clients experience profound changes in their nervous system responses, thoughts, and emotions. Such changes, in turn, often lead to changes in behaviors, actions, and relationships.

Breath awareness of location, space, and distribution, especially as related to subtler dimensions of vitality (or *Prana*), typically needs to be nurtured deliberately over time to help clients develop answers to these questions. Chap. 8, in the section about breath awareness, is very useful in guiding this particular aspect of breath assessment—hence, the relative brevity of this section here. This choice serves as another reminder that assessment and treatment go hand in hand. While described linearly and separately, they coexist and interrelate. This is a beautiful way to remind ourselves and our patients that everything we do, whether it involves paying attention or taking deliberate action, makes a difference and supports our growth and evolution.

6.3.5 Assessment of Breath Texture and Sound

Texture and sound are explored by directing students' attention to these breath features *and* by teachers observing students' breath textures and sounds. It does not require sophisticated apparatuses or deep knowledge to begin to attune to whether breath is smooth, gentle, free-flowing versus choppy, jerky, or erratic. Similarly, breath sounds become easily self-evident. Sound assessment records whether breath is silent or noisy; if breath is noisy, assessment investigates whether the sound was intentionally created with breath (e.g., because the individual believes that breath *should* have a certain sound or resonance). Chapter 4 presented a table of descriptors that can be used to define various breath textures, from smoothness to roughness. This table is very useful for helping students begin to pay attention to the moment-to-moment unfolding of their breath. The breath awareness portion of Chap. 8 also provides more context that can be used as much for assessment as for intervention. Finally, Table 6.11 provides additional suggestions about how to proceed with texture and sound assessment.

Sleep sounds and textures can also be noted. It is helpful to have another person observe sleep to note whether there are breathing-related sounds and textures during sleep. Snoring, gasping, choppy breathing, and other issues can be noted. In a general breathwork practice in a yoga context, it is not typical to make a specific assessment of sleep sounds and textures. However, if these are known, it is helpful to make

Table 6.11   Examples of texture-related assessment questions or observations

How often does your breath texture feel:
- Smooth, buttery, feathery, gentle, free, comfortable
- Rough, jerky, heavy, hoarse, restricted, uneasy

How often does your breath feel:
- Rapid, erratic, agitated, strong, quick
- Very slow, tight, barely notable, weak, timid
- Restful, silent, smooth, rhythmic, easeful
- Full (lots of air moving in and out)
- Shallow (little air moving in and out)
- Urgent (with a sense of hungering for air or a mild fear of suffocating)

How often does your breath sound:
- Noisy and probably audible to others
- Relatively quiet
- Completely silent—inaudible to you and others

How often do you make other breath-related sounds:
- Gasping, snuffling, panting, or sounding winded
- Sighing, yawning, or otherwise audibly heaving the breath
- Clearing the throat, coughing, hoarse voice, or breathy speech

Do you create breath sounds intentionally and for what purpose:
- No, never
- Yes, sometimes—explain why
- Yes, all the time—explain why

How do the above observations change, depending on:
- Activity (e.g., during rest, with gentle physical exertion, with cardiovascular workouts, during walking).
- Body position (e.g., standing, walking, sitting, lying down)

How do the above observations change, depending on:
- Mental and emotional state (e.g., when you are confused, mentally taxed, distracted, focused, stressed, sad, anxious, or angry)
- Contextual circumstances (e.g., when you are alone… with a loved one... With boss or someone who is difficult, challenging, …)

a note of them. In a healthcare context, formal assessment of sleep sounds and textures may be highly appropriate—with commensurate referral and collaboration.

Much of the exploration and assessment of texture and sound characteristics are about creating more self-understanding about breath, breathing habits, and respiratory pattern-locks, even about patients' preconceived notions about how breath should unfold or sound. Students and clients, and even yoga professionals, are often very surprised to learn that a natural breath is smooth and feathery, gentle, and silent. Thus, this assessment can be of profound help in setting goals and planning interventions.

6.3.6   Assessment of Breath Phases

Assessment of breath phases explores the manifestations of inhalations, exhalations, retentions at the top, and suspensions at the bottom of each breath. It is focused on noting what is naturally present rather than what can be achieved with maximal effort. It is important to explore whether students have awareness of breath pauses and a sense of when inhalations and exhalations begin and end. It is not uncommon for patients not to realize exactly when inhalations or exhalations have started or ended. They may be able to sense a rising and falling of the abdomen or an increase or decrease in pressure or tension on the chest. However, they may not be fully aware of the entire span of each of the four phases of breath. Retention and suspension, in particular, are often beyond the awareness of clients early on during breathwork. Once again, awareness assessment and intervention interact. Initial assessment may be less about exploring the four phases than exploring *whether there is awareness* of the phases. As time passes and awareness grows, clients may make amazing discoveries about their breath cycles that were completely inaccessible to them early on.

Assessment with regard to breath phases has three possible foci of exploration, typically assessed or observed in the following order:

1. Awareness and nature of each phase of the breath
2. Awareness and nature of the transitions from phase to phase
3. Awareness and nature of relative proportions of the four phases of the breath to each other

Accuracy and utility of all assessments, of course, rest on whether clients have sufficient awareness of all of four phases of the breath and whether clinicians can gather sufficient visual and auditory data via observation to draw their own conclusions. These assessments are excellent preparations (even initial practices) for specific breathing techniques related to four-part breathing (covered in Chap. 10). They increase awareness that a breath cycle has four distinct phases and that the phases interact with one another, as well as with nervous system state, psychology, anatomy, and physiology.

As was true for assessing other breath characteristics, assessment of the four breath phases starts with observation and awareness while at rest and then moves through various other conditions, such as different body positions (e.g., standing, walking, sitting, lying down), activities (e.g., during rest, with gentle physical exertion, with cardiovascular workouts, during walking), mental and emotional states (e.g., when confused, mentally taxed, distracted, focused, stressed, sad, anxious, or angry), and contextual circumstances (e.g., when alone, with a loved one, or with a boss or someone who is difficult, challenging). Since students by now have already observed breath sounds, textures, rates, and volume, all of these aspects of breathing are possible to discern separately for each breath phase. Clearly, this work unfolds over time and proceeds from assessment to breath awareness to breath intervention.

Understanding the Four Breath Phases

With regard to recognizing and assessing the four breath phases, it is helpful to define them via the course each takes, its muscular actions, and its physiological and nervous system reverberations. These aspects are defined in Table 6.12 for each breath phase—a graphic display that can be shared with clients to help them begin to have awareness and recognition that each breath cycle is more nuanced than they may ever have imagined.

Table 6.12 Four phases of the breath

Inhalation

Course
- Lasts from the moment when the breath naturally begins to travel into the body until the moment when the inward voyage of the breath ends naturally—with beginnings and endings being triggered by various chemical and mechanical signals from the body

Anatomy
- The diaphragm contracts into abdomen and lower ribs lift outward and upward, resulting in intra-abdominal pressure that supports posture and spinal stability; decreased pressure in the lungs invites air to flow into the lungs

Energetics
- Air traveling into the nose is purified and cleansed; nitric oxide increases; air travels toward and into the alveoli; a sympathetic shift occurs in the nervous system as the vagal brake lifts lightly; energy lifts

Retention at the top of the breath

Course
- Lasts from the moment when the inward voyage of the breath has ended to the moment when the outward voyage of the breath begins

Anatomy
- Postural stability is maintained by diaphragmatic action and increase in intraabdominal pressure; inhaled air is retained in the lungs

Energetics
- O_2 diffuses from the alveoli into the blood; CO_2 diffuses from the blood into the alveoli; sense of fullness, perhaps of attachment or holding on

Exhalation

Course
- Lasts from the moment when the breath naturally begins to travel out of the body until the moment when the outward voyage of the breath ends naturally—again, with beginnings and endings being triggered by chemical and mechanical signals from the body

Anatomy
- The diaphragm relaxes upward toward the lungs, and lower ribs move inward and downward; intrathoracic pressure increases and invites air to flow out; core muscles may lightly contract to support the movement of air and to create stability

Energetics
- Air leaves the alveoli and travels upward and outward; air traveling out of the nose remoisturizes and cleanses the airway; a parasympathetic shift occurs in the nervous system as the vagus nerve is stimulated and puts the brakes on the SNS; energy settles

Suspension at the bottom of the breath

Course
- Lasts from the moment when the outward voyage of the breath has ended to the moment when the inward voyage of the breath begins

Anatomy
- Light core contraction continues to support postural stability; a residual volume of air is retained in the lungs

Energetics
- Arterial CO_2 increases and facilitates CO_2 release into tissues, resulting in enhanced oxygenation of tissues, including the brain; sense of emptiness, sometimes with a sense of need or relief

Exploring the Transitions Across Phases

With regard to the transitions from breath phase to breath phase, it is helpful to inquire about or observe whether each phase is distinct from the others and complete before the next phase starts. For many students, recognition of retention and suspension is particularly difficult. For some, this difficulty reflects a lack of awareness of the pauses. For others, it reflects an accurate observation that no such pause exists. Of particular interest are patterns that emerge related to where the breather's focus lies. Some clients are observed to hasten to certain aspects of the breath. For example, some breathe in quickly, have no pause at the top of the breath, and then release the breath more slowly with a long pause at the end. They seem to be more focused on letting go than inviting in. In quite the opposite patterns, other patients barely (or do not) complete the exhalation and do not suspend the breath, being in a great hurry to quickly draw in the next breath. Their energy may be one of need, of grasping and holding on—perhaps leading to hyperventilation. There are innumerable breathing patterns based on the four phases, and it takes a bit of observing and experimenting to begin to gain a full understanding of what they signal physically, energetically, and psychologically—for client and clinician. In fact, understanding the four phases and their interactions in this way is therapeutic breathwork in and of itself, often very helpful for creating breath attunement and changing breathing rhythms and patterns.

Exploring the Proportions of the Phases

With regard to proportions of the phases to each other, several dimensions can be explored. A great starting point is the relative length of the inhalation compared to the exhalation, with consideration of the reality that inhalations are linked to the sympathetic nervous system and exhalations to the parasympathetic nervous system. Also of interest are the relative lengths of naturally preexisting pauses at the top and bottom of the breath. Observation is *not an invitation* to increase these pauses—at this point, we are simply assessing what is naturally present. It may be important to recall the difference between a natural pause (*stambha* in Sanskrit) and a deliberate breath hold (*kumbhaka* in Sanskrit). Assessment is concerned with the natural pause (*stambha*); deliberate breath holds (*kumbhaka*) are explored in the context of measuring the controlled breath pause (see above) and in the context of intervention (i.e., as tailored or intentional breathing techniques). Many patterns are possible, with some students having no discernable or very short retention and having a longer suspension; others have the opposite pattern. It is helpful to begin to observe and assess the energetic reverberations of the proportions of the four phases, as they all have different impacts on energy, psychology, muscular effort, and so on.

   A *special note about pauses*: Natural pause assessments can be useful in creating awareness of breath apneas (i.e., moments when the breath stops involuntarily), including daytime apneas, such as stress apnea. Stress apnea occurs in a significant proportion of the human population in response to stressful events. It refers to a sudden holding of the breath, often at the top of the breath and sometimes in the form of a paradoxical breath, in response to a particular emotional cue. For example, it has been noted in the research literature as related to opening email [14]. It has been observed that workers hold their breath as soon as they open their email in clear anticipation of a stressful event. This breath-holding as a response to stress can become conditioned; it can become habitual and pattern-locked. Habitual breath holding is of great interest in the context of assessing breath on the mat (where it can occur during difficult postures or instructions), during healthcare or breathwork visits, and especially in daily life. If clients know that they stop breathing during sleep in the form of sleep apnea, this can also be noted under this assessment. However, in general breathwork practice, primary focus is on daytime breath holding and daytime distribution of the four phases across each breath cycle. Sleep apnea assessment typically requires specialized laboratory conditions and the involvement of a qualified healthcare provider. Addressing sleep apnea is beyond the scope of this book and the typical practice of a breathwork guide. Once again, referral and collaboration can become essential.

6.3.7   Assessment of Body, Breath, and Mind Patterns Reflecting Nervous System State

Breathing assessment in this context refers to observations of breath and related physiological and anatomical self-expressions that provide clues about patients' nervous system state (or *guna*). Recognizing whether students are in a state of chronic sympathetic arousal or dorsal collapse versus resiliently moving across the three polyvagal states can be helpful in understanding patient needs and creating intervention plans. Breathing instructors and clients benefit from being able to observe and read signals that suggest whether there is a nervous system default that can be rebalanced via breathwork. Following are a few tips on how to recognize pure gunas or polyvagal states. The chart in Chap. 4 that elucidates mixed states can be helpful for inferring the signs and symptoms of intersections and co-occurrence of these nervous system states. A standardized measure is now available to provide self-reports of clients' nervous system states. This measure is the *Neuroception of Psychological Safety Scale* (NPSS [15]; available in the public domain for free use (https://www.traumascience.org/neuroception-of-safety-scale). Table 6.13 overviews a few helpful signs and signals that may help identify various nervous system states.

6.3.8   Assessment of Breathing-Related Symptoms

Breathing symptoms can be explored via an intake form, intake interview, or brief questionnaires that are either self-constructed or available in the clinical literature. It is important in assessing breathing-related signs and symptoms to stay within our own scope of practice. In a yoga or breathwork-related setting, it is likely most appropriate to ask students about known breathing-related issues, perhaps using a brief questionnaire or a structured (i.e., questions-based) interview. If significant breathing issues exist that involve physical or mental health causes or

Table 6.13   Signs and signals of various neural platforms using polyvagal theory

Signs and signals of a resilient ventral vagal state	Signs and signals of an activated sympathetic state of arousal	Signs and signals of a collapsed dorsal vagal state
Sense of safe emotional connection and commitment	Focused on self-protection and protection of the tribe; disconnected from "other"	Emotional disengagement, numbness, or disconnection—even dissociation
Balanced and harmonized in body, energy, and mind	Braced (hypertonic), tense, and agitated in body, energy, and mind	Collapsed in body (hypotonic), energy, and mind
Resilient, optimal functional breathing—smooth, nasal, diaphragmatic, quiet, slow-paced	Rapid and voluminous OR shallow breath; gasping for air; noisy and rough; mouth and chest breathing	Shallow, disrupted, or irregular breathing; mouth and under-breathing; breath holding
Adaptable heart rate and increased heart rate variability	Increased heart rate	Slowed heart rate
More typically undisrupted sleep	Insomnia, disrupted sleep	Fatigue and/or lack of energy or vitality; impaired or excess sleep
Capacity to express and receive empathy, compassion, and joy	Inability to rest or relax—physical and energetic nervousness	Fear-, threat-, or shame-based emotions and reactivities
Calm and collected presence	Inability to sit still or focus; anxious or angry presence	Emotional overwhelm or lack of emotional resilience; dissociative
Energetic and motivated	Hypervigilance and hyper-alertness; excessive worry; ready for action	Sense of lack of control; energetically withdrawn; possible fainting spells
Resilience and strong capacity to cope with challenges	Environmental scanning for danger; chronically alert	Sense of being alone in the world, of abandonment, of despair
Relaxed and toned muscles with adaptability as situations demand	Muscular activation with a strong urge to move, run, fight, or flee	Slowed movement and possible lack of coordination
Curious and interested	Nervousness and jitteriness; chronically stressed	Impaired processing speed and/or memory
Mental clarity and creative problem solving	Increased sweating and blood flow, perhaps with skin reddening	Concrete, incoherent, or slowed thinking
Mindful and concentrated presence	Intermittent concentration; reactive	Poor concentration; mentally absent
Joyfulness, playfulness, hopefulness, and optimism	Irritation, frustration; aggression and defense	Hopelessness, helplessness, stagnation, heaviness

(continued)

Table 6.13   (continued)

Signs and signals of a resilient ventral vagal state	Signs and signals of an activated sympathetic state of arousal	Signs and signals of a collapsed dorsal vagal state
No predictable health pattern—more likely to be in good health and well-being	Digestive problems, weakened immunity, heart disease (e.g., high blood pressure and cholesterol); longer-term physiological effects of decreased functioning in many physiological systems, including physical and mental exhaustion and adrenal burn-out	Digestive problems, challenged immunity, chronic pain; other longer-term physiological effects of decreased functioning in many physiological systems
No predictable mental health pattern—more likely in good mental and emotional health and well-being	Fear, panic, anxiety, agitation, and other longer-term mental health effects of hypervigilance and hyperarousal	Depression, anxiety, PTSD, dissociative states, and other longer-term mental health effects of social/emotional disconnection and physiological shutdown

manifestations, it is essential to collaborate with a primary healthcare or mental healthcare provider who can help support the patient and inform the breathwork. However, not inquiring about breathing-related symptoms can be a significant omission in working with clients (and in our own breathing practices). It is helpful to know which symptoms are preexisting, which symptoms may arise during breathwork practice, and which symptoms may be ameliorated by the practice.

Dysfunctional Breathing Symptoms

Table 6.14 lists a few symptoms that can be explored explicitly. It is followed by a description of a few questionnaires that can be used in a breathwork context, as they have been used for that purpose in the research literature. Breathing-related symptoms are important to measure, so they can be tracked to learn how breathing affects us in each moment and across time. Breathing-related symptom assessment is also helpful because it draws attention to the reality that some breathing-related experiences and characteristics that we may consider general health challenges but that may actually be related to breathing patterns or even breathing exercises. Knowing that signs and symptoms may find relief through committed breathwork practices may become a powerful motivator to practice breathing formally and to continue assessing and observing our breathing in daily life. Symptom measurements, as is true for assessment of all breath characteristics, yield great outcome measures that can be tracked across time, signal progress, and indicate when breathwork has served its purpose and when the formal therapeutic collaboration can end.

Dysfunctional Breathing Questionnaires

Extant formal questionnaires of breathing-related symptoms tend to include symptoms that are associated with various characteristics of breath, such as signs and

Table 6.14 Breathing-related symptoms assessment questions

How often do you experience the following:
- Shortness of breath
- Breath moving in and out freely and smoothly, without hitches or glitches
- Holding the breath
- Stuffiness or blockages in the nose and/or sinus cavities
- Congestion in the lungs
- Tightness in the chest or rib basket
- Tightness in the jaw or neck, especially on awakening or after exertion
- Forward head or rounded shoulders

How often are the following true for you?
- I need to drink water during the night
- I snore during sleep
- I have been diagnosed sleep apnea
- I wake up with a dry mouth
- I wake up with a sore or dry throat
- I have stress apnea

How often do you make other breath-related sounds:
- Gasping, snuffling, panting, or sounding winded
- Sighing, yawning, or otherwise audibly heaving the breath
- Clearing the throat, coughing, hoarse voice, or breathy speech

symptoms related to breathing rate, volume, texture, sound, and phases of breath. Symptoms related to these aspects of breath, as well as additional breathing-related symptoms listed here, are all of interest to better understand clients' (and our own) breathing. The Breathing Assessment sample at the end of this section is an example of a useful addendum to an overall intake and assessment process that can be used by practitioners and teachers, who are always careful to stay within an appropriate scope of practice. As noted, and yet important to mention again in this specific context, breathwork guides stay faithful to their defined role with their patients, not overstepping their area of expertise and skillfulness.

One example of an extant questionnaire that includes all breath dimensions is the *Self-Evaluation Breathing Questionnaire*, a quick and easy standardized and self-administered scale of functional versus dysfunctional breathing [16]. This instrument has 25 items assessing various breathing-related symptoms, each of which is rated on a four-point Likert scale (ranging from 0 = *Never or not true at all*, 1 = *occasionally, a bit true*, 2 = *frequently, mostly true*, to 3 = *very frequently, very true*). Endorsement of symptom presence on 11 items or more is considered indicative of breathing challenges. Sample symptoms include items about sighing, yawning, irregular breathing, fast breathing, breath holding, breathlessness, mouth breathing, effortful breathing, and more. The scale reportedly is reliable and valid with good utility for ongoing assessment and reassessment to evaluate treatment outcomes [17]. The questionnaire is available in the public domain: https://static1. squarespace.com/static/5979d7fa9de4bb0311b000a1/t/60d9bd58931c7740e 8f17d5b/1624882585688/Self-Evaluation+of+Breathing+Questionnaire.

The *Nasal Obstruction Symptom Evaluation Instrument* (NOSE [18, 19]) provides a quick and easy measure of nasal congestion and obstruction via five

questions rated on a 5-point Likert scale. The questions inquire about nasal congestion or stuffiness, nasal blockage or construction, trouble breathing through the
nose, trouble sleeping, and inability to get air through the nose during exercise or
exertion. Individuals endorse each item on a scale ranging from 0 (*not a problem*) to
5 (*severe problem*). A total score above 30 is clearly indicative of nasal obstruction,
with a rating of moderate for 30–50, severe for 55–75, and extreme for 80–100. The
scale is in the public domain and can be retrieved at various sites online (e.g., https://
www.jnjmedtech.com/en-US/nasal-obstruction/nao-quality-of-life).

Other easily administered questionnaires and self-assessments for dysfunctional
breathing exist in the public domain, and new ones are added regularly. Following
are links to a few more examples. Clinicians are well-served to check online every
so often to discover new assessment resources as they become available.

- The *Breathing Pattern Assessment Tool* [20, 21] was developed to support the
  identification of breathing pattern disorders. It is a quick and easy assessment
  tool that is available in the public domain at this link: https://www.physio-pedia.
  com/Breathing_Pattern_Assessment_Tool
- The *Nijmegen Questionnaire* [22] was developed to detect possible hyperventilation and is available in the public domain: https://hgs.uhb.nhs.uk/wp-content/
  uploads/Nijmegen_Questionnaire.pdf

6.3.9   Ongoing Assessment and Inquiry

Assessment does not have an end—it continues the entire time student and teacher
or client and clinician are working together. It is as essential in the middle phase of
intervention as it was at the beginning; it is as useful toward the end of the work
together, as it was at the outset. Assessment and self-inquiry can be repeated regularly throughout breathwork as they are quick, easy, and unobtrusive; they make
great outcome or impact measures of a breathing practice on our anatomy, physiology, psychology, and breathing rhythms. On an ongoing basis, as clinicians or
teachers, we can ask our clients the most relevant of the following sample questions
(and, of course, many others) after any breathwork practice to assess its immediate
and distal impact:

- Has your breath rate changed? How about breath volume? Are you breathing
  harder or gentler now?
- How did breath texture evolve? How about sound?
- Do you feel a change in body temperature? Warmer? Colder?
- Is the nose less or more blocked? Do the sinuses feel clearer or more congested?
- Is there more or less saliva in mouth?
- Do you feel a greater or lesser sense of ease? Where? In the body? Energy or
  vitality? Mind, thoughts, or emotions?
- How has your energy or vitality changed? Do you feel more present?
  Alert? Active?
- Where is your attention? How has your attention shifted? In the body, breath,
  mind, emotions?

- Has your level of alertness changed? What is your level of tiredness now?
- Have your emotions changed? How?
- Has your mind state changed? How? (e.g., from distracted to focused? from disorganized to clear?)
- Is sustaining speech, chanting, or singing easier?

Self-assessment remains a helpful way for clients to conduct self-check-ins once breathwork is moved into home practice, without a teacher or clinician. Cultivating consistent and ongoing self-assessment skills is useful in daily life as it provides immediate feedback about anatomy, physiology, nervous system state, and psychology. It is an excellent way to remain connected to what is happening in all layers of self so that we begin to have choices in each moment—choices to stop, make conscious decisions; choices to respond rather than react; and choices to pick a breathing strategy that will help us re-regulate our nervous system before we act.

6.4   Where We Go from Here

Once assessment is complete and motivation for breathwork has been established, breathwork can begin. Clinician and client have created clarity about their goals for the joint work, understand the greater context, and are ready for the journey toward resilient breathing in daily life. They have established which types of changes are most necessary for the patient and where to enter treatment—whether there is a need for biomechanical interventions, practices to transform biochemistry, and/or practices that address polyvagal states and psychological causes and conditions related to breath and breathing. Assessment results guide all breathwork from here. As clinicians now have a clearer understanding of their patients, they can discern the types of physical preparations that are necessary, the mental and emotional work that may need to be integrated, and the types of breathing practices that are foundational and immediate, versus offered later in the course of intervention or treatment.

Chapter 7 addresses physical practices and vital, affective, mental, and emotional preparations that support breathwork and breathing, practices that help clinicians shape interventions to focus on the most relevant change mechanisms that will be propitious for the client. These practices are not separate from breathwork; they are deeply integrated into it, from beginning to end of each session and across time. They are addressed in a separate chapter for clarity about how body, emotions, and mind are integrated into breathwork proper. In practice, however, they are an essential and *integrated* aspect of breathwork, breath, and breathing. Physical and emotional preparations are extremely useful for many biomechanical, biochemical, and psychological interventions. Defining their role in breathwork and in relationship building between clinician and client is the aim of Chap. 7.

Breathe – Feelings come and go like clouds in a windy sky.
Conscious breathing is my anchor.—Thich Nhat Hanh

6.5   Sample Breath Assessment Form

Part one—Breathing assessment
Collated by Christiane Brems, PhD, ABPP, ERYT500, C-IAYT based on many resources in the research literature

Heart rate measurement
- Find your pulse in your wrist or at your neck.
- Once you can reliably locate your pulse, start a timer set for 1 min.
- Count your pulse.
- Your total count when the timer runs out, is your heart rate. _____

Breaths per minute (BPM) measurement
- Take a few moments tuning into your breath, becoming familiar with sensing the breath to be able to count how often it moves through you in a given time period. You might do this by counting the number of inhalations, the number of exhalations, the number of inhalations and exhalations, or the number of times you feel your abdomen rise and fall.
- Once you can reliably locate or identify a breath cycle, start a timer set for 1 min.
- Count the number of breaths while the timer is running.
- Your total count when the timer runs out, is your rate of breaths per minute.

_____

Controlled breath pause measurement (aka control pause)
Purpose
This assessment is a proxy measure of CO_2 tolerance in the medulla. Higher controlled breath pause indicates that the body is tolerant of higher levels of CO_2 in the blood. Lower levels are indicative of CO_2 sensitivity, the likely consequence of chronic hyperventilation and commensurate chronic hypocapnia (i.e., low CO_2 levels in the blood).

Instructions
- Be prepared with a stopwatch
- Inhale gently through the nose
- Exhale lightly through the nose
- Pinch the nose shut (optional but preferable) and start a stopwatch at the same time
- Hold the breath after the exhale until the first sign of air hunger (i.e., the desire to inhale)
- Check the stopwatch, noting the duration of the breath hold in seconds
- Open the nose, inviting an inhalation ➔
  - This inhalation should be normal and comfortable
  - If it is a gasp, the breath hold was too long
  - Wait a few minutes (allowing the breath to resettle) and repeat at a lesser level of desire to breathe
- The time on the stopwatch represents the length of your comfortable pause.

_____

Interpretation
- <=10 s: very low CO_2 levels with likely CO_2 hypersensitivity and commensurate dysregulated or dysregulating breathing patterns (hyperventilation, chest breathing)
- >10–15: low CO_2 with likely vulnerability to CO_2 hypersensitivity and the tendency to be triggered into reactivity in breathing patterns
- >15–20: healthy CO_2 levels and a stable and resilient respiratory system
- >20–30: good vitality and health with near optimal tolerance and levels of CO_2
- >30: mild to no breathlessness during exercise; excellent vitality and CO_2 tolerance

Part two—Qualitative observations of breath

Answer the following questions to the best of your current ability. You may not yet know the answers to some of these questions as some characteristics of the breath may be out of your typical state of breath awareness.

Answer the following questions based on your TYPICAL experience:

How often does your breath sound:

Noisy and probably audible to others	Seldom	Often	Usually
Relatively quiet	Seldom	Often	Usually
Completely silent—inaudible to you and others	Seldom	Often	Usually

How often do you make other breath-related sounds:

Gasping, snuffling, panting, or sounding winded	Seldom	Often	Usually
Sighing, yawning, or otherwise audibly heaving the breath	Seldom	Often	Usually
Clearing the throat, coughing, hoarse voice, or breathy speech	Seldom	Often	Usually

How often does your breath feel:

Rapid, erratic, agitated, strong, quick	Seldom	Often	Usually
Very slow, tight, barely notable, weak, timid	Seldom	Often	Usually
Restful, silent, smooth, rhythmic, easeful	Seldom	Often	Usually
Full (lots of air moving in and out)	Seldom	Often	Usually
Shallow (little air moving in and out)	Seldom	Often	Usually
Urgent (with a sense of hungering for air or a mild fear of suffocating)	Seldom	Often	Usually

How often do you experience the following:

Shortness of breath	Seldom	Often	Usually
Breath moving in and out freely and smoothly, without hitches or glitches	Seldom	Often	Usually
Holding the breath	Seldom	Often	Usually
Stuffiness or blockages in the nose and/or sinus cavities	Seldom	Often	Usually
Congestion in the lungs	Seldom	Often	Usually
Tightness in the chest or rib basket	Seldom	Often	Usually
Tightness in the jaw or neck, especially on awakening or after exertion	Seldom	Often	Usually
Forward head or rounded shoulders	Seldom	Often	Usually

How often do you feel the breath in the following locations:

Shoulders (e.g., lifting or rising upward)	Seldom	Often	Usually
High chest or region of the clavicles (e.g., a subtle lifting or outward movement)	Seldom	Often	Usually
Mid chest or the thoracic region (e.g., a sense of expansion and contraction)	Seldom	Often	Usually
Abdomen (e.g., a rising and falling)	Seldom	Often	Usually
Low rib basket (e.g., moving slightly outward and inward)	Seldom	Often	Usually

How often are the following true for your tongue?

It rests at the bottom of the mouth	Seldom	Often	Usually
It rests at the roof of the mouth	Seldom	Often	Usually
It presses against the hard palate of the mouth	Seldom	Often	Usually
It is strong and toned	Seldom	Often	Usually
It is weak and flaccid	Seldom	Often	Usually

How often do the following describe your breathing?

I breathe through the nose most of the day	Seldom	Often	Usually
I breathe through the mouth most of the day	Seldom	Often	Usually
I breathe through the nose most of the night	Seldom	Often	Usually
I breathe through the mouth most of night	Seldom	Often	Usually
I breathe through the nose during exertion or exercise	Seldom	Often	Usually
I breathe through the mouth during exertion or exercise	Seldom	Often	Usually

How often are the following true for you?			
I need to drink water during the night	Seldom	Often	Usually
I snore during sleep	Seldom	Often	Usually
I have sleep apnea	Seldom	Often	Usually
I wake up with a dry mouth	Seldom	Often	Usually
I wake up with a sore or dry throat	Seldom	Often	Usually
I have stress apnea (i.e., catch myself holding the breath during stressful situations)	Seldom	Often	Usually
I talk a lot (e.g., teachers, actors, etc.)	Seldom	Often	Usually
I laugh a lot	Seldom	Often	Usually

References

1. Miller WR, Rollnick S. Motivational interviewing. 3rd ed. Guilford Press; 2013.
2. Farhi D. Yoga mind, body & spirit: a return to wholeness. Owl Books; 2011.
3. Mitchell J. Yoga biomechanics.. Handspring; 2019.
4. Porter K. Natural posture for pain-free living. Inner Traditions International; 2013.
5. Schiffmann E. Yoga: the spirit and practice of moving into stillness. Gallery Books; 2013.
6. Brule D. Just breathe: mastering breathwork for success in life, love, business, and beyond. Atria/Enliven Books; 2017.
7. Parkes MJ. The limits of breath holding. Sci Am. 2012;306(4):74–9. https://doi.org/10.1038/scientificamerican0412-74.
8. Rothenberg R. Restoring prana: a therapeutic guide to pranayama and healing through the breath for yoga therapists, teachers, and healthcare practitioners. Singing Dragon; 2020.
9. McKeown P. Oxygen advantage: the simple, scientifically proven breathing techniques for a healthier, slimmer, faster, and fitter you. William Morrow; 2015.
10. McKeown P. Buteyko instructor training manual. Oxygen Research Institute; 2020.
11. McKeown P. The breathing cure. Humanix; 2021.
12. Skaggs SA, McCarthy M, Shelledy DC. Physical assessment. In: Shelledy DC, Peters JI, editors. Respiratory care. Jones & Bartlett Learning; 2022. p. 151–202.
13. Scott JB, Kaur R. Monitoring breathing frequency, pattern, and effort. Respir Care. 2020;65(6):793–806. https://doi.org/10.4187/respcare.07439.
14. Stone L. Just breathe: building the case for email apnea. https://www.huffpost.com/entry/just-breathe-building-the_b_85651. Updated 2008. Accessed 18 March 2024.
15. Morton L, Cogan N, Kolacz J, Calderwood C, Nikolic M, Bacon T, et al. A new measure of feeling safe: developing psychometric properties of the neuroception of psychological safety scale (NPSS). Psychol Trauma. 2024;16(4):701–8. https://doi.org/10.1037/tra0001313.
16. Courtney R, Greenwood KM. Preliminary investigation of a measure of dysfunctional breathing symptoms: the self evaluation of breathing questionnaire (SEBQ). Int J Osteopath Med. 2009;12(4):121–7. https://doi.org/10.1016/j.ijosm.2009.02.001.
17. Mitchell AJ, Bacon CJ, Moran RW. Reliability and determinants of self-evaluation of breathing questionnaire (SEBQ) score: a symptoms-based measure of dysfunctional breathing. Appl Psychophysiol Biofeedback. 2016;41(1):111–20. https://doi.org/10.1007/s10484-015-9316-7.
18. Stewart MG, Witsell DL, Smith TL, Weaver EM, Yueh B, Hannley MT. Development and validation of the nasal obstruction symptom evaluation (NOSE) scale. Otolaryngol Head Neck Surg. 2004;130(2):157–63. https://doi.org/10.1016/j.otohns.2003.09.016.
19. Lipan MJ, Most SP. Development of a severity classification system for subjective nasal obstruction. JAMA Facial Plast Surg. 2013;15(5):358–61. https://doi.org/10.1001/jamafacial.2013.344.

20. Hylton H, Long A, Francis C, Taylor RR, Ricketts WM, Singh R, Pfeffer PE. Real-world use of the breathing pattern assessment tool in assessment of breathlessness post-COVID-19. Clin Med. 2022;22(4):376–9. https://doi.org/10.7861/clinmed.2021-0759.
21. Todd S, Walsted ES, Grillo L, Livingston R, Menzies-Gow A, Hull JH. Novel assessment tool to detect breathing pattern disorder in patients with refractory asthma. Respirology. 2018;23(3):284–90. https://doi.org/10.1111/resp.13173.
22. van Dixhoorn J, Folgering H. The Nijmegen Questionnaire and dysfunctional breathing. ERJ Open Res. 2015;1(1):1. https://doi.org/10.1183/23120541.00001-2015.

Preparing for Body and Mind for Breathwork

7

> *Breathing is not merely an in-drawing and out-streaming of air, but a fundamental movement of a living whole, affecting the world of the body as well as the regions of the soul and mind.*
>
> *Karlfried Graf Durckheim*

7.1 Overview: Preparing All Layers of Self for Breathwork

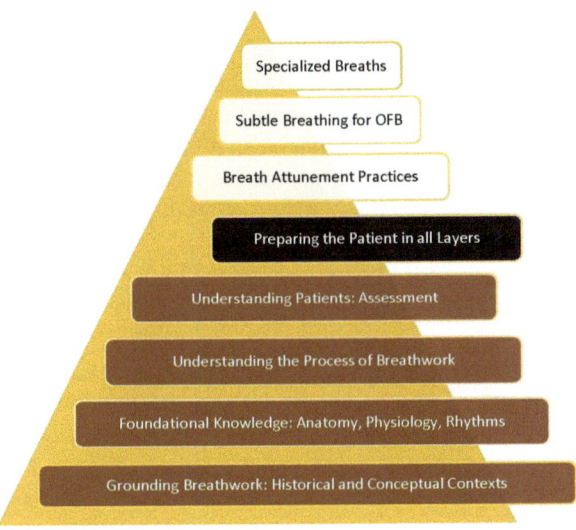

Before we explore the practices included in a breathwork session, it is helpful to remember that we always work with all layers of self—body, energy and vitality, mind and emotions, intuition and wisdom, connection and relationships, even joy. We honor all yogic and mindfulness practices so even when we focus on one, we

C. Brems, *Therapeutic Breathwork*,
https://doi.org/10.1007/978-3-031-66683-4_7

remain aware and respectful of the others, however, subtly or implicitly. Given that frame, movements and forms in a breathing practice are integrated aspects of breathwork. They may be taught or sequenced distinctly, but they are part and parcel of the breathwork—in the same way we carefully prepare the environment (honoring nonviolence, truthfulness, moderation) and clarify intentions and commitments. Form (e.g., yoga *asana*) and movement (e.g., *kriya*, *vinyasa*) support breath and breathing; likewise, breath and breathing support form and movement. Similarly, no matter in which portion of a breathing practice we find ourselves, mindfulness, concentration, and a deep guarding of our energy are helpful and fully integrated. With each movement, with each breath, we honor connection, union, interdependence, and co-arising. We do so with joy and wisdom in all experiences of self.

This chapter explores vital, mental, and physical preparatory practices that ensure that clients can optimally benefit from breathwork. It opens with preparations targeted to helping patients find ease and peacefulness in their vital and mental layers of experience, offering sample scripts for opening centering practices and exercises to calm the nervous system and achieve a sense of calm before and during physical and breathing practices. This type of vital and mental preparation is included to help clinicians welcome and support most, if not all, aspects of sensations, mind stories, and strong emotions that may arise for clients during breathwork. With that context in place, this chapter explores physical practices that support healthful postural alignment and offers movement explorations that help with physical awareness and readiness for breathwork. For example, the chapter offers practices for neck and shoulder releases, rib basket resilience, vital heart opening, and core stabilization. It explores the connections of nasal clearing and tongue strengthening to optimal breathwork practice, as well as breathing in daily life.

Many samples of the preparatory practices discussed here are offered in a YouTube playlist by this author. Clinicians can feel free to access this exclusive playlist with the following link and may share it with their patients: https://www.youtube.com/playlist?list=PLzvkZpUGjwIGxil7eP9j41Zw4PALDm6yx.

7.2   Energetic and Mental Preparations in Breathwork

Just as we attend to physical preparations that can support breathwork, so too do we attend to energetic and mental preparations. Energetically, it is optimal if we invite clients to settle into stillness and ease before, during, and after breathwork. An opening centering that invites grounding, expansiveness, and harmony into all *koshas* can feel particularly settling for the nervous system. It can help clients begin the breathwork session more fully and with open focus. The extra time spent on an opening centering can magnify the impact of the breathing practice and is well worth the time investment. Closing with a calming practice can be helpful as well, especially if strong affects or emotions, overwhelming sensations, or mental stories emerged during breathwork. It is useful for client and clinician to realize that strong sensations, affects, arousal, and emotions may emerge during breathwork. As clinicians, we can feel more able to support our patients and welcome their difficulties if we have prepared ourselves mentally and with concrete strategies for how to deal with such challenges. With preparation for language, attitudes, and cuing in place ahead of time, clinicians are able to offer clients strategies and tools to experience sensations and fluctuations of mind and emotions with an open heart and open mind. The mental and energetic practices presented in this chapter are appropriate for all clients, regardless of what the assessment revealed, as long as they are appropriately tailored to specific in-the-moment needs.

7.2.1   Energetic Preparations in Breathwork

Cultivating Calm and Centered Presence with an Opening Centering Practice

Although relaxation is not the actual goal of breathwork, breathing practice is well-served by inviting a few moments of deliberate fostering (or at least invitation) of gentleness, easefulness, release, and quietude before moving into breathing practices (this is in line with the session sequencing ideas suggested in Chap. 5). This recommendation holds true whether breathwork is offered in the context of yoga and/or physical practice or in healthcare or mental healthcare settings. Many strategies exist to help clients move toward ease, tranquility, and relaxed presence. An opening centering approach is offered here as a means of inviting easeful energetic preparation for clients in all their layers of experience at the beginning of a breathwork session. Opening centering practices help set the stage for ease *before* a breathing session; calming practices may be used at the end of a breathing session, especially with patients prone to anxiety or sympathetic nervous system states. As appropriate, calming strategies can also be used throughout a session if signs of dysregulation or anxiety emerge in a client. Practices such as *kosha* meditations, progressive muscle relaxations, or yoga *nidra* may be helpful [1, 2]. Many other possibilities exist for inviting patients into easeful attention before (and possibly after) breathwork.

Following are three sample scripts for energetic preparation and debriefing via suggested sample interventions. The scripts offered below are not meant to be used exactly as written. They are simply examples, mere invitations for clinicians to be creative and to develop their own language and way of offering centering, tension-releasing practices before and after physical practices and breathwork. The main take-away from the sample scripts is to invite patients into practices that move them into awareness of all layers of experience; releasing tension, holding, or gripping; and scanning or attending to body, vitality, and mind. In all scripts, attention is drawn first to tangible, easy-to-access *body parts and physical sensations*. This is followed by invitations to notice the presence and perhaps accessing a calming of energy, *vitality, arousal,* and affect. Finally, each sample script gently attends to non-attachment to *thoughts and emotions*. All tangible layers of self are acknowledged without judgment and invited to yield with ease and open-heartedness into the present moment and circumstances to the greatest degree possible. It is important to be clear that all offered guidance is only an invitation—invited practices are not meant to trigger an inner fight to release tension. Some clients defeat the purpose of centering practices by over-efforting in an attempt to create tranquility. Language that invites easeful presence and accepting openness to what emerges can help such clients surrender their (likely broader pattern of) over-efforting and simply be with experience as it unfolds in each moment.

Opening Centering—A Sample Script

This script is most appropriately used at the beginning of class and may optimally last no more than 5–7 min. It is offered as an invitation, with many additional phrasing and action options. The script does not cover all possibilities, or it would simply be too long to use. It is an example of how an opening centering on all of the layers of self-experience can be offered in a manner that is calming for the nervous system, settling for the mind, and grounding for the body. While it is framed as an opening centering, a very similar practice could be offered at the end of a session. Slight changes in wording and emphasis may be necessary. Clinicians are encouraged not simply to read a script, but to understand its essence and to put its essence into their own words. Scripts are best not used as offered below because each patient is different. Only the clinician who knows the client can determine what kinds of language, pacing, and invitations are most appropriate for each individual.

Opening Centering
A Brief Sample Script—To be adapted as needed

I invite you to take a moment to get settled on the earth, either in a seated or a lying-down position that serves your body and your vitality in this moment … Notice if there are any supportive props that might help bring greater ease into your body, your breath, even your mind, and find them now… for example, it might be lovely to sit slightly elevated on a blanket or a cushion… it might be helpful to cover up with a blanket or to put on an extra layer of clothing if your environment is cool… be deliberate in your choices about the kinds of support you can offer yourself as you settle into the earth…

[Pause]

Once you have found a comfortable position, please know that you can always gently move and readjust if something begins to feel uncomfortable… Simply do this with awareness and move slowly and mindfully so that you don't disrupt the calmness you are cultivating… You might also make a gentle decision about whether you would like to keep your eyes open or closed; perhaps taking stock of your nervous system to see what feels safe and appropriate in this moment and given the environment in which you are practicing…

[Pause]

Gently move your attention into your body, making note of how your physical being is arriving in this moment… What is your body bringing with it this morning? … Notice any sensations that are arising within you… maybe you are noticing whether you are feeling warm or cool … maybe there are little aches or pains… maybe some tingling or pulsing …

[Pause]

Perhaps some of these sensations are pleasant ... others may be unpleasant ... others may be neutral or even a bit confusing ... simply take note of your body and greet whatever sensations are arising from your physical being ... making no judgments but meeting your body and sensations in this moment with compassion and with an open loving heart...

[Pause]

Keeping your body in the background of your awareness, gently shift your attention to your energy in this moment ... what are you bringing with you today as with regard to your breath ... your vitality ... maybe even your affect ... do you feel calm or a bit agitated ... or maybe, on the other hand, a bit tired ... worn out or lethargic ... how is your energy or vitality showing up for you ... perhaps the breath is a helpful indicator of just how settled or activated your energy is ... invite yourself to meet the signs and signals of your vitality with an open heart ... with compassion ... there is no need for evaluation or judgment ... can you open your heart to whatever sense of energy emerges in this moment ...

[Pause]

You might note for a moment how your inhalations and exhalations are moving through you ... perhaps noticing just how much breath is moving ... or how quickly the breath is moving ... what the texture is like ... is the breath rough and choppy ... or smooth and buttery ... meet whatever you are noticing with an open heart and an open mind ... there is no need to change anything or judge or criticize ... you are simply meeting your vitality and energy in this moment, just as it is ...

[Pause]

Continuing to hold your body and your energy in the background of your awareness, gently shift your attention to what is happening in your mind ... meet any thoughts that are present ... perhaps preoccupations with what has already happened today ... or planning for what still needs to unfold ... perhaps there are thoughts that are judging or confused about what is happening in this moment ... whatever thoughts appear, gently make note of them ...

[Pause]

There is no need to change anything ... simply be clear about the thoughts that are present for you .... without following the storyline ... nor trying to make these thoughts go away ... thoughts are a natural reality of the human brain ... you can simply acknowledge them ...

[Pause]

Then, perhaps turn your attention to notice what emotions are present for you today ... in this moment as you settle into your chosen shape ...

[Pause]

Holding your body, your energy, and your mind with its thoughts and emotions, in the background of your awareness, let yourself become aware of this capacity you have to meet yourself … to watch yourself … to pay attention to what is happening in your physical being … in your energy … what thoughts and emotions are unfolding coming and going … perhaps you can rejoice in this capacity to pay attention to what is happening … right here, right now …. within you and even around you … perhaps you can rejoice in the wisdom of sitting still … remaining compassionately settled and calm even as you watch this unfolding in and around you …

[Pause]

This very wise intuitive intelligent part of you is always there for you … you may simply lose track of it at times … and so in these moments when you become aware of your wise capacity … take a moment to take a breath … perhaps you can connect to the joy of this human life that you have … that allows you to make conscious choices … discerning decisions … that allows you to learn new things and to be in the world in new ways …

[Pause]

[for patients who are lying down, cue them to rise to a seated position]

I invite you now to bring your hands to your heart … as you bow your head to your heart to invite an intention for your time in this session today … your intention might come to you as a simple word or a phrase … it could be a felt sense that has no words … invite your intention to help you find meaning and purpose in your practice … perhaps guiding your work in the session today …

[Pause]

If something meaningful arose for you, I invite you to seal your intention, however tangible or intangible, into your own heart as you draw a breath in … and then I invite you to release that intention silently outward as you let go of a breath out…

[Linger for a few moments, attentive to what may emerge nonverbally from the patient]

Scan of Layers of Experience—A Sample Script

This script walks patients through all of their layers of self, inviting a noting of sensations and experiences in each layer. It is a calming script in the sense that the pacing is slow and comfortable. There is no long lingering on any single aspect part of a patient's experience. It is a touching-in with all that is present in the given moment and space. This script can be made more nurturing by adding invitations to convey compassion, breath, lovingkindness, and other self-nurturing actions and intentions to any region of a patient's experience that are presenting significant challenges for the individual. The practice thus moves beyond an opening calming practice to evolve into a contemplative practice of selfcare. Sometimes it is difficult to know at the beginning of a session where a patient needs to go with an opening centering. In one-on-one sessions, it is possible to let the guidance evolve into a more self-nurturing, rather than opening or calming, practice. Only the clinician who is with the patient can notice exactly how to let the experience unfold for each individual. As noted earlier, it is crucial that clinicians understand the essence of a script and then put it in their own words and in language that is most accessible to their particular clients.

Scan of Layers of Experience

A Brief Sample Script—To be adapted as needed

I invite you to get settled … *[offer choices of sitting or lying down, based on observation]* … allow yourself the pleasure of using supportive props to achieve a sense of comfort and ease in your physical being as you settle yourself in … *[offer options that are available]*

[Pause]

Gently begin to take note of how your body is arriving in this space and in this moment … check in with your physical being overall and note the energy that is present … note any sensations that are speaking up most noticeably …

[Pause]

Then, very gently begin to scan your body … starting by noticing sensations in your feet … perhaps there is warmth or tingling … maybe there is a bit of tension … simply note what is present in your feet … receiving the feedback from that part of your body … with an open heart and an open mind … without judgment …

[Pause]

Gently begin to sweep your attention upward … through your ankles … into your calves … noticing sensation along the way … accepting whatever sensations arise … as your attention moves further upward through your knees … your thighs … noticing sensations in both legs …

[Pause]

As your attention moves upward into your hips … the entire pelvic girdle … as you meet whatever is present in this part of your body … in this moment … meeting sensations with compassion, with kindness … without judgment, without a desire to change anything … settling into the reality of the sensations in both legs and your hips …

[Pause]

As your attention moves upward into your lower abdomen … your waist … the upper abdomen … as you meet sensations here … maybe there are sounds … maybe there is a sense of movement … simply notice what is present here … meeting all sensations arising from this part of your body without judgment … with compassion …

[Pause]

As you gently sweep your attention further upward … into your torso … into the upper chest … all the way upward toward your shoulder girdle … noticing sensations … meeting whatever is present in this part of your physical being … open-heartedly and open-mindedly … no matter how pleasant … or unpleasant … or neutral … or perhaps confusing the sensations are that you are meeting …

[Pause]

Gently invite your attention to sweep through the entire shoulder girdle … and into the arms … noticing sensations in both upper arms … both elbows … and your forearms … your wrist … your hands … all the way into your fingertips … fully aware of any sensations … pulsations … vibrations … that are emerging in your arms …

[Pause]

Then, gently sweep your attention toward your neck … through the throat to the base of your skull … across your scalp … toward your face … noticing sensations in your forehead … your temples … your cheeks … noticing anything that is present in terms of physical sensation in your eyes … your nose … the outer part of your nose … the inner part of your nose … your mouth … your lips … your jaws … your teeth … your tongue … the back of the throat … becoming very aware of sensations that are present in your face …

[Pause]

As you then move your attention inside your head … sensing into the center of your brain … as you notice what is present here … being with the sensation … tuning into the inside of your head … the inside of your throat … the inside of your chest … the inside of your abdomen … the entirety of your inner being … meeting sensations from the inside out … calmly receiving the feedback about your body in this moment … being compassionate and kind … responsive to everything you encounter … perhaps sending compassion … to parts of your body that need a bit of attention …

[Pause]

Perhaps sending the nourishment and vibration of an inhalation in the direction of strong sensation in your body … perhaps releasing sensation with a conscious breath out as you gently begin to note the rhythm of your breath … the inhalations … and the exhalations … traveling in and out … as you perhaps note the presence of thoughts … and emotions that are emerging … being with whatever arises … returning to the breath … over and over … inhaling and exhaling compassionately … with dedication to being fully present in this moment … and in the space … take another moment to sense into the entirety of your being

[Pause]

[for patients who are lying down, cue them to rise to a seated position]

And then when it feels appropriate, bow your head to your heart, as you perhaps place the hands at the heart to invite an intention for your session today…

[Pause]

If something meaningful arose for you, I invite you to seal your intention, however tangible or intangible, into your own heart as you draw a breath in … and then I invite you to release that intention silently outward as you let go of a breath out…

[Linger for a few moments, attentive to what may emerge nonverbally from the patient]

Table 7.1   General cuing for scans and centering

- Create ease in the face—letting go of holding or gripping in the forehead, temples, eyes, eyeballs, lips, corners of the mouth, jaws, tongue
- Find a gentle inner gaze, inviting the muscles around the eyes and even the eyeballs to soften and let go
- Bring ease into the throat and neck
- Release tension from the shoulder, hands, and fingers
- Invite gentleness or serenity into the heart, chest, and abdomen
- Soften the grip of the hands or fingers
- Let go of any unnatural, excessive holding or bracing in the hips
- Invite any unnecessary efforting in the hips, legs, and toes to release
- Meet body and breath with a peaceful openness
- Notice your energetic or vital presence and meet it with compassion, gentleness, and gratitude for all sensations you encounter
- Release any sense of trying to <u>make</u> relaxation happen—soften into the moment instead
- Open up to the possibility of accessing an easeful energy and peaceful presence
- Invite serenity or peace into the entirety of your being
- Soften into an open-hearted, tranquil state of being
- Meet your physical and vital state of being peaceful, without expectations or judgment
- Allow the mind to let go of any obsessive or compelling thoughts, simply letting them be what they are—not attaching to them, not trying to force them out
- Notice straining or overthinking in the mind and invite peacefulness and grounding
- Softly allow thoughts to come and go … noticing that you neither have to cling to them nor chase them away
- Release tension even in the face of what might emerge in body, breath, and mind—it was already there; you are simply meeting it consciously
- Gently, compassionately meet any emotions that emerge—holding them lightly, neither immersing in them, nor trying to make them go away

Table 7.1 provides additional general cues that can be embedded in the scans offered earlier, adding language about releasing strong or difficult sensations or experiences. These possible prompts are invitations to find creativity in using the aforementioned scripts with a slightly stronger focus on letting go, rather than simply being with. Notable for their absence are prompts that use language such as "melting" or "dissolving." These words can be problematic for individuals who are prone to dissociation and not worth the potential downsides, given that many other options exist.

Opening or Closing Progressive Muscle Relaxation—A Sample Script
This script requires slight tensing and subsequent releasing of physical body parts to help clients move into more intimate experiences of their anatomy. For some patients, this is the only way that they can begin to get in touch with physical sensations. The script is offered mostly with such individuals in mind. For patients who are already very braced and over-efforting, this may not be an ideal choice. That said, sometimes increasing gripping is the only way strained or constricted clients can notice that they are bracing habitually. As always, clinicians are encouraged to review the essence of the script and then to vary its intention and language based on the people in front of them.

Progressive Muscle Relaxation

A Brief Sample Script—To be adapted as needed

Welcome to this moment and this space. I invite you to find a comfortable seated or lying-down position with whatever supports or props that serve you today. *[offer choices based on observation]* Make a discerning choice about how you would like to place your hands and whether it feels appropriate to close your eyes. *[offer options for both]*

[Pause]

Gently become aware of your breathing—perhaps gently notice how the breath travels through your nose … how it collaborates with your belly and side waist… remain with a gentle breath … inviting each inhalation to nourish you and each exhalation to bring an increasing sense of ease and presence …

[Pause]

Acknowledge any thoughts or emotions that are with you in this moment … simply notice—no need to engage or to try to chase them away. Let them be what they are … thoughts may come and they may go … that is the nature of our human mind. Simply let them be and when you notice that they draw your attention away, gently bring yourself back to my voice and into your body…

[Pause]

Gently move your attention to your feet. Curl your toes gently for a few seconds … hold … then release and invite the toes to let go completely. Can you sense the experience of tension transforming into greater ease as you release the toes …

[Pause]

Gently move your attention upward to your calf muscles. Slowly engage the calf muscles by pointing your toes towards your body… hold for a moment … and release… let go of any holding or gripping. Can you notice a shift in sensations … perhaps of warmth or ease or release spreading through your calves …

[Pause]

Gently guide your attention upward to your thighs. Engage the muscles in your thighs by pressing your knees toward each other… hold for a moment … then let go … release …. Can you notice change in the experience of your thighs as muscular tension releases … is there perhaps a sense of warmth or letting go …

[Pause]

Very gently and compassionately draw your attention to your hips. Create a sense of engagement here, perhaps gently squeezing the glutes … hold … and then release … let go … As you release, can you note the sensations in this part of your body as it lets go … as it releases into a sense of ease…

[Pause]

Moving your attention now to your abdomen, take a gentle breath in and, as you exhale, draw the belly muscles inward, reaching your belly button toward your spine … hold for a moment … then release and allow a natural breath to flow in and out … can you sense into your abdomen … is there perhaps a softening or a sense of letting be …

[Pause]

Now, gently direct your attention to your hands. Clench your fists gently, feeling tension in your fingers and palms … hold for a moment … then release … let your hands rest gently and notice any difference … note what has changed as the hands have let go …

[Pause]

Moving up your arms, flex your biceps by bringing your fists toward your shoulders, tightening the muscles in your upper arms … hold briefly … then release … what do you notice … is there a greater sense of ease … perhaps a sense of warmth spreading down your arms …

[Pause]

Gently shift your attention to your shoulders. Gently shrug them up toward your ears, feeling engagement in your shoulder muscles … hold for a moment … then invite the shoulders to drop … to release … to find ease. What do you notice as tension drains away … is there a sense of ease that follows …

[Pause]

Finally, gently move your attention to your face. Scrunch up your face gently, wrinkle your forehead, close your eyes, grip your jaw … hold for a moment … and release and let go … allow your face to soften and notice— notice any sensations that enter this part of your body as you release and let go …

[Pause]

Gently tune into a sense of ease in your face, your shoulders, your arms… your abdomen, your hips, your legs, and your feet. Absorb any sense of release and ease that is present … invite yourself into this moment of letting go … of simply being present with what is … of being without any doing …

[Pause]

Enjoy the sensation of letting go … of ease and release flowing through your entirety of your being. Notice your body, your breath, even your mind— are there any changes in how you experience your body, your breath, our mind … now compared to just a few minutes ago…

[Linger for a few moments, attentive to what may emerge nonverbally from the patient]

[gently guide the client back to an upright position, ready to engage in the breathwork session]

Maintaining Calm and Centered Presence Through the Session

Once ease and tranquility have been accessed via present-moment self-experience, stillness and calmness can be invited into body and vitality throughout the breathing session. Sample facilitating cues that can be inserted into breathwork instructions are provided in Table 7.2. Many other pathways exist to support easeful energy, adaptive arousal, and tranquil affect during a breathwork session. Understanding our clients (via assessment and relationship building) and considering their current circumstances and needs guide how and when we insert cues (such as the examples that follow) as needed during physical preparation practices and breathwork proper.

Once clients' energy settles (typically in an observable way), we can begin to add work with the mind—addressing emerging thoughts and emotions. It may take a few breathing sessions to move explicitly and persistently into the mental layer of experience. Patience is key to maintaining ease and a sense of not needing to accomplish anything, especially not quickly.

7.2.2 Mental and Emotional Preparations in Breathwork

Breathing practices, especially integrated holistic breathing that involves a multitude of practices (i.e., commitment to integrating values, intention, movement, and focus) and honors all layers of consciousness, can bring with them strong reactions in body, affect, mind, emotions, and psyche. It is best if we enter breathwork knowing that strong sensations and reactions may emerge and to be prepared with strategies and tools for being with sensations and the mental and emotional reactivity that may result. We are most likely to gain access to the benefits of breathing practices if we are prepared to embrace sensations with open hearts and open minds, with compassion, friendliness, and lovingkindness. A few suggestions follow about how to help clients move into sensation with a sense of calm, collected, and equanimous presence. These suggestions are grouped by intention. However, in actual clinical or

Table 7.2 General cuing to invite ease and calm during breathwork

- Invite the body to become still so that the only major movement left is the movement of the inhalation and exhalation
- Collect your attention into the breath, noticing breath traveling in and breath traveling out gently, naturally, lightly
- Invite energetic tension and emotional worry to flow away with each exhalation to the degree possible—do not stress if this does not work right away
- Prevent energy from moving outward to the senses—invite energy and attention inward instead, continuously returning to the breath to inner sensation
- Stay compassionately connected to your inner vitality and vibrancy
- Allow yourself to tune into your aliveness, as signified by the pulsation of breath moving through you gently and freely
- Meet your breath, energy, and vitality with openness and without expectations or judgment
- Allow your vitality, radiance, and energy to move through all of your experiences and into your life
- Remind yourself that regardless of what emerges in your physical or breathing practice—it was already there; you are simply meeting it consciously and with an open heart

teaching practice, it is quite likely that clinicians choose to mix these categories based on client observations, needs, and preferences. Such adaptations are not only natural and appropriate, but important for maintaining a tailored and person-centered relationship with each patient. Separate listings are offered simply as a variety of ideas about how particular intentions can be cued. As always, clinicians translate offered cues into their own voice and vocabulary, choosing words and phrases that are authentic for them and accessible and inviting for their clients.

Moving into Acceptance of Experiences Emerging from All Layers of Self

Clients need to understand that breathing can evoke various sensations across all aspects of self, including stories of the mind and strong emotions. They are encouraged to embrace the full spectrum of possibilities that may arise. Patients are invited to observe physical sensations without urgency or bias, whether pleasant, unpleasant, or neutral. They are emboldened to resist the urge to cling to or push away sensation; instead, viewing sensations as opportunities to understand their breath and its movements through the body and effects on the mind. Clients benefit from learning to stay present with discomfort—whether in the form of physical sensations, affective arousal or reactivity, mental judgments or stories, or strong emotional reactions, acknowledging these phenomena without wishing for them to change. As patients begin to approach sensations and experiences in all layers of experience without judgment or aversion, they recognize that experiences ebb and flow—they arise and they leave; even if they persist, they change and transform. Through this observation, patients realize that rather than creating narratives around sensations and other phenomena, they can greet each fluctuation or experience with curiosity and openness of heart and mind. They can trust themselves to embrace whatever emerges, understanding that these sensations, fluctuations, and emotions already exist and that welcoming them allows for growth, understanding, and transformation over time.

To assist clients with developing strategies for staying present with sensation, experiences, fluctuations, and emotions that may emerge during breathwork, they can be guided toward developing open-heartedness, self-compassion, lovingkindness, curiosity, and open-mindedness. They are guided into mindful and equanimous presence repeatedly until curiosity, compassion, and equanimity replace reactivity, fear, or shrinking back from sensation, affective arousal, mind stories, and emotions. A few guiding principles for encouraging patients or students to embrace these characteristics of emotional resilience are offered next.

Finding Openheartedness

Nurturing openheartedness is about embracing the present moment fully, welcoming the breath in its entirety across all layers of being. It encourages patients to allow whatever is already present to naturally come into their awareness, understanding that nothing needs to be feared or resisted and that whatever emerges during breathing practices existed prior to a client's noticing. Patients are invited to release preconceived notions about how a practice should unfold or what it should invoke.

Instead, they are encouraged to allow experiences and breath to unfold organically, moment by moment. If they find themselves striving in their practice, clients are encouraged to let go gently and refocus their attention on the instructions provided by the care provider, returning to the simplicity of each breath invitation. Table 7.3 offers sample cuing.

Cultivating Self-Compassion and Lovingkindness

To help clients develop self-compassion, they are encouraged to prioritize self-nourishment and self-compassion, recognizing the time for breathwork as a time for healing that fosters inner strength and resilience. Patients are invited to approach their breathing practice and the experiences it may stimulate with boundless lovingkindness and compassion, extending compassion toward every aspect of their being, from bodily sensations, to energy or vitality, to mind states, to thoughts and emotions. Clients are encouraged to approach their breath and its reverberations with kindness, even if what arises does not align precisely with their expectations or the instructions they received from the clinician. Maintaining a nonjudgmental and gentle attitude toward themselves is of utmost importance, regardless of what arises physically, energetically, mentally, or emotionally. Clients learn to embrace discomfort encountered during breathwork with deep compassion and an open heart, rather than with judgment or fear. They allow lovingkindness and acceptance to arise naturally; they meet themselves and their breath with compassion and trust, acknowledging the inherent process and wisdom within each breath—even if that wisdom is not yet self-evident. Table 7.4 offers sample cuing.

Creating Curiosity and Open-Mindedness

To help create an open mind, clients are heartened to approach each breath with a genuine sense of curiosity, remaining open to every sensation and experience that arises from breath, body, and mind. They are asked to embrace the act of breathing without passing judgment or forming preconceived notions; instead, they develop open-hearted curiosity and inquisitiveness. They understand that there is no predetermined "right" way to perceive or be with their breath; each breath—no matter what shape it takes or consequences it has—is met with reverence, curiosity, and kindness, regardless of its nature. Clinicians thus help clients approach breathwork with a spirit of exploration, avoiding attachment, aversion, fear, or confusion, and instead meeting themselves and their experiences with openness and curiosity.

Table 7.3 Possible cues for open-heartedness

- Open yourself to what is already present; the practice is about meeting your breath in all of your layers exactly as you are in the present moment
- Invite what is already present to come to your attention or awareness; there is nothing to fear or fight: whatever emerges in your breathing was already there; you did not create it by attending to it
- Recognize that there is no agenda or intention that has to define you—open yourself up to the unfolding of experience and breath moment after moment after moment
- If you notice striving in your practice, invite yourself to let go and return your full attention to the instructions or invitations for breathing as offered by the care provider

Table 7.4 Possible cues for self-compassion and lovingkindness

- Remind yourself that this a time for self-nourishment, a time that invites a breath for healing, and a time for breathing that supports inner strength and resilience
- Practice with unconditional lovingkindness and compassion for yourself and everything that shows up in body, breath, and mind
- Be kind to your breath even if it is not unfolding exactly as you would like it to or are instructed to by your breathing instructor
- Stay nonjudgmental and kind toward yourself regardless of what emerges in body, energy, mind, or emotions—regardless of how your breath initially unfolds or evolves; have faith that over time the breath will find a natural and healthful rhythm
- Be gentle with yourself, your breath, your sensations, your opinions; you might encounter unpleasantness while breathing; open your heart to it with deep compassion
- Lovingkindness and acceptance emerge spontaneously—try not to force them as this tends to create mental and physical tension, and may impair the natural breath
- Compassionately meet yourself and the breath where you are—trust the process; trust the breath

Table 7.5 Possible cues for curiosity and open-mindedness

- Stay interested in anything and everything that is experienced or arises from breath and body
- Breathe without judgment, valuation (or evaluation), or prejudice; simply breathe with openhearted curiosity
- Remember that there is no right way to feel, sense, think, or experience the breath—instead, meet every breath, regardless of its nature or characteristics, with respect and gentleness
- Explore every breath without getting attached, averse, scared, or confused—meet yourself with open-mindedness and curiosity
- Invite variation into your breathing practice rather than routinizing it; routinizing may lead to a mechanized practice that bears little fruit
- Try new methods of breathing or try the same type of breathing in a new way—come to the breath with beginner's mind

Curiosity and a beginner's mind can be greatly supported by introducing variety into offered breathing practices to prevent breathwork from becoming mechanized and stagnant, as this may limit its effectiveness. Experimenting with new breathing techniques or approaching familiar methods with a beginner's mind invites continual growth and discovery. Table 7.5 offers sample cuing.

Staying Present with Mindfulness

To support ongoing development of mindfulness and its generalization to daily life, clinicians encourage their patients continuously to bring their attention fully to each breath, while recognizing that mind wandering is a natural aspect of the human experience. Instead of judging the mind, clinicians remind their patients that when the mind strays into thoughts of the past, visions of the future, or simply into imagination, it is gently guided back to focus on the breath, on the rhythm of each inhalation and exhalation. It can be helpful to remind clients that mindfulness occurs in the moment of realizing that the mind has wandered away. In other words, clients can learn to deeply appreciate it when they catch their mind wandering. They can use this emerging awareness to return to the breath and their present-moment

Table 7.6 Possible cues for mindfulness

- Collect all of your attention into each breath; and yet, understand that the mind will wander—this is natural and human
- Do not judge the mind when it strays into the past, the future, your imagination, stories, opinions, or judgments; instead gently invite your mind back to attend to and focus on the breath; gently remind your mind to come into each inhalation and exhalation, the rhythm and characteristics of each breath unfolding
- Mindfulness happens in the moment when you notice that the mind has strayed; thus, when you notice the mind has wandered, express gratitude that you noticed and created the opportunity to return to the breath
- Imagine mindfulness as a mirror that reflects the truth of your life and your experience; meet what emerges with an inquisitive open mind without allowing it to disrupt the breath
- Stay mindful of your breath not just on the mat, but (especially) in life

experience. They consider mindfulness as a mirror reflecting the truth of their life, meeting distracting or recursive thoughts or emotions with an open and inquisitive mind, without disrupting their breath. Through mindfulness during breathwork, clients begin to extend mindfulness beyond the session, integrating it into daily life for deeper awareness and presence. Table 7.6 offers sample cuing.

7.3   Physical Practices in Breathwork

With energetic settling or centering, and emotional and mental supports firmly in place, we turn toward physical practices (grounded in yoga asana, kriya, and vinyasa) that serve to enhance the experience and impact of breathing practices. Physical practices prepare body and mind for breathwork; they support optimal functional breathing and movement off the mat, supporting a state of health and well-being in all layers of consciousness (i.e., *koshas*). The primary categories of physical movement that prepare us for breathwork are those that honor healthy biomechanics of breathing and that work with the relationship between breath and movement. We utilize physical practices that support healthful postural alignment, rib basket resilience, neck and shoulder release, and heart-opening. The physical practices highlighted in this chapter represent a sample of possibilities for how body and breath can deliberately interact to support and nurture each other, and how they can affect one another in a health-promoting and resilience-supporting manner. Before delving into this section, review of Chaps. 2 and 6 about biomechanics of breathing and postural assessment is recommended to recall fully why physical preparation is important to resilient breathing and how the offered physical practices are particularly valuable. Review of Chap. 6 is a great reminder to assess relevant anatomy first to plan the physical practice from there—tailored based on assessment findings related to posture and movement characteristics.

Ideally, breathwork guides have familiarity with yoga *asana* and sufficient experience and training to guide clients into breathwork from a solid postural foundation. Although this chapter provides guidance about alignment and instructions, it assumes that yoga and movement arts knowledge or experience are already important aspects of the clinician's life. It is especially helpful for breathing guides to know how to support clients in the physical shapes in which breathwork takes place, with the most common shapes being reclining and seated. While it is often asserted that all breathwork needs to occur while seated, beginners are extremely well-served by reclined and supported reclining positions [3, 4]. Those new to breathing practices often do not have the muscular stability to sit upright without back support for an extended period of time. Their struggles with maintaining posture can interfere with the intentions of offered breathing practices. Lying supine, on the other hand, invites release, tranquility, and relaxation. The downside may be that sleep might overcome the patient. The clinician needs to discern which choice is most tailored for each individual. Options for many types of positions for breathwork are offered below.

In all cuing—regardless of shape, it is crucial that instructions for physical practices that precede or support breathwork are *offerings, not directives*. We are each the owners and agents of our practice—whether we are practicing alone, in a group, or with a guide. In our practice, we own the decision-making about what is or is not supportive for our body, breath, mind, or emotions; we are each the only person who can sense the reverberations of the practice in our body, vitality, and psyche. This means that we, as clinicians, make only *invitations* to clients—we give *choices* about how clients might sit, stand, or lie; whether to shift positions; how to breathe; and whether to change breathing rhythms. This is not to say that clients should ignore or discount directions and wisdoms of their clinicians or breathing guides. However, it is up to each patient to test their teacher's suggestions and to decide how to use and apply them.

The following suggestions for teachers and breath guides are offered in the spirit of inviting clients and students to be the agents of their own life and practice. It is beyond this book's scope to help clinicians learn how to teach *asana*. However, the following principles are crucial though not always applied in general yoga classes. The guidelines shown in Table 7.7 are offered as essential strategies for breathwork guides who offer physical preparatory practices.

7.3.1 Postural Alignment Practices

As discussed in Chaps. 2 and 6, posture and breath are closely aligned and related. Posture affects breath; breath affects posture. Mention of this is already made in the yoga sutras, which assert that for ideal breathing to emerge, posture needs to be optimized. Thus, a breathwork session is well-served—time permitting—by attention to wholesome posture while standing, seated, walking, and moving, before engaging in breathing practices.

Focus is placed on aligning the spine in its natural curves and assembling the base, whether on the sitz bones, tops of femurs, feet, or other body parts. Guidance is offered about aligning the spine in standing and seated positions, *in general*. Then, several typical forms or shapes are presented that are conducive to natural breathing, breath observation and awareness, and many types of breathwork. Recommendations are offered as inspiration and guidance—not as strict rules for how to sit, lie, or move. It is important to invite patients into self-agency and

Table 7.7 Guidelines for inviting agency during physical practice

- Provide patients the pleasure of and guidance for using props and supports that help balance effort and ease
- Give clients reminders about finding ease in body and breath many times during the practice
- Encourage students to experience *from the inside* what is helpful versus hurtful
- Invite clients to make adjustments, according to interoceptive and neuroceptive feedback
- Allow clients to experience the joy of persistence and of balancing effort and ease by not giving up to soon, but also not persisting with a practice that seems less than useful in a given moment
- Let patients know that they can shift and move if there is significant physical discomfort and a change in body position might bring greater ease to body or breath
- Reminds patients to move and adjust slowly and mindfully, with clarity and intention, not automatically or reactively.
- Remind clients that the choice about how to move and hold still is always theirs—that they get to experiment with each shape and movement to discern what is optimal for them
- Introduce clients to the idea that they are their best inner teacher when they learn to listen inward and to guide movement and shapes based on their deep appreciation of arising sensations and energies

empowerment in each shape and movement, using variations, props, and adaptations that best serve the individual given current states of body, vitality, psychology, relationships, and environment. Clinicians who want additional expert advice on postural work will benefit from *Natural Posture* by Porter [5], *Complete Guide to Postural Training* by Patel [6], and *Sit Up Straight* by Pham [7].

Assembling from the Feet Upward to Support a Natural Spine in Standing Postures

Before moving into standing shapes for breathwork, it is useful to awaken the feet with footwork to assure that the stance rests on *alive, grounded feet and strong ankles*. Awakening the feet can include ball rolling, toe twining, and toe grasping. Awakening and strengthening the ankles can be invited via ankle rolls and unilateral squats that move the ankles through their range of motion. These exercises can be completed while clients are seated on a chair or even lying down. Once feet and ankles are ready for action, mountain pose serves as the quintessential standing shape from which to assemble the body in alignment with a natural spine.

Cuing tips to help students into a standing practice are offered in Table 7.8. These invitations are relatively standard for cuing standing shapes. Notably, extra attention is given to pelvic alignment as this is often misunderstood. Specifically, there are significant disadvantages to pelvic tucking that are avoided in the offered cuing [8]. Pelvic tucking while standing upright interferes with freedom of movement of the diaphragm and hence the breath. It can flatten lumbar lordosis and the cervical spine (due to lumbar-cervical sympathetic movement), distort the SI joint, and drop the weight of the trunk onto the intervertebral discs, increasing compression. It may drop the weight of the organs onto the pelvic floor, potentially weakening it. It may disengage the abdominals and result in a posture that fights gravity. These factors often combine to make pelvic tucking unwholesome for breathwork.

Table 7.8 Guidance for helping clients with alignment in standing shapes

- Attend to the *corners of the feet*: acknowledge that not all students feel the same number of corners; invite students to lean side to side and front to back gently to feel the corners more concretely; point out that some students feel three corners, others feel four
  - *Three corners*: big toes and little toe ball mound, and heel as a whole
  - *Four corners*: big toe and little toe ball mounds and inner and outer heel
- Mention and explore the *four arches*: although this is not essential to cue, it is worthwhile observing in students; it is helpful to note each arch and how it meets its primary function; sensitivity and information about the arches often automatically activate them; extra activation can be achieved by lifting the toes and planting the feet while very gently engaging the external rotators around the ankles, knees, and hips.
  - *Medial arch*—the primary shock absorber
  - *Lateral arch*—the super stabilizer or outrigger
  - *Distal transverse arch*—the assistant for weight distribution
  - *Proximal transverse arch*—the great weight bearer
- Invite *engaged legs*—wake up the leg muscles with creative movements, tailored to the shape of the leg bones as necessary or engaging in both directions:
  - If the *knees tend to buckle inward*, engage the legs muscularly outward (e.g., leg abduction with a strap or exercise or elastic band around the thighs)
  - If the *knees tend to buckle outward*, engage the legs muscularly outward (e.g., leg adduction with a yoga block, Pilates ball, or even a pillow squeezed between legs)
  - If there is balance, *hypermobility*, or no way to individualize, engage the legs in both directions (e.g., could use a strap and a block at the same time—squeezing in and pushing out)
- Activate the legs further by drawing knee caps toward the hips; draw attention to the ensuing stabilization of the patella
- Find a *natural pelvis:* note the slight anterior tilt (the sacrum is not vertical) and remind students that the pelvis is made for stability primarily and mobility secondarily; it is supported by strong hip rotators, and activating the glutes is essential to standing (especially standing on one leg by preventing the hip from dropping out from under us)
- Ground (perhaps slightly internally rotating) the tops of femurs into the back plane of body to find an engaged yet soft stance
- Feet, knees, and hips are aligned in such a way as to *maximize knee health*, not foot position
  - Align the knee to the optimal position, and let the feet follow by either turning out, in, or neutral
  - Cue optimal sensation in the knee joint over aligning the feet with the edges of the mat (often done backward in yoga classes)
- Find a *natural thoracic spine:* the thoracic spine has light kyphosis, and the entire rib basket rolls slightly anteriorly; avoid standing at attention:
  - Low ribs are neither tucked deeply into the abdomen nor flaring out
  - A slight kyphotic curvature of the upper back will be visible
- Adjust the *head to rest naturally* on top of the cervical spine, ensuring slight lordosis of the cervical spine and a very slight anterior rotation of the head; the chin is tucked ever so slightly and then drawn back to align the openings of the ears with the center of the tops of the shoulders

Assembling from the Pelvis Upward to Support a Natural Spine in Seated Shapes

Before moving into seated positions for breathwork, it serves to note how the base of the spine, pelvis, and legs are best supported for the emergence of natural spinal curves. A general guideline is that if the lumbar spine loses its natural lordosis and/

or the sacrum loses its natural slight anterior slant, a prop is placed under the sitz bones and upper portions of the femurs. Ideally, the iliac crest is higher than the knees. If this is not yet achieved, more supports may be needed. Blankets, bolsters, and yoga blocks are useful in this regard. Sitting on a chair and using a meditation bench are excellent options. It is beneficial to remind clients using chairs not to rely (exclusively) on the backrest to remain upright. Excellent guidance on helping patients access seated postures is offered in *Yoga Myths* by Lasater [8]. Table 7.9 offers helpful suggestions for cuing.

Table 7.9 Guidance for helping clients into healthful alignment while seated

- *Use appropriate props under the seat to support the spinal natural curves*, including the slant of the sacrum, when seated:
  - Use a prop under the seat
  - Use a prop between the wall and the top of the sacrum
  - Use a prop between the back of a chair and the sacrum
  - In a neutral pelvis, the sacrum naturally wedges down against the ilia for maximum sacroiliac (SI) joint stability
  - Pelvic tucking decreases sacroiliac joint stability and has other drawbacks (see standing postures)
  - Any movement in a seat (or forward fold, twist, or standing pose) ideally brings minimal movement into the sacroiliac joint and pubic symphysis, as these are built for stability, not flexibility
  - Move the pelvis as a unit (most sacroiliac pain is caused by ligament laxity around the joint, not lack of flexibility)
  - If the lumbar spine flexes (i.e., loses its lordosis) in a seat and the pelvis cannot adjust forward successfully (i.e., the spine cannot neutralize for any reason of compressive or tensile restriction), increase the angle at the hip joint by lifting the sitz bones and tops of femurs onto a prop
- *Use the upper leg bones, not just the sitz bones, to help support the seat*:
  - Grounding into a seat is facilitated by grounding the torso's weight into the tops of the femurs, just forward of the sitz bones
  - Internal rotation of the femur helps plant the femoral head in a more neutral position in the acetabulum; this facilitates:
    1. Grounding the femur to the back plane of the body
    2. Anterior tilt of the pelvis, which invites the natural forward slant of the sacrum and natural lordosis into the lumbar
- Note that *some seats start with the hip joint in neutral or adduction, and some start in abduction*—shape and orientation of acetabula and femoral heads, as well as width of pelvis, affect ease and effort differently in these two types of seats:
  - Staff, hero, and cow face poses start in adduction or neutral; it may be easier to ground the femur to the back plane in these seats, as it is easier here to actively engage internal rotation of the femur
  - Easy seat and bound angle (and all lotus variations) start in abduction; it may be more difficult to sense or achieve grounding of the femur, although any degree of engaging internal rotation may help achieve more ease
  - Opening the legs (e.g., butterfly seat) is limited by bony structures of the hip socket or acetabulum, and femur; range of motion is determined by depth and anterior orientation of the acetabulum and/or the angle of the femoral neck—do not force legs open; instead, use supports under the knees as needed
  - Either way, make a healthful link between hip and knee joints—tight hips present more risk to the knees in very externally or very internally rotated seats as any limitation in the hip joint's range of motion transfers to the knees; use supports under the hips and/or knees as appropriate
- *From the pelvis up, assemble the spine as described in standing postures*

Seats come in a great variety of shapes. For breathwork, it is key to identify a natural upright seated posture that grounds the body with ease and comfort by exploring the utility of props or supports (e.g., chairs, zafu, benches, blankets, bolsters, and even walls). A wholesome seat allows patients to ground into the earth, expand toward the sky, and stabilize at the core. It is enhanced by consciously choosing how to place the hands (e.g., in the lap, on thighs, palms up or down; with hands placed in the lap, a lift (e.g., pillow) can bring ease to the arms and maintain an open heart). A seat can be enhanced by conscious choices about whether to close the eyes to withdraw attention from outer sense impressions or to keep them open (e.g., at half-mast with a soft gaze point). The following illustrations provide examples of seats that work well for breathwork; many other options exist (Illustrations 7.1, 7.2, 7.3, and 7.4 show upright seats; Illustrations 7.5, 7.6, 7.7, and 7.8 show reclined seats).

Upright Seats

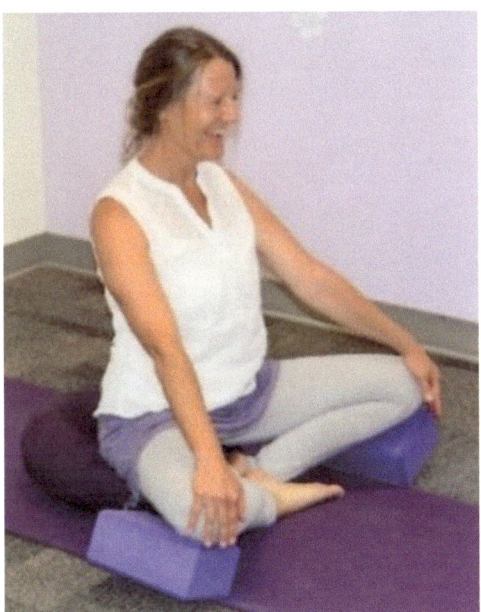

Illustration 7.1 Sweet seat with supportive props

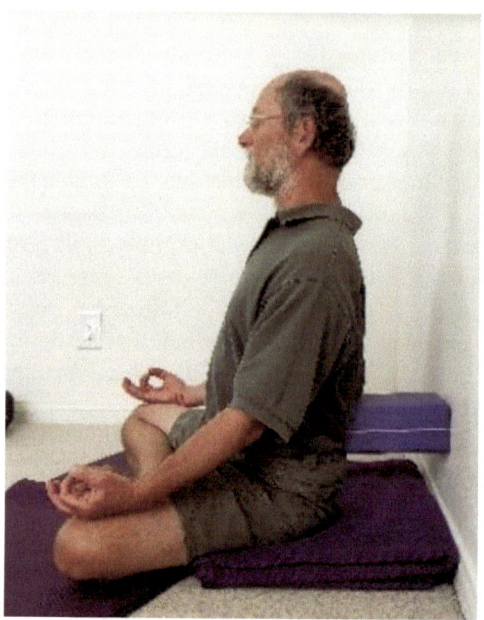

Illustration 7.2   Sweet seat at the wall with back support

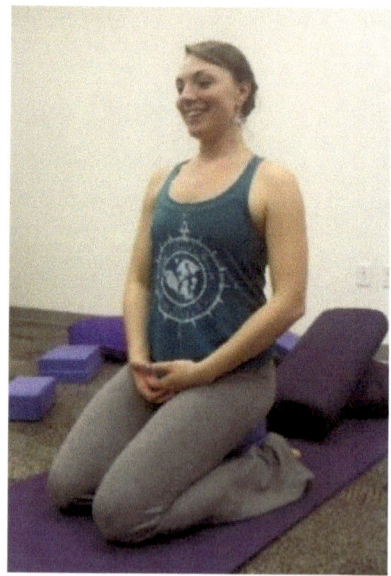

Illustration 7.3   Hero's seat with support under the sitz bones

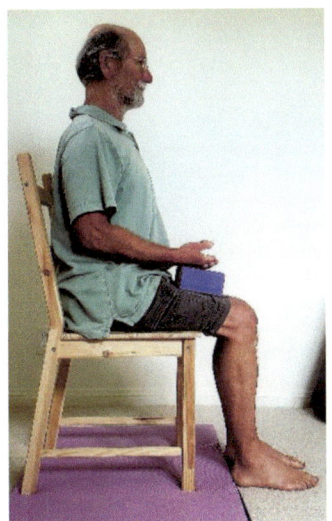

Illustration 7.4 Hero's seat on a chair

Reclined Seats (Illustrations 7.5, 7.6, 7.7, and 7.8)

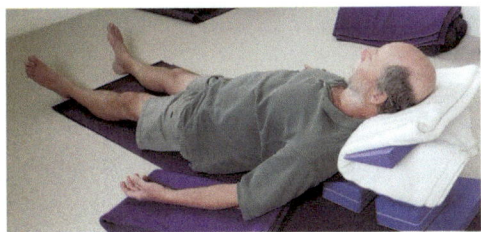

Illustration 7.5 Reclined supported relaxation shape

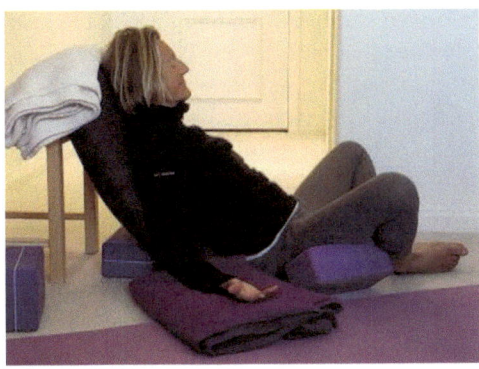

Illustration 7.6 Reclined supported butterfly seat

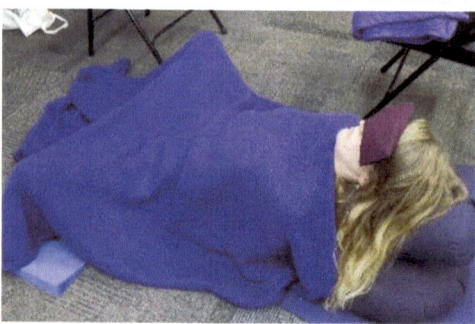

Illustration 7.7   Reclined supported butterfly seat with blanket

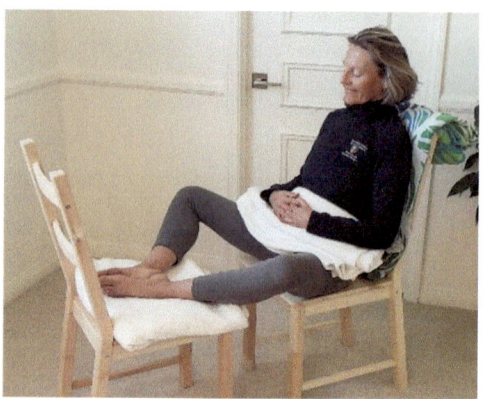

Illustration 7.8   Supported butterfly seat on a chair

Assembling the Body in Other Positions Used in Breathwork

For some individuals, starting breathwork in seated, standing, walking, or yoga posture practices is not possible. The demand of breathwork is such that the additional strain or muscular efforts of sitting or standing may be too distracting or preoccupying for some. For such individuals, it can be advantageous to rest on the back (fully supine) or belly (prone). We will take a brief look at positions assembled in physical shapes other than sitting or being upright, looking at supine (on the back) and prone (on the belly) options. The offered possibilities are meant to inspire the imagination about how to practice breathing more fully supported and closer to the earth. Many other options exist, and it can be quite enlightening for clients to be invited into free experimentation with patience and compassion. Additional ideas are offered by restorative yoga traditions, including *Restore and Rebalance* by Lasater [9] and *Restorative Yoga* by Baginski [10].

Supine Positions

To access a natural spine in a supine posture, it is helpful to use props to support the spine. Even while lying down, it is essential to consider maintaining the natural curves in all spinal sections. Props may be required under certain body parts, from head to neck, to back and pelvis, to knees and feet. We ensure that the student's back body is grounded or rooted to the earth; that the spine is naturally elongated; and that there is a sense of stability at the body's center even in supine, supported positions. Supine shapes often benefit from arms and hands by the side, as far away from the side body as feels most comfortable for the shoulders. Palms can be turned up or down depending on what feels most supportive, unless directed otherwise (e.g., as might occur in particular breathing practices, such as alternate nostril breathing). To lengthen the spine and invite its natural curves, it can be useful to lengthen through the legs and let the feet fall open. In these shapes, as in seated shapes, conscious choices are invited about whether to close the eyes to withdraw from outer sense impressions or whether to keep them open. While closed eyes reduce distraction by the senses, if tired, especially in a supine position, it may be necessary for clients to keep their eyes open to avoid falling asleep. Finally, while supine, it can feel caring for the patient to cover up with a blanket to reduce a sense of vulnerability or create warmth in a chilly environment (Illustrations 7.9, 7.10, 7.11, and 7.12).

Illustration 7.9   Reclined relaxation shape with back body ad head supports

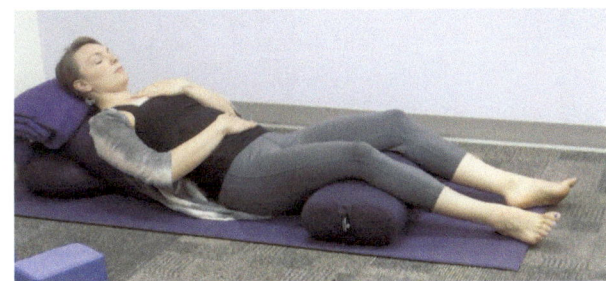

Illustration 7.10   Legs up the wall with props and weight

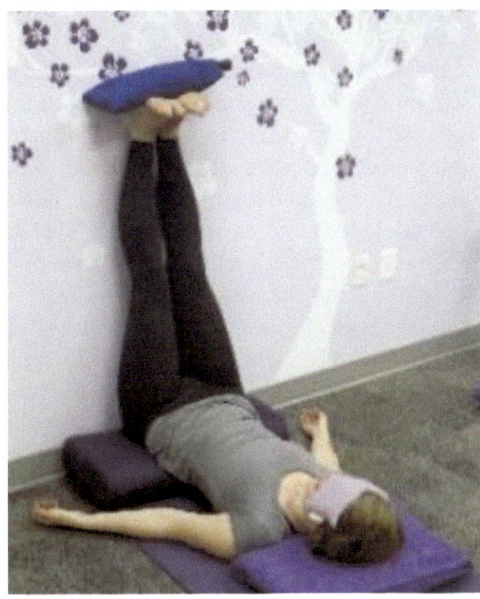

Illustration 7.11 Legs up
the wall with flexed knees
for low back relief

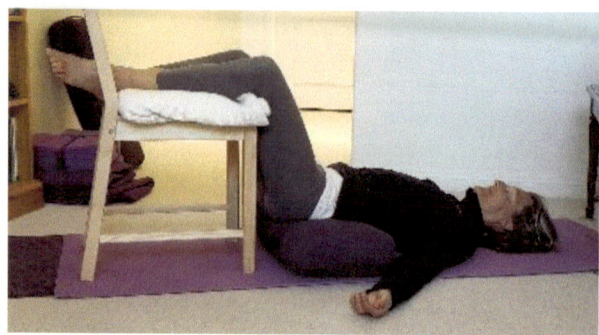

Illustration 7.12
Relaxation shape with knee
and head supports

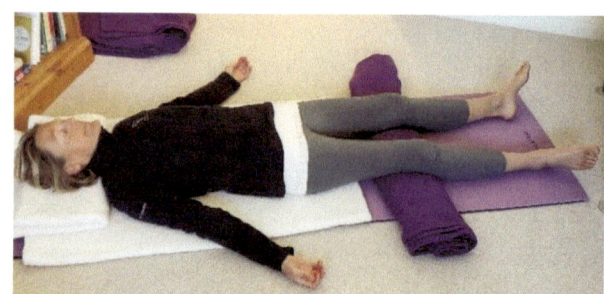

Prone Positions

To find a natural prone posture, it is typically essential to use props to support the
front body as needed for the desired effects on the breath. Key supporting portions
of the front body need to feel grounded and stable; all spinal sections, especially the
neck, stay naturally elongated and curved. Stability at the core is ideally palpable
even in a supported prone position. Arms and hands rest by the side or forward,
depending on shape and props. Palms can be turned up or down depending on what
feels most compassionate. Given that the eyes are facing the floor, prone positions
can be a wonderful opportunity to close the eyes if the patient's neuroceptive sense
of safety permits. As in supine positions, a blanket to cover the body can reduce
perceived vulnerability and provide warmth and comfort. Prone shapes invite
expansiveness and resilience into the side waist and back body, as the front body is
constricted by the earth or props. This can be difficult early on in breathwork.
However, it is worth returning to prone postures regularly, as they are very useful in
expanding the breath into underutilized sections of the lungs and in creating rib
basket resilience (especially reducing rib flare). If a patient is willing to stay with
shape for a little while, even if it is uncomfortable (yet not so long as to cause distress), the amount of time lying prone can slowly increase across sessions.

Patients with large breasts or ample abdomens need special attention to ensure
that they can find comfort in prone positions. Some clients are well served with
extra props that elevate the shoulders and create space for the belly and breasts to
prevent excessive compression of tissue. Others may benefit from a prone shape
with a slight rotation to create more space for the front body. Following are a few

possibilities for breathing with the front body facing or grounded into the floor or props. Many other prone options exist to help draw attention to the back body during breathing. Testing what works for given body anatomies, as well as emotional needs and challenges, requires patience, gentleness, and compassion (Illustrations 7.13, 7.14, 7.15, 7.16, 7.17, 7.18, 7.19, and 7.20).

Illustration 7.13 Child's pose

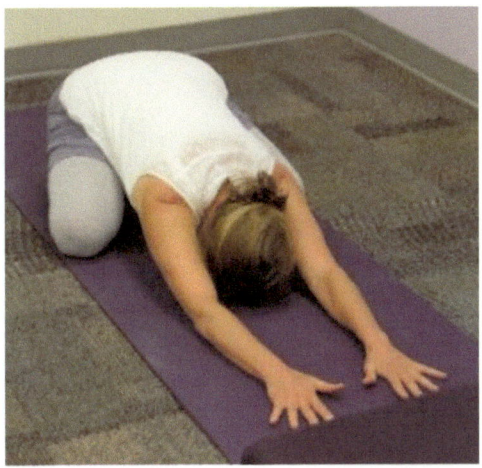

Illustration 7.14 Supported child's pose propped for knee and head support

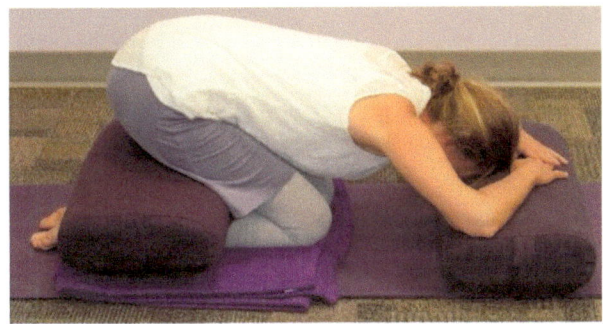

Illustration 7.15 Supported child's pose propped for support under the entire front torso

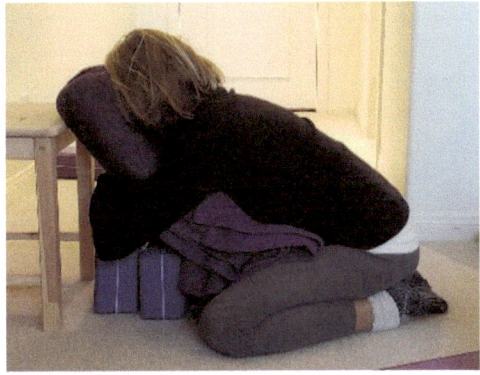

Illustration 7.16 Supported
wide-legged seat

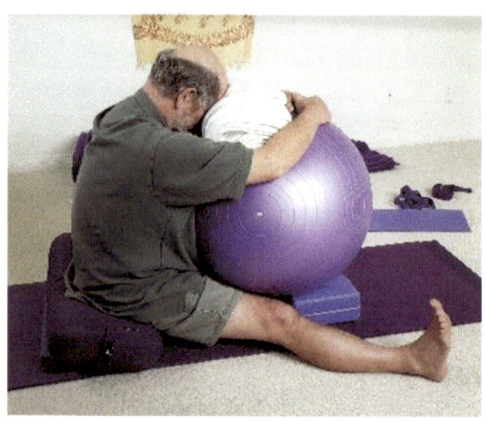

Illustration 7.17 Seated
supported wide-legged
forward fold on chairs—
arms could also rest on
chair next to head

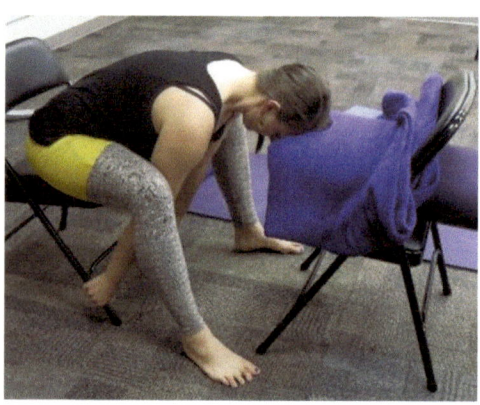

Illustration 7.18 Seated
supported wide-legged
forward fold

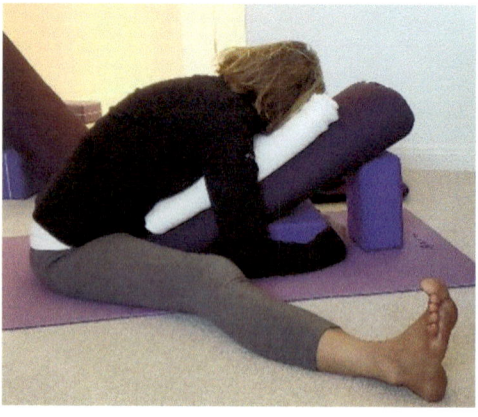

Illustration 7.19 Seated supported twist

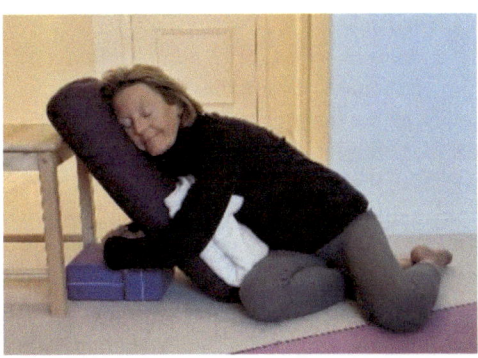

Illustration 7.20 Supported prone relaxation pose

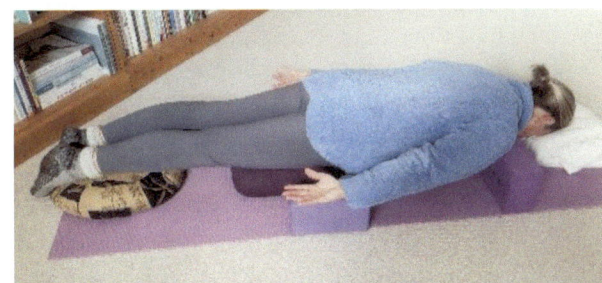

Helpful Postural Enhancement Practices

The following brief practices are focused on creating physical resilience that serves natural breathing. Most address natural spinal alignment, attention to natural curves in various spinal sections, strengthening the body's muscular backline while opening the frontline muscularly and fascially, and taking the spine through its natural movements. These mini practices prepare patients well for the physical demands of breathwork and tend to create mental presence that enhances attentiveness and concentration. The intention is not to suggest that all of these practices are necessary in each breathing session; quite to the contrary. They are offered as possibilities and inspirations for creativity—as an acknowledgement in each breathing session to honor the biomechanics of breath. Further, they are wonderful daily practices for patients to use at home. In all categories, yoga and other disciplines offer many more options and variations. Choices included here are based on their ease of use and accessibility. They are not meant to discourage experienced yoga teachers from using alternative shapes and movements that provide similar benefits but may need more nuanced cuing.

Neck Preparations

Primary foci for chin tucks and neck strengtheners are healthful neck alignment, healthful head placement atop the spine, and cervical spine resilience. These practices can be done anytime, anywhere—including at a desk to counter forward head posture. Neck preparations begin to encourage proper alignment, coupled with releasing fascial tension and muscular strengthening in the neck region for free flow of nasal breath.

Chin Tucks
- Stand or sit with the natural curves of the spine, grounding through the tops of the femurs if seated
- Rise up through the crown of the head
- Use the fingers of the dominant hand and bring them to the bottom of the chin
- Use the fingers to urge the chin downward (without exerting pressure—this is a nudge, not a command) as the head slightly nods forward (nodding "yes")
- Then, use the fingers to urge or nudge the chin back so that the head moves toward the back plane of the body until the openings of the ears align more closely with the tops of the shoulders (they may not reach the destination, but the importance rests in the fostering of the *movement direction*)
- Hold the chin tuck for a few moments
- Repeat this process often throughout the day, especially while standing or sitting for a long time
- Use this chin tuck movement every time before doing neck stretches or heart openers, including all of the following movements

Neck Strengthening
- Come to standing or to a comfortable seat with natural curves in the spine as described for mountain pose
- Tuck the chin and draw the head back as described above in *chin tucks*
- Place a flexible band around the back of the head so that it spans across the region of the occiput
- Hold one end of the flexible band in each hand and use the hands to draw forward on the band while resisting the forward movement of the band with the head (remaining in the chin tuck position throughout) (Illustration 7.21)

Strengthening in Thoracic Spine Region
Seated and quadruped rows (on hands and knees) are a great choice for the creation of strength and resilience in the thoracic spine. Rows create strength in the back body while opening the front body. They are a great practice that can be done daily and as a warm-up for breathwork, yoga asana, or other physical activity.

Illustration 7.21 Neck strengthening with chin tuck and resistance band

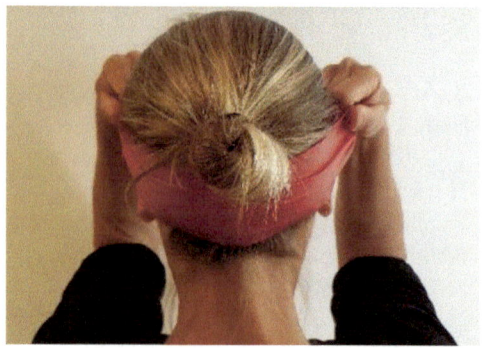

Seated Row Version

- Sit on the floor with both legs outstretched in staff pose
- Wrap a resistance band around the balls of the feet and hold one end of the band in each hand
- Draw the bands back, bringing the elbows as far behind the back as possible
- Repeat 10–20 times
- Can be done without the resistance band depending on the needs of the individuals

Quadruped Row Version

- Come to table top (on hands and knees)
- Take a small hand weight (or other weighted object such as a bag of rice) into your right hand
- Lift (or row) the right elbow up toward the ceiling and then down toward the floor, to lift and lower the weight
- Alternatively, place one end of a flexible band under the left hand, and grab the other end with the right hand; row the right elbow up toward the sky as high as possible, then release back down
- Repeat 10–20 times; then switch sides and repeat on the other side (Illustrations 7.22 and 7.23)

Illustration 7.22 Seated row

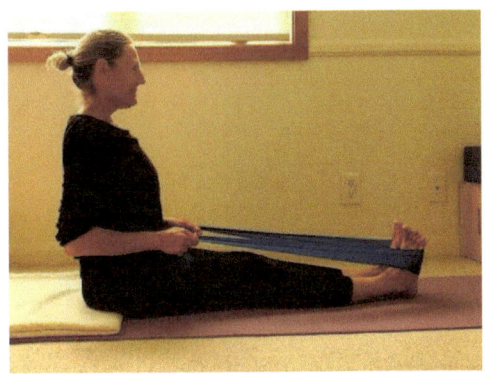

Illustration 7.23 Row in table top

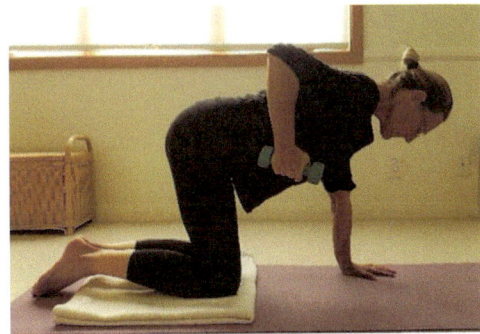

Shapes and Movements with a Shoulder V

Shoulder V is an excellent mobilization of the shoulder blades and scapulothoracic junction. It strengthens several sets of back muscles (including mid-trapezius and rhomboids) while encouraging resilient opening of the clavipectoral fascia. Creation of strength and mobility around the rib basket translates into resilience in breathing.

Scapular Squeezes—the Shoulder V

- Come to standing or sitting with a natural curve in the spine
- Bring the arms to goal post
- Draw the arms toward the back plane of the body, careful not to overextend
- Draw the shoulder blades toward each other and down the back
- Pulse gently with the breath, opening the heart with the inhalation and releasing the stretch with the exhalation; or inhale to open and hold for a few breaths, release with the exhalation
- Repeat 5–20 times (Illustrations 7.24 and 7.25)

Illustration 7.24 Scapular squeezes with cactus arms

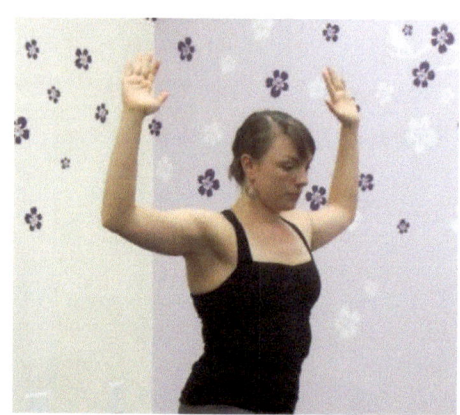

Illustration 7.25 Scapular squeezes with alternative arm placement/movement

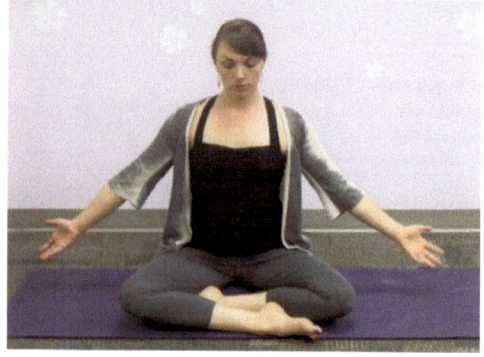

Cat-and-Cow Flow with Shoulder V

- Come to table top to move through cat-cow with the following variations:
- Extension and flexion occur high in the shoulder girdle
- In cow, make a strong V with the shoulder blades drawing them toward each other and down the back
- In cat, move into flexion drawing the shoulder blades outward and slightly upward
- The lower back and neck stay relatively still
- Repeat 5–10 times
- Variation: do this standing anytime, anywhere

Elastic Band Pull-Apart with Shoulder V

- Stand or sit with a natural curve in the spine
- Take one end of the elastic band in each hand
- Stretch the arms out wide, stretching the elastic band across the front of the body
- Maintain a strong V in the shoulder blades, drawing them toward each other and down
- Either open and close the arms (loosening the band) with the breath (opening while inhaling; closing while exhaling) or open the arms (tightening the band) with an inhalation and then hold for a few breaths; release with an exhalation
- Repeat 10–20 times

Heart Opening for Posture

Opening the front line in the upper torso invites resilience into clavipectoral fascia and rib basket. Rib basket resilience contributes to easeful and efficient breathing. If used as a passive stretch (i.e., doorway version), it is important not to overdo this particular preparation, especially if clients tend toward hypermobility (if this is a diagnosed condition, doorway stretching is contraindicated). Concurrent work in the back body is crucial, essentially adding a *shoulder V* with all its benefits. This is a spinal extension movement, and it is helpful to ensure that the low ribs do not flare during this practice. Drawing the low ribs in adds to rib basket resilience and contributes to strengthening the intercostal muscles. The opening of the heart (while strengthening the back) can be greatly facilitated with two prompts that can be used anywhere, anytime. Once clients have learned these two tricks, they can be helpfully used for postural alignment in all contexts and especially during breathwork.

- *Manubrium maneuver*—rather than reaching the whole sternum up to open the heart, the opening is invited to come from the manubrium (top part of sternum); this prevents the low ribs from splaying out too much and maintains some core stability; to employ this maneuver, take the ring and middle finger of the dominant hand and bring it to the manubrium and give a directional prompt upward and backward—this is not a strong push, but a very gentle guidance for the heart region to open without flaring the low ribs
- *Suspender move*—this move is a nice reminder to roll the shoulders up and back to open the heart; it asks the scapulae to move down and back; to utilize this move, place the thumbs into the axilla and point/move the fingertips upward

toward the ceiling—this will invite the heart to open; be sure to contract the rectus abdominis to draw the low ribs toward the hips to prevent flaring; if the thumbs cannot wrap into the axilla, the palms of the hands can be placed to the side ribs, as high up the chest as possible to prompt the same opening motion

Doorway Heart Opener (passive)

- Come to standing, directly behind a doorway
- Bring the arms into goalpost or cactus position
- Please one forearm (elbow, length of the ulna, wrist, and hand) on each side of the doorway
- Lean the chest forward to open the heart through the center while keeping the low ribs tucked; release after a short hold
- Repeat 3–5 times

Shoulder W movement with back at the wall or seated

- this movement opens the chest, helps with forward head (see next bullet), strengthens traps and rhomboids
- for this movement, stand with the back ant the wall and bring the arms into a W shape
- then slide them up and down
- the arm movement can be combined with flexing the knees toward a wall seat

Plank/cobra at the wall

- Lean into the wall, moving the axilla toward the wall and sliding the arms up and down (in a way this is a reverse W movement) (Illustrations 7.26, 7.27, 7.28, and 7.29).

Illustration 7.26 Shoulder W arms at wall—starting position

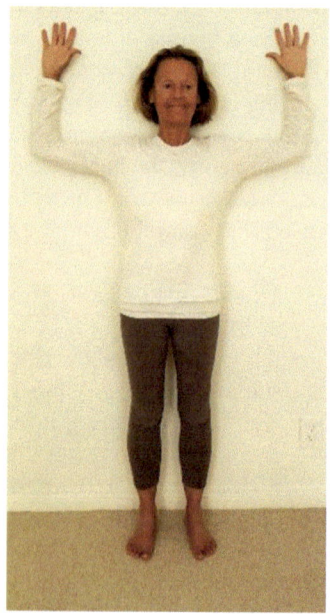

Illustration 7.27 W arms
at wall—with squat

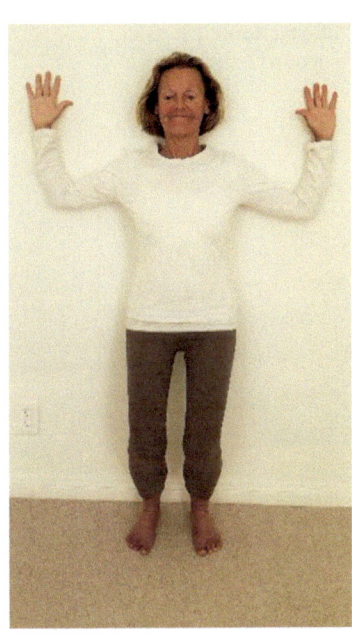

Illustration 7.28 Wall
plank

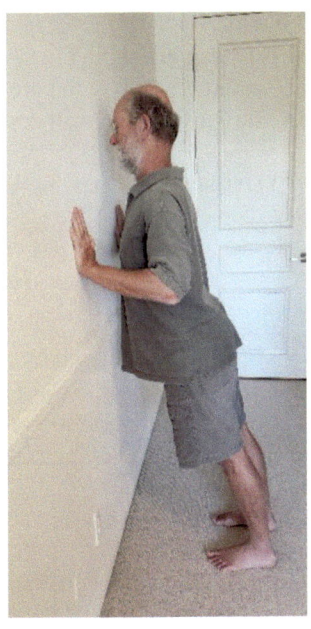

Illustration 7.29 Wall
cobra with slight chin tuck

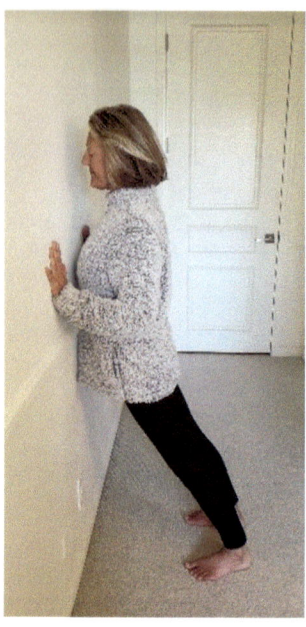

Wall twist
- opens the heart and stabilizes the shoulders
- stand with the side body to the wall
- turn toward the wall and press the hands into the wall from this slight rotation OR
- start the wall twist by bringing the side of the body to reach both arms forward along the wall
- then, slide the outer arm open as the thoracic spine moves toward the wall with arms in a T-position and upper back at the wall

Cow face arms
- opens the chest and mobilizes the shoulders; requires strap
- reach one arm forward and supinate the wrist to face the palm, thumb pointing out (external rotation of shoulder)
- reach the arm up and overhead; bend the elbow and bring the palm to the upper middle back
- bring the other arm forward and turn thumb in and down (internal rotation of shoulder)
- reach the arm behind and slide the hand up the back
- connect the two hands directly with a strap—the latter is highly recommended
- pressing the lifted hand and/or arm into the back of the head, shoulder, or back adds strength and stability (Illustrations 7.30, 7.31, and 7.32)

Illustration 7.30 Wall twist

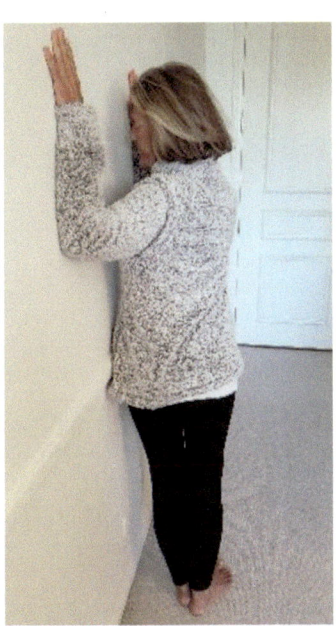

Illustration 7.31 Cow face arms—front view

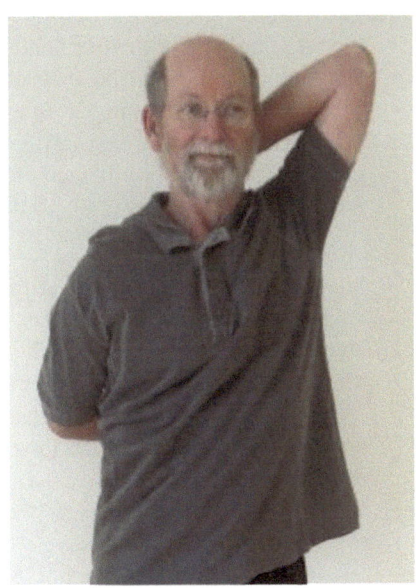

Illustration 7.32 Cow
face arms—back view

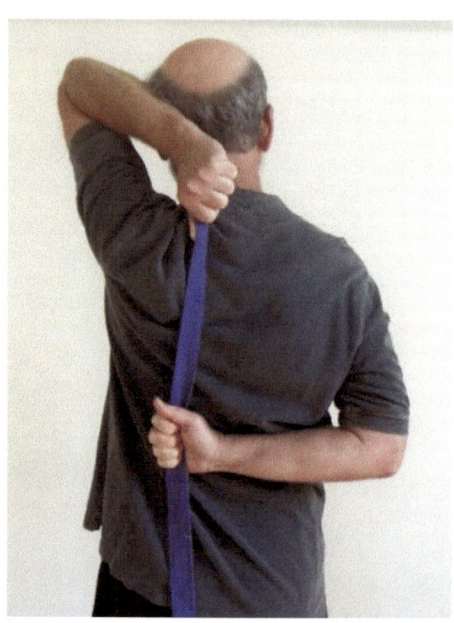

Angel Wings
- Lie on your back with your hands by your side with palms up
- With inhalation, slide the arms along the floor until the arms are reaching overhead on the floor, making an imaginary angel wing
- With exhalation, draw the arms back down to your side—be sure to keep the scapulae drawing toward each other and down the back
- Repeat this movement up to 10 times

Snow Angel at the Wall
- Stand with your back flush at the wall—if you have significant postural challenges, it is possible that the feet may need to be away from the wall a bit for the buttocks, the upper back, and the back of the head to touch the wall
- Make these adjustments with care and tuck the chin
- Then draw angel wings at the wall, lifting the arms along the wall up and overhead with the inhalation and lowering the arms back down to your sides with the exhalation
- Can also use angel wings at the wall from a wall squat position for a little extra effort

7.3.2 Neck and Shoulder Release Practices

Neck and shoulder releases are helpful for breathwork not because they open the upper rib basket (a common misconception) but because they reduce tension and tightness in this region's tissues that result from slumped sitting, standing, walking, and moving—often related to staring at devises, especially cellphones. Shoulder circles and undulation are extremely helpful, as is scapular mobilization. Neck circles are used with great care to move within the natural range of motion of the cervical spine. The neck is not designed to make full circles. Half-circles toward the chest are fine; circling the head along the back body is counter to the natural construction of cervical vertebrae and should be avoided.

Better than neck (half-) circles are neck undulations (e.g., such as pretending to draw shapes or letters in the air with the tip of the nose). Dangling or undulating the head from forward folds with hands on blocks or a chair can also release tension from neck and shoulders. Gentle side stretches of the neck can also bring relief. Such side stretches can be directly to the side (ear to top of shoulder) or can include a gentle rotation (ear to top of shoulder and then a slight turn of the head as if looking up toward the ceiling over the other shoulder). Proper alignment of the head on top of the cervical spine before initiating side stretching in the neck is key to success (see the *chin tuck* above). Other practices that help bring healthful range of motion to the neck include several vagus nerve resets developed by Rosenberg [11] and described in Table 7.10.

Table 7.10 Vagus nerve resets and neck health

Pre-test: Check range of motion of neck rotation
Basic polyvagal reset exercise
- Come to a comfortable supine position
- Interlace hands and place them behind the head with thumbs at occiput
- Without moving the head at all, turn both eyes to the right and look to the right for at least 30–60 s (or until a deep sigh or yawn escapes)
- Then return eyes to center and take a moment to notice
- Repeat with eyes turned to gaze to the left for at least 30–60 s (or until a deep sigh or yawn escapes)
- Then return eyes to center and take a moment to notice

Salamander exercise
- Come to standing or to a comfortable upright seat; make sure head is in line with spine (e.g., tuck chin and draw head back)
- Sidebend neck only to the right; gaze left with the eyes; hold for 30 s or so
- Bring head upright; release the eyes; notice your sensations and reactions
- Now sidebend neck only to the left; gaze turns to the right; hold for 30 s or so
- Bring head upright; release the eyes; notice your sensations and reactions

Post-test: Recheck range of motion of neck—note if there is a difference; typically there is a lot more ROM

Trapezius release exercise
- Come to standing and make ragdoll arms (hands to opposite elbows)
- Let the arms hang naturally in front of the low abdomen; rotate right and left approximately 3–5 times (see Illustration 7.33a)
- Lift ragdoll arms to shoulder height; rotate right and left approximately 3–5 times (see Illustration 7.33b)
- Lift ragdoll arms to above the head; rotate right and left approximately 3–5 times (see Illustration 7.33c)

Credit for these practices goes to Rosenberg [11]

Illustration 7.33 Trapezius
release exercise

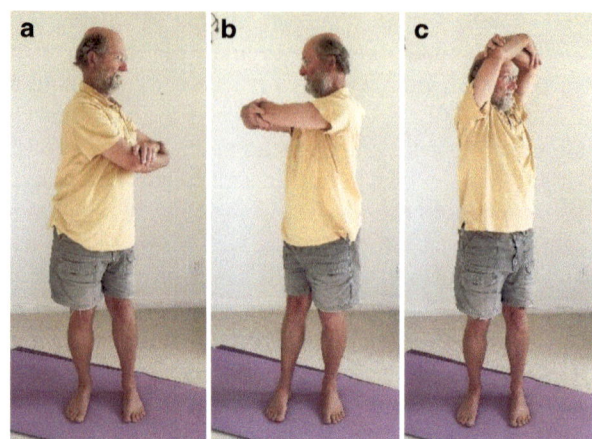

7.3.3   Rib Basket Resilience Practices

Like posture, resilience in the rib basket can make a significant difference to healthful breathing. Rib baskets tend to become stiffer with age, especially in the absence of targeted work on maintaining their pliability. Often, this stiffness is in the direction of slightly flared low ribs, which impairs the capacity to exhale optimally (see Chap. 2). Flared ribs decrease the zone of apposition in which the diaphragm moves, making the diaphragm less effective at expelling air from the lungs with the exhalation. Form and movement practices that integrate gentle side bends and natural-range (*not* torqued or forced) spinal rotations along the body's axis can be very supportive of maintaining rib basket resilience. Practices that involve moving rotation and side-bending above the waist and into the ribcage itself are particularly helpful. Heart-opening practices, especially with focus on the upper thoracic spine, can be useful; however, it is important to neutralize this type of opening of the rib basket with contractions inward to avoid aggravating any extant flaring of the ribs. Twists and side bends are therefore the preferable choices for working with resilience in this body region.

Despite breathwork's focus on creating resilience in the rib basket, knowledge of natural ranges of motion in all spinal sections is key to teaching twists and side bends successfully (as twisting in one spinal section often reverberates into others). The greatest amount of rotation is possible in the cervical spine, followed by the thoracic spine; the lumbar region has limited rotation. Lumbar rotation is easiest when the lumbar spine is in its natural lordosis—lumbar flexion limits rotation further. There is no rotation, flexion, or extension in the sacrum *independent* of the pelvis. It is crucially important to allow natural rotation of the entire torso without excess strain. This means that the pelvis moves in the direction of the twist; we *do not anchor the sitz bones or tops of the femurs* when twisting in a seated shape. It is important to rotate with resilience and without bracing, gripping, or forcing. This is because the sacroiliac joint (between the ilia of the pelvis and the sacrum) is made for stability, not mobility (via very strong ligaments). It is important not to work counter to this natural function. Table 7.11 provides important guidance for this concept as many yoga classes instruct the opposite. Clinicians who need or want more advanced

Table 7.11 Special notes and instructions for twisting shapes

- Let the pelvis and sacrum move as one unit—the SI joint is made for stability via very strong ligaments; do not torque or rotate the sacrum inside the ilia lest you weaken the ligaments over time (repetitive strain) and destabilize the SI joint
- The iliolumbar ligament (from L4 or L5 to the top of the iliac crest) can be injured by forcing spinal rotation (twists) too low into the spine—twist from L1 and up
- Weight-bearing of the sacrum and SI joint is best when the sacrum is at a 30-40° angle as this creates a wedging action of the sacrum in the ilia by the weight of the trunk bearing down on the SI joint—the sacrum is locked down into stability by this diagonal wedging action
- Give freedom to the pelvis to rotate into the direction of the twist—this is a completely natural movement
    - Let the hip joint opposite the side you are twisting toward move forward and up or down (depending on posture) into the twist
    - Let the buttock of the side away from the twist lighten, maybe even lift off the ground (if seated)
    - Let the shoulder that moves in the direction of the twist gently move downward
    - If you anchor from the sitz bones, the rotation will either be very limited OR there is great risk of injury to the SI joint
    - Do not keep the pelvis level during standing twists—let the side of the pelvis and shoulder move naturally

Table 7.12 Invitations for moving into rotation from side-lying

- Lie on the left side in a slightly more open version of a fetal position
- Leave the lower body where it is, and with inhalation, open the right arm up and over to the other side of the floor, opening the heart and drawing the scapulae toward each other and down the back
- If the right shoulder floats in the air, lift the knees off the ground and support them with a prop so the shoulder can be grounded
- Either pulse with the breath, opening like a book with the inhalation and closing like a book with the exhalation <u>or</u> hold the heart open, with both arms outstretched in line with the shoulders and hold the shape with gentleness for a few breaths
- Repeat on the other side; repeat both sides for 2–3 rounds

understanding of the functioning and healthy movement of the sacroiliac region are well-served by *Pathways to a Centered Body*, by Farhi and Stuart [12].

Open Book Side-Lying Twist

This gentle spinal rotation creates excellent resilience in the rib basket and thoracic spine. The specific transition into this twist *from side lying* (rather than from supine position) is important to note (see Table 7.12). It is chosen because it creates rotation (and thus resilience and strength) in the thoracic spine, instead of the lumbar spine, which does not undergo much rotation and often is overly stressed when this shape is entered into and exited from lying supine.

A few additional twists are shown in the illustrations as additional alternatives for accessing rotations in a natural way. The basic principle of creating the movement in the thoracic, rather than the lumbar, spine applies to all (Illustrations 7.34, 7.35, and 7.36). Illustration 7.37 demonstrates natural reaching with rotation to demonstrate the intuitive movement of the pelvis and the shoulders. The shoulder moving into the rotation lowers; the opposite shoulder lifts (Illustrations 7.38 and 7.39).

Illustration 7.34 Side-lying rotation with legs supported

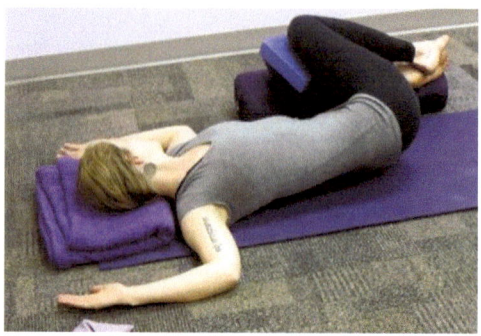

Illustration 7.35 Side-lying rotation with head turned and cactus arms

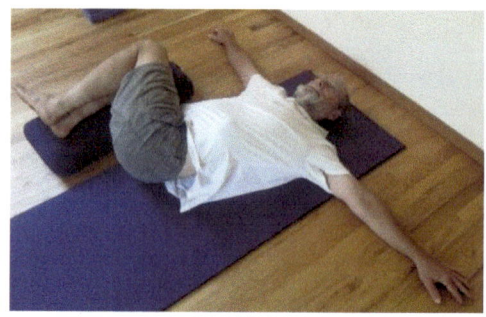

Illustration 7.36 Windshield wiper release

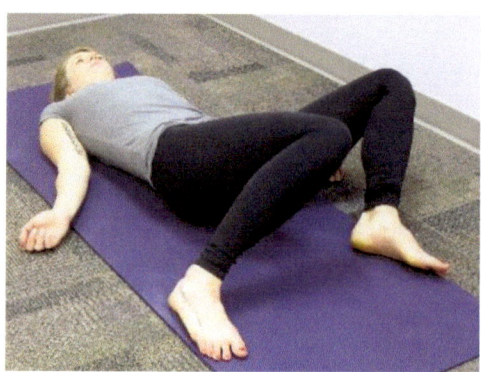

7.3.4   Heart-Opening Practices

Heart-opening preparations for breathwork are not backbends in the usual sense; they are neither large in range of motion nor wide open. They are gentle extensions and flexions of the spine that always end up in a state of postural balance. Heart-opening preparation for breathing involves sensing the upward and outward openings of the (low) rib basket via inhalation and its inward and downward movements via exhalation. There is no focus on large ranges of motion; quite the opposite. Focus is on creating spinal balance, extending and flexing the spine to contribute to resilience, neither to laxity nor deep opening. It is ideal to integrate the vagus nerve

Illustration 7.37 Seated rotation with hip support

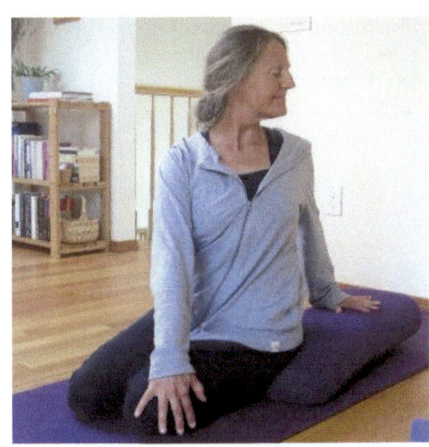

Illustration 7.38 Natural rotational movement to the right demonstrating hip mobility and shoulder movement

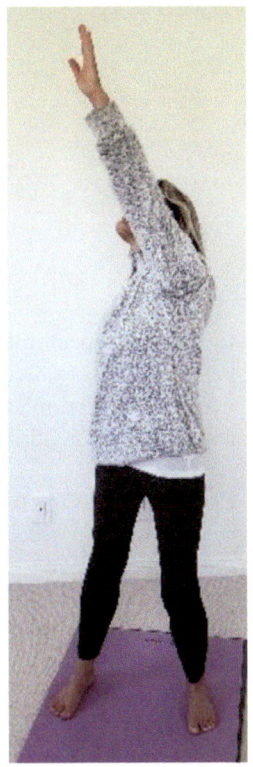

resets (see Table 7.10) with heart-opening practices to ensure that we are not over-taxing our patients' nervous system.

Pectoral muscles and clavipectoral fascia (i.e., upper chest muscles and connective tissues) must be resilient and balanced by strong back muscles (e.g., trapezius muscles and rhomboids) for the heart to open [13]. Shoulders that roll forward due

Illustration 7.39 Natural rotational movement to the left demonstrating hip mobility and shoulder movement

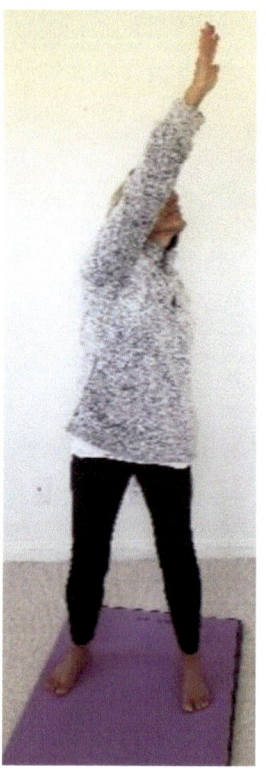

to tight clavipectoral fascia and short pectoralis minor muscles impede an open heart and are avoided to the extent possible. A few examples of heart-opening practices are offered to stimulate ideas and creativity about how to create this type of resilience for breathing in and out.

Prone Heart Openers

- *Cobra and related supine shapes*: even while lying prone on the floor, care is taken take care to have a sense of drawing the low ribs inward; the core is drawn inward and the thighs and tops of the feet press into the ground; the inhalation helps lift the chest and head (keeping the neck in line with the spine, not hyperextending it) either into cobra, seal, or upward facing dog—favoring handless cobra early on to avoid overextending (Illustration 7.40 and 7.41).

  Variation: resting prone, come onto the forearms to move into sphinx—watch out for appropriate movement in the low ribs as flaring is common here; sphinx is a *harder* variation than cobra!

- *Puppy and chair-supported puppy shape*: this shape can be misunderstood as being passive; be sure to press the floor away with the hands as the back muscles make a shoulder V and the front body yields with resilience; if on the floor, slight side-bending can be added by walking the hands along the floor to the right and left; in a chair version, the arms rest on a chair with elbows flexed or straight (Illustrations 7.42, 7.43, 7.44, and 7.45).

Illustration 7.40 Handless cobra—great starting point for spinal extension

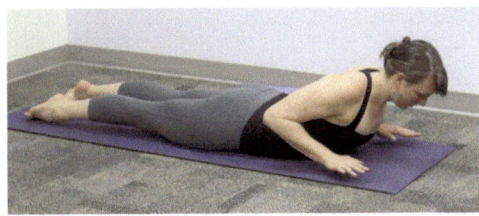

Illustration 7.41 Seal shape with strong core engagement—use with caution

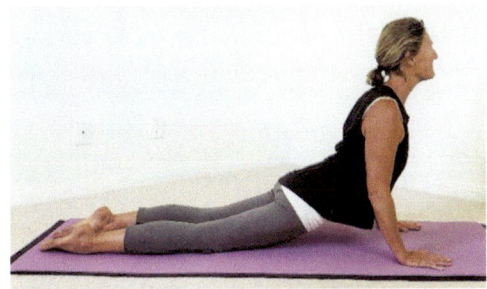

Illustration 7.42 Puppy on floor with (optional) head support

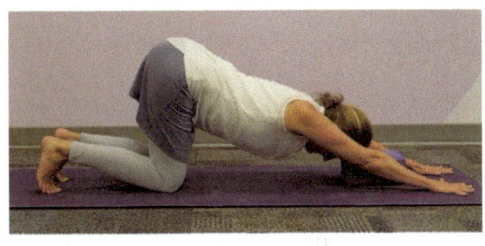

Illustration 7.43 Puppy on floor with lateral flexion

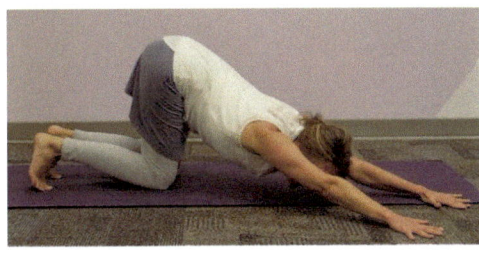

Illustration 7.44 Puppy on chair with elbows flexed

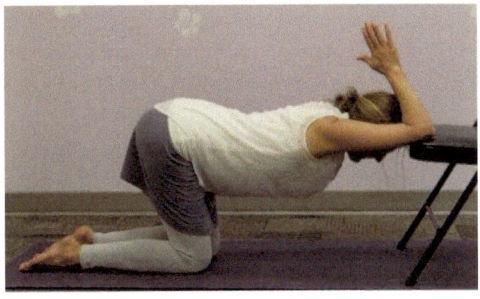

Illustration 7.45   Puppy
on chair

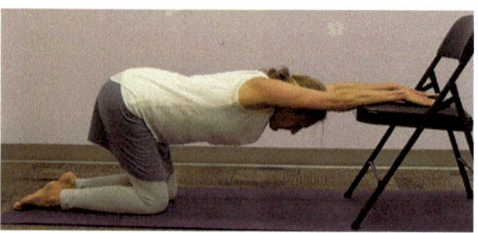

Table 7.13   Instructions for moving through yoga mudra

- Come to standing or sitting with natural curves in the spine and proper pelvic rotation
- Interlace the fingers behind your low back
- Draw the scapulae toward each other and down the back, lift the arms away from the region of the sacrum as high as possible without rounding the shoulders in front
- Keep the low ribs tucked gently
- Stay here or begin to bend at the hip joint to come toward a half lift with the interlaced hands resting on the sacrum to begin with
- Once in a half lift, raise the arms up toward the ceiling and, if appropriate for your body in the moment, lower deeper into a forward fold; it tends to be most helpful to bend the knees
- In a variation, come into yoga mudra while in hero's pose; then move toward child's pose with the top of the head placed on the floor and arms reaching up
- Can repeat once or twice

Yoga Mudra

Yoga *mudra* is a combination of several healthful spinal movements that support strength and resilience in the thoracic spine and rib basket. It can be a somewhat demanding shape for some patients and is offered once shoulder Vs and heart openers have become easeful and pleasant. Yoga *mudra* combines shoulder V, heart opening, and spinal flexion. It is complex yet very powerful as a spinal health practice. Instructions for yoga mudra are complex, thus a little more detail is offered in Table 7.13. It is best to receive instruction from a skilled teacher if this is an unfamiliar flow and shape.

Supine Heart Openers

- *Bridge*—this shape is a great transition and combination of heart-opening and core stabilization as it opens the heart region, strengthens the back, and strongly stabilizes core and pelvic floor muscles—all key to healthful breathing; a resistance band around and block between the knees can be helpful in achieving optimal muscular contraction to lift the hips from a supine position; a strap in the hands under the back body can support healthful opening in front and strengthening in back; lying on blankets is key with older patients or individuals with osteoporosis (Illustration 7.46 and 7.47).
- *Candle stick*—evolves out of a supported bridge pose and can be added for strengthening the diaphragm (Illustration 7.48).

Illustration 7.46 Bridge—
may add band around and
block between knees for extra
engagement

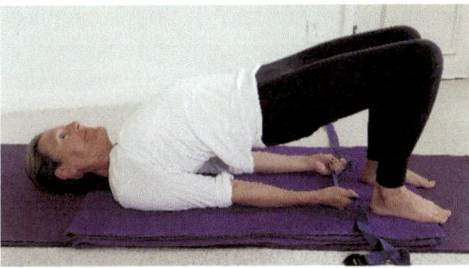

Illustration 7.47 Supported
bridge with a block under the
sacrum and between the
knees

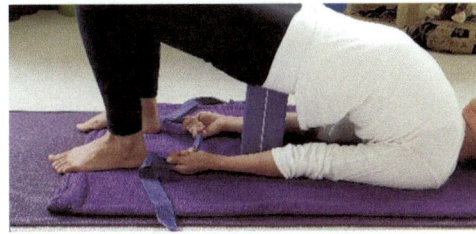

Illustration 7.48
Supported candlestick with
a block under the sacrum
and straps linking the
hands

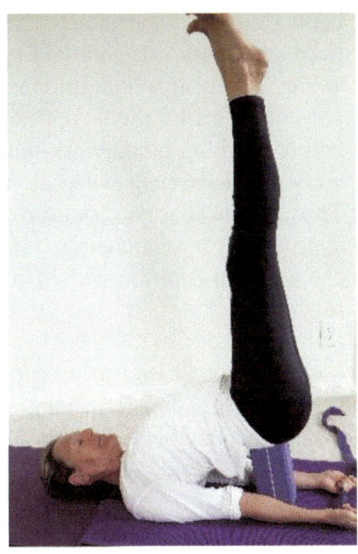

7.3.5   Core and Pelvic Floor Stabilizing Practices

Core and pelvic floor stabilization and diaphragmatic engagement go hand in hand. When the diaphragm contracts downward during inhalation, core and pelvic floor release. During the exhalation, the diaphragm releases and the deep core and pelvic floor contract (upward), stabilizing intraabdominal pressure. If we do not have the capacity to contract deep core and pelvic floor muscles, effectiveness of the diaphragm is reduced. For those who have difficulty accessing the diaphragm during breathing, core and pelvic floor strengthening can greatly enhance sensitivity to and effectiveness of the diaphragm. Without coordination of deep core and pelvic floor muscles, natural diaphragmatic breathing is challenging. As noted earlier, a central differentiation between abdominal breathing and natural diaphragmatic breathing is co-engagement of transverse abdominis and pelvic floor muscles in diaphragmatic breathing (especially on exhalation—while contraction of these muscles is absent or minimal in abdominal breathing [14]). Individuals who have difficulty activating the pelvic floor (i.e., in yogic terms, who cannot seem to find root lock) or the transverse abdominis often have a weaker, less efficient natural diaphragmatic breath and less intraabdominal pressure on the exhalation. Relatedly, patients who do not breathe diaphragmatically often have pelvic floor dysfunctions. Of course, all breathing involves the diaphragm to some degree. However, diaphragmatic range of motion and strength are not givens; co-contraction of core and pelvic floor is also not easily accessed by all. In particular, chest- and reverse breathing patients can have difficulty coordinating these muscles as they breathe—being habituated to (overly) use their chest muscles instead.

Core and pelvic floor stabilization practices support activation and coordination of these muscle groups. Once patients understand core coordination, this work can be integrated into almost all form and movement work and many breathwork practices, although some cautions and guidance are useful to ensure that offered or practiced core work does not end up interfering with optimal functional breathing (see Table 7.14 for tips and guidance). Integration of core stabilization and breathwork presents a bit of a chicken-and-egg conundrum: Do we teach core stabilization before teaching breathwork that requires core engagement? Or can we use breathwork practices, such as *kapalabhati* (rapid breathing), to support core stabilization? This puzzle has no definitive answer—different clients may need different approaches or sequencing. Interoceptively aware practices and mindful teaching can make the difference in identifying the most patient-tailored approach and sequencing.

Stabilization of core, back, and pelvic floor muscles is practiced and cued in such a way as not to lead to interference with natural breathing and digestion—active focus happens during exhalation; ease during inhalation. *Natural* tone of the core means that neither core nor pelvic floor muscles become hypertonic (or permanently contracted); they do not need to fire at full strength. The key is to develop *tone* in the core, pelvic floor, and diaphragm that is not tense or hard: the tone we look for is *neither braced, nor collapsed,* but *supportive and yielding.* Diaphragmatic breathing education is key to a healthy pelvic floor.

Stabilization is *the* major job for the abdominal muscles. Core stabilization has many benefits beyond strength and tone in the abdominals:

- It stabilizes the spine in particular and the torso as a whole.
- It stabilizes the ribs and pelvis.
- Stable and toned abdominal muscles hold the organs (or organ column) in place and support the vertebral column (especially at L4–L5).

Table 7.14 Practice and teaching tips for core stabilization

- Laugh, cough, or clear your throat—these actions engage the core and can help develop interoception of the muscles we seek to strengthen and awaken
- Place a block between the thighs or knees to awaken the adductors in the legs—they are often helpful in kick-starting transverse abdominus and pelvic floor engagement as they are fascially linked; squeeze and release quickly for several repetitions
- Practice squats—inhaling downward into the squat and exhaling upward out of the squat— focus on upward and inward movement from the pelvic floor on up when rising out of the squat
- Come to table top; slowly, slowly, slowly move the shoulders ahead of the hands—at some point, when you are just about to lose your balance, the deep core muscles will naturally kick in
- Come to table top and move into bird dog —one arm and the contralateral leg raise; sway forward and back and/or side-to-side, challenging your balance; yet again, the core will kick in spontaneously
- Come to table top and move into bird dog—one arm and the contralateral leg raise; tap the lifted elbow to the lifted knee under your chest
- Come to table top and find a natural spine with gentle core and pelvic floor engagement; with the exhalation lift the knees off the ground and hover for a few rounds of breath
- Come onto your back, fully outstretched with all limbs on the floor; lift one leg to make a 90° angle at the hip joint; then lower the leg slowly; if this is very difficult, bend the knee of the lifted leg
- Come onto your back with legs raised up in the air; slowly lower one leg toward the floor—if this is too difficult place your hands under the buttocks till the core strengthens
- Sit in boat pose with both feet on the ground; straighten one knee to raise that leg upward in a diagonal; make sure to maintain the natural spinal curves, especially in the lumbar region
- Lie prone; with an inhalation, let the movement of diaphragmatic contraction lift the chest and shoulder off the ground in a hands-free low cobra; with the exhalation return to the floor and hugs the low ribs into the abdomen; suspend the breath until you feel the urge to inhale; repeat twice
- Find bridge pose and candlestick as appropriate for conditioning, using blankets under the torso for comfort and adequate props for emotional and physical support (e.g., contraindicated for osteoporosis)

For a sample of a basic core stabilization practice, check out Brems's *YogaX Core Stabilization* class at https://youtu.be/We6gIj-EWJw

- Together, the spine, organ column, and abdominal muscles stabilize us during movement. For more details, see this amazing link: https://youtu.be/AsS1zXoIABA).

In practicing and teaching core and pelvic stabilization, it is helpful to attend especially to the deepest of the four layers of abdominal muscles, namely transverse abdominis, for deep inner stability. Activation of transverse abdominis and upward contraction of the pelvic floor are natural on exhalation; on inhalation the abdomen remains soft and resilient (with some gentle slow-twitch muscle action). Activation of external and internal obliques (the second and third layers of the abdominal muscles) is especially accessible when adding rotation or side-bending to standing, seated, or other postures. If activation of the diaphragm is the primary teaching goal, *pranayama* practices such as slow-motion *kapalabhati* may be helpful. Tricks and movements for discovering core stability are presented in Table 7.14.

7.4   Nose and Tongue Practices for Breathwork

It can be helpful in teaching breathing to attend to practices that support nasal breathing. Switching to nasal breathing can be a significant initial hurdle for some clients as they adapt their breath and breathing to new realities. Congested nasal passages and sinuses can become such a significant obstacle that patients give up trying to retrain and optimize their breath. Preparatory exercises that prepare nose and tongue can help remove this obstacle and lead to better progress.

7.4.1   Nasal Clearing and Preparation for Nasal Breathing

Since nasal breathing is essential, the importance of nasal clearing and decongestion exercises cannot be overstated. Various types of obstructions can block the nose and interfere with nasal breathing. Anatomical obstructions (e.g., polyps and severely deviated septa) may need to be corrected medically, even surgically. However, often obstructions are related to mucus or habit and can be addressed with the practices listed below. Even once nasal clearing exercises have taken effect, they remain helpful to maintaining resilient breathing (as is the regular practice of subtle or reduced breathing; see Chap. 8) to keep the nasal passages clear. Assessment for measuring nasal blockage and dominance was offered in Chap. 6 and can be integrated with nasal clearing practices as concrete biofeedback about changes in the freedom of breath flow that arise from these particular practices. Of course, other biofeedback can emerge spontaneously, such as the subjective experience of more easeful breathing or reduction of collateral symptoms associated with mouth breathing.

To begin with, nasal clearing practices are best explored in collaboration with the patient, with careful observation and monitoring of the client's reactions. We do not want to put a patient into a respiratory crisis by choosing nasal clearing practices that are beyond their current level of comfort. At the same time, these exercises are inherently stressful, which may be part of their effectiveness. When we move into a sympathetic nervous system state, our body does what it can to clear the nose to prepare for a self-protective response. One exercise that can help clear the nose that is not covered here in any detail is sex. Sexual intercourse tends to decongest the nose due to the physical activity involved and its effect on breathing in the heat of the moment.

If the nasal clearing practices outlined in Table 7.15 are not successful, it may be necessary to seek medical consultation. Such referral and consultation are necessary if there is constant nasal obstruction or congestion, especially in the context of other breathing-related symptoms.

Table 7.15 Practices for nasal clearing

Maximum breath hold and movement for clearing the nose for nasal breathing [15, 16]
1. Take a few gentle natural breaths; then take a gentle inhalation and release a natural exhalation
2. At the end of the exhalation, pinch the nose closed with thumb and index finger, making a tight seal
3. Nod your head up and down and/or rock the head side to side for as long as you can hold the breath—make sure to use gentle movements that do not jeopardize the neck
4. Hold the breath for as long as possible; this is a *maximum breath hold*, not a comfortable or controlled breath pause
5. When you feel the need to breathe, *inhale through the nose* to utilize the nitric oxide that was produced during the breath hold*
6. If the nose is not clearer, *repeat these steps a few times until the nasal passage feels less obstructed* (up to six repetition of 5 min each, with at least 30 s in between repetitions)**

The movements that are part of the breath hold phase of this nasal clearing exercise are largely a way to distract and maintain the greatest degree of relaxation. Gentle swaying or gentle movements of the head may be equally helpful as more vigorous movements. This can be tailored to each student.

*It is hypothesized that at least part of the effectiveness of this exercise is the production of nitric oxide during strong breath holds. The increase in NO, transported into the body via the inhalation, supports the opening of the airway.

**If this exercise does not result in any degree of nasal clearing, there may be an anatomical obstruction that is interfering with free airflow. A medical consultation may be indicated.

Minimum breath hold and gentle movement for clearing the nose for nasal breathing [15, 16]

For patients with contraindications for maximum breath holds, gentle breath holding—repeated several times—can be used to acclimate them to nasal clearing and breath holding. This practice can also serve as a *breath recovery practice*.
1. Take a few gentle natural breaths; when energetically ready, gently inhale and release a natural exhalation
2. At the end of the exhalation, pinch the nose closed with thumb and index finger, making a tight seal
3. Hold the breath for a *comfortable pause* (perhaps 2–5 s)—there should be no strain or gasping
4. If desired and accessible, add gentle undulations of the head that do not jeopardize the neck
5. After releasing the breath hold, breathe natural for several rounds of breath to recover a natural breath
6. Then start the cycle again and repeat for approximately 5–6 min at a time; repeat several time per day

(continued)

Table 7.15 (continued)

Using a neti pot or nasal irrigator for nasal clearing

This simple device is easy to use and can be helpful in clearing nasal obstructions due to congestion from allergies, particulates in the air, dust, and more.

- Fill the neti pot with distilled water of body temperature or slightly warmer
- Add about ¼ tsp of natural, finely ground sea salt—stir well until all the salt is dissolved
- Tilt the head into a position that allows water that is being poured in one nostril to exit via the other nostril
- If the water runs into the throat, change the head position until that problem is resolved
- Use one full neti pot rinse per nostril
- Clean your neti pot thoroughly after each use
- Follow the manufacturer's instructions

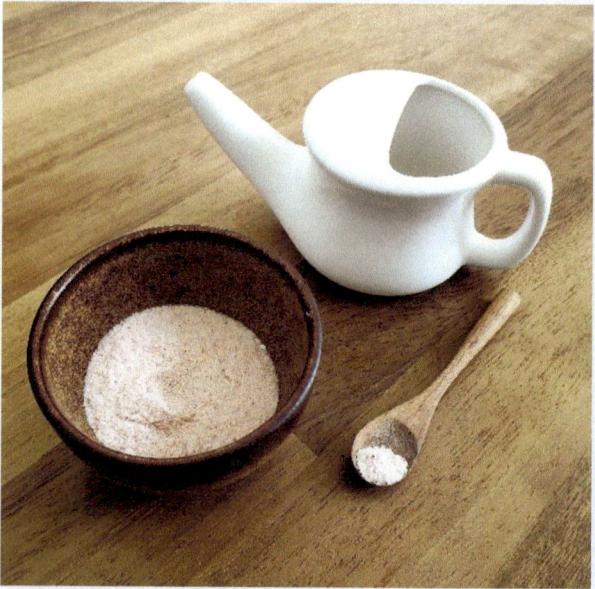

(continued)

Table 7.15 (continued)

Mouth taping for nasal breathing [16, 17]

Nighttime mouth taping is used to support nasal breathing at night, to reduce snoring, create a slower and lighter breath, and recalibrate the medulla to normal CO_2 levels. The process is easy but takes some getting used to for most clients. Some individuals benefit from shorter taping episodes (rather than the whole night) when they first attempt this practice. 3M micropore surgical tape appears to be used successfully by most clients. However, some individuals do better with a specialized MyoTape that does not cover the lips, but surrounds the mouth. This latter type of mouth taping is highly recommended for children to prevent choking.

The same taping procedures can also be used during the day. This may be helpful as training prior to nighttime taping to get used to the idea of taping. It can also be useful as a reminder to breathe nasally during the day until the habit has been established. If the mouth is moist and fresh in the morning upon awakening, nighttime taping is likely unnecessary.

1. Prepare a strip of medical tape of desired length (this can vary widely from person to person—anywhere from 1 to 7 in.)
2. Close the mouth and place the strip across the lips—you can either go vertically or horizontally, whichever feels more comfortable; vertical taping leaves the option of some mouth breathing (which can be good and bad)
3. If it feels too overwhelming to do this at night initially, test taping during the day for short time periods
4. Remove the strip carefully in the morning or after use; a folded-over edge can help
5. Check in with how you feel, comparing morning symptoms with and without taping (note difference in dryness of mouth, soreness of throat, level of thirst)

If mouth taping at night does not result in better sleep and clearer breathing even with the use of the specialized MyoTape), a nasal dilator may need to be worn at night. We can mimic the action of a nasal dilator to see if it would be helpful by taking our fingertips on the cheekbones just below each eye and moving/stretching the facial skin outward and upward, away from the center of the nose. If we feel significantly enhanced airflow into the nose, nasal dilators may serve to enhance sleep.

In time, if used successfully, taping at night can become a conditioned stimulus for better and deeper sleep.

7.4.2 Tongue Training

It is important to remember that the tongue is myofascially integrated with the deep myofascial frontline that connects a multitude of structures and muscles from the feet, through the legs, to the pelvic floor, diaphragm, core muscles, lungs, throat, and tongue. As discussed in Chap. 2, a strong and well-placed tongue can reduce jaw pain, ameliorate tension headaches, prevent dental misalignment (in children), and support easeful nasal breathing. A well-placed tongue supports healthful spinal and head alignment, supports optimal posture, contributes to balance and stability, and enhances gait and other movement dynamics.

Through physical proximity, the hypoglossal nerve—the 12th cranial nerve, which carries sensory and motor signals to and from the tongue—is intimately connected to the vagus nerve. Through this relationship as well as its strong connection to the brainstem, the tongue has also been linked to our capacity to quiet the mind and to move into meditative or contemplative states. Thus, the importance of tongue training cannot be overstated, a fact that was not lost on ancient yogis who were strong supporters of creating a healthy tongue via specific tongue exercises, cleansing, and respiratory practices. Ancient yogis already recommended what science is now affirming, namely the optimal placement of the tongue is on the upper (hard) palate, with the tip resting against the back of the upper front teeth (i.e., against the retro-incisor buds) [18]. This placement of the tongue has many concrete advantages, from enhancing spinal alignment, to preventing dental malocclusion, supporting nasal breathing, and enhancing movement dynamics and balance. A tongue that is able to stay in this position at the roof of the mouth can help ameliorate snoring and sleep apnea. Tongue placement on the upper palate, with the tip at the back of the upper front teeth, also supports healthful actions related to swallowing, chewing, speaking, and—most importantly, in our context—breathing.

Options for strengthening, mobilizing, and retraining placement of the tongue are numerous. Any practices that strengthen core, diaphragm, pelvic floor, and hyoid muscles can support tongue health, and vice versa. This can be easily felt in a variety of fun ways. Using a yogic breath called lion's breath is a particularly effective way to experience this relationship. In this practice, we take a few rounds of natural breathing. Then, we inhale a bit more fully than typically, and with the exhalation, we open the mouth wide and stick out the tongue forcefully. There will be a strong co-contraction of all core stabilizer muscles. Additional examples of tongue exercises based in the yoga tradition and on modern recommendations can be found in Table 7.16 as inspiration for more creativity. Even eating unprocessed food that requires a large amount of chewing is a great way to (re)train and strengthen the tongue—think about the chewing required for a big bowl of salad with chunks of carrot, cabbage, and celery; a crunchy apple; a handful of nuts. In other words, patients can be encouraged to become creative in discovering their tongue as a strong and supportive muscle. Tongue exercises can be done anywhere and anytime;

Table 7.16 Recommended daily tongue exercises

Kechari Mudra—the tongue lifts and curls backward with the mouth closed
• With a closed mouth, extend the tongue to the hard palate (touching the roof of the mouth and sweeping the tongue back)
• Then slowly move the tongue back along the hard palate toward the soft palate
• Move the tongue as far back as you can reach; the distance will change over time
• Hold until the tongue is fatigued
• Repeat often throughout the day
Tongue Push Up—press the tongue up against externally created resistance
• Open the mouth and place a spoon on the tongue
• Press the spoon down on the tongue and at the same time press the tongue up against the spoon, creating isometric action
• Hold for 5 s and repeat several times
Tongue Push Forward—with the tongue sticking out, press against externally created resistance
• Open the mouth and stick out the tongue as far as possible
• Press a spoon against the tongue and at the same time press the tongue against the spoon, creating strong isometric action
• Hold for several seconds and repeat a few times

(continued)

Table 7.16 (continued)

Tongue Side Push—tongue presses against the inner sides of the cheeks against external resistance
- Close the mouth and place several fingers against the side of one cheek, approximately an inch from the corner of the mouth
- Move the tongue to side of the mouth where the fingers are resting
- Press the fingers into the cheek and resist with the tongue by pressing the tongue against the fingers
- Hold for several seconds and repeat on the other side
- Repeat several times, alternating between both sides

Tongue Sucking—this movement mimics babies' motion of sucking on a pacifier and trains the tongue, as well as strongly stimulating the vagus nerve
- Nestle the tongue to the hard palate with the tip of the tongue resting at the inside of the front teeth
- Pretend you are sucking on a pacifier (if you can make this happen, actually suck on your thumb for a moment to learn how—then go back to the sucking motion without a thumb)
- Add smacking sounds and motions to intensify

Roof-of-Mouth Push Ups—press the tongue up against the hard palate
- With the mouth closed, press the tongue against the roof of the mouth as hard as possible
- Press and hold the resistance for at least 5 s
- Repeat several times in a row and throughout the day

Tongue Swooshing—swoosh the tongue over all the teeth in a circular pattern
- Start with the outside of the upper teeth, then the inside; then the outside of the lower teeth, followed by the inside
- Do this a few times starting clockwise
- Then repeat a few times in the opposite direction

Tongue Pops—tongue strengthening and habituation to roof placement
- Press the top of the tongue against the roof of the mouth
- Release it with a popping or clucking sound—the mouth may open reflexively with the release of the tongue; however the breath moves nasally
- Repeat till the tongue feels fatigued
- Practice several times a day
- *Special note*: When a location is found for the tongue so that a nice popping sound is created by this tongue exercise, that placement of the tongue tends to be the ideal resting spot for it in daily life

Tongue Retraction and Protraction—tongue strengthening and habituation to roof placement of the tongue
- Start with the top of the tongue pressed to the roof of the mouth and the tip of the tongue pressing against the inside of the front teeth
- Retract the tongue toward the back of the throat until you feel the urge to curl it under
- Then protract the tip of the tongue back forward to the lower front teeth
- The top of the tongue remains in contact with the roof of the mouth the entire time
- Repeat till tongue feels fatigued
- Practice several times a day to increase tongue range of motion and strength

Tongue Side-to-Side Swooshes—tongue strengthening and habituation to roof placement
- Start with the top of the tongue pressed to the roof of the mouth and the tip of the tongue pressing the palate just above the top of the upper front teeth
- Slide the whole tongue to the right, maintaining full contact with the roof of the mouth
- Then slide the whole tongue to the left, maintaining full contact with the roof of the mouth
- Repeat the side-to-side movement till tongue feels fatigued
- Practice several times a day to increase range of motion and strength

(continued)

Table 7.16 (continued)

Lion's Breath Preparation—stick the tongue out and move it in the following directions, holding for approximately 10 s in each direction
- Straight forward
- To the front and up toward the nose
- To the front and down toward the chin
- To the far right
- To the far left

Lion's Breath—tongue activation with heavy exhalation (use only if advanced in functional breathing); as noted, this breath encourages contraction of the deep abdominal muscles and can be used to help clients locate and activate these important core stabilizers
- Inhale gently through the mouth
- On the exhalation, open the mouth wide, stick out the tongue as far as you can, slightly angled downward toward the chin—forcefully exhale along with the tongue movement
- At the end of the exhalation, retract the tongue, close the mouth, and gently inhale nasally
- Take at least one full round of gentle nasal breathing
- Repeat if that feels appropriate energetically and physically

Sitali Breathing—tongue roll-ups (use only if you are already an adept nose breather as this is an oral breath); the idea is to strengthen the tongue and/or to cool the physical heat of an agitated mind)
- Stick out the tongue and curl up the sides
- Breathe in through tongue curl as if breathing through a straw
- At the end of the inhalation, close the mouth and touch the tongue to the backs of the upper front teeth
- Breathe out through nose and repeat a few times

they can be used frequently over the course of the day. Because of the ease and accessibility of these practices, success can occur quickly. The more often we practice, the more quickly we may begin to see changes in tongue strength, mobility, and placement—the more easily we will gain access to healthier breath rhythms.

7.5   Where We Go from Here

With the assessments offered in Chap. 6 and the many possible preparations to choose from that were offered in this chapter, breathwork emerges from an integrated holistic context that increases the likelihood that clients will experience a beneficial practice. With careful assessment, preparation, and intention-setting, auspicious changes in breath and breathing are likely to occur. In other words, careful preparation and sequencing of a practice within and across sessions are worth the time and patience. That said, each clinician needs to make the final decision about what is possible and appropriate for a specific context in which breathwork is unfolding. If time does not permit protracted preparation in each session, useful work can still be done by directly jumping into breathwork. Decision-making is then based on which breathing practices can be offered in a time- and context-limited manner. Breath awareness and optimal functional breathing are typically great choices for most clients and students. This is where we will turn our attention in the next two chapters.

Breath is the bridge which connects life to consciousness, which unites your body to your thoughts. Whenever your mind becomes scattered, use your breath as the means to take hold of your mind again.—Thich Nhat Hanh

References

1. Brems C. Basic skills in psychotherapy and counseling. Brooks/Cole; 2001.
2. Miller R. Yoga nidra: the iRest meditative practice for deep relaxation and healing. Sounds True; 2022.
3. Iyengar BKS. Light on pranayama. HarperCollins; 2013.
4. Rosen R. The yoga of breath: a step-by-step guide to pranayama. Shambala; 2002.
5. Porter K. Natural posture for pain-free living. Inner Traditions International; 2013.
6. Patel K. The complete guide to postural training. Bloomsbury; 2015.
7. Pham V, O'Connell J. Sit up straight. Scribner; 2022.
8. Lasater JH. Yoga myths. Shambhala; 2020.
9. Lasater JH. Restore and rebalance: yoga for deep relaxation. Shambhala; 2017.
10. Baginski C. Restorative yoga: relax. restore. re-energize. Alpha Books; 2020.
11. Rosenberg S. Accessing the healing power of the vagus nerve. North Atlantic Books; 2017.
12. Farhi D, Leila S. Pathways to a centered body. Embodied Wisdom Publishing; 2022.
13. Myers TW. Anatomy trains. 4th ed. Elsevier; 2022.
14. Coulter D. Anatomy of hatha yoga. Body and Breath; 2001.
15. McKeown P. Oxygen advantage: the simple, scientifically proven breathing techniques for a healthier, slimmer, faster, and fitter you. William Morrow; 2015.
16. McKeown P. The breathing cure. Humanix; 2021.
17. Nestor J. Breath: the new science of a lost art. Riverhead Books; 2020.
18. Gil H, Fougeront N. Tongue dysfunction screening: assessment protocol for prescribers. J Dentofac Anom Orthod. 2015;18(4):408. https://doi.org/10.1051/odfen/2015026.

Part IV

Toolbox for Breathwork

Creating Attunement with Breathwork 8

> *To breathe correctly is to hear the secret language of life.*
>
> *Michelangelo (1475–1564)*

8.1 Overview: Breathing Optimally through Mindful Presence

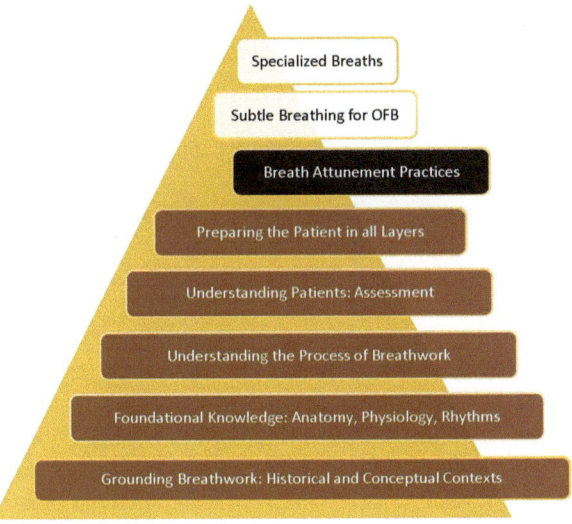

Specialized Breaths

Subtle Breathing for OFB

Breath Attunement Practices

Preparing the Patient in all Layers

Understanding Patients: Assessment

Understanding the Process of Breathwork

Foundational Knowledge: Anatomy, Physiology, Rhythms

Grounding Breathwork: Historical and Conceptual Contexts

Breathwork is always embedded in a larger context of safety, compassion, ethical care, loving kindness, and deep respect. It relies on creating an environment that optimizes the opportunity for patients to feel safe, to feel heard and understood, to have autonomy and agency, to exercise options and explore variations, and to be

© The Author(s), under exclusive license to Springer Nature Switzerland AG 2024
C. Brems, *Therapeutic Breathwork*,
https://doi.org/10.1007/978-3-031-66683-4_8

honored and respected with regard to their unique biopsychosociocultural context. Breathing practices are conducted in a safe and compassionate context, always grounded in the first two limbs of yoga, that is, in ethical and engaged ways of practicing that involve self-assessing, changing, learning, unlearning, and relearning. Principles of non-harming, truthfulness, moderation, and ease are deeply ingrained in each session. Within this context, discipline with clear intention and purpose is invited, as well as self-reflection and commitment to the practice. Intention and purpose are linked to a realization of the potential benefits of the practice, supporting and encouraging motivation and commitment.

The breathwork covered in this chapter is focused on attunement to the breath and represents an important step toward resilience, coherence, and adaptability in daily life. This chapter grounds attunement practices in purposeful and intentional design and sequencing. It recapitulates breath characteristics in the context of how to help patients become familiar with the quality of their breath and how to use attunement practices to develop interoception, neuroception, and a calmer state of mind and nervous system. To that end, this chapter provides instructions, cuing suggestions, and sample scripts; recommends sequencing options within and across sessions; and provides guidance about variations and adaptations for patient-centered tailoring of breath observation and awareness. The goal for these attunement practices is integrated attention to and impact on all layers of being, via the following:

- Attunement to and refinement of the manifestation of breath in the physical body
- Attunement to and refinement of energy, affect, and arousal in the vital experience
- Recognition of the breath's impact on mental, emotional, or cognitive experiences
- Recognition of the breath's reverberations into nervous system states and psychological presence
- Insight into how breath can guide wise choices and enhance a sense of connection
- Openness to the possible emergence of spontaneous joy and a deep sense of well-being simply through being with the breath in a conscious and mindful manner

8.2 Breath Attunement

This set of breath-based interventions, ranging from observation to awareness, may be the most useful method for exploring and refining breath and breathing, especially for patients who are new to breathwork. Attunement practices tend to automatically facilitate quiet, light, and slow breathing, which can have positive effects on heart rate variability, calm the nervous system, invite a state of relaxation, reduce stress perception, and lower blood pressure, among other profound physical, energetic, and affective or emotional influences. In fact, many breathwork experts believe that breath attunement practices, in their function as meditative or contemplative practices, are more effective in settling the breath and nervous system than specific breathing exercises, even increasing bottom-up top-down integration [1, 2].

Breath attunement practices are even effective with regard to recalibrating disturbed breath biochemistry, reducing hypocapnia and hyperventilation.

Breath attunement supports the development of physical, somatic, energetic, and affective mindfulness [3, 4]. Applications can range from observation (or attention) to awareness, can transition from one to the other, or can intermingle both. It is imperative that clinicians understand their intention for a given patient and focus the practice accordingly. If the goal is to learn more about the breath, how it appears in the moment, and how it may evolve over time, breath observation may be most appropriate (e.g., attending to rate, volume, texture, space, and resting pauses). If the goal is to increase spacious experience of breath as energy and vitality, focus (and cuing) can emphasize awareness (e.g., "knowing that you are inhaling while breathing in; knowing that you are exhaling while breathing out"). Breath attunement practices are embedded in a context of nonjudgment and compassion. The mental and emotional preparations offered in Chap. 7 are essential to breath attunement practices and can be very successfully interwoven with them. Breath attunement honors present-moment experience; it may bring forth reactivities that need attention and support. Due to this focus, attunement practices can also facilitate *insight*—bringing to light personal and intimate reactions in response to certain inner or outer stimuli and experiences. In that sense, breath attunement practices are powerful means of learning more about ourselves in an effort to transform reactivity into responsiveness, perhaps discovering our capacity for emotional, mental, and relational self-regulation. Breath attunement practices also have profound psychoeducational value, in that instructions and cuing during the practice can incorporate anatomical, physiological, and psychological background information.

Differentiating Attention (or Observation) and Awareness

Attention or Observation: Concentration on a specific point of focus related to the breath—such as its texture, sound, location, cadence, or phase in the present moment. Attention in daily life is a focus on a particular set of stimuli, which may lead to thought or action. Such attention tends to shift to whatever seems most salient to the intention we bring to a situation.

Awareness: In the context of a breathing practice, awareness is spacious and open; it is more inclusive than a single point of focus and yet fully absorbed in the experience of the breath's many dimensions and reverberations in all layers of experience. In daily life, awareness is the background of our experience—we strive to be aware of the sights, sounds, textures, tastes, smell, and other sensations of our inner and outer world.

Their Relationship: Attention, or focus on a specific input or set of inputs, arises out of awareness as something *catches our attention* and invites us to observe a salient inner or outer stimulus. Awareness can arise out of attention when we broaden our focus from being exclusive (attending to a single stimulus or set of stimuli) to becoming inclusive (being spaciously and openly present without a specific focus).

Awareness is primary and always diffusely present in the background of our experience. It may be more or less conscious, depending on circumstances. In other words, *sometime we are aware that we are aware; other times, we are not aware that we are aware—and yet awareness is always present*. From awareness arises sensation (i.e., sensory experiences received via neuroception, interoception, and exteroception), which interacts with intention. The combined experience of sensation and intention helps direct attention. Where and how the focus of our attention is directed contributes to our mental and emotional experience of what it is we are observing. In essence, there is a chain of events that moves from spacious or broad awareness to an interaction with intention and sensation to attentional focus and attentional shifts to thoughts and emotions.

Breath attunement practices of all types have tremendous potential for supporting healthful biomechanics and biochemistry [5, 6]. They shine, however, with regard to nervous system or psychological impacts [3, 7, 8]. They are key practice for clients whose assessment reveals that they tend toward extreme expressions of the polyvagal states, either living chronically in a sympathetic state of arousal or a dorsal vagal state of collapse [9, 10]. They are powerful means to shift clients toward a ventral vagal state, especially helping to reduce the fight-or-flight-based stress response [11, 12]. When embedded in a supportive and compassionate social presence with the clinician, even patients in a dorsal vagal state can be supported with breath attunement practices. Cuing is adapted, as will be explored in the *Variations* section, depending on whether nervous system regulation is in the direction of activation or calming. Breath attunement practices improve vagal tone and invite the vagus nerve to engage the brake on the sympathetic nervous system. Along the way, these practices increase heart rate variability, regulate blood pressure, and promote the recovery of emotional well-being and physical health [3].

Samples of breath observation and awareness practices are offered on a YouTube playlist by this author. Clinicians can feel free to access this exclusive playlist with the following link and may share it with their patients: https://www.youtube.com/playlist?list=PLzvkZpUGjwIGxil7eP9j41Zw4PALDm6yx.

8.3   Breath Observation

Breath attention or observation is just that—a practice of observing naturally existing breathing to become more familiar with how its various features are unfolding moment to moment. Attention can be directed to any breath quality, from breath rate and volume, to texture and sound, location and space, or phases. Resting pauses are observed without any intention of creating longer pauses or breath holds. Breath observation, while being an attention-honing and calming practice, is nevertheless breathwork. The first step in the process of freeing or restraining breath (the definition of *pranayama*; see Chap. 1) is to know what is already present. Breath observation, once learned, has many positive impacts when practiced not only in sessions with a breathing instructor but also, more importantly, while immersed in daily life. Observation of breath helps us recognize when we have lost our natural and optimal breathing rhythm, inviting us to investigate why, and how to return to resilient breathing and with that, to physical, mental, and emotional balance.

Breath observation is linked to healthier biochemistry of breath and a calmer state of mind, with a parasympathetic shift in the nervous system. It is hopefully self-evident by now that it is not a good idea to dive into complex breathing practices with patients without having first developed their skill to observe and become aware of breathing. The capacity of observation is foundational to all breathing practices that alter the breath. It helps clients have a sense of self-agency when they begin to create and feel the related impacts of changing the breath. Therefore, breath observation is used throughout all breathwork sessions, being interwoven with all other breathing practices. This interweaving or breath observation (and awareness) supports an easeful approach to breathwork that may otherwise be challenging or even dysregulating for patients' nervous systems.

Breath observation practices are helpful for almost all clients. They are especially useful for patients for whom assessments suggest that they need to start with very gentle breathwork due to significant dysregulation in breath (e.g., poor biochemistry; very low controlled breath pause) or vitality (e.g., in dorsal collapse) or due to significant physical challenges related to breath health (e.g., very poor biomechanics, such as mouth breathing, poor posture, lack of resilience). Contraindications may include acute psychosis or trauma reactivity, panic and anxiety disorders, lack of cognitive capacity, or acute breath dysfunction [13]. Observing breath pauses is the most challenging aspect of breath observation and may be reserved for some clients until they have developed adequate capacity for nasal breathing.

8.3.1 Instructions and Cuing Tips for Breath Observation

In an office or yoga setting, observational practices are ideally preceded by an opening centering if time permits. In daily life and in session, they can happen seated, supine, prone, walking, standing, moving, waiting in line, sitting at a desk, and attending a meeting—really anytime, anywhere, under any circumstance. Observation employs nonjudgmental curiosity to collect data about the breath to understand how it emerges in each and every moment. It uses beginner's mind— each time we notice the breath, we do so as if, for the first time, we are free of preconceived ideas, open and receptive to what is present. Observation of breath dimensions can include a scanning into these features' reverberations into body, affect, arousal, and mind. Such noticing lays important groundwork for understanding how ultimately to apply breath to recalibrate the nervous system.

In cuing breath observation, it is best to favor the word "natural" over "normal" for any breath dimension or quality to which we are drawing patients' attention or focus. No invitation is made to alter the breath; there is only watching and observing with curiosity and an open mind. It is helpful to remind clients that observed breath may change simply from receiving attention. Such changes reflect the breath's natural capacity to adapt to new demand characteristics and remind patients that changing the breath (e.g., in daily life or under stress) can be as simple as paying attention to it. Cuing invites attention to any or all of the dimensions of breath with frequent reminders that there are no expectations about what will emerge. Table 8.1 provides a few general cuing suggestions; additional cuing examples are offered later in the chapter for each specific breath characteristic. Clinicians are invited to note the open-hearted cuing that is often phrased in the form of a question, an invitation into exploration, or a reminder to stay present-focused and nonjudgmental. Agency is offered to the patient throughout observational practices.

Table 8.1 General cuing examples for breath observation

The invitation is to gently begin your natural breathing just as it unfolds in this moment … there is no need to change anything …

Can you gently meet your breath, however it emerges in this moment—without judgment or analysis …

Invite curiosity about how you are breathing right here and right now … what emerges?

What kind of breath are you bringing with you today? Is it … [offer sample adjectives based on clinician observations]

I invite you to notice your breathing without any expectation about what you might find out … staying open …

How does your breath reflect the energy that you are bringing with you today? Can you sense what it tells you about how vital or tired you feel?

Observe without expectations about what you will meet as you welcome your breath just as it is …

Can you give yourself permission to observe the breath without any intention or attempt to change anything

Even when there is no attempt or intention to change the breath, you may notice changes simply from being observed—this is natural … just notice and keep watching …

Can you witness your naturally emerging breath (texture/space/location/sound/etc.) with curiosity and open-mindedness

Witness the breath without judgment (rhythm/sound/texture/speed/volume) as it flows through you in this moment

How is the breath unfolding in this moment?

Which quality of the breath is most pronounced right now? What aspect of the breath capturers your attention?

Notice if the breath changes … without expecting anything in particular … or anything at all …

Are there any reverberations of the breath into your body/vitality/mind/thoughts/emotions?

Does the breath seem to transform? If so, can you notice what changed? How do you perceive this new breath?

Can you stay with the breath regardless of what you notice, not judging what emerges … simply staying present …

8.3.2 Breath and Practice Aspects of Focus

Breath observation is the key practice that begins to familiarize patients with breath dimensions or characteristics. Any guided breath observation can focus on a single dimension or characteristic of the naturally preexisting breath, it can touch on all of them briefly, or it can highlight a relevant subset. Patient or student needs and session intentions guide these choices. To make the practice more subtle, observations can be parsed further for each explored characteristic by comparing its manifestation during various breath phases, for example, comparing texture or sound during inhalation versus exhalation.

Attending to Breath Cadence

Many ways exist to help clients observe and explore breath cadence. For example, patients can be asked to count the number of breaths per minute or within some other timeframe (likely measured by the clinician for the patient and as explained in Chap. 6). More commonly, they are invited to make a slightly less objective note of breath speed. For example, they can be invited to count how long it takes them to inhale and how long it takes them to exhale. If counting is not desirable for the patient, alternative ways of "measuring" breath length include exploring how many times clients can recite a mantra, how many letters of the alphabet they can recite, or how many times they can say their name during inhalation and then during exhalation. If this method for tracking the length seems too tedious to the patient, it is also fine simply to invite them to note subjectively how long it takes to inhale versus exhale (i.e., if one is seemingly longer than the other).

Related cadence dimensions can be explored by inviting clients to note whether breath feels rushed or pressured versus slowed or decelerated. Simple questions about noting whether breath seems to be fast or slow, long or short can be enough to foster a subjective sense of breath speed. Sometimes it is helpful to inquire about breath-rate-related symptoms the clinician may be observing in the breathing patient. For example, if breathing appears too fast for the task at hand, the clinician may ask whether the patient feels as though they are hyperventilating. Patients may also be invited to notice experiences such as cold extremities, muscle tension, breathlessness, emotional reactivity, irritability, and other signs and symptoms that breath cadence may not be optimal in the moment.

Attending to Breath Volume

With regard to breath volume, patients can be asked to observe whether their breath seems full or shallow. Synonyms can be offered that may be more accessible to a given client, asking whether the breath seems to feel ample or scant, deep or shallow, strong or weak, heavy or light, expansive or restricted. Another way to help patients observe volume subjectively may be through the use of questions in attunement practices. Such questions can be based on what the clinician is observing, yet they neither lead the patient to a particular conclusion nor suggest that there is need to change anything. The questions are there to guide the patient into a personal experience of the volume of their breath and to offer assistance if there seems to be confusion or lack of interoception. At times, questions can redirect if the patient seems to be making efforts to change the volume of breath.

Examples of guiding, but not leading or suggestive, questions include the following:

- How much air seems to be moving through you?
- What is the volume of the inhalation versus the exhalation?
- Does the breath seem shallow or ample?
- Would a feather near the nose be moved by the exhalation?
- Are you reaching for more air?
- How far away from your nose can you feel the exhalation with your hand?
- Are you taking big, gulping, greedy breaths?
- Is the breath frozen and collapsed with very little movement of air?
- Is it difficult to get enough air?
- Is it possible that you are making more effort than needed to simply *sense into how much breath* is flowing?
- Does it seem as though more/less air is flowing in than out?
- Does your breath feel as though it is bringing enough air into your body?
- Can you notice if the breath is ample or not quite enough or perhaps a bit too full?
- Can you notice how much air is moving in and out without trying to change anything?

Attending to Breath Texture

To help patients observe their breath texture, it may be helpful to invite synonyms for the two extreme manifestations of texture, providing options for its smooth and supple expression versus its choppy and irregular expression. For example, the clinician may invite clients to observe whether the breath is choppy, smooth, regular, even, irregular, tense, heavy, light, hesitating, jerky, harsh, labored, tight, rough, buttery, uneasy, scratchy, feathery, uneven, and so on (see Table 4.6 for many anchors and synonyms). Clients can also be asked to notice if the breath catches anywhere or if it flows unencumbered. It is helpful to offer a variety of adjectives and to intermix the two ends of the texture spectrum so as not to lead the client toward a particular experience simply based on the words that are offered. Enough choices are provided so that students *understand* the concept of breath texture and explore it from the inside out without being led to a particular conclusion by the phrasing. Invitations can be added to notice any differences in texture of the inhalation versus exhalation. Some patients present with profound differences in breath texture by the phase of the breath.

Breath texture can be difficult to discern, and patience is key to helping patients develop interoceptive skills to notice this breath dimension. For some individuals, texture is more observable in the context of movement when they have a clearer sense of the shift in the nature of their breath as some exertion is added. Creativity can be expressed in how this observation skill can be honed. For some patients, it may require the clinician to share what they are observing in the patient's breath outside of a breath observation context, but in the context of a conversation or during movement when texture seems particularly notable. If the patient can sense into the texture in such a moment, this insight can then be creatively woven into cuing during an observational practice (e.g., remember when… how does the breath compare now…).

Attending to Breath Sounds

Clients can be initiated into the concept of breath sounds simply by asking them to observe whether they can hear themselves breathe. From there, they can begin to observe whether they believe that they breathe loudly enough that others can hear them or silently enough that others cannot. Of course, as is true for texture, clinicians may be aware of breath sounds that are emerging from the patient. If this is the case, it may be appropriate to inquire about specific sounds. For example, it may be possible to ask whether the patient notices sounds of gasping or snuffling or of being winded. Clients' attention and observational capacity may be directed to whether they can hear other breathing-related sounds, such as rasping or whistling sounds in their nose or throat. It is not uncommon for clients not to be aware of their own breath sounds when they first begin to observe this breath dimension. Thus, occasionally, it is helpful, when clinicians note specific sounds, to invite specific observations during or outside of the attunement practice. In other words, if a clinician notes a rasping sound of which the patient is unaware, there can be an invitation to note that sound to help the client become aware that this is happening. Following is a brief sample script for observing breath texture and sound; it can be easily adapted for other breath dimensions.

Observing Breath Texture and Sound
[side notes in italics and brackets]
   [transition from another practice aspect …]
   From here, I invite you to notice the sounds of your breathing … in this moment, are sounds almost absent or is your breath noisy or loud right now … is it raspy or wheezy … or very silent, very quiet … can you witness the sound of your breathing …
   [pause—then perhaps repeat some of the prompts]
   Notice if there is a texture to the breath … is there perhaps a sense of jerkiness or does the breath seem smooth … maybe the breath feels almost buttery and soft … or maybe it catches and or is a bit raggedy … is it relaxed and unlabored … or are there little hitches and glitches … observe what is present …
   [pause—then perhaps repeat some of the prompts]
   Sound and texture are wonderful biofeedback mechanisms—not just about the breath in and of itself, but about the state of body and mind … can you give yourself this moment to experience, to observe … to really hear and sense into the textures and sounds of your breathing

[pause]

Do you notice whether there is a difference in the texture of the inhalation as compared to the exhalation … is one perhaps easeful and unblocked … while the other is strained or sticky … observe compassionately … *[give more examples/adjective as appropriate]* … without any desire to change anything …

[pause]

Maybe you detect if there is a difference in the sound of the inhalation versus the exhalation … is one silent and calm … and the other croaky or loud … simply notice … without judgment … *[give more examples/adjective as appropriate]* listening to your own breathing … sensing into each inhalation … each exhalation … inviting a noticing of any sounds in the breath …

[pause]

We know from physics that everything that is observed is likely to change simply from the act of being observed … are you noticing any changes in your breath texture and sound … can you let yourself observe, not expecting anything … yet knowing that even though you are not trying to create change, change may happen … can you explore with curiosity …

[pause]

I invite you now to let exploration fade into the background … keeping the breath in the background of your awareness so that you can continue to sense the texture and sound of your breath as you ready yourself for movement …

[session moves to a different focus from there, yet inviting continued awareness of texture and sound]

Attending to Breath Location

With regard to breath location, clinicians can invite patients to notice where in the body breath is sensed most easily, noticeably, or tangibly. If clients appear unsure about open-ended instructions, clinicians can suggest specific body locations in which to observe the presence or absence of any movement or sensation related to breath rhythms. For example, they may direct patients' attention to the rising and falling of the abdomen, coolness or warmth in the throat, outward or upward movement of the low rib basket, expansion and contraction in the side waist, temperature of air in the nostrils, or movement in the back body.

It is helpful for clinicians to observe whether clients are breathing high into the chest, perhaps as high as the clavicles, whether the abdomen moves within a healthful range of motion, and whether there is visible movement in the side waist or low rib basket. If movements are discernable, clinicians can choose to inquire about them specifically. Such explicit direction toward a particular body location might facilitate observation and attention for clients who have difficulty sensing into locations where breath can be perceived. Even with such direct cues, however, some patients initially have difficulty noticing their breath locations. As noted in Chap. 6, it can be helpful to give such patients external feedback into their bodies' movements with breath. For example, they may be offered an resistance band around the low rib basket, hands or a light weight (e.g., a stuffed animal, small pillow) on the abdomen, or hands on the chest or at the side waist. Patients can be invited to observe their body in different orientations in space to tune into breath locations that are more difficult to access. For example, some clients may not be able to sense breath moving in their back body. They can be invited into a child's pose with a cushion under the abdomen and perhaps a blanket or light pillow on their back body. They can then be invited to sense movement in the back body as breath travels in and out while the lungs in the front body are compressed.

Observation of breath location is helpful in working with clients collaboratively to identify whether they are breathing diaphragmatically, thoracically, clavicularly, or abdominally. Even reverse breathing can be identified through observation of breath location. If less than optimal breathing patterns are identified via observation practices, clients are well served by the physical preparation exercises offered in Chap. 7 to slowly evolve their breath to become diaphragmatic. Although breathing practices that emphasize diaphragmatic breathing are useful, they assume that the client has enough self-awareness to be able to shift their strong preexisting pattern. For those who cannot reset through breathing practices (such as cadence breathing, alternate nostril breathing, abdominal breathing, or four-part breathing; all covered in Chaps. 9 or 10), a few more tailored practices are offered in Table 8.2. In all cases, the client is first encouraged to notice existing breathing patterns (e.g., reverse or chest breathing). Then, strategies are offered to help create a different flow of breath in the body.

Observing breath locations also helps clients discern whether they are breathing nasally or orally. Many people are completely unaware that they are breathing mostly through the mouth. Helping them develop attentional skills to notice mouth or nose breathing supports their shift to nasal breathing over time. If observation of breath locations leads client and clinician to conclude that the client breathes through the mouth most of the time, nasal clearing exercises offered in Chap. 7 facilitate the transition to nasal breathing, especially if one reason for oral breathing is congestion. Creating motivation through education may also be indicated, and some of this information can be woven into breath attunement exercises, moving a bit beyond observation into supporting insight and transformation. Following is a longer sample script that can be used for observing breath location, particularly in the abdomen and chest. It deliberately integrates an educational component by adding commentary about breath biomechanics. Integration of observation and psychoeducation can enhance patients' capacity to observe and notice what is happening with the breath. The script can be easily adapted for other breath dimensions.

Table 8.2 Helping clients shift toward diaphragmatic breathing

Noting and transforming reverse breathing
- Reverse breathing can be explored and ultimately corrected by inviting clients to:
  - Press on the belly during the exhalation and free the compression on the inhalation
  - Exaggerate outward movement of the abdominal wall on the inhalation by breathing into a hand or a light sandbag placed on the belly
  - Place their hands on or tie an elastic band around the low ribs, with encouragement to make the hands or band move upward and outward with deliberate action of the ribs
  - Over time, such deliberate actions to invite expansion of the midriff and upward and outward movement of the low ribs will help clients retrain their muscles and develop new neuromuscular pathways.
- It can also be helpful to ask clients to imagine that they are forcefully blowing dust out of their nose. This spontaneous action can help reset reverse breathing [14].
- A similar action can be engaged via a forceful lion's breath (see Table 7.16) or spontaneous laughter.

Noting and transforming chest breathing
- Relaxation practices (see samples in Chap. 7) may help clients achieve a more relaxed and open posture to receive the breath in the mid-torso with a gentle expansion of the abdomen and upward-outward movement of the low ribs.
- Adding relaxation practice may be necessary repeatedly during retraining as clients are likely to revert to their strong patterns. Relaxing before shifting to a new pattern helps recondition the nervous system as well as the anatomy.
- Chest breathing is often stress related or posture related, with clients having a rounding in the thorax, with low ribs pressing inward and impairing expansion of the mid-waist on inhalation, forcing the air high into the chest.
- Postural work (described in Chap. 7) can be very helpful with explicit invitations to help the client to relax the shoulders and upper back; to release the belly, waist, and low ribs; and to open the heart and find a more upright posture.
- Sometimes, clients attempt to hide their belly posturally, resulting in excess engagement of the core muscles that forces the inhalation high into the chest. In this case, the above practices will be helpful. However, it may also important to consider the need to loosen tight-fitting clothing or belts to allow the breath to drop easily into the belly without meeting external resistance.

Observing Natural Breath Location—Abdominal and Chest Emphasis
[side notes in italics and brackets]

I invite you to draw inward to begin to observe how your breath is flowing through you in this moment, being completely open to whatever you find out … becoming very curious about how your breath is traveling into and how your breath is traveling out …

[pause]

You might choose to notice your breathing at the level of your belly, noticing perhaps the slight movement in the abdomen as you breathe in and out …

[pause]

If this is a new experience for you, to try to feel your breath more keenly, you could place your hands at the side waist … placing the part of the hands between the thumbs and the index finger so that it is hugging around your waist … fingers pointing forward and thumb pointing back … this may help you receive some external feedback about the movement that is happening at the point of the low rib basket—the side waist just above the pelvis …

[pause]

What are you noticing in this part of your body with each inhalation and exhalation …. Can you notice how the hands are being moved by each inhalation … and how do they move with each exhalation … Is there a notable movement outward or upward as breath draws … and perhaps inward and downward as breathe releases out …

[pause]

Can you be present with what is noticeable with each present in your low ribs and side waist … this may be a very subtle movement … or it may be a very pronounced movement … every body is different … every moment may bring a new sensation or experience … simply notice if you have a sense of outward movement at the side waist … if you perceive this movement, know that it is inspired by your diaphragm … not in the sense that you are feeling your diaphragm move per se … but in the sense that you are perceiving the response of other muscles and tissues in this region of your body to the movement of your diaphragm…

[pause]

Keep noticing … observing with curiosity … how your waist region is pulsing with the breath …

If you prefer, you can drop your hands now *[if clients has not already done so]* and explore if you can sense this movement from the inside out … noticing how your diaphragm is moving your waist region … your belly … your side waist as you inhale and exhale …

[pause]

Let this be a gentle observation … there is no attempt to change anything … this is just a way for you to observe how you can sense your breathing in your body … in this particular region … in this particular moment … sensing movement in the belly … in the side body … sensing the effects of the diaphragm contracting downward as you breathe in … and the reverberation of the gentle relaxation of the diaphragm back toward the lungs as you breathe out …

[pause]

Can you sense in this movement the resilience of your organs and your muscles in your abdomen as they respond collaboratively to the contraction and relaxation of the diaphragm …

[pause]

If you are seated upright, without anything to lean against, can you perceive a slight contraction that happens in the deep belly as you exhale … can you sense that those same muscles deep in your belly relax slightly when the diaphragm contracts downward with the inhalation … can you perceive this a very smart system … when the diaphragm contracts, the deep belly muscles relax … as the diaphragm relaxes, the transverse abs contract ever so slightly ... helping you maintain your posture ... helping maintain healthy pressure in the abdomen ...

[pause]

Sense into yourself to see if you can get an inkling of this collaboration between your diaphragm and your abdomen ... can get a sense of this mutuality ... or is it perhaps too subtle to note ... maybe over time your interoception will become keener and you begin to sense the collaboration that is happening in your body ...

[pause]

Can you perceive the slight outward and upward moving movement of the low ribs ... the gentle movement in the low rib basket created mostly by the movement of the diaphragm ... can you image the diaphragm being attached all around the bottom edge of your rib basket ... as well as to your spine ... can you sense that this movement in the low rib basket or the greater region of the body ... is guided by the contraction and relaxation of the diaphragm ....

[pause]

There may be some collaboration by some small muscles between the ribs called the intercostals but when

Sitting still, breathing naturally ...softly ... and gently ... these little muscles do not have to do a lot of work ...

[pause]

I invite you to gently sweep your attention a bit higher into your chest ... do you detect any movement in the high chest ... perhaps observing all the way up toward the shoulders ... just notice ... you are not trying to create any changes ... you are simply noticing what movement is present for you as you sit and breathe easily ...

[pause]

If you are not sure if there is any movement in this part of the body, you could choose to place your hands in the region of your chest ... maybe the fingertips touch the high ribs ... maybe the clavicles ... be curious if there is any discernable movement here ...

[pause ... observe the degree of agitation or calmness in the patient's breath and adapt the next sentences accordingly]

[if calm] If your breathing seems very calm and quiet, it is likely that there is no movement above the low rib basket at all ... there is no need for the upper rib basket ... or the clavicles ... or the shoulders to support a natural breath, a gentle breath .... openheartedly notice what is present for you ...

[pause]

Sometimes, maybe in high anxiety situations, when stressed, or during strenuous exercise situations, you might feel strong sensations or movements in the upper chest ... we only recruit the muscles in the upper chest when we really have to ... when there is some reason ... some strain or stress that requires or creates more work to move air into and out of the lungs ... can you sense the relationship between the nature of breath and the movement ...

> *[pause]*
> If your hands are still on your chest or at your waist, I invite you to release them now … gently ponder if maybe you learned something new about your breath … about how breathing feels when you are collected … when you are calmly settled into the present moment … and then, if your eyes are closed, invite them to open … if your gaze was lowered, perhaps lift it … take a moment to tune into the entirety of your being … as you gently return your awareness to the outer world …

Attending to Breath Space

Although related to exploring breath location, observing the breath's distribution within the physical body has a slightly different focus and can serve as preparation for breath awareness exercises that invite a more spacious exploration of subtle energetic flow or distribution. Breath space explorations invite clients to observe whether there are uneven patterns of breath and energetic flow. For some patients, breath may flow freely into the right lobes of the lungs (and body) but not the left; for others, energy may be notable at the center of the body, but not the extremities. Some clients sense pulsation of *breath and energy* throughout their physical being and are attuned to more subtle signs of breath vitality. They may even sense energy entering their physical being through the skin. For others, subtle flow of breath and energy is not accessible because they can feel the flow of breath and vitality only via tangible external cues (such as hands on the abdomen or rib basket; coolness of air in the nostrils). For some, this exploration is not useful early on in breathwork as it may simply lead to frustration or be met with doubt, even cynicism, about the capacity to experience subtle dimensions of breath and vitality. This way of observing the breath does not have enough functional utility to persist with such invitations if clients are not able or ready to perceive these subtleties quite yet. However, it is worthwhile to return to these types of observations if the patient develops greater capacity for interoception over time.

Energy's distribution in the inner space of the body can be invited via some of the following possible cues:

- How does the breath/energy/vitality distribute throughout the body?
- Is breath notable as a flow or air/energy/vitality into all physical spaces?
- Does more breath/vitality/energy seem to flow into one side of the body than the other?
- Does breath or vitality flow differently in the right half of the body versus the left?
- Do you perceive energy/vitality/breath differently at the top or bottom of the body?
- Can you sense vitality/pulsation/vibration of breath in your finger tips or toes?
- Can you soften into your physical experience of the pulsation and energy of the breath?

- Can you invite the breath to open the body from the inside out?
- Can you invite the breath's energy to open the body in all directions (360°)?
- Can you imagine energy/vitality entering the entire surface of the body?
- Can you notice subtle vibrations of breath in your being? Where are they most notable?

Attending to Breath Phases

Observation of breath phases is an important preparation for breathing practices related to four-part breathing (see Chaps. 9 and 10). To be able to use breathing practices that differentially invite changes in various breath phases (e.g., inhalation versus exhalation; pauses at top versus bottom), patients have to be able to perceive and understand these four parts of the breath cycle. Breath observation is excellent for this purpose. It is helpful to have explanatory or educational language embedded in the cuing of breath phases to help clients who were not aware (especially of breath pauses) learn about this complexity (similar to the location script above). Materials offered in Chap. 4 (e.g., Table 4.8) are helpful to clinicians as they offer psychoeducation about breath. Once clients understand the breath phases, their observation can be invited regularly. Cuing for all breath characteristics offered earlier can now be offered selectively for each breath phase. For example, exploration of texture may be invited separately for the inhalation versus exhalation. Noticing breath location may be differentiated by tangible sensations in the body as breath travels out versus in. Breath sounds may be very different at the end of a breath suspension as compared to the end of breath retention.

Observation of breath pauses tends to be the most unfamiliar experience for patients. This exploration can be useful in identifying unconscious breath-holding as might occur in the case of stress apnea throughout the day. Clients are often unaware that they have spontaneous breath holds, especially since such holding patterns tend to be autonomically driven (e.g., in patients who have dorsal vagal neural defaults). Some patients have never experienced breath pauses before and are greatly appreciative of the gap in energic movement that can be accessed while exploring gentle suspension and retention. For many clients, beginning to notice breath pauses is a powerful experience with calming effects on the mind and nervous system states. Observing breath pauses can be a powerful aspect of calming mind states—the gaps in the breath become linked to gaps in thinking, creating a sense of calmness and serenity.

Particularly useful, breath phases can be tangibly linked to movement, with movement gently pausing as the breath pauses. For example, patients may explore breath phases by lifting their arms with inhalation, gently holding their arms up while their breath is retained, lowering their arms with the exhalation, and gently resting their arms by their side while their breath is suspended. Any two-part movement that allows for a conscious pause offers an excellent opportunity to help create attention and focus on breath pauses (e.g., cat/cow; rising from a forward fold to a half lift; rotating into a twist with the exhalation and rotating out with the inhalation and many other movement patterns where a pause can be perceived somatically and energetically).

A few examples of straightforward cuing about breath pauses are as follows:

- Do you notice a natural gap in the breath—as the inhalation ends and the exhalation has not yet begun?
- Do you notice a natural gap in the breath—as the exhalation ends and the inhalation has not yet begun?
- Are there natural pauses in the breath—either at the top or the bottom or both?
- Can you notice the shift that happens when the inhalation has ended and the exhalation has not quite yet begun?
- Do you notice a moment of quietude when the exhalation is complete and before the inhalation begins to flow in?
- Can you perceive a slight moment of no movement at the cusp of the inhalation?
- Is there a possibility of a brief pause, a brief lingering at the end of the exhalation?
- How long are the pauses when you do not try to expand them but let them emerge naturally?
- How similar or different are pauses at the top and bottom?
- After suspending the breath at the end of an exhalation, are you reaching or gasping for the next breath?
- Are you impatient in reaching for the next part of the breath cycle, or can you linger with the pause?
- Are the rests or pauses gentle or stressful?

Recognizing and Dealing with Daytime Stress (aka Email or Screen) Apnea
Step-by-Step Recognition of Stress Apnea:

1. Observe breath pauses or holds in session to gain greater ability to identify pauses versus holds of the breath
2. Observe breath pauses in daily life that nurture (not deplete or stress) energy
3. Notice spontaneous emergence of breath holds (versus pauses) during daily life, especially in stressful situations
4. Learn to recognize environmental triggers of stress apnea (e.g., opening email, walking into a boss's office, encountering a difficult conversation)

Inoculation Against Stress Apnea:

1. Anticipate situations that may induce stress apnea
2. Engage in calming breathing practices right before an environmental trigger is anticipated
3. Continue to use calm breathing rhythms as the triggering situation unfolds—notice any stress reaction in breath rhythm and consciously regulate
4. Make conscious note of success or lack thereof—use this information for enhanced stress inoculation the next time the stressful trigger is anticipated
5. Engage in regular practices of stress management—such as calming breathing practices, centering and relaxing practices, yoga nidra, mindfulness, and similar strategies

8.3.3 Sequencing Breath Observation Practices

Breath observations are appropriate from early on during breathwork, both with regard to sequencing across time and within sessions. They are safe to suggest for home practice right away, except in unusual circumstances (e.g., severe symptoms from complex trauma; uncontrolled seizure disorders). They can be offered at any time during a breathwork or yoga session and are very auspiciously placed at the beginning and/or end. When offered at the beginning of a session, they are powerful practices that help regulate the nervous system and hone interoception, for some patients even neuroception. Applied after a vigorous physical or breathing practice, observation serves to help clients witness breath and nervous system re-regulation, interoceiving and neuroceiving their body's and mind's capacity to self-regulate affect and arousal. Observation practices remain useful across time, being introduced in the first session and never abandoned. They can be engaged within the context of teaching and practicing specific breathing practices focused on changing breathing patterns and quality.

8.3.4 Additional Variations and Intentions

As noted earlier, one way to vary observation is by which dimensions or qualities are explored in any given practice, as well as by exploring dimensions separately during inhalation versus exhalation. Additional variations are available to meet specific physical, emotional, and mental needs and circumstances. Three categories of variations are offered further, namely observation during movement, in the context of polyvagal states, and in daily life. However, many other possibilities exist—in fact, they are virtually endless and optimally designed through the clinician's understanding of each patient. The following offerings are meant to inspire ideas and creativity for tailoring breath observation to patient needs.

Variations Involving Physical Shapes and Movements

Breath observation can occur in a variety of shapes as well as during movement. Each shape or type of movement provides new opportunities for attention and insight. A few interesting variations that tend to yield valuable and meaningful information include, but are not limited to, the following possibilities:

- Seated fully upright or slightly reclined
- Standing in mountain or extended mountain; standing in warrior or similar more demanding shapes
- Partly or fully supine, possibly with hands or a weight (e.g., sandbag or bag of rice) on the lower to mid abdomen
- In any position with an elastic band tied around the lower ribcage
- Prone or in in child's pose to feel the breath in the back body
- With eyes open, open with a soft focus, partially closed, or fully closed
- During gentle flows (e.g., cat/cow), kriya (e.g., dynamic side-bending or rotation), or vinyasa

Variations Based on Nervous System Defaults

Breath observation can be useful in helping patients identify their nervous system platform (or polyvagal state). This can occur in any of the aforementioned shapes or movements and involves cuing clients to note their level of arousal and affect while observing the breath. Such observation of breath can bring awareness to current level of arousal and provide insight into how the nervous system may be rebalanced to access a more ventral vagal space. For example, if upregulated breathing is observed while attending to rate, volume, texture, or sound, this information can be used to select subsequent movement or breathing practices that help calm the nervous system, shifting it toward a ventral vagal or *sattvic* state. Similarly, identifying breathing patterns during a state of calm (or ventral vagal connection) can help clients find ways to re-regulate to such a pattern when they notice that they are moving away from it, either into dorsal collapse or sympathetic states of fight or flight. This concept of using breath observation to tune into a polyvagal state or *guna* will be explored again in the context of all breathing practices offered in Chaps. 9 and 10.

Variations That Take Breathwork into Daily Life

It can be helpful and illuminating to invite patients to observe their breath in various life situations and relationships. Such explorations help patients identify balanced and resilient versus stressed or challenged breath patterns. Such differentiation can then be used to promote breathing patterns that reconnect clients to social engagement and overall well-being.

Patients can be encouraged to attune to their breath quality when they feel physically or emotionally hurt, offended, cared for, hugged with consent and compassionately, touched without consent in a way that invades their space, and similar situations. They can be encouraged to note their breathing in work contexts, such as while under stress, while being praised, while receiving a new assignment, or after turning in an important piece of work. Observation is possible while exercising, including during aerobic, endurance, strength-building, or balancing physical practices, or while holding a yoga shape. Observation while experiencing difficult emotions, such as anger, hopelessness, helplessness, anxiety, fear, or grief, can provide important feedback. Similarly, observing the breath while experiencing joy or excitement can begin to link breathing patterns with affective and emotional states. Observation can be helpful while solving problems, to begin to link breath patterns to flow states, during struggle, while confused, or when a solution appears. The possible applications of mindful observation in daily life are endless. Such observation can create insight that leads to agency as patients learn to employ specific breathing practices to reshape their breathing upon noticing its dysregulation. Thus, observation leads to energetic, somatic, and mental shifts that have behavioral and relational implications, with empowering effects for the patient.

8.4   Breath and Vital Awareness

Breath observation is about focusing attention and creating a better understanding of how breath unfolds moment to moment in a variety of circumstances. Breath awareness is a practice of being with the breath as it unfolds in the present moment. It invites staying with the current state of being and thus nurtures the capacity to develop a wider bandwidth or window of tolerance for inner sensations. Breath awareness is an exceptional practice for helping clients refine interoception and neuroception, honing their capacity to notice, tend to, and accurately interpret inner signals. Most clients can engage in breath awareness; exceptions might be clients experiencing dorsal collapse or high arousal, who cannot tolerate the more open-ended nature of breath awareness. Specific contraindications may include acute psychosis, acute symptoms of posttraumatic stress, panic or anxiety disorders, or acute breath dysregulation.

Awareness can be directed to the same breath characteristics explored via observation, as well as to subtler energies to become familiar with how breath and vitality (or lifeforce) reverberate through all layers of experience. Increasing awareness of current-moment breathing (*prana*) and vitality (*Prana*) leads to awareness of the subtlest energies associated with breathing, inviting patients into a relationship with the pulsations and vibrations of life, with bottom-up signals from their autonomic nervous system. Listening to the subtle energies of breath and breathing—perhaps in the form of sensing vitality within body and mind—can reset hypersensitivity of the medulla to CO_2 and reduce chronic mild hyperventilation.

Breath awareness can be developed in many ways; we will explore awareness at three levels:

- *Tangible spacious awareness*: At the most tangible level, spacious or open awareness can be fostered for all breath dimensions explored in breath observation, but without cuing *attention* to any particular type of experience within that dimension. Instead, clients are invited to notice breath textures without offering specifics (as is done in observation), but rather with an open invitation to be spaciously aware of how breath textures unfold and reverberate into layers of experience. Similarly, awareness of breath locations can be invited without any guidance as to what might emerge or where—simply with an invitation to notice where breath is felt in the body, how breath moves through the body, where in the body pulsation of breath can be noticed, and similar open-ended cues. Even breath rate and volume are experienced spaciously, with an invitation to sense the pulsation of breath more so than to assess or observe for the purpose of measuring or information.
- *Subtle awareness*: This level of awareness invites opening to sensations arising from subtle expressions of breath and may add visualizations that move beyond observation. Expressions of vitality at cellular level are invited; visualizations guide awareness to vitality, pulsation, and rejuvenation of breath and energy. Examples may include invitations to connect to the subtle energy associated with

exchanging oxygen and carbon dioxide at the alveolar-capillary interface or to connect to the pulsation of energy as notable at the extremities.

- *Pranic awareness*: Awareness at this level is less clearly directed to somatic, arousal, and affective aspects of breath and more about sensing vitality and life-force as it courses through the body and affects thoughts and emotions [15]. It connects to the concept of *Prana*, or vital energy or lifeforce, in its five yogic forms called *pancha vayus* (five movements of vitality; explained below). Awareness of these subtlest of energies is an inner practice (yogic limbs 5 or 6) more so than a breathing practice; yet, it is helpful to integrate into breathwork, as it invites clients into a relationship with their sense of energy and vitality (arousal and affect) without judgment or expectation. It invites an open heart and mind to experience *Prana*. Awareness of the subtlest energies invites a state of *being*, rather than *doing*. It can be a powerful practice to help clients read neuro-ceptive signals. From this understanding, patients can learn to transcend or at least recognize and accept nervous system states and to move beyond preoccupa-tions with attachment, aversion, fear, ego, and anxiety. A bit of definition is nec-essary before we explore sample cuing for this aspect of breath awareness.

8.4.1   Definition of Prana's Rhythms of Vitality

Thus far, this book has focused on grounding breathwork in anatomy and physiol-ogy—informed by research and clinical practice. We now turn to exploring *Prana* from the perspective of the ancient traditions of yoga, diving into the *fourth pranayama*—namely lifeforce beyond the breath. *Prana* (as lifeforce) transcends the coming and going of inhalations and exhalations, moving beyond tangible expe-riences of breath quality into the inner experience of vitality—its psychological, emotional, relational, and mental reverberations. This complex lifeforce moves through us in each moment, connecting us to experiences in all of our layers and connecting us to the greater rhythms of life. *Prana* is multifaceted, integrated, and reflective of enormous complexity, profound interpersonal connection and interde-pendence, and humans' resilient and ever-evolving nature. It is not a singular energy; rather, it has five separate, subtle dimensions that collaborate and interplay to create moment-to-moment experiences to create insight, wisdom, and transfor-mation. *Prana* is the force that connects body and mind; arousal and emotion; inten-tion and impact; sensation and reaction; discernment and response.

These five energies reflected within *Prana*, or *pancha vayus* (Sanskrit for "five winds"), are present in all aspects of nature, not just the human body [15–17]. *Vayus* are important in Ayurvedic medicine and yoga psychology, with strong links to well-being and health in all layers of experience. *Vayus* are important to life balance and vitality; they remind us to take in only as much as we need, to use energy wisely, not dissipating or scattering it frivolously. When we scatter, disperse, or otherwise compromise (and create deficiency in) the presence of *Prana*, we lose resilience and encounter illness or unease. The five winds of *Prana* are *prana vayu*, *apana vayu*, *samana vayu*, *udana vayu*, and *vyana vayu*.. Although it may be easy to dismiss the five *vayus* as yogic esoterica, they actually have a profound link to modern science related to breath and breathing, vitality, the polyvagal state, stress resilience, and householding energy. The *vayus* are invaluable for helping patients begin to become more aware of how they are taking in energy, how they use it, and how they expend it. Awareness of the vital airs fosters interoception and neuroception, inviting patients to become keenly aware of subtle inner sensations and outer stimuli, as well as of their influences on the nervous system. It invites recognition of profound connections and interdependence between body, affect and arousal, thoughts and emotions, social connection and responsibility—it connects body, mind, heart, and spirit.

Tuning into the vital airs supports gaining access to bottom-up (interceptive and neuroceptive) signals from the body that tend to drive reactivity. As clients become more aware of the subtle energies within, they attune to inner signals, learn to recognize them, notice their reactivity to them, and develop the capacity to become responsive rather than reactive. Working with the *vayus* reminds us that breathing practices, just as movement practices, are preparatory to and meant to integrate with practices that create transformation and integrated holistic well-being and that create compassion and social connection. Breathwork is not just a matter of working with our body; perhaps even more importantly, it awakens us to and transforms the fluctuations of our mind. Subtle breath awareness is contemplative in nature and promotes the recognition that we are whole, multilayered complex systems that depend on social connection, depend on nourishment for all layers of self, and evolve toward compassionate action that supports the entire web of life in which we are embedded. The five airs of vitality remind us of the profound connection between all inner and outer layers of experience. Through honing recognition of bottom-up signals, *pranic* awareness makes experiences more available to top-down processing, giving humans a foundation on which to build strategies for regulating the nervous system, affective reactivity, physical and emotional arousal levels, actions in daily life, and interactions in relationships.

Following is a detailed description of the five *vayus* that make the connection of the subtle energies to physical, vital, mental, emotional, and relational processes, insights, compassion, and transformation. Awareness of the vital airs fosters a calm nervous system to create resilient ventral vagal or *sattvic* ways of being, with the capacity to up- or downregulate energy as needed for daily life. Pranic awareness practice stimulates the vagus nerve, moderates energy expenditure in all layers of self, invites self-regulation, supports moderation and generosity, and connects us to the abundance and sharing inherent in our human connection to a greater web of life. It awakens us to our social responsibility, compassionate presence in all relationships, and deep interdependence with life as it unfolds on this planet all around us.

Prana Vayu

Prana vayu, often translated as forward-moving wind, is the most central of the five winds of *Prana*, setting life in motion and moving us forward. It is life-giving and always present—from the moment we draw the first breath, to the moment we release the last breath. *Prana vayu* is the aspect of *Prana* that brings vitality and motivation. It sustains life through absorbing energy, sensations, impressions, and nourishment from the outside to the inside. *Prana* draws in physical nourishment, in the form of food and water; it draws in breath and energy (sometimes framed as moving us forward), especially to the head, heart, and lungs. *Prana* supports the respiratory and circulatory systems (along with *vyana*) and receives sensory stimuli and inputs (with *udana*). It nourishes the brain and our wisdom and provides energy for the other four winds of *Prana*.

This taking-in may be most notable in body and breath, but applies to all *koshas*. *Prana* is about receptivity in all layers of consciousness. It feeds and nourishes our body with food and water. It feeds respiration with air, especially oxygen. It feeds mind and emotions with sensory inputs, mental impressions, and information. It feeds heart and wisdom with interpersonal experiences, including in our closest emotional relationships as well as more distant social interactions. For *prana* to be taken into our being, we encourage openness and still spaces where *prana* can go. We develop an open heart, open mind, and general openness to experiences and nurturance. We become receptive and open in all layers of consciousness, entrusting ourselves to the world and community around us. If we are closed off to inputs, *prana* can become deficient. We may experience a sense of lethargy, fatigue, malaise, or illness in the body; we may sense a lack of vitality, energy, and arousal in our energetic being; we feel a restriction in openness to new information and input in our life in general and in our relationships in particular. Deficiency translates into lack of physical vitality, mental clarity, emotional receptivity, relational openness, and behavioral flexibility.

Apana Vayu

Apana vayu, often translated as the wind that moves away or downward, relates to vital energy in our abdomen that supports downward or descending flows of energy that are calming and cleansing; as such, it is central to the excretory system, supporting elimination. Secondarily, *apana* is related to the reproductive system, including childbirth. *Apana* grounds breath, attention, movement, and energy downward, to the lower half of the body. *Apana* is connected to the water element, to a sense of letting go and letting things flow in all *koshas*. It moves mass and energy downward and outward, inviting the release of anything that no longer serves. Via physical elimination, it supports the obvious (i.e., defecation, urination, and sweating). Via exhalation, it invites release of carbon dioxide. Via emotional and mental letting-go, it supports release of sensory, mental, and emotional experiences and preoccupations that impede well-being. Interpersonally, it supports letting go of relationship experiences that hold us back, have harmed, or otherwise did not nourish us. Physical letting go also supports childbirth and menstruation.

Downward energy of *apana* is stabilizing and grounding; anchored and supported. It liberates unhelpful emotions and upsetting affects, even supporting the clearing of past trauma. *Apana* helps release mental ruminations and worries; it can help free us of relational habits and patterns. If *apana vayu* does not flow freely, there is a sense of physical, emotional, mental, and energetic blocking (most literally, constipation), an inability to let go, to release suffering. We hang on to experiences, feelings, beliefs, attitudes, and emotions, rather than releasing and freeing ourselves from all that no longer serves us. We are weighed down by excess that does not nourish, but hinders. A major hindrance that arises from deficiency in *apana* is that *prana* cannot travel in. If we do not let go of the old, we cannot receive and be nourished and renewed by the new.

Samana Vayu

Samana vayu, translated most typically as balancing wind, relates to stabilizing and nourishing energy that helps digest physical nourishment as well as experiences (or inputs) and all *koshas*. Commensurately, it is associated physically with the digestive system and enteric nervous system. *Samana* stabilizes body, breath, energy, attention, and emotions, especially the region of the navel—literally in the digestive tract and figuratively at the core of being. *Samana* is at the center of what and how much we take in and how much and what we release. It creates balance between *prana* and *apana*. It equalizes and balances experiences by metabolizing and processing them to extract what is useful and sort out what is not. Physically, it does this through digesting food and utilizing water, separating nutrients from waste products. Energetically, it does this by helping with optimal gas exchange during breathing (steering gas exchange at the level of the tissues, absorbing O_2 and releasing CO_2) and by processing affect and arousal. It helps us digest, process, and metabolize emotional experiences, inputs, sensations, and interactions. It helps us digest mental inputs, new learning, information, and impressions, including those arising from relationships, and social and educational exchanges.

For *samana* to do its job, we need to slow down, decompress, and create space. While *prana* helps us take everything in and *apana* helps us eliminate what no longer serves, *samana* processes what is received to discern what serves and what does not. It helps us learn from experiences, processing everything that arrives in all *koshas* and allowing the releasing and cleansing energy of *apana* to take away what does not serve us. Through discerning processing of experiences by *samana*, we develop personal power and agency, motivation, and self-esteem—the capacity to discern what to accept and what to reject, what to keep and what to release, and what to honor and what to dismiss. *Samana* provides us the energy to sustain health and well-being; it lights the internal fire to process experiences in all *koshas*. Without the fire of *samana*, there may be stagnation and lack of balance in all *koshas*. *Samana* may help explain the profound connection between physical and emotional health. It is the balance between *prana* and *apana*, stabilizing and balancing us, inviting us into intuition, and helping us access wisdom.

If the heat of *samana* is deficient or blocked, we do not process what we take in. Most concretely, we do not process and digest food properly and may experience illnesses related to poor digestion and nutritional deficiencies. Breath is less efficient as we may overbreathe and yet lack in proper oxygenation of tissues, including skeletal muscles, heart, and brain. We may fail to learn from experiences; we may be drawn into craving and clinging (greed), dull mind states, and emotional stagnation. We may experience blockages in relationships, persisting in relationships that do not foster well-being or health. We may hang on to patterns, habits, routines, and ruts that no longer serve.

Vyana Vayu

Vyana vayu, typically translated as outward-moving wind, is central to expansion, coordination, and distribution—or inner transport—in all *koshas*. It spreads nutrients, water, breath, energy, emotional nourishment, and attention outward to the periphery, to the far reaches of body and beyond. *Vyana*, in essence, envelops the wholeness of our being and is closely related to movement and flow in all *koshas*. It is associated with blood circulation and the nervous system, imparting movement and vigor in the physical body, energetic body, and mind and emotions, even reaching into relationships and groundedness and integration into community. It is related to flow of blood, lymph, and energy, and the radiance and contagion of affect, arousal, and emotion into our relationships and communities. It relates to our sense of wholeness and integration; it creates a sense of shared vibration or pulsation. It includes the energetic sense of exchanging *Prana* through all pores of the body.

Vyana vayu invites integration, coherence, synchronization, radiance, and cohesion. It includes focus and precision necessary for coordination within and outside the body, within the mind and in relationships, within emotional states, and in collaboration with others' affective contributions. *Vyana* integrates all parts and functions into a whole that is greater than the sum of its parts. It is spacious awareness of pulsations and movements in the *koshas*, from the pumping of blood, beating of our heart, flow of our lymph, to movement of energy, firing of neurons, to resonance with others. It utilizes what is taken in via *prana*; it relinquishes what is released via *apana*. It soaks in processed and metabolized experiences from *samana*; it stimulates uplifting and transformative powers of *udana*. It allows us to absorb life experiences and transform them into growth and wisdom.

If *vyana* is blocked, there may be numbness, poor circulation, and lack of coherence in all layers of self. Blockage can lead to disconnection and isolation and to a sense of separateness and false independence. It can lead to feeling scattered, unintegrated, and separated from the world and from others. This separation disconnects us from our responsibility and compassion for ourselves, other beings, and even this planet. *Vyana* is deficient in most Western cultures that live in a state of confusion, clinging, aversion, ego, and fear.

Udana Vayu

Udana vayu, translated as upward-moving wind, relates to positive, uplifting energy that invites life to unfold with meaning and purpose. Its energy supports insight, transformation, and growth—especially growing, caring, and thinking beyond the individual self. *Udana* draws breath, energy, and attention upward to the throat, neck, and head, energizing the senses of hearing, seeing, tasting, smelling, and interoception, inviting us to process inputs via discernment so that consciousness can evolve to a higher, more perspectival and compassionate layer. *Udana* is associated with the nervous system and prefrontal cortex. It reflects and guides the capacity to regulate and balance bottom-up sensation with top-down control, wisdom, and guidance. The ascending nature of *udana* energizes and brings clarity to thoughts, communications, and relationships; it brings discernment to speech, actions, and relational self-expression. It supports new learning and memory consolidation. *Udana* is said to open the central channel, inviting the radiance of wisdom, perspective, and transformation.

Udana's light and uplifting energy is related to thoughts, speech, and actions that create positive, compassionate, kind, and joyful connections with others. It allows us to exchange information and caring for the growth and healing of relationships, for the betterment of social contexts and realities. *Udana* relies on gathering inputs from *prana*, processing those inputs by *samana*, eliminating what does not serve by *apana*, and integrating coherence of *vyana*. From these energetic supports, *udana* invites energy to move upward to a broader, more perspectival level of understanding and caring. *Udana* sustains and transforms us by connecting us to mature emotions of compassion, loving kindness, altruistic joy, and equanimity. It invites a sense of calming and balance, especially in the autonomic nervous system by engaging the vagal brake on the sympathetic nervous system. From a polyvagal perspective, it invites a ventral vagal (connected, compassionate, aware, and discerning) state of deeply-caring connection with our community and entire biopsychosociocultural matrix.

When in balance, *udana* allows us to assert ourselves and values without aggression, to share knowledge and wisdom without arrogance, and to speak with heartfelt capacity, while listening and learning. It allows us to take our place and to express our opinions and to openly exchange ideas, beliefs, and attitudes. *Udana* is the energy that gives us the open-heartedness and open-mindedness to learn, unlearn, and relearn—not to freeze into opinions or habits. *Udana's* uplifting energy facilitates growth and transformation that serve the greater good. *Udana* cannot exist if it is not fed by *prana*, energized by *samana*, freed (untethered) by the letting go of *apana*, and nourished wisely by *vyana*.

When applying the concepts of the vital airs to hone awareness of subtle energy, of interoceptive and neuroceptive bottom-up signals, it is not necessary to use *Sanskrit* terminology. Table 8.3 can be used to guide breath awareness exercises focused on the subtle airs, by providing language for how these different energies can be experienced and explored. Although each *vayu* is presented individually, these subtle energies need to be understood in terms of their interdependence, collaboration, co-arising, and interactions to create a human experience that feels whole, integrated, healthy, and wise.

8.4.2 Instructions and Cuing Tips for Breath Awareness

As with breath observation, breath awareness can occur while seated, supine, prone, walking, standing, moving through asana, waiting in line, sitting at a desk, or attending a meeting—really anytime, anywhere, under any circumstances. It depends on nonjudgmental curiosity, an open mind and heart not guided by expectations or desire for a particular way in which body, energy, or mind ought to show up. Its

Table 8.3 Subtle manifestations of vitality to which awareness can be directed

Prana Vayu	Apana Vayu	Samana Vayu	Vyana Vayu	Udana Vayu
• Vitality, sensitivity	• Groundedness	• Peacefulness	• Expansiveness	• Lightness, joy
• Associated with the inhalation and uptake of oxygen into lungs	• Associated with the exhalation and release of CO_2	• Associated with breath pauses and distribution of oxygen via the blood	• Associated with balance across the full breath cycle and internal respiration	• Associated with the top of the inhalation and top of the exhalation
• Strong inhalation can energize (release the vagal brake); soft inhalation can calm	• Long and gentle exhalation invites calming of the nervous system	• Balance supports overall physical and emotional wellbeing	• Invites nervous system regulation and resilience	• Invites ventral vagal, compassionate connection
• Moves energy inward, upward, even forward	• Moves energy downward and outward	• Moves energy from edges to the core, especially the region of navel	• Moves energy outward from center to periphery, downward	• Moves energy upward, all the way to the head, senses, & mind
• Most central of the five energies; sets everything in motion, moving us forward	• Vital energy of release that supports elimination and reproduction, as well as letting go	• Central stabilizing energy that imbues heat and warmth, especially at the center of our being	• Circulation and distribution of energy through all *koshas*	• Primary positive energy that invites life to unfold—Inviting growth and transformation
• Central to receptive vitality and openness			• Central to distributing benefits of what we take in	
• Able to direct energy for growth and development	• Able to withdraw energy	• Able to contract and hold steady	• Able to expand and absorb what serves us	• Able to ascend, grow, rise up
• Provides energy to the other *vayus*	• Connected to the water element	• Relates to the fire element of the body	• Envelopes the wholeness of being	• Supports growth and transformation
	• Is a calming and cleansing energy of release	• Relates to spirit and regulates inner fire	• Creates our aura	• Invites consciousness to evolve; most important to spiritual growth
	• Protects from outer negativity	• Stimulates the vagus nerve	• Clears energy throughout	
			• Invites self-regulation	

purpose is to better understand how experience presents itself in each and every moment and, even more importantly, to connect us to deeper pulsations of life in all *kosha*s. Awareness brings us home to the entirety of our being; it attunes us to the pulsations of life through body, mind, emotions, relationships, and the world—all layers of experience. In applying tangible, subtle, and pranic awareness, we draw special attention to the witnessing or observer function, honing skills to support our intuitive sense of how to meet life in any given moment. Through awareness, patients learn about themselves without the pressure of trying to create change. However, awareness also creates the recognition that body, energy and breath, as well as mind and emotions, may change despite the intention not to change anything—this is natural (and in line with the laws of physics) because anything that is observed is influenced by the observer.

Cuing Tangible and Subtle Awareness

Possible cuing may begin early in breathwork practice with a focus on creating awareness of the breath and its many characteristics, followed by awareness of breathing as a vital process that provides the energy for coping, healing, and thriving in all layers of self. As patients progress toward greater awareness, coupled with an opening of their mind and heart to more subtle energies, cuing can shift along the three dimensions of tangible, subtle, and pranic manifestations of breath and vitality. Possibilities for cuing tangible spacious awareness and awareness of the subtler energies are offered in Table 8.4.

Table 8.4 Tangible and subtle breath awareness cues

Tangible breath awareness cues
- Can you sense into the texture of the breath overall?
- Where do you notice the footprints of the breath in your body?
- Bring your mindful attention/mindful presence/awareness to the breath as it naturally flows in and out
- Do not seek to alter the breath—watch and observe with curiosity and openness of heart and mind
- You may notice that even when there is no attempt to change the breath, it may change simply from being observed—this is natural
- Experience the breath with curiosity and open-mindedness
- Attend without expectations about what you will meet as you breathe
- Witness the unfolding of each breath without judgment
- Be fully present for each inhalation as it travels in
- Be fully present for each exhalation as it travels out
- Become aware of your breathing rhythm without attempt to define or label it
- Become aware of any pauses/gap/resting points in the breath
- Become aware of the fullness or subtlety of the breath
- Become aware of the texture of your breathing without any attempt to define or label it
- Become aware of any sounds associated with your breath and breathing

Subtle breath awareness cues
- Where do you sense the breath in the body/the mind/your intuition/your being?
- Are there reverberations of the sound of your breathing into your body or mind?
- Is there a connection between the flow of breath and your experience of warmth or comfort?

(continued)

Table 8.4 (continued)

- How do the different phases of the breath affect your experience of your body/the stories in your mind/your emotional presence?
- How do you sense the breath in body/mind/emotions?
- Invite the exhalation to support the natural expelling of carbon dioxide
- Sense into the power of the inhalation/breath retention to brings oxygen (vitality) into your blood/tissues
- Can you sense your vital being, perhaps as warmth or pulsation in the fingertips?
- Do you perceive the calming influence of the exhalation on the mind?
- Can the inhalation convey a sense of nurturance of your physical and emotional being?
- Can you notice the sense of release as the breath travels out?
- Is there a sense of urgency at the end of a breath suspension?
- Can you sense into the feeling of having let go of everything at the end of the exhalation, before the inhalation travels in?
- How does your vitality shift when you stop the breath for a moment?

Following is a sample script of breath awareness. The focus of this script is on a general overview of the breath and its various qualities—not paying attention, but becoming aware. Of course, language for attention versus awareness can overlap. The subtle difference emerges from the overall intention of the practice and the type of priming of the patient with regard to the aim of the exercise. Breath awareness, as with all breathing practices, is always embedded in this larger context of setting intentions, being clear about an aim that is related to the treatment goals overall, and a debriefing of the experience once the practice is complete. Debriefing awareness can focus on highlighting experiences related to enhanced interoception, neuroception, and exteroception and the realization that the awareness exercise most likely created a shift in the patient's nervous system and mind state, although this was not intentionally cued or attempted. This can be a very empowering experience for patients as they learn a strategy for self-agency and self-regulation.

Breath Awareness Sample Script
[side notes in italics and brackets]
I invite you to find a comfortable reclined seat, carefully supporting the back body, the legs, the arms, and the head, paying attention to settling the body into this moment and into this space to make it as comfortable as possible... feel free to use a blanket to cover yourself up to feel warm and comforted … the more compassionately you settle your body into this moment, the more settled your nervous system can be as you begin the practice of spacious breath awareness…
[pause until the patient seems settled; adding prompts as needed]
With your body settled, the invitation is to move into spacious and open-hearted awareness of the rhythms … the quality … the nature of your breathing … no need to focus attention on any single dimension of the breath … simply being aware of breath traveling in … breath traveling through …

breath traveling out ... nothing in particular needs attention ... no focus on any particular aspect of the breath ... unless something *draws* your attention or focus... if so, perhaps lingering with the observation for a moment to take note ... then gently shifting to being spaciously aware ... curious about the nature of the breath ...

[pause]

Spaciously present with the pulsation of breath as it moves through your being ... perhaps sensing the speed of the breath ... rapid or settled or slow ... speed or hurriedness ... patience or calmness ... reflected in the pulsation of inhalations and exhalations ... as they travel in and out ... lingering perhaps when the breath pauses for a moment ... spaciously, openly aware of breath unfolding ... coming ... and going ...

[pause]

Spaciously sensing air moving with each breath ... maybe being aware at some level ... of the breath as shallow ... or full ... aware ... open ... attuned to pulsations of breath right here ... right now ... receiving feedback from the breath ... its vibration .... its quality ... its nourishing presence ...

[pause]

Staying aware of pulsation ... vibrancy of breath moving in and out ... sensing perhaps a quality of texture ... or sound ... noisiness or silence ... ease, smoothness, or softness ... or a sense choppiness or hesitation ... open to the quality of vitality pulsing through your being ...

[pause]

Remaining open and aware ... watching breath unfolding in this moment ... simply being with sensation ... of breath moving in and out ... without expectation ... without judgment ... with a deep compassion for this pulsation ... appreciation for this vibration of vitality ... energy, breath moving through you ... meeting the breath ... the energy within you just as it is ...

[pause]

Perhaps sensing pauses or gaps ... however subtle ... between inhalation and exhalation ... gentle openings between drawing in nurturance ... vitality ... and letting go of what can be released ... feeling no need ... no urge ... to attempt to change anything ... simply aware of how breath unfolds ... how vitality dances ... in this moment ...

[pause]

compassionate ... content with however life is moving through you .... right here ... right now ... continuing to maintain spacious awareness of the entirety of each breath .... one after the other ... patient... open-hearted ... open-minded ... moving now into a couple of minutes of spacious ... silent ... open awareness.... until my voice calls you back ...

[invite the client to linger as appropriate for a brief period of time, observing and gauging whether the individual can persevere for a full 2 min or if an earlier end of the practice is indicated—e.g., dysregulation is noted]

> Gently reconnecting now to the full range of inner sensations … noticing your body … its sensation …. your mind …its thoughts … its emotions … noticing external stimuli and impressions … sounds, temperature, air on your skin …
>
> *[and similarly cues to bring an end to the practice; then move into a debriefing of the experience]*

Cuing Pranic Awareness—Vitality (*Pancha Vayus*)

Possibilities for cuing pranic awareness include, but are not limited to, the bulleted ideas in Table 8.5. The listing provides a few quick hints; not every breathing instructor chooses to cue this level of experience; not every student is ready for it. It takes discernment to know when and with whom exploration of pranic energy is appropriate. When in doubt, do not. The suggestions are not all inclusive; this would be an impossible endeavor. The goal is to stimulate creativity in how subtlest energies may be cued in an integrative way within breathwork that is evidence-based and honors proper biomechanics and biochemistry. Additional inspiration can come from the definitions of each *vayus* in Table 8.3.

As can be noted from these cuing examples, deeper awareness of pranic vitality that infuses all experiences can occur without specific mention of the *prana vayus*. It can invite a spacious awareness of energetic pulsations and reverberations of breath in all layers of experience. Pranic awareness invites clients to experience the notion of *householding* energy, of moderating how energy is taken in and how vitality is expended. Pranic exploration of breath and vitality is deeply tied to the belief that energy, like food, needs to be taken in a measured and mindful way. It needs to be drawn in and released out with equal care to achieve balance and harmony in the way we collect, utilize, and expend our vital resources.

Awareness practices invite patients into a new relationship with their experience, opening them up to perceiving subtle pulsations and vibrations, and in the process honing interoceptive and neuroceptive skills. It is this link to the autonomic nervous system that underlies at least some of the value of this type of work. For some patients, connecting to subtle pranic energy opens doors into awareness of vitality that increases curiosity and motivation about how they can shift their experience of breath and life. For such patients, a more nuanced journey into the five *vayus* can be offered. Discernment is invited in offering these practices, as they are not crucial to other breathing practices and may be difficult for some patients to accept, especially early during breathwork (as opposed to outright inner yogic practices). Table 8.6 offers cuing tips specific to each of the five *vayus*.

Table 8.5 General cues for awareness of pranic energies

- Is there awareness of energy or vitality beyond the breath?
- Are you aware of vibration/energy/pulsation in your being?
- Bring your mindful attention/mindful presence/awareness to your vital energy/affect/arousal as it naturally emerges in this moment/in this space/in these circumstances
- Can you sense the nourishing and nurturing quality of the breath traveling in?
- There is no attempt or intention to change your energy/vitality/affect/arousal and yet it may change simply from being observed—this is a natural law
- Can you be with your energy/vitality with curiosity and open-mindedness, allowing it to transform your experience
- Become aware of the reverberations of breath energy/vitality in your body/vitality/mind/thoughts/emotions
- Are you aware of your central energy that impels you to move/motivates you/gives you vitality/brings you a sense of direction (*prana*)?
- Is there a sense of energy moving outward from your center to your edges? Nurturing you from the inside out?
- Can you sense a central stabilizing energy at the center of your being? Holding you steady and ready?
- Is there awareness of a downward energy that is grounding, calming, cleansing?
- Can you find a sense of positive energy that is transformative, inviting, optimistic, and light?
- Can you nurture a sense of receptivity? Of being open to something new?
- Can you meet the breath with open heartedness and a deep sense of appreciation? Of gratitude?
- Can you tap into a sense of gratitude with each inhalation and exhalation?
- Is there awareness of a sense of abundance or fulfillment?
- Can you meet the breath as a way of finding balance … harmony?
- Invite a sense of being open to processing your experience with an open heart and a curious mind
- Can you invite a willingness to let go and release?
- Release the exhalation with the faith that what you need is still present
- Find a sense of non-clinging as you as you release out the exclamation
- Explore if there is a sense of lightness as you give away the breath
- Invite a sense of sharing your resources as you release out your exhalation
- Settle into a very grounded and nourishing energy
- Can you be with your breath calm with calm abiding in the experience in the experience of this moment?
- Can you release any energy of wanting or of being afraid or of being averse to

Table 8.6 Cuing vital energies of transformation

Ideas to guide cues for forward-moving, receptive energy (Prana)
Cued as a smooth inward and forward flow of energy:
- Breathe in softly and gently through the nose
- Sense the nourishing quality of each inhalation
- Receive the newness and freshness of each new breath
- Open the breath, open the mind, open the heart
- Invite incoming energy to nourish, support, and guide you forward
- Invite vitality and clarity to enter with each inhalation
- Cherish and absorb what is taken in by lingering in the pause at the top of the breath
- Find a smooth texture for the inhalation, neither striving for more … nor depriving the flow of breath
- Breathe into the full circumference of the body—right, left, up down, forward, and back
- Receive the inspiration and newness or freshness that flows in with each inhalation
- Receive the vitality of the breath and let it inspire you to be open to the new, the innovative, the creative

(continued)

Table 8.6   (continued)

Ideas to guide cues for downward-moving, grounding energy (Apana)

Cued as a descending and releasing energy:

- Invite a sense of letting go or releasing with each exhalation
- Notice a grounding and settling as you release the breath and let go
- Invite a sense of lengthening the exhalation, of releasing energy outward … downward …
- Free the breath, the mind, your emotions … of any gripping or holding on
- Suspend the breath at the bottom of the breath, being with the freedom of having let go
- Invite a sense of eliminating, of releasing and letting go of that which does not serve
- Descend, rejuvenate, and ground your energy
- Let go of the unskillful or unhelpful to make room for the skillful, for the helpful
- Let go of emotional or affective gripping or hanging on
- Release excess arousal, accessing a grounding and settling energy and way of being
- Invite a cleansing downward energy

Ideas to guide cues inward-moving, stabilizing energy (Samana)

Cued as stabilizing and sustaining energy:

- Guide vitality to your core, supporting and nourishing its warmth, its fire
- Feel the stabilizing and warming presence of your breath
- Settle peacefully into the pause at the top of the breath—lingering with the sensation of taking in nurturance
- Can you hold steady as vitality is drawn to the center of your being, from the edges inward to the core
- Tune into the amazing balance between inhalation and exhalation, between taking in and letting go
- Absorb and digest the current moment experience
- Allow yourself the space to integrate and absorb inner and outer sensations and stimuli
- Breathe with peacefulness and patience, receiving what is offered … drawing it inward to your core
- Invite gently pauses and stillness at the top and bottom of the breath
- Sense into the grounding, stable warmth at your navel
- Find your stable presence and groundedness in the peacefulness of each cycle of breath
- Notice warmth of vitality at your core that cleanses and nourishes, that releases blockages and obstacles
- Sense into your perfect temperature for wellbeing, lucidity, and joy
- Sense into the experience of steadiness that can grow from a fiery energy that is patient and peaceful

Ideas to guide cues for outward-moving, coordinating energy (Vyana)

Cued as pulsation, integration, absorption, resonance, and coordination:

- Tune into your deep inner expansiveness and vitality
- Notice vital pulsations spreading outward to the very edges of your being
- Sense inner pulsation … aliveness … all the way to the fingertips via upper arms, elbows, forearms, hands
- Feel an expansive coordinating energy all the way to your toes via thighs, knees, lower legs, feet
- Imagine breathing in and out through the pores of the body … feeling expansive and cohesive …
- Invite your energy to move outward … connecting you to the outer world … to your community … your family…
- Sense a flow from your core to your edges … sending nurturance and vitality through the entirety of your being …
- Feel connected to something greater … sense into your connection with your community … your planet … your web of relationships
- Notice your integration with the world … realize your part/role/responsibility in creating community …
- Rest in the spacious awareness of absorbing what you need where you need it
- Experience the resonance with …
- Absorb the practice—allow it to integrate into your nervous system and your tissues
- Soak in all that you experience and transform experience into wisdom

(continued)

Table 8.6 (continued)

Ideas to guide cues for upward-moving, inspiring energy (Udana)
Cued as ascending and uplifting energy that transforms
- Invite a sensation or breath of uplifting or lightness
- Invite a subtle and silent natural breath with smooth, buttery and light texture
- Move into spaciousness but not spaciness
- Open to inner sensations and understand their reverberations within and around you
- Notice bodily and energetic sensations—pleasant, unpleasant, neutral—accepting what shows up
- Tune into your body … your breath sounds … your heart beat … what do they teach you
- Notice sounds in your surroundings … how do they reverberate within you …
- Observe scents and aromas … what do they stir in you …
- Pay attention to mind—thoughts, judgments, plans, etc. … how can they support your wisdom and decision-making
- Invite your energy and breath to stay light, ascending, inspiring, uplifting
- Cultivate growth and transformation for yourself and your family, community, world …
- Make wise and discerning choices
- Live life from a larger perspective that considers the greater good
- Live with purpose and meaning
- Settle into your compassion, patience, joy, and generosity

8.4.3   Sequencing the Practice

Breath awareness is introduced later in a course of breathing sessions than breath observation, and its point of introduction depends on the client. Some clients may not do as well with breath awareness, being better served by breath observation and resilient, coherent breathing. Breath awareness is a form of inner practice that can be very powerful. For clients who resonate with such an open-ended, intangible practice, breath awareness is safe to suggest for home practice except in unusual circumstances (e.g., extreme symptoms from complex trauma; seizure disorder). Breath awareness, if deemed appropriate for context and client, can be implemented anytime during a breathing, yoga, or mental health-focused session, but especially after either *asana* that has invigorated and moved energy, such as in *kriya* or *vinyasa*, or after nervous system dysregulation due to having had a difficult experience or having touched on an emotional topic. Breath awareness can be useful toward the end of a breathing session to (re)regulate the nervous system; it is also helpful early in a session to hone interoception and neuroception. Breath awareness always progresses from open awareness of breath characteristics, to subtle awareness of vitality in body and mind, and only if appropriate for a given client, to the most subtle vital energies of the *vayus*.

8.4.4   Variations and Intentions of Breath Awareness

As noted earlier, one way to vary observation is by level of subtlety, from tangible to subtle to pranic. Additional variations are available to meet specific physical, emotional, and mental/emotional needs and circumstances. The typical categories of variations are offered (in the context of movement, the polyvagal states, and in daily life). Other possibilities exist and are optimally designed by clinicians for the individual needs of each patient. The following ideas are intended to inspire creativity.

Variations Involving Physical Shapes and Movements

Breath awareness, especially at the tangible and subtle level, can happen in a variety of shapes as well as during movement. Each shape or type of movement provides new opportunities for awareness of the breath and insight about how its reverberations affect body and mind. The same physical and movement variations offered for breath observations apply—always in the specifically tailored context of each patient and the clear intention of the practice. Offering breath awareness practices within movement practices hones skills of interoception and neuroception as patients begin to discern different energies across diverse situations.

Connection Breath as an Example of Breath Awareness During Movement

This movement is accessed either from standing in mountain, or from a comfortable seat without leaning back, with arms resting comfortably at the side of the body. The flow invites inward focus and full awareness of each breath and its specific link to movement that helps underscore the breath phase. The flow consists of three sets of movements, each choreographed with a breath cycle that attends to all four breath phases.

Set 1:

- Inhale naturally while lifting arms out to the side and then up, traveling "around the world"
- Pause naturally, holding arms and body steady
- Exhale, touching the palms together above the head, then drawing joined palms down through the midline to the heart
- Pause naturally, resting palms at heart

Set 2:

- Inhale naturally, moving the arms out to the side at shoulder height
- Pause naturally, holding arms open in a receptive stance
- Exhale, drawing the palms to the heart
- Pause naturally, resting palms at heart

Set 3:

- Inhale naturally, lifting the arm forward and up "reaching for the sky"
- Pause naturally, keeping arms lifted
- Exhale, lowering the arms down to the side "traveling around the world" and then in toward the heart
- Pause naturally, resting palms at heart

Repeat at least twice and as many times as eight (for a set of nine connections breaths)

Variations Based on Nervous System Defaults

Breath awareness, even more so than breath observation, is useful in helping patients identify and gain access to their polyvagal state. It hones not only interoception, but also neuroception (especially at the subtle and pranic levels), and can help create clarity about current levels of arousal and affect, as well as laying the groundwork for insight into how the nervous system may be balanced with breathing practices to access a more ventral vagal space. Breath awareness can be used to help patients identify when they are shifting from ventral vagal social connection into perception of signals of danger or life threat. It connects patients to diffuse bottom-up signals and affective reactivities, enabling them to shift themselves back to a responsive and socially connected state [2]. The capacity to become attuned to inner neuroceptive signals, to employ strategies to deal with these signals and to transform them can help create new neural defaults over time.

Variations That Take Breathwork into Daily Life

The same variations offered for breath observation can be offered for practice of subtle breath awareness. For patients who resonate well with honing and understanding awareness of subtle energies, taking the practice off the mat is worthy of cautious exploration. Tuning into awareness in daily life becomes increasingly appropriate as patients embrace and refine strategies for shifting their neural platform effectively in life and relationships. It is quite likely that such patients move beyond breathwork into *inner work*, either through yogic inner practices, such as concentration and meditation, or psychotherapeutic approaches.

8.5   Where We Go from Here

This chapter emphasized that breath observation and awareness precede other breathing practices to familiarize patients with their breath and its many dimensions and implications. Practices offered in this chapter draw heavily on the psychoeducational (didactic) information presented in the science chapters, especially in Chap. 4. All are preparatory for and part and parcel of practices offered in Chaps. 9 and 10. For most patients, breath rhythms and patterns can become more healthful simply by engaging in breath attunement. Breath attunement practices are intentionally interwoven into almost all other breathing practices. As patients are introduced to practices such as subtle breathing, four-part breathing, or alternate nostril breathing, their learning can be greatly enhanced by invitations to observe and become aware of breath and vitality while shifting to new breathing patterns. As patients discern shifts in their energy when they try out a new way of breathing, this biofeedback from observation and awareness can become a strong motivator to change respiratory habits and patterns.

Now that breath observation and awareness skills have been introduced, it is time to shift patient education and breathwork practice to an emphasis on optimal functional breathing (OFB) in daily life. Breathwork for coherent, slow-paced breathing is offered with an invitation to release stressful exertion by balancing effort and ease. Chapter 9 invites patients to develop new breathing habits that transform the biomechanics, biochemistry, and psychology of their breathing. They are invited to embrace subtle breathing as a transition to more slow-paced breathing in daily life, ultimately moving toward resilient, coherent, and situationally adapted breathing. Chapter 9 encourages a baseline of optimal functional breathing that is nasal, slow, smooth, quiet, rhythmic, and conducive to a ventral vagal nervous system state. Promoting optimal functional breathing during regular daily activity lays the foundation for resilient, adaptable resilient breathing during situations that demand more effort than necessary during a typical day. In that way, practices mentioned in Chap. 9 naturally lead to more specialized and demanding breathing practices offered in Chaps. 10 and 11.

To awaken, sit calmly, letting each breath clear your mind and open your heart.—
The Buddha

References

1. Gerritsen R, Band G. Breath of life: the respiratory vagal stimulation model of contemplative activity. Front Neurosci. 2018;12:1–25. https://doi.org/10.3389/fnhum.2018.00397.
2. Herrero JL, Khuvis S, Yeagle E, Cerf M, Mehta AD. Breathing above the brain stem: volitional control and attentional modulation in humans. J Neurophysiol. 2018;119(1):145–59. https://doi.org/10.1152/jn.00551.2017.
3. Goleman D, Davidson RJ. Altered traits. Avery; 2017.
4. Khalsa GDS, Stauth C, Borysenko J. Meditation as medicine: activate the power of your natural healing force. Simon & Schuster; 2011.
5. Bhanushali D, Tyagi R, Limaye (Rishi Nityapragya) N, Anand A. Effect of mindfulness meditation protocol in subjects with various psychometric characteristics at high altitude. Brain Behav. 2020;10(5):e01604. https://doi.org/10.1002/brb3.1604.
6. Wielgosz J, Schuyler BS, Lutz A, Davidson RJ. Long-term mindfulness training is associated with reliable differences in resting respiration rate. Sci Rep. 2016;6(1):27533. https://doi.org/10.1038/srep27533.
7. Zaccaro A, Piarulli A, Laurino M, et al. How breath-control can change your life: a systematic review on psycho-physiological correlates of slow breathing. Front Hum Neurosci. 2018;12:353. https://doi.org/10.3389/fnhum.2018.00353.
8. Tellhed U, Daukantaitė D, Maddux RE, Svensson T, Melander O. Yogic breathing and mindfulness as stress coping mediate positive health outcomes of yoga. Mindfulness. 2019;10(12):2703–15. https://doi.org/10.1007/s12671-019-01225-4.
9. Schwartz A. Applied polyvagal theory in yoga: therapeutic practices for emotional health. Norton; 2024.
10. Dana D. The polyvagal theory in therapy: engaging the rhythm of regulation. Norton; 2018.
11. Porges S. The pocket guide to the polyvagal theory: the transformative power of feeling safe. Norton; 2017.
12. Porges S. The polyvagal theory: neurophysiological of emotions, attachment, communication, and self-regulation. Norton; 2011.
13. Rossman ML. Guided imagery for self-healing. 2nd ed. New World Library; 2000. http://www.books24x7.com/marc.asp?bookid=12914
14. Devi NJ. Secret power of yoga. Harmony/Rodale; 2022.
15. Sterios P. Gravity and grace. Sounds True; 2019.
16. Rosen R. The yoga of breath: a step-by-step guide to pranayama. Shambala; 2002.
17. Rothenberg R. Restoring prana: a therapeutic guide to pranayama and healing through the breath for yoga therapists, teachers, and healthcare practitioners. Singing Dragon; 2020.

Breathwork for Optimal Breathing

9

*A recognized fact which goes back to the earliest times
is that every living organism is not the sum of a multitude of
unitary processes but is –
byvirtueofinterrelationshipsandofhigherandlowerlevelsofcontrol–
an unbroken unity.*

Walter Hess, Nobel Prize Winner for Work on the Brain, 1949

9.1 Overview: Breathing Optimally Through Creating Subtlety

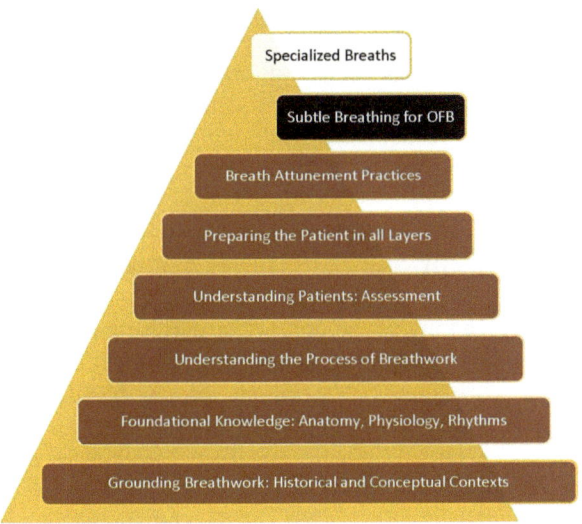

Almost as soon as breath observation and awareness skills have been introduced, it is helpful to provide education about optimal functional breathing (OFB) in daily life. In fact, the two practices (attunement and OFB) go hand in hand. Breathwork to foster coherent, slow-paced breathing is offered with an invitation to release stressful exertion by balancing effort and ease. Over-efforting during breathwork can lead to injury, including damage to the heart muscle. Underefforting may not lead to the full benefits of an energetically tailored practice. From that perspective, some *pranayama* and Western breathing practices are not consistent with optimal functional breathing. They are best used with intention to facilitate a particular interoceptive, neuroceptive, or other somatic or emotional experiences. For example, they may be used deliberately as a form of stress inoculation (or hormesis) or high-intensity interval training for the breath—stressing body and nervous system, only to recalibrate them consciously to foster resilience in preparation for meeting real-life stressors and demands. They may be appropriately accessed for particular life circumstances, to help breathing remain coherent and resilient as suitable for context and need. Many clients present with chronic heavy or overbreathing— sometimes inadvertently because of modern life's biases toward hyperventilation, erratic breathing, gasping, and grasping; other times, because they misunderstand the biochemistry and biomechanics of breath, perpetuating personal breathing habits and patterns.

This chapter offers a four-pronged process toward helping patients develop breathing patterns that support them most helpfully during regular daily activities and life situations. It emphasizes subtle breathing practices that slowly but surely help shift the biomechanics, biochemistry, and psychology of the breath. Cuing suggestions and sample scripts bust many myths about how to teach breathing and how to invite natural breathing. Language is shifted toward slow-paced and light breathing with a rhythmic cadence, smooth texture, and no sound. These concepts about natural breathing are often misunderstood, especially in the context of yoga. This chapter hopes to create insight into the need to help patients access a breathing cadence that optimizes biochemistry while supporting a calm and socially connected state of the nervous system.

9.2   Cultivating Optimal Functional Breathing

Optimal functional breathing in the context of daily life supports a ventral vagal state and is nasal, diaphragmatic, slow, subtle, and rhythmic (see Table 9.1 for a summary). It reflects a rhythmic, peaceful, and easeful breath that calms and heals when we are stressed; that vitalizes and nourishes when we are tired; and that promotes resilience and balance. Coherent, resilient breathing is linked to the autonomic nervous system via important somatosensory feedback from the entire body. As noted previously, inhalation is linked to the sympathetic nervous system, as is the right nostril [1, 2]. Exhalation is linked to the parasympathetic nervous system, as is the left nostril [3, 4]. If we understand these basic concepts, we realize that emphasis can change the seemingly same breath in radically different ways.

Table 9.1 Optimal functional breathing is defined by the following traits[a]

- *Nasal*: Silent breathing in and out through the nose at all times (including at night and during exertion; mouth breathing in emergencies only)
- *Biasing the diaphragm*: When breathing is diaphragmatic, movements are notable primarily in the abdomen and low rib basket; upper chest, shoulder, and neck muscles stay relaxed and passive (unless purposefully or intentionally contracted)
- *Slow*: 5.5–10 breaths per minute
- *Light, silent, and subtle*: Inhalation is neither shallow nor forced—tailored to move just the right amount of air given the circumstances, leading to a normal volume of 5–6 L of breath per minute; exhalation is easeful and quiet
- *Rhythmic*: Breath oscillates with a soft texture and rhythm that is neither rigid nor too relaxed—reflecting a balance of ease and effort; resting pauses at the top and bottom of breath may be notable but their length is natural not forced; there is no gasping or grasping

[a]See Chap. 4 for a complete review

Attention and deliberate focus on inhalations may deliberately or inadvertently stimulate and activate; focus on exhalations may deliberately or inadvertently create a sense of slowing and calming. Given our propensity to overbreathe, for most humans, it is more helpful to favor slow, light breathing over fast or deep (i.e., voluminous) breathing, in daily life, during rest and sleep, and even during light to moderate exercise.

Virtually all patients, clients, or students benefit from being exposed to the concepts and practice of optimal functional breathing. It is a universally helpful way to breathe and a cornerstone in health and well-being. There are few if any contraindications to teaching patients strategies that invite them to achieve optimal functional breathing. Assessment results are necessary, however, to understand how best to broach OFB with individual patients, to ensure that they are invited into the practice in a manner that is based on their current state of breathing. As shown in Table 6.9, patients who are chronically overbreathing, with an extremely low controlled breath pause, breathing through the mouth and into the chest, and medullas that are hypersensitive to CO_2, need to be exposed to the preliminary practices that teach OFB gradually and with clear intention and guidance.

9.2.1   Steps in Teaching Optimal Functional Breathing

Anatomy, physiology, psychology, and rhythms of healthful breathing, covered in Chaps. 2, 3, and 4, are woven together to teach clients resilient and coherent breathing patterns. Interweaving and applying breath science to teach clients optimal breathing can be approached as a multipronged process. Much education occurs across the various foci, and clinicians are encouraged to provide patients with as much verbal and written information as they can handle. Titrating information is as important as titrating the dosage of medications or breathing practices. The four prongs of the approach to cultivating OFB are summarized further for guidance; breath attunement has already started this journey. The prongs reflect the primary change mechanics that have been addressed throughout this book thus far. Specifically, they address:

- *Psychology and nervous system defaults*, refining neuroception, interoception, proprioception, and exteroception, as well as facilitating psychoeducation, motivation, and bottom-up, top-down self-regulation by enhancing the vagal brake and reducing either sympathetic or dorsal reactivity;
- *Biomechanics*, integrating attention to nasal and diaphragmatic breathing, postural alignment, tongue placement, and breath qualities related to location, texture, and sound;
- *Biochemistry*, integrating subtle breathing and breath qualities related to rate and volume, as well as breath phases; and
- *Generalization into daily life,* encouraging the practice to be applied as life unfolds with all its challenges, stressors, and tasks.

Breathwork typically unfolds in the order in which the prongs are presented, starting with making patients comfortable and safe, and moving onward from there. As the prongs are introduced to the patient, they build on and augment each other; they become interwoven and interdependent. Once introduced, safety and comfort, biomechanics, biochemistry, and generalization are never abandoned; they become a way of practice and a way of life.

Prong One: Addressing Awareness, Polyvagal Defaults, and Self-Regulation

This prong must be mentioned despite being amply explored in prior chapters. It is concerned with creating a context of safety, co-regulation, social connection, and personal transformation. Clinicians work with great care to accommodate the autonomic nervous system of each patient with patience, compassion, and insight. Through assessment, they identified clients' neural defaults (for sympathetic arousal, dorsal collapse, or ventral vagal connection). They now unfold the breathing practice in this context, offering an environment, relationship, and practice sequencing that is molded to the types of affective, vital, mental, and emotional reactivities and responses most likely for a given individual. The practices in this prong are as follows:

- Creating a safe environment and supportive compassionate relationship between clinician and client (Chap. 5)
- Providing support, information, and compassion to the patient as assessment leads to a greater understanding of symptoms, etiologies, prognosis and goal-setting, and specific intervention choices (Chaps. 5 and 6)
- Careful preparation that helps support social connection, a positive clinician-client relationship, the capacity to stay regulated and calm, and practices that facilitate relaxation and recovery at the beginning, middle, and end of a breathwork session (Chap. 7)
- Self-observation and increasing self-awareness of patterns and impacts of breathing via attunement practices (Chap. 8)
- Adapting breathwork to polyvagal state, inviting activation when energy is flagging, inviting calming when energy is excessive, taking in nourishment when

energy is depleted, and seeking resilience and moderation in all practices and life circumstances (variations sections in this chapter and Chap. 10)

Once a clinician assesses that a positive relationship with the client has been established, that the patient understands the intention and goals of breathwork, that the client can (co-)regulate body, vitality, and mind through calming practices and the relationship with the clinician, specific breathwork can begin. The next step in the process is to move into practices that begin to alter extant breathing patterns, challenging patients to begin to embrace respiratory behavior changes that can be as profound as they may be difficult. For most clients, this journey begins with the biomechanics of breath.

Prong Two: Addressing Breath Biomechanics

As clients have come to understand their breath from observation and awareness, they are ready to explore how breath and biomechanics interact to create diaphragmatic breathing. This focus supports nasal breathing over mouth breathing and invites patients to let go of unnecessary chest breathing by emphasizing and (re-) training physical expressions of the breath in the mid-torso, abdomen, and low side ribs. The physical practices offered in Chap. 7 can now be brought to bear, as some clients need to learn new physical patterns and need to prepare for this shift via guided physical movements that train core and pelvic floor engagement, as well as rib basket resilience.

Nasal Breathing

Biomechanically, nasal breathing is introduced as essential to health before teaching diaphragmatic breathing. Nasal breathing in and of itself can support diaphragmatic breathing and hence is a preliminary practice for diaphragmatic breathing. Clients are invited to embrace the strategies offered in Chap. 7 for clearing the nose and training the tongue. They can be offered information about the positive impacts of nasal versus mouth breathing (perhaps by sharing the summary offered in Chap. 2) during all waking and sleeping hours. Breath observation and awareness are key to helping patients shift from oral to nasal breathing and from chest or reverse breathing to diaphragmatic breathing.

Central strategies for nasal breathing have already been addressed and are summarized here, with references to relevant prior chapters where more information can be reviewed as needed. Nasal breathing is promoted via all of the following practices:

- Providing psychoeducation about the advantages of nasal breathing over oral breathing (Chaps. 2, 3, and 4)
- Developing motivation for nasal breathing (Chap. 6)
- Identifying the most accessible nasal clearing practices (e.g., neti pot, movement with nostrils closed, mouth taping during the day and/or at night) (Chap. 7, especially Table 7.15)

- Creating attunement to oral versus nasal breathing via breath observation and awareness, with focus on location, texture, and sound related to the breath's journey through the nose and airways (Chap. 8)
- Using subtle breathing practices (addressed below)
- Encouraging nasal breathing during exertion via exercise and in daily life (e.g., nasal breathing while walking, one of the subtle breathing practices; see further and Chap. 10)

Diaphragmatic Breathing

As nasal breathing takes hold, many patients begin to shift toward diaphragmatic breathing very naturally (this may be notable by a longer controlled breath pause—an indicator when a client is ready to shift from an exclusive focus on nasal breathing to integrating diaphragmatic breathing; see Table 6.9). As diaphragmatic breathing takes hold, patients often experience naturally enhanced posture and movement dynamics [5]. They begin to shift biomechanical patterns beyond the breath, which is not surprising given the profound connection of the diaphragm to core and pelvic floor muscles and its profound relationship with the psoas complex during walking and moving. A shift to diaphragmatic breathing can result in profound reverberations into the chest and shoulders, reducing back and neck pain [6]. As patients begin to move beyond noticing (via attunement practices offered in Chap. 8) to altering the breath, they often experience profound shifts in their nervous systems as well—simply because of the reverberations of anatomical and biomechanical changes into all layers of experience [7].

In many contexts, including yoga and meditation, cuing or talking about the breath revolves around the up and down movement of the diaphragm. Unfortunately, the way in which many clients hear this description is as strictly chest and belly movement. This misperception is reinforced by frequent focus on feeling the belly rise and fall with the inhalation and exhalation and on instructions to breathe like a baby (something we now know from Chap. 2 is not really possible for adults). Although none of this is (entirely) incorrect, it is incomplete. The movement of the diaphragm and related structures (via muscular attachment points, connective tissue, and fascia) is not just up and down, but also in and out to the sides. The movement of the low ribs and resilience in the rib baskets, when optimal, are upward and outward with the inhalation and downward and inward with the exhalation. The abdomen does not simply rise and fall with the breath; it also travels outward and inward to both sides of the waist, even at the back body, as breath comes and goes.

It is helpful to cue and talk about all of these directions—up and down, in and out, front and back—movement that can be perceived in the body in 360°. The upward and downward movements are as, if not more, important as the rising and falling of the belly and greatly contribute to breath health. We do not want a heaving chest; we want a resilient rib basket. We want resilient movement in the side body, the capacity to allow the diaphragm's motion to distribute throughout the entire mid-section of the body.

Experiencing the Movements of Diaphragmatic Breathing
Experiencing the combination of movements can be helpful to understanding diaphragmatic breath:

- Sit in a comfortable position
- Wrap the thumb and index fingers around the low waist (just above the hip bones), with fingers pointing forward and palms parallel to the floor
- Breathe in and notice—the hands likely are being pushed outward to the both sides by the inhalation
- Breathe out and notice—the hands release inward toward the center as the exhalation travels out
- Place the hands on the back body (wherever you can reach—notice the reverberation of breath as movement even in the back portion of the torso

Many strategies for supporting diaphragmatic breathing have already been described and are summarized here, with references to relevant prior chapters where more information can be accessed as needed. In using these practices, it is important to understand that the diaphragm needs to be able to release as well as contract. Contraction invites inhalation; release supports exhalation. Both aspects of diaphragmatic functioning are addressed by the summarized practices. Clinicians choose specific physical strategies based on whether they observe excessive bracing or too much laxity or collapse in the client's body, energy, or even emotions.

Diaphragmatic breathing is developed via all of the following practices:

- Encouraging nasal breathing in a variety of ways (see previous text)
- Providing psychoeducation about the advantages of diaphragmatic breathing over chest breathing (Chaps. 2, 3, and 4)
- Developing motivation for diaphragmatic breathing (Chap. 6)
- Identifying the most needed physical practices for training the diaphragm (Chap. 7, ranging from postural alignment, to spinal mobilization, neck and shoulder releases, rib basket resilience practices, heart openers, to core stabilizing practices—adapted to patient needs based on physical assessment findings)
- Focusing physical practices on release *and* strength, first emphasizing and teaching the missing component, attending to excessive laxity or excessive bracing and cuing movement accordingly (Chaps. 6 and 7)
- Creating attunement to diaphragmatic versus chest breathing via breath observation and awareness, with significant focus on location and space related to notable movement in the torso (Chap. 8, especially Table 8.2 which provides specific exercises to reduce chest and reverse breathing)
- Using subtle breathing practices (addressed below)
- Breath with strong movement practices that create diaphragmatic strength (this chapter and Chap. 10)
- Encouraging diaphragmatic breathing during exertion via exercise and in daily life

Addressing Breath Texture and Sound

Focus on nasal breathing is a logical segue into exploring textures and sounds of breath to create change (unlike in observation, where no change is cued). Attunement to and alteration are part of this process, proceeding from texture to sound. Unlabored, stable, fluid, and relaxed textures are invited and may naturally result in quieter, even soundless breathing. Patients are invited to cultivate smoothly textured and silent breathing, emphasizing avoidance of habitual sighing, frequent yawning, and *deep* breaths (one "deep" breath can keep a human being hyperventilating for 10 min). Information can be offered about noticing habitual patterns in the breath, as psychoeducation helps clients understand that a natural breath is a breath without sound and with an easeful, buttery texture. During breathing sessions, clinicians take the role of monitor and coach, giving feedback when patients' breath dysregulates, becomes choppy or labored, noisy or wheezy, or otherwise reflects compromised nervous system states. Over time, clients learn to identify their tendencies and begin to take smooth and silent breathing into daily life, internalizing the monitoring and correcting functions.

Texture and sound are excellent biofeedback mechanisms that are easily noticeable to patients once they are aware of them and understand the importance of altering habits and patterns. As patients learn to quiet and smooth out their breath, their emotions and well-being are altered as well. The profound reciprocity between breath textures and sounds and nervous system states helps shift patients' self-perceptions and perceptions of stress. Working with texture and sound is a great bridge to work on biochemistry. To make texture smooth and sound subtle, the breath must become subtle. This moves us to the work with Prong Three.

Prong Three: Addressing Breath Biochemistry

The third prong reshapes breathing habits toward subtle and phase-related breathing, drawing attention to refining respiratory biochemistry. Often, as breath biomechanics and texture are altered, biochemistry naturally begins to reset [8]. However, for most patients, deliberate attention to subtle breathing is beneficial (including some phase-related breathing practices), first in collaboration with the clinician and ultimately in daily life. Controlled breath pause assessment and reassessment (see Chap. 6) are an important part of this prong and supply quick information about breath biochemistry in session and in life. Subtle breathing, including breathing related to breath phases, is the focus of the remainder of this chapter once the four prongs have been summarized. Tables 6.8 and 6.9 can guide choices of subtle breathing practices, although it is important to use controlled breath pause measurement with caution, as some clients can become obsessed with measuring their scores, rather than open-heartedly embracing a new way of breathing.

Deliberate changes to breath rate and volume are central practices that reset breath biochemistry. It is vital to start subtle breathing practices *in session* (rather than as homework) to observe how clients respond to these practices autonomically, affectively, and emotionally. Patients with conditions that directly affect breathing (e.g., anxiety, panic, asthma, and other breathing disorders) especially need the support of careful monitoring and co-regulation. Resetting biochemistry can be uncomfortable as it involves the creation of air hunger by reducing breath rate and volume.

Psychoeducation about subtle breathing can be helpful, as knowledge is motivating and helps clients persevere. The bulk of this chapter is dedicated to teaching subtle breathing. There are many variations and options, creating access for most patients. It may be necessary to explore which subtle breathing practices work most effectively with each individual client, rather than using all practices indiscriminately with all patients. This process requires some trial and error, and careful collaboration and co-regulation with the client, as ideal subtle practices are identified.

Once subtle breathing becomes easier and slow-paced breathing becomes accessible without nervous system dysregulation (i.e., as the length of the controlled breath pauses increases), resilient breathing is integrated by adding practices that include attention to four-part breathing, alternate nostril breathing, breathing with force and sound, and similar more demanding types of breathing (covered in Chaps. 10 and 11).

Prong Four: Integrating Optimal Breathing into Daily Life

The final prong for teaching resilient breathing involves taking the offered teachings into daily life. Patients are encouraged to recognize signs and symptoms of disordered breathing and to check their controlled breath pause regularly but not obsessively in their home and work environments. They can use all the practices of self-assessment that they learned in session, including measuring breaths per minute, control pauses, proper biomechanics (diaphragm, nose, posture), optimal biochemistry (e.g., reduced, soundless breathing; short breath holds), and capacity to shift breath rhythms resiliently based on circumstances. They can begin to apply subtle and slow-paced breathing during a variety of life circumstances, at work, in relationships, during easeful states, and during challenging times. They can be invited to use optimal functional and light breathing during light to moderate exercise, often transforming their endurance and conditioning.

The entire thrust of helping patients access subtle breathing to transform their biochemistry and biomechanics of breath is to bring these skills into daily life. Breathwork is not about changing the breach while being in the office with a breathing coach. It is about accessing healthful and adaptive breathing everywhere and under most circumstances. This breath is strongly linked to a ventral vagal state and facilitates a state of calm and social connection. It has the power to shift patients' experiences in their body, vitality, thoughts and emotions, relationships and social contact, and even in their athletic endeavors. If clients who have mastered OFB in daily life want to learn how to apply subtle and optimal breathing to athletic performance, they can be referred to extant excellent resources [9].

9.3 Cultivating Optimal Functional Breathing via Subtle Breathing Practices

Specialized breathwork that is not offered on a foundation of optimal daily breathing may not achieve its goals as effectively and successfully as breathwork that begins with and always returns to soft, slow, rhythmic, subtle, nasal, and diaphragmatic breathing that optimizes the anatomy, physiology, and psychology of the breath. Since breath dysregulation is commonly associated with a tendency to hyperventilate given stressful and demanding lifestyles, the art of subtle (reduced or slow-paced) breathing is key to promoting OFB. Subtle breathing emphasizes nasal and diaphragmatic breathing. It increases breath efficiency, reducing either volume or rate without affecting the other; in effect, it reduces the amount of air breathed in any given time period [10]. It alters extant breathing rhythms to make them soft, smooth, silent, and light. Subtle breathing invites a sense of ease and helps reveal reactivity, over-efforting, or emerging symptoms of panic or breath dysregulation.

Subtle breathing employs various strategies, introduced further in *Forms of Subtle Breathing*, for making breath slower, lighter, silent, smooth, and/or directed low into the abdomen. Most strategies involve combinations of several of these qualities, cutting across biomechanics, biochemistry, and psychological and nervous system factors. To recap, breathing lightly and quietly invites a gradual increase in CO_2 in the blood and moves the individual toward tolerable air hunger, which over time adjusts chemosensitivity of the medulla [8]. It also increases the amount of nitric oxide in the nasal cavity and airways, resulting in increased breath efficiency. Breathing low into the abdomen, allowing breathing to occur via the diaphragm, over time supports healthier biomechanics, supporting core stability, posture, and other functional movements while also supporting enhanced gas exchange due to better perfusion. Breathing slowly and smoothly is calming for the nervous system, supporting a ventral vagal state that allows for supportive co-regulation and connection. Of course, it also has positive effects on respiratory biochemistry. Finally, subtle breathing likely will cause a temporary drop in oxygen saturation in the blood. This is due to the fact that it increases carbon dioxide in the blood, which in turn allows hemoglobin to release oxygen into the tissues (via the Bohr effect). This temporary decrease in oxygen saturation has similar benefits to training at high altitudes and can enhance breath (and athletic) performance.

9.3.1 Special Notes and Cautions About Subtle Breathing Practices

Some risks can emerge with subtle breathing that require vigilance on the part of the clinician. Ideally, clients have been cleared by their medical provider if they have conditions that may represent a contraindication for these practices, including (but not necessarily limited to) pregnancy, respiratory conditions (such as asthma, COPD, respiratory infection), cardiovascular conditions (such as hypertension, arrhythmias), or psychological conditions (such as PTSD, panic disorder, anxiety disorders). A history of fainting suggests caution, as this can be a risk of subtle breathing with clients who are susceptible to loss of consciousness (e.g., patients with dorsal vagal neural defaults).

The general rule of thumb for subtle (and many other) breathing exercises is to start slowly, gradually increase intensity, and pay close attention to clients' physical, vital (arousal and affective), mental, and emotional responses as the practice

Table 9.2   Signals of breath dysregulation during subtle breathing

- Constricting or contracting stomach muscles
- Straining neck muscles
- Forced breathing
- Involuntary contraction (spasm) of the diaphragm
- Chest breathing, especially paradoxical or reverse breathing
- Tensing, spasms, twitches, or other signs of increasing tension in any part of the body
- Obvious discomfort that the client seems to ignore or fail to notice (often because they are very used to discomfort related to their breathing—a lack of sensitivity they need to relearn)

unfolds. Subtle breathing may initially aggravate hyperventilation, increase anxiety or induce panic, and cause dizziness or tingling. Clinicians keenly observe their patients during subtle breathing and are vigilant for signals that the breath is dysregulating, so that clients can be directed to return to natural breathing as appropriate. It is helpful to teach clients how to watch for these signals themselves, as their recognition is vital to safe home practice. As soon as certain signals appear (see Table 9.2), subtle breathing is gently discontinued (taking care not to create panic or sense of vulnerability), and natural breathing is invited. A break from the practice is indicated until tension dissipates and clinician and client feel co-regulated; then return to the practice can be explored.

It is important to use caution when teaching subtle breathing to individuals with known diagnoses of anxiety, panic, PTSD, or asthma so as not to disrupt their breathing or cause emotional dysregulation [11, 12]. These individuals will most likely greatly benefit from these practices in the long term; we simply need to use caution and be careful not to suggest home practice of subtle breathing prematurely. Thus, with such individuals, subtle breathing techniques are (at least initially) best used only in closely monitored (ideally one-on-one) sessions. Embedding practices in a context of relaxation and relational support is crucial and means starting breathwork once the patient has accessed a sattvic or ventral vagal nervous system state. It is best to stay connected to the client, check in regularly about the effects of the practice, ensure that no significant symptoms emerge, and ensure that the student does not begin to hyperventilate. For patients who are mouth breathers, nasal breathing in and of itself already feels like subtle breathing in the beginning. With these clients, it is best to stick with relaxation and nasal breathing for several sessions. The more demanding subtle breathing practices offered here can be titrated in as appropriate.

How quickly this prong can be taken outside of the office and into daily life will depend on the patient. Once clients begin to breathe in a way that resets their biochemistry, especially on their own, it is important to track their progress and have regular check-ins. One issue to monitor is whether students develop detoxification symptoms (see Table 9.3). If present, such symptoms may worsen for a while but then improvement will follow quickly [13]. According to Ayurvedic medicine, detoxification symptoms can be alleviated by drinking one glass daily of warm water with a ½ tsp of natural sea salt.

Table 9.3 Possible acute
detoxification symptoms
to monitor

- Insomnia
- Feeling as though having a head cold
- Loss of appetite
- Runny nose
- Increased frequency of urination
- Slight headache
- Emotional upset

9.3.2   Instructions and Cuing Tips for All Subtle Breathing Practices

This book offers many summary tables; clinicians are welcome to share these resources with clients. The YouTube playlist offered in the Preface is another resource for the multipart process of reshaping breathing. All sessions support OFB; the first five sessions are dedicated explicitly to subtle breathing and may be a helpful resource for patient homework. Subtle breathing practices are best initiated once a state of ease, even relaxation, is present in body, vitality, mind, and emotions. Centering practices that invite attunement to all *kosha*s, the present moment, and current space are useful preambles. Softness, ease, and release in body, breath, and mind are key. It is helpful to cue relaxation repeatedly throughout subtle breathing practices.

General Principles

Subtle breathing practices are nasal and diaphragmatic and follow the biomechanics outlined in Prong Two. Subtle breathing creates air hunger in the attempt to recalibrate the medulla's sensitivity to CO_2. Air hunger is a sense of urgency to breathe that is maintained until an inhalation is needed to prevent breath dysregulation, distress, or tensing of the musculature. Subtle breathing, despite its intention to create air hunger, is gentle, soft (to modulate tidal volume), and light (to modulate respiratory rate). It is quiet and silent, with a smooth texture and easy flow; it is nasal and diaphragmatic. Cues or reminders to that effect can be repeated often. In using subtle breathing practices, it is helpful to engage the student in several rounds of subtle breathing with resting periods in between that invite breath recovery and relaxation. Each round of subtle breathing can last for up to (although typically no longer than) 4 min; it is recommended to work up gently to that length of time. If the practice is too long for a given patient, it will move them into a sympathetic, rather than a parasympathetic, state. Ongoing monitoring for symptoms of dysregulation, tension, or stress is indicated and necessary to help adapt the practice to patient needs.

Let us start this section with *what not to do*. It is best to avoid cuing for a particular lower breath rate, as this often results in increased breath volume and does not actually alter biochemistry. Instead, the cues that will be offered below create subtle breathing without naming breath rate explicitly. Similarly, it is best to avoid prede-termined breath counts early in sequencing. Over time, as clients are more facile with subtle breathing, practices such as box breathing may become feasible. It is best to avoid asking students to inhale, exhale, or hold for a particular period of time. A natural evolution into a slower breath cycle, less volume, and increased pauses is preferable to externally imposed rhythms.

Subtle breathing practices can be cued in a variety of ways and can be easily adapted as the client is observed to shift focus in a more appropriate and useful way. Cuing can be extremely powerful if it integrates education—explaining why certain cues are offered and what patients can attend to. Following are categories of cues that support the teaching of subtle breathing, namely biomechanical cues, biochem-ical cues, and cues related to breath rhythm and characteristics. For each of the three categories, the first two sets of cues can be used freely; the third set of cues is best avoided unless there is a specific intention (e.g., to demonstrate what not to do; to use a breath of hormesis).

Biomechanical Cuing

Table 9.4 provides useful hints for clinicians to guide clients toward optimal breath-ing from a biomechanical perspective. These are suggestions about phrasing the biomechanics of breath, especially as taught in healthcare settings. The ideas are not meant to be all-inclusive; this would be an impossible endeavor. Positive cues are followed by examples of how not to cue breath biomechanics. These imprecise cuing examples are included because they are often heard in yoga classes despite their inaccuracy and lack of clear utility.

Table 9.4 Helpful and unhelpful biomechanical cues

Helpful nasal breathing cues—Use freely
The invitation is to breathe exclusively through the nose
- Can you invite the breath to flow in and out of the nose only?
- How does it feel to breathe only through the nose?
- How does the breath want to flow naturally—through the nose or the mouth? Can you invite only nasal breathing?
- What happens if you only breathe through the nose? How does your mind react? What emotions emerge?
- Nasal breathing has many important advantages that oral breathing cannot offer:
  - Filters the air of particulates via cilia
  - Moistens and warms the air on the way
  - Cleanses the air of toxins via cilia, mucus, and nitric oxide
  - Pressurizes the air and slows it down
  - Releases nitric oxide
  - Over time it is decongesting
- Breathing through the nose activates the diaphragm

(continued)

Table 9.4 (continued)

Helpful diaphragmatic breathing cues—Use freely
The invitation is to breathe diaphragmatically rather than breathing into the chest
- Can you invite more movement into the lower part of the torso and less into the chest?
- How can you support belly breathing?
- Can you feel the low rib basket expand in 360°?
- Notice if the abdomen not only rises and falls, but also expands out laterally
- Can feel the breath in your back body?
- Notice where in the body you can feel the movement of the breath
- Notice how posture affects where you feel the breath in the body
- Notice the low ribs—are they drawing inward and downward on the exhalation?
- Notice the low ribs—are they moving outward and upward—like a bucket handle—on the inhalation?
- Notice the amount of effort/engagement in your belly/abdominal muscles as you breathe in/out
- Notice the amount of effort/engagement in your upper chest/neck muscles as you breathe in/out
- Can you keep movement of the upper chest and neck to a minimum?
- Can you keep the upper chest, clavicles, and neck still as you breathe in and out?
- Does it feel okay to place one hand on the lower abdomen and one hand on the chest to minimize movement under the hand on the chest, while the hand on the lower abdomen rides with the wave of the breath?
- Chest breathing is a like a piston forcefully moving up and down, exerting excessive force on your heart
- Diaphragmatic/abdominal breathing is like a graceful jelly fish that is pulsing its way gently through the water—there is only pulsation, not force
- Can you place the hands to the sides of the low rib basket to notice the pulsation outward and upward?

Unhelpful biomechanical cues—Avoid unless there is clear intention or purpose
- Bring as much air into your lungs as you can
- Clear all the air out of the lungs
- Breathe out all of your air
- Release the breath completely
- Empty your lungs completely
- Breathe your heart wide open
- Move the inhalation from the belly to the chest, all the way to the clavicles
- Open the chest with the breath
- Breathe the air all the way to the top of the rib basket
- Fill your chest/lungs completely
- Inflate your lungs like a balloon
- Inflate the belly as you breathe in .... Draw the belly in strongly/forcefully as you breathe out ...
- Feel the breath only/mostly/deeply in the rising and falling of the navel
- Engage your core strongly to support the exhalation (this is only necessary during strong exertion but not during rest or light-moderate exercise)

Before moving on to explore biochemically advantageous cues, a brief side note is offered about abdominal versus diaphragmatic breathing. Abdominal breathing can seem like diaphragmatic breathing (in that the chest does not move), but it lacks the muscle tone and contraction of the pelvic floor and abdominal muscles (especially the transverse abdominis and inner and outer obliques). Therefore, abdominal breathing does not create as much intra-abdominal pressure, is less stabilizing, and has fewer respiratory and functional benefits. Its value arises from its relaxing and refreshing nature during deep supine relaxation.

Biochemical Cuing

Table 9.5 provides useful hints for clinicians to guide clients toward optimal breathing from a biochemical perspective. These suggestions about phrasing the biochemistry of breath, especially as taught in healthcare settings, are not all-inclusive. Many more possibilities exist. Positive cues are followed by a few examples of how not to cue breath biochemistry. These misguided cuing examples are included because they are often heard in yoga classes despite their inaccuracy and lack of clear utility.

Table 9.5 Helpful and unhelpful biochemical cues

Helpful light breathing cues—Use freely

The invitation is for light breathing, softened breathing, reduced breathing, or use similar such invitations, emphasizing words such as subtle, gentle, easy, silent, quiet, soft…

- Is it possible to make the breath more subtle? To move less volume?
- Can you gently invite the breath to soften/to be very light/to be quiet/to be peaceful/to be easeful?
- Can you invite a sense of ease as you breathe out?
- What happens of you invite a gentle and light flow of air in and out?
- Can you breathe so softly that the hairs in your nose don't move?
- Can you allow the breath to be soft and gentle—compassionate and kind?
- Is it possible to invite a breath so soft that it is barely perceptible?
- Can the exhalation become a tiny bit longer?
- Can the inhalation with minimal, the exhalation relaxed?
- Can you release any sense of efforting or striving in the breath?
- I invite you breathe in only what you need … and then a little bit less than that …
- Invite yourself to breathe with ease
- How can you create a breath that is easeful … relaxed … quiet … silent … light …?
- Can you invite a breath so light or subtle that it results in a mild air hunger?
- Invite a subtle breath—a breath that is hardly noticeable … hardly audible …
- Quieter … calmer … softer … gentler … easier …. Subtler …. More delicate…

Helpful CO_2-related cues—Use freely

The invitation is to add CO_2-regulating efforts if this type of language seems appropriate for the patients' interest and ability level

- CO_2 is needed in optimal amounts in the blood for oxygen to be absorbed into the tissues
- Optimal levels of CO_2 open our airways and reduce chest tightness
- CO_2 in optimal levels increases circulation and warmth, especially in the hands and feet
- It is less important to bring a lot of air into the lungs than it is to create the right conditions for oxygen to be released into your tissues—this requires the presence of CO_2 in the blood
- It is the level of CO_2—not the level of O_2—that triggers the medulla to initiate a new breath
- The right amount of CO_2 stimulates the vagus nerve and shifts us into a parasympathetic state
- We are a culture of overbreathers—natural breathing that creates mild breath hunger can reset the sensitivity of the medulla to become more tolerant of CO_2
- Natural breathing allows us to create ideal sensitivity to CO_2 levels
- Air hunger is a sign that CO_2 is increasing in the blood
- Breathe so softly, lightly, and subtly that you have a sense of mild air hunger—just as we wait to feel hungry before we eat again

(continued)

Table 9.5 (continued)

Helpful air hunger and other cues—Use freely

Gentle cuing can be added about the possibility of a sense of air hunger—of not getting quite enough air—often along with an urge to return to the natural breath. Students are encouraged to stay with this sense of air hunger as long as possible and yet *not so long* as to create tension, panic, unease, or breath dysregulation. (Adjust the length of time for which subtle breathing is used, recognizing that air hunger without tension may take some time to learn.)

- Can you breathe so lightly that the breath feels subtle and that there may be a sense of hunger for more air before you allow the next inhalation to travel in?
- Can you breathe so slowly that a sense of air hunger is notable just before you inhale again?
- Can you notice some of the cues that your biochemistry is shifting? Maybe there is a sense of:
  - Increased production of saliva
  - Warmer hands and/or feet
  - A pink glow in the face
  - The nose draining
  - Profound calmness or ease
  - Greater alertness

Unhelpful biochemical cues—Avoid unless there is clear intention or purpose

- Take a big cleansing breath out/exhalation
- Breathe so that O_2 can replace/displace CO_2 in the blood
- Take a deep/big/complete breath in/inhalation
- Rid your blood of CO_2/toxins/toxic chemicals/toxic CO_2
- Breathe out all of your carbon dioxide/air
- Breathe out forcefully/as forcefully as you can
- Breathe rapidly in and out and then hold for at least XXX seconds
- Notice your breath expanding the chest all the way to the collar bones

Cuing of Breath Rhythms, Texture, and Sound

Table 9.6 provides useful hints for clinicians to guide clients toward optimal breath rhythm and characteristics. These are suggestions about phrasing rhythmic, textural, sound-related, and spatial or location characteristics of breath, especially for healthcare settings. Positive cues are followed by a few examples of how not to cue breath rhythms. These misleading cuing examples are included because they are often heard in yoga classes despite their inaccuracy and lack of clear utility.

Table 9.6 Examples of helpful and unhelpful texture and sound cues

Helpful sound-related cues—Use freely
- Can you invite your breath to become completely quiet?
- Can you quiet the breath so much that not even you can hear it?
- Can you breathe in such a way that I/the person next to you can no longer hear it?
- Can you tell what is happening that creates the noise in your breathing?
- How can you invite your breath to become a little more silent/less audible/less obvious?
- Do you notice any sighing in the breath? While sighing can feel cleansing or calming in a moment of stress, as a *habit* or used long-term, it can lead to hyperventilation and loses its calming effect

Helpful texture-related cues—Use freely
- Can you invite the breath to become smooth and gentle?
- If the breath is choppy, with little hitches and glitches, what can change to make it less so?
- How can you even out the texture of the breath? Perhaps it can slow down? Perhaps it can become quieter/less labored/less effortful?
- Can you tell what is happening that is disrupting the buttery and easeful flow of breath?

Helpful rhythm-related cues—Use freely
- If you decrease the number of breaths per minutes, can you keep the breath subtle and light?
- Can you decrease the rate of breathing without getting to the point of gulping air?
- Can you keep the breath subtle and light even as you are increasing its length?
- Increasing the volume of the breath when you start taking fewer breaths in per minutes is like drinking fewer glasses of alcohol but making the glass bigger …
- Can you sense the rhythm of your breath from the inside out and adjust based on your sense of what you need in the moment?
- Can you attune to your interoceptive skill to notice if your breath is calming or agitating you and then adjust the rhythm accordingly?
- I invite you not to copy another person's/my breathing rhythm—honor your own breath rhythm
- Can you breathe in a way that feels light, subtle, and optimal for you?
- Can you sense that hard and fast breathing reduces blood flow to the brain and can make you dizzy or light-headed?
- You might sense inward to intuit that hard and fast breathing can interfere with oxygen delivery into the tissues even though you are taking in a lot of air …
- Breathing is not a competition/performance—can you allow yourself not to strive for the perfect breath or the breath you observe in another person?
- Beware of getting obsessed with finding the *perfect* breath—find a gentle and calming rhythm instead…
- Breathe in a way that supports for sense of calm, even during challenge or stress …
- Use your experience of the breath as biofeedback about your vitality and adjust it according to your needs in this moment?

Unhelpful cues—Avoid unless there is clear intention or purpose
- Make your breath loud/heard/audible
- Always breathe with sound
- Maintain ujjayi breathing throughout your yoga practice
- Let me hear you breathing
- Take as few breaths as possible
- Slow down your rate of breathing (*without* reference to reducing its volume)
- Sigh out a long, deep breath
- Make your breath strong and forceful
- Breathe into the chest
- Make your exhalation as long as possible
- Hold your breath as long as you possibly can
- Regularly measure the length of your breath hold (control pause) to train your breath (*a really bad cue*—CP is an *assessment*, not a *practice*)

9.3.3   Sequencing Subtle Breathing Practices

Subtle breathing is introduced early in breathwork—once breath attunement, especially breath observation, has been successfully introduced. It is introduced embedded in a practice that includes relaxation or centering (see Chap. 7), both *before and after* the subtle breathing exercise. Subtle breathing can be recommended for regular home practice once it can be performed in session without nervous system or affective dysregulation. Subtle breathing is most effective at altering chemosensitivity of the medulla and enhancing biochemistry if practiced regularly throughout the day (e.g., for 5–10 min every hour). Gentle cautions about remaining attuned to emotional or physiological reactivities (such as symptoms of anxiety or breath dysregulation) are key to successful home practice. During in-session practice, clinicians can help monitor reactivity, as evidenced by dysregulating breathing rhythms, straining in the neck muscles, or fear reactions, and can help clients begin to attune to signs that they need to end subtle breathing. Home practice is most successful if attention is given to creating a state of relaxation before, during, and after subtle breathing.

9.3.4   Forms of Subtle Breathing

Numerous forms of subtle breathing can be used to help patients move toward optimal functional breathing. Choices are tailored to the specific physical, emotional, and mental needs and circumstances of each patient. Early in the work, many options are offered so that patients may access the form of subtle breathing that best serves them as they strive to reset their biochemistry. After exposure to the options, some patients may develop a strong preference for one variation over others. Instructional guidance and commentary follow for the most commonly and helpfully applied subtle breathing practices. Some forms of subtle breathing are easier in a supine position than others; with new patients, it is helpful to start with supine subtle breathing unless they are able to sit with skillful ease.

All of the breaths described below are carefully sequenced, generally offered after initial practices such as an opening centering and intention-setting, breath attunement, any needed assessment, gentle preparatory movement, and natural breathing. As noted in the general cuing instructions earlier, all subtle breathing practices require nasal and diaphragmatic breathing, favoring gentle movement in the abdomen and side waist (with low ribs moving outward and upward, if at all). All invite smooth texture, silent breath, and slow-paced breathing. The general instructions offered earlier are universal and applied to all subtle breathing practices that follow—even if all of these features are not always repeated in specific instructions for each given style of subtle breathing.

Basic Subtle Nasal Breathing
Basic nasal breathing can be accomplished in any position, including lying down, sitting, standing, or even walking. The focus is on directing the breath only through the nostrils by keeping the mouth closed. For some clients, this may require taping of a mouth, as their urge to breathe orally is so strong and habitual that they cannot overcome

it. Basic nasal breathing begins with the client's natural breath rhythm. Nasal breathing, in and of itself, is likely already a subtle breath for many patients who are used to breathing through the mouth, even if just on occasion. Many individuals do not realize how often they recruit oral breathing to supplement nasal breathing, especially if nasal clearing is still an issue for them. Once clients are comfortable breathing naturally through the nose, additional instructions invite a slight slowing of the breath to create more subtlety via a longer breath rate. It is important to emphasize that the slowing of the breath is not accompanied (made up for) by an increase in breath volume. It is not recommended to dictate a particular cadence or number of seconds for either the inhalation or the exhalation. Clients are simply encouraged to make their current nasal breath slightly slower than their natural breath. The slowing of the breath can be increased until a point may be reached when the client feels excessive air hunger and the breath begins to dysregulate. Clinicians remain vigilant about signs of breath dysregulation as described earlier and support the client with cues about returning to natural breathing.

Cautions Specific to Basic Nasal Breathing

If slow nasal breathing is not possible for the patient, it is important to return to earlier steps in the journey toward changing breath biomechanics. It may be necessary to return to nasal clearing exercises, beginning with the gentlest versions. The strong nasal clearing exercise offered in Table 7.15 may not be possible for clients who cannot access subtle nasal breathing. They may need to find a much briefer (perhaps 2–5 s) breath suspension; then, they return to their natural breath rate— still through the nose. If possible, these shorter breath holds are repeated until there is a perception of some clearing in the nose. If the client never feels comfortable breathing through the nose, despite prior medical clearance that ruled out physiological or anatomical reasons, wearing a nasal dilator strip may be helpful.

Variations for Basic Subtle Nasal Breathing

The most basic procedure for subtle nasal breathing at the beginning of breathwork is as described earlier, with a focus on slowing the breath cycle, without increasing breath volume. An alternative approach can be a focus on lengthening only the exhalation, rather than lengthening all phases of the breath. The advantage of an extended exhalation is that exhaling is linked to the parasympathetic nervous system and typically helps engage the vagal break. Thus, a focus on the extension of the exhalation rather than the entire breath cycle may be more accessible for some patients who might otherwise quickly move into a sympathetic nervous system arousal state.

It is important to understand that extension of the exhalation in this version of breathwork is not the same as (the significantly longer and more demanding) extension of the exhalation used with four-part breathing. That particular type of breathwork is covered in Chap. 10 and has stronger demand characteristics for patients than does embedding extended exhalations in the context of subtle breathing. It is important not to prescribe a particular cadence or count for this practice. This is often offered, especially in the context of yoga and mental health practices. However, when working with subtle breathing, the goal is to simply extend the exhalation slightly beyond what is typical for the patient. No need exists to achieve externally imposed criteria for how long exhalation should take. Clients decide what is possible for them to remain in a regulated nervous system state.

Hands-on-Belly-and-Chest Breathing

Hands-on-belly-and-chest breathing can be accomplished in any position and is a wonderful practice for people who are not yet able to sit with ease. Starting in a restful position, patients are invited to place one hand at the region of the umbilicus and the other hand low on the chest (or rib basket). Practice begins with gentle nasal breathing into the hands and feeling the breath under the hands. The placement of the hands is then used to ensure that the client is supporting the breath with diaphragmatic movement. If chest breathing is noted, the first step in this exercise becomes finding ways to help the patient breathe diaphragmatically by discontinuing chest and/or reverse breathing using the suggestions offered earlier and in Table 8.2 in Chap. 8.

Once the patient has been able to engage in several rounds of nasal *and* diaphragmatic breathing, an invitation is issued to press the hands firmly into the front body to begin to feel a sense of constriction physically, and by extension, in the breath. Clients can slowly exert increasing pressure until they find the breath constriction stronger than they can tolerate physically or emotionally. It is crucial to track whether a client's breath is dysregulating, for example, by noting changes in texture and sound or reverting to mouth breathing. If signs of anxiety or excessive air hunger emerge (e.g., gasping or grasping for air, spasms of the diaphragm), the client is invited back to natural breathing, with hands removed from the body until breath, arousal, and affect have recovered. Then, as appropriate, subtle nasal and diaphragmatic breathing can be restarted.

Variations for Hands-on-Belly-and-Chest Breathing

Instead of using the hands, an external weight can be used. If the client provides consent, the clinician places two weights on the abdomen, one in the region of the belly button and one on the low chest. Amount of weight is determined collaboratively by clinician and client. It can be helpful to start with lighter weights and then increase the amount of pressure exerted on the body over the course of a few sessions. It is easy to have various weights available by using bags of uncooked rice or beans. These can be purchased in 1-pound and 5-pound weights (5-pound bags can easily be cut open to be adjusted to intermediate weights and then carefully resealed). Sandbags work very well, but are less readily available. Some patients much prefer external weights to their own hands to create constriction; others prefer to feel the additional biofeedback in their hands.

Cautions Specific to Hands-on-Belly-and-Chest Breathing

Even if external weights are to be used, natural breathing is used first with hands on the low chest and belly. Once clients are observed to be in a peaceful rhythm, with smooth texture and silence, weights can replace the hands. Of course, patients must be prepared for exactly what is about to happen during the breathing practice before the clinician places the weights. Thus, clinicians request consent again from clients when the time comes for the first set of weights to be placed. Vigilance is needed by the clinician in this approach; furthermore, clients are encouraged to move the weights anytime they feel dysregulated or if air hunger becomes intolerable.

This breath is not only a subtle breath; it is also a wonderful mechanism for redirecting clients who are chest breathers into becoming abdominal breathers. The weight on the chest can be made heavier than the pressure on the abdomen, inviting the breath to flow naturally lower into the body, moving the abdomen and the low rib basket.

Brief Sample Script for Hands-On-Belly-And-Chest Breathing

[start with calming and relaxation, followed by breath observation; then introduce the subtle breath, emphasizing nasal breathing]

Gently place one hand on your belly at about the region of your belly button and one hand low on the chest, really on the low rib basket ... notice the feedback on your body from your hands ... now breathe into your hands ... perhaps noticing the hands moving with the breath...

[wait a few minutes as the client breathes naturally]

Now that you have a sense of your natural breathing, begin to press the hands into your body... breathe and notice the impact of the pressure of the hands ... As you breathe several rounds of breath ... pressing inward with the hands ... you may begin to feel a sense of constriction in the breath... That is the goal...

[pause]

Your hands are making the breath a little more subtle ... you are moving a little bit less air for a few moments... press the hands into the low chest and belly and notice how this shifts your experience of the breath...

[pause and observe—cue as appropriate based in observation]

If at any point, this feels overwhelming ... or causes anxiety ... gently and calmy return to natural breathing without pressing the hands into the body... letting them rest there if that feels okay.

[wait a few cycles as the client breathes subtly or naturally]

Check in with your nervous system to notice if you can take a few more rounds of breath in this very subtle way ... breathing through the nose ... noticing movement created by the diaphragm, especially under the hand on your belly ...

This subtle form of breathing might also give you a sense of how the body accommodates constriction in the front body ... by directing breath into the side waist ... even the back body ... what do you notice under the hands now ...

[pause]

After your next exhalation you can release your hands and once again tune into your natural breathing ...

Back Body Breathing

Back body breathing is a practice that straddles breath attunement, diaphragmatic breath retraining, and subtle breathing. Breathing occurs while in child's pose (or another seated forward-folding shape), with the front body compressed either against the folded legs or against a prop or pillow that is placed between or on top of the legs (see Illustrations 7.13–7.18 in Chap. 7 for sample positions). Resistance, either from the legs or from the prop, serves to create a similar experience to breathing with a belly weight or with the hands pressing on the abdomen and chest. However, the compression is slightly stronger, and there is less capacity to compensate for the compression in the front body. Therefore, subtle breathing now is experienced as breathing into the back body. Breathing in this position has profound effects on the internal organs and the musculature of the torso. It tends to create a gentle self-massage of the organs as well as a releasing of the fascia, energy, and unnecessary contraction in the front body. As such, it is a wonderful practice for people who are chest breathers and who need to learn how to develop new breathing habits. This practice is also helpful for improving rib basket resilience and increasing the use of lung tissue in the back body, potentially increasing lung capacity as well as breath efficacy.

Variations for Back Body Breathing

Variations for this breath are essentially modifications to child's pose. Chapter 7 can be consulted for more information. Illustrations 7.13–7.15 in the *Prone Positions* section of Chap. 7 show variations of child's pose that create more accessibility for most clients and are conducive to back body breathing. Illustrations 7.16–7.18 offer variations with legs in a wide-legged forward fold, a helpful option for some clients, especially if their knees do not allow them to be in a flexed, weight-bearing prone shape.

If patients become comfortable with back body breathing in session, they can be invited to make this a home practice. Back body breathing can be a lovely morning or evening practice, as it contains within it breath attunement work that can be calming for the nervous system.

Cautions for Back Body Breathing

Although this breath accomplishes the intentions outlined above, it is a subtle breathing practice *and* a prone practice—both of which can be triggering for some patients. Careful monitoring of clients is necessary. Patients have to be able to handle the constriction of the breath as well as the downward facing position. For some individuals, this can be an overwhelming request. Careful preparation with clear instructions and invitation about how to release from the practice are key to successful initial attempts.

Care needs to be taken in using this breathing practice with individuals who have trauma histories or significant psychopathology. Careful investigation and observation are necessary to ensure that the practice is not contraindicated for a given patient. Observation can ensure that any signs of emotional distress are ameliorated by inviting the patient to rise up for a few rounds of natural breathing. Then, the client is given a choice about whether to return to the practice.

Feather Breathing

Feather breathing requires a seated or partly reclined position (a supine position is difficult because of the hand positions that are required). It is accomplished by holding a feather or the palm of the hand a few inches away from the nose. Instructions begin by directing the client to move the feather or the hand to a distance from the nose where they can *just* begin to notice their exhalation—either as a gentle stream of air on their hand or as slight movement in the feather. Breath is maintained at this volume for a few rounds. The client is then asked to move the hand or feather a little bit closer and to reduce the breath enough that they notice the same amount of air on their hand or the feather as before, when the hand or feather was farther away. In other words, the feather or hand is moved closer and closer to the nose; however, the amount of air that reaches the feather or the hand is adjusted to stay the same. This process slowly makes the breath increasingly more subtle and/or slower. As with all subtle breathing, it is important to track whether clients are becoming reactive. If their breath dysregulates (e.g., they are gasping for air upon inhalation), they are asked to move their hand or feather away from the nose, resting the hands for a while and returning to a few rounds of natural breathing. When the breath has recovered, feather breathing can resume. It is helpful to repeat several cycles as time permits. If the client does well with the practice, it can be assigned as homework, with a recommendation of repeating the practice as often as 5 min every hour with vigilant self-monitoring and a preplanned calming practice before and after the practice.

Variations for Feather Breathing
For clients who do not have a feather but cannot make feedback on their hand work, the screen of a turned-off cell phone or a small handheld mirror can be used. The external feedback is then the slight footprint of the breath's vapor that is noticeable on the screen or mirror on exhalation. The initial distance is determined by moving the screen or mirror closer and closer toward the nose until the breath leaves a tiny bit of condensation. Breathing starts a little bit farther away than that, and the goal is to leave no footprint on the screen or mirror, even as it is slowly brought closer and closer toward the nostrils.

Brief Sample Script for Feather Breathing
(using hand or cell phone screen; explanation of the process has already been given)
[start with calming and relaxation, followed by breath observation; then introduce the subtle breath, emphasizing nasal breathing]
Now that you have observed your natural breath for a while, we will go ahead to begin with feather breathing…

Bring the back of the hand or the screen side of your turned-off phone under your nose a few inches away, far enough that you do not think the breath can reach the hand or the screen…

Bring the hand or screen closer until you feel the footprint of your exhalation … feel the warmth of breath on your hand or notice the moisture ring from the breath on your screen …

[pause]
from here gently create just enough additional distance until you reach point when you can no longer feel [or sense … or see] the footprint of the breath … take your time …

[pause]

Breathe nasally for a few rounds … just hold your hand or your screen under the nose and breathe naturally … if you need to shift hands or hold the phone with the other hand, feel free to do that at any time …

[pause]

Now gently make your breath more subtle … lighter … so that you can move the hand or the screen a little bit closer to the nose … yet there is still no footprint of the breath … this is called feather breathing and if you had a feather you could use a feather instead of a screen or a hand … the goal being for the feather never to be moved by the breath …

Now see if you can move the hand a little bit closer … still without feeling the breath … or bring the screen closer, adjusting the breath so there is no moisture on the screen … you are slowly making the breath more and more subtle …

[pause]

You might create a sense of air hunger here … that is deliberate and will ultimately serve your capacity to breathe optimally …

[observe and cue accordingly]

If you feel as though you are suffocating or you start to panic, move the hand or screen farther away and let the breath become more natural …

[pause and observe]

When you feel recovered, slowly start again, never overdoing … never forcing … being very patient … your hand or screen may never get close to the nose today … that is perfectly fine … this is a practice that best happens regularly

[pause]

The next time you exhale you can release the hand or the screen … return to your natural breathing …

[wait for client to recover]

If you noticed any gasping when you tried to recover, then maybe you tried a little bit too hard … the recovery from feather breathing should only take one or two breaths … you should be back to your natural cycle …

[pause to observe and cue accordingly]

How is the natural breath unfolding now … how would you like to approach the next round of feather breathing … perhaps go a little easier during the next round …

Hands-Cupping-Face Breathing

Hands-cupping-face breathing is most easily accomplished in a seated or partly reclined position. However, clients who cannot yet manage to sit still without tensing or collapsing can access this practice by lying comfortably on their back, with adequate propping. The practice requires that the two hands are used to form a cup over nose and mouth. This is most easily accomplished by bringing the left hand to the left side of the face and the right hand to the right side, covering nose, cheek, mouth, and jawbone. Most likely, the index and middle fingers come to rest at the side of the nose, with ring and little fingers of the two hands touching each other above the bridge of the nose. The thumbs will most likely come to rest on the cheek and palms will lightly rest on the jawbones. The little-finger sides of the hands touch one another, making a gentle seal across the bridge of the nose, mouth, and chin. The seal of the hand is light and somewhat incomplete, which allows some air to move in.

Once the cupping has been described and understood by the client, the practice proceeds as do most subtle breathing practices (noting the following cautions first). The patient is invited to breathe naturally; once settled, the invitation is to move into cupped breathing. Clinicians closely monitor patients' breath and affective/arousal responses, adjusting the length of cupped breathing as necessary. As needed, natural breathing can be used to recover from excessive air hunger, gasping or grasping, shutting down, or other signs of nervous system dysregulation. Well-timed within-practice recovery moments make several repetitions of cupped breathing possible. If the patient can easily recover from cupped breathing, it can be assigned as homework with a recommendation of repeating the practice for 5–10 min every hour or two.

Cautions for Cupped Breathing

Cupped breathing is a more demanding practice than feather breathing or hands-on-body breathing. Careful attention is necessary to titrate the practice to patient capacity. Clients with significant complex trauma or assault histories may have strong reactions to hands cupping over the face and mouth, as this is a position they may have encountered during an assault. It is important to talk with clients about this position of the hands and its connotations for the individual before actually utilizing this practice. Caution is also necessary with individuals with panic or anxiety disorders, as well as individuals with respiratory conditions. As is true for all subtle breathing, prior explanations, slow progression, and regular debriefing will help clinician and client explore with safety and co-regulation.

Brief Sample Script for Hands-Cupping-Face Breathing
(give an explanation first; then practice)
   [start with calming and relaxation, followed by breath observation; then introduce the subtle breath, emphasizing nasal breathing]

In this version of subtle breathing you will take your hands and cup them across the nose and mouth *[show this cupping position]* … then you will breathe through your cup … the cupped hands will help carbon dioxide slowly accumulate a little bit because you are not letting the breath move freely … it is a little bit like breathing into a brown paper bag but not quite because you are allowing fresh oxygen to come in …
   [pause]

This is a way of working with the breath's biochemistry … if at any point you feel panicky, light-headed, or dizzy, please release the hands and come back to natural breathing until the breath has recovered …

Once the breath has recovered, you could try a different form of subtle breathing like feather breathing or hands to the belly and the chest … then perhaps try to take a couple more rounds of subtle breathing with hands cupping the face …

[pause]

Allow yourself to take a break and breathe naturally, releasing the hands and noticing if it feels like an easy or difficult recovery … if it feels like a difficult recovery, then for the next round, try a shorter time period;

if you recover quickly then you can take another round and experiment with how long you want to breathe with hands cupped over the nose and mouth …

[pause]

At the end of your next exhalation, return to the natural breath and notice your recovery … release the subtle breathing and notice if there is any gasping or grasping for breath … or if recovery seems to happen naturally within a breath or two … perhaps let that feedback guide your future practice …

As you come back to a comfortable natural breathing rhythm, begin to ready your nervous system for a shift in position … and then in the next 20–30 s, take all the time you need to rise to a seated position ….

[debrief]

If this subtle breath was tolerable, it may be helpful to take this practice into daily life …

[assign homework: e.g., great breathing exercises to do once an hour or once every 2 h for about 5–10 min; this will slowly help you recalibrate the biochemistry of your breathing—you can measure your control pause occasionally to notice if anything is changing—but not expecting or striving for a particular outcome…]

Variations for Cupped Breathing

Hands-cupping face can be used while standing and moving. It is a subtle breathing practice that can be applied in combination with light to moderate physical exertion, unlike the prior practices that use particular shapes or implements (e.g., feather, screen, mirror; supine or prone positions). Adding movement to cupped breathing turns it into a more demanding practice and hence is not used until later, perhaps once clients are ready for more demanding breathing practices.

Interestingly, another use for cupped breathing is as a recovery breath. The nature of the seal makes cupping different from breathing into a brown paper bag when patients are hyperventilating. Cupped breathing is actually a superior version of recovery breath and can be used instead of a brown paper bag if a client moves into a state of hyperventilation (typically expressed as panic, anxiety, or asthma symptoms). This is because cupping allows CO_2 to accumulate while still inviting in sufficient oxygen.

Single Nostril Breathing

Foreshadowing single nostril breathing, which becomes an important focus in Chap. 10, single nostril breathing in the context of subtle breathing is offered as a transitional practice into more challenging breathwork. In the context of subtle breathing, single nostril breathing arises from the successful practice of shifting clients to predictable nasal, diaphragmatic, light, smooth, and quiet breathing. Once patients are able to maintain a healthful subtle breathing practice for an extended period of time and under a variety of circumstances (e.g., during home practice, during movement, during exercise), more demand can be introduced by inviting them to close one nostril, using slight pressure of a finger on the side of the nostril. The invitation typically begins by asking the client to note which nostril is the clearer, less congested nostril. The assessment practice offered in Chap. 6 can be used for this purpose. The client is then invited to close the more clogged nostril to breathe only through the clearer nostril.

Once breathing through the clear nostril has become comfortable, the client can be asked to explore what might happen during a shift to breathing only through the more clogged nostril. While this may cause some dysregulation for some clients (as more air hunger is triggered and more effort is necessary to breathe through the clogged nostril), this practice can be profoundly helpful in supporting the clearing of the clogged nostril. The practice is most successful if clients can remain relaxed and socially connected, in a ventral vagal state. If indications of dysregulation emerge (e.g., gasping or spasming; anxiety or panic), the individual is encouraged to return to natural nasal and diaphragmatic breathing through both nostrils. A nasal clearing practice may then be used before single nostril breathing is attempted again.

Cautions About Single Nostril Breathing

Most contraindications or cautions about single nostril breathing are self-evident. If a patient has not yet reached some facility with other subtle breathing strategies, shifting to single nostril breathing is premature. Clients with severe congestion, either due to respiratory illness or allergies, or with untreated high blood pressure are also not ready candidates for this practice. Single nostril breathing is a more challenging practice than most of the other subtle breathing practices, perhaps with the exception of breathing subtly during physical exertion. Single nostril breathing can result in discomfort, including dizziness or lightheadedness, especially if the client cannot breathe slowly or gently. Any indications that the individual is moving into hyperventilation suggest the practice be discontinued. Single nostril breathing can be anxiety-provoking or agitating. Being stressed and in a state of sympathetic arousal is a contraindication for this practice.

Subtle Breathing with Physical Exertion

Subtle breathing with physical exertion is premised on the idea that the client has developed the capacity, while seated, lying down, or otherwise at rest, to breathe nasally and diaphragmatically, finding a light breath that is smooth in texture and without sound. All previously defined subtle breathing practices are wonderful pre-requisites for taking subtle breathing into a movement or exercise context. Since physical exercise or movement in and of itself increases CO_2 levels in the blood, breathing nasally while during light, moderate, or even intense exercise or movement can be a profoundly helpful and challenging subtle breathing practice. Breath combined with movement, exertion, or exercise can be especially challenging for individuals who have a history of chronic mouth breathing, or of respiratory or anxiety disorders. Although such clients may have learned to breathe in a subtle way while at rest and under particular conditions (e.g., during a breathwork session), they may find themselves reverting to oral and/or chest breathing with sound or disrupted texture when placed into situations requiring more physical (or even mental or emotional) exertion.

As with all subtle breathing practices, the goal of subtle breathing with physical exertion is to create tolerable air hunger and healthful breath biomechanics, while remaining in a socially connected, ventral vagal nervous system state. The primary difference compared to other subtle breathing practices is that this time, the focus is less on changing breath dynamics and more on adding physical activity to create an increase in carbon dioxide levels in the blood and to create challenges to maintaining healthful biomechanics. Nasal and diaphragmatic breathing for the entire time period of exertion remain, nevertheless, the key to this practice being *subtle* breathwork. Subtle breathing under exertion may be a significant challenge for some clients, and they may need to start this practice with a taped mouth, as the urge or habit to breathe through the mouth while moving, especially exercising, may be strong. Clinicians need to use their judgment to determine whether mouth taping in this context is appropriate. It may be possible to observe clients while they are in a movement practice and to give necessary verbal reminders to breathe nasally and low into the abdomen.

Cautions for Nasal Breathing with Physical Exertion

Simply while moving and breathing nasally, clients may begin to feel air hunger. If the breath dysregulates or other autonomic reactions signal that the physiology or nervous system is overly challenged, pauses in movement can be offered to allow the breath to recover. On the other hand, if clients are already used to nasal breathing, simply walking or doing a light yoga practice may not be sufficient to make this a subtle breathing practice. For them, closing one nostril may create sufficient extra demand to result in air hunger. Alternatively, patients can be invited to jog, rather than walk, or to choose a challenging yoga vinyasa. If the urge is felt to breathe orally or into the chest or if breath or nervous system dysregulate, level of exertion can be lessened. If lessening the demand is not enough to reregulate clients' physiology, a break is taken from the movement altogether until a natural rhythmic breath reemerges.

Variation of Subtle Breathing with Physical Exertion
Slow, light, smooth, and soundless nasal and diaphragmatic breathing during exertion offers almost endless varieties within breathwork sessions and as homework in daily life. The practice can be kicked off with walking in an office or outdoor setting, accompanied by the clinician. It can be used during yoga vinyasa or kriya. Even a postural yoga practice with emphasis on combining breath with movement as students move in and out of various yoga shapes can be sufficiently demanding to increase CO_2 levels and challenge habitual biomechanics. Clients can be encouraged, once somewhat successful with the practice (and evidence of appropriate self-awareness), to take subtle breathing with exertion into daily life. They can use this approach for daily walks, typical exercise (e.g., while jogging), housework or gardening chores, and work settings. When appropriate, they can tape their mouth if they note that they revert to oral or dysregulated breathing, to help themselves break old habits. Generalizing subtle breathing to these various situations outside the context of breathwork or yoga sessions is key to the ultimate success in altering breathing patterns under all types of conditions.

9.4   Where We Go from Here

This chapter has presented foundational breathwork appropriate for the majority of patients in healthcare settings or beginning yoga clients anywhere. It emphasized staged intervention approaches that help people foster resilient and optimally adaptive daily breathing. As was true for Chap. 8, all practices offered in this chapter are founded on the psychoeducational (didactic) information covered in Chaps. 2, 3, and 4—information that is freely shared with patients to motivate them to change respiratory habits and pattern locks. All practices are preparatory for more specialized practices offered in Chaps. 10 and 11. For many breathwork clients, the practices of Chaps. 10 and 11 are not necessary; they are supplemental. Most patients' breath rhythms and patterns will become more healthful simply via the breath attunement practices described in Chap. 8, and the optimal functional breathing cultivated via the practices offered in this chapter.

Chapter 10 is a logical continuation of this chapter and branches out into more specialized and specifically intentioned breathwork. It begins with an exploration of breathwork focused on the four breath phases. These practices continue to decrease breath rates without increasing volume, while adding more demand via longer extensions of breath phases, adding breath holds, and inviting specific cadences applied to the inhalation, retention, exhalation, or suspension. Going beyond four-part breathing, Chap. 11 then explores single nostril breathing and finally ends with practices that use sound and force to create more advanced breathwork.

> *What the bodily form depends on is breath (ch'i)*
> *and what breath relies upon is form.*
> *When the breath is perfect, the form is perfect (too).*
> *If breath is exhausted, then form dies.*—from the Chinese Taoist Canon Tao Tsang

References

1. Bhavanani A, Ramanathan M, Balaji R, Pushpa D. Differential effects of uninostril and alternate nostril pranayamas on cardiovascular parameters and reaction time. Int J Yoga. 2014;7(1):60–5. https://doi.org/10.4103/0973-6131.123489.
2. Raghuraj P, Telles S. Immediate effect of specific nostril manipulating yoga breathing practices on autonomic and respiratory variables. Appl Psychophysiol Biofeedback. 2008;33(2):65–75. https://doi.org/10.1007/s10484-008-9055-0.
3. Pal GK, Agarwal A, Karthik S, Pal P, Nanda N. Slow yogic breathing through right and left nostril influences sympathovagal balance, heart rate variability, and cardiovascular risks in young adults. N Am J Med Sci. 2014;6(3):145–51. https://doi.org/10.4103/1947-2714.128477.
4. Birdee G, Nelson K, Wallston K, et al. Slow breathing for reducing stress: the effect of extending exhale. Complement Ther Med. 2023;73:102937. https://doi.org/10.1016/j.ctim.2023.102937.
5. Nelson N. Diaphragmatic breathing: the foundation of core stability. Strength Cond J. 2012;34(5):34–40. https://doi.org/10.1519/SSC.0b013e31826ddc07.
6. Shah S, Shirodkar S, Deo M. Effectiveness of core stability and diaphragmatic breathing vs. core stability alone on pain and function in mechanical non-specific low back pain patients: a randomised control trial. Int J Health Sci Res. 2020;10(2):232–41. https://www.ijhsr.org/IJHSR_Vol.10_Issue.2_Feb2020/36.pdf
7. Chen Y, Huang X, Chien C, Cheng J. The effectiveness of diaphragmatic breathing relaxation training for reducing anxiety. Perspect Psychiatr Care. 2017;53(4):329–36. https://doi.org/10.1111/ppc.12184.
8. Bilo G, Revera M, Bussotti M, et al. Effects of slow deep breathing at high altitude on oxygen saturation, pulmonary and systemic hemodynamics. PLoS One. 2012;7(11):e49074. https://doi.org/10.1371/journal.pone.0049074.
9. McKeown P. Oxygen advantage: the simple, scientifically proven breathing techniques for a healthier, slimmer, faster, and fitter you. William Morrow; 2015.
10. McKeown P. The breathing cure. Humanix; 2021.
11. Meuret AE, Ritz T, Wilhelm FH, Roth WT, Rosenfield D. Hypoventilation therapy alleviates panic by repeated induction of dyspnea. Biol Psychiatry Cogn Neurosci Neuroimaging. 2018;3(6):539–45. https://doi.org/10.1016/j.bpsc.2018.01.010.
12. Meuret AE, Rosenfield D, Hofmann SG, Suvak MK, Roth WT. Changes in respiration mediate changes in fear of bodily sensations in panic disorder. J Psychiatr Res. 2009;43(6):634–41. https://doi.org/10.1016/j.jpsychires.2008.08.003.
13. McKeown P. Buteyko instructor training manual. Oxygen Research Institute; 2020.

Breathwork with Phases of the Breath

10

*Breathwork is integrated into an overall approach to healthcare –
carefully coordinated and sequenced.
Breathing practice happens in session – carefully embedded
and sequenced.
Breathing application happens in real life – carefully, and
increasingly spontaneously,
adapted moment-to-moment to personal and relational needs as
life unfolds
in its many surprising, challenging, and beautiful ways.*

10.1 Overview: Creating Accessibility Working with Breath Phases

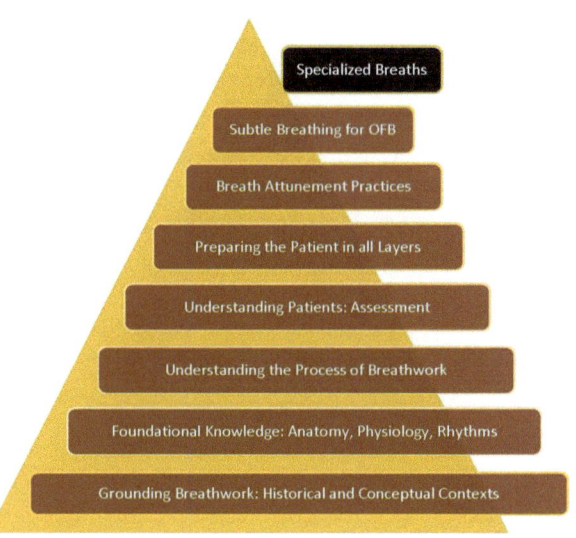

All breathing practices provide opportunities for bottom-up awareness and top-down self-regulation to access emotional and physical balance or equanimity. They provide access to inner awareness via neuroception and interoception via stimulation of somatosensory afferent vagal fibers; they enhance emotional self-regulation, attention, and memory via balanced autonomic nervous system states, changed stress perceptions, greater intentionality and discernment, increased mental clarity and mindfulness, and other top-down pathways. Breathing practices stimulate the vagus nerve, include humming and sounding breaths, happen in a co-regulated interpersonal context, and invite relaxed yet engaged muscles—all in the service of creating resilience in the nervous system. Optimal functional breathing (i.e., low, nasal, slow, light, silent, and smooth) in and of itself, and even more so specific breathing practices, can be utilized to move the practitioner—clinician and client alike—toward more resilient states of being, engaging the vagal brake, increasing vagal tone, and enhancing heart rate variability. Breathing practices interact profoundly with physical movement and mental fluctuations and thus open doors into all the tangible layers of experience. Breathwork is a wonderful foundation for resilient breathing practice and application that is adaptive to the needs of the moment, for example, allowing for more energy when activity level demands and less energy when quietude is the goal.

This chapter and Chap. 11 present several essential categories of specialized breathing practices that have specific purposes and can be tailored to needs and contexts in a multitude of ways. The two chapters emphasize that specialized breathing practices are purposeful—they are not offered in a generic way to a generic group of clients or students. It is essential to understand each client individually and then to select and apply breathwork in the most patient-centered and appropriate way. All specialized breathing practices can be individualized in thoughtful ways to support resilience, coherence, and adaptability in the breath for each and every patient.

To help choose specific practices and their adaptations and variations, for each type of breathing taught, studied, practiced, and analyzed, Table 10.1 provides an overview of all specialized practices offered in this chapter and Chap. 11. Both

Table 10.1 Specialized breathing practices for healthcare and therapeutic yoga

Type of breath	Purpose or intentions	Important consideration
Working with the breath phases (this chapter)		
Equal breathing	• Calms mental fluctuations and emotions • Reduces stress perception • Increases focus and attention • Enhances blood pressure regulation • Resets chemosensitivity	• Can function as a subtle breathing practice • Can lead to hyperventilation or dizziness

(continued)

Table 10.1 (continued)

Type of breath	Purpose or intentions	Important consideration
Extended exhalation	• Calms nervous system and emotions • Increases mental clarity and attention • Is emotionally & physically grounding • Improves cardiovascular function • Resets chemosensitivity • Enhances internal respiration	• Can function as subtle breathing practice • Not helpful with clients in chronic dorsal disconnection • Safe for most other clients due to its deeply calming and grounding effect
Extended inhalation	• May help counter dorsal collapse • Can reset chemosensitivity • Enhances external respiration • May enhance lung capacity	• Not helpful with clients in chronic sympathetic arousal • Can lead to hyperventilation or dizziness
Breath suspension	• Increases number of red blood cells • Resets chemosensitivity • Supports core & diaphragm strength • Decreases chronic pain perception • Supports nitric oxide production and absorption • Supports relaxation for most	• With short comfortable pauses, can serve as a recovery breath from panic or asthma attack • With long holds, creates hypoxia • Not appropriate during pregnancy and many chronic illnesses • Can be emotionally challenging for some
Alternate and single nostril breathing (Chap. 11)		
Channel purifying	• Balances nervous system & emotions • Promotes hemispheric integration • Lifts mental wellbeing and mood • Boosts attentional focus • Improves cardiovascular functions, especially heart rate variability • Enhances respiratory functions • Resets chemosensitivity • Decreases mental fluctuation	• Can be used as a subtle breathing practice • Generally safe and accessible for most clients • Contraindicated during head colds or sinus infection or while experiencing severe headache • Can be used as a concentration practice and hones focus
Moon piercing	• Calms, grounds, and cools the body and nervous system • Promotes sleep and relaxation • Decreases blood pressure • Sharpens mental focus and attention • Enhances physical and emotional wellbeing	• Can be used as a subtle breathing practice • May be contraindicated for individuals with low blood pressure • May be less appropriate for individuals in dorsal vagal collapse

(continued)

Table 10.1 (continued)

Type of breath	Purpose or intentions	Important consideration
Sun piercing	• Energizes and vitalizes the nervous system • May increase body temperature • Lifts mood and wellbeing • Supports digestion and circulation • Improves alertness and mental clarity • Clears the nasal passages	• Can be used as a subtle breathing practice • May be too upregulating for clients with sympathetic hyperarousal • Best avoided during fever and heat • May be contraindicated with hypertension
Breathing with sound (Chap. 11)		
Bumblebee	• Enhances mental wellbeing and mood • Enhances concentration and focus—related to theta waves • Enhances cardiovascular functions • Resets chemosensitivity • Encourages diaphragmatic breathing • At low frequency, increases nitric oxide—clears & opens the airways • Relieves headaches • May relieve tinnitus	• Can be used as a subtle breathing practice by increasing the length of the exhalation—it then shares the benefits of subtle breathing practices • Generally safe and accessible for most clients • Excellent practice for boosting nitric oxide
Silent *ujjayi*	• Increases mental focus and attention • Calms nervous system via vagal brake • Increases peacefulness and ease • Enhances respiratory efficiency • Enhances cardiovascular health	• Often overused in yoga contexts • Should be silent, not noisy • Not for general breathing in daily life • Can lead to excessive efforting
Breathing with force (Chap. 11)		
Skull-shining	• Supports core strength and stability • Can cleanse & detoxify (moves lymph) • May enhance lung capacity and rib basket resilience • Energizes the nervous system • May increase mental clarity • May improve digestion • Lifts depressive mood and sluggishness	• A kriya of hormesis—hyperventilation • Not appropriate for individuals in chronic sympathetic arousal • Can create dizziness & lightheadedness • Has caused heart attacks in some • Has many contraindications (e.g., glaucoma, hypertension, detached retina, vitreous detachment, hernia) • Use only the slow-motion variation
Against-the-grain	• Can enhance overall wellbeing • Can invite uplifting energy and joy • Energizes the nervous system and may uplift dorsal collapse • Can reset shallow breathing, strong emotions, and stress	• Can cause hyperventilation & dizziness • A favorite *viloma* application is breath-of-joy kriya • If taught with against-the-grain action on the inhalation, is akin to physiological sighing, a helpful reflex

chapters, while focused on different types of breathwork, provide details about the intention of each breathing practice; associated techniques, intentions, cautions, and—where applicable—contraindications; teaching principles and cuing considerations; sequencing of each technique within and across sessions; and potential physical, emotional, and mental effects and benefits of each specific practice. Variations are invited for all offered practices with focus on three variables, namely breathing with physical movement or in a particular body position, breathing for discerningly affecting polyvagal state, and generalizing breathing practices into breathing application in daily life.

10.2 Foundations of Variations for All Specialized Breathing Practices

For each breathing practice covered in this chapter and Chap. 11, at least three categories of variations are possible and encouraged. The first category of variations incorporates physical movement or exploration into the particular type of breathing. This can occur in the form of a particular shape in which to explore the breath, in the context of a particular flow (e.g., within a sun breath or breath of joy), or in the context of exercise applications. The second category of variations is based on patients' polyvagal states, adapting breathing practices to be calming, energizing, or balancing to best serve patients' needs in the moment. The third category of variation concerns itself with generalization of breathing practices to daily life, inviting ways in which an altered breath can be incorporated in the context of home life, relationships, work, and more.

10.2.1 Variations Based on Integration with Physical Movement or Activity

Linking breath with physical movement or posture encourages both to become mindful and smooth and supports the mind in maintaining focus and attention. The union of breath, movement, and mindful presence develops inner wisdom and intuition, guides physical actions and breathwork within safe limits, enhances proprioception, creates interoception and neuroception of changes in the nervous system, supports the capacity to re-regulate, and creates emotional and mental resilience. It helps patients recognize the impact of breath and movement on mind and emotions, inviting keen recognition of that connection while offering strategies for developing a concentrated mind and more easeful emotions. Mental concentration supports the flow of postures and breath. It also helps clarify the impact of a dysregulated, non-attentive, or distracted mind on our daily life.

Connecting breath and movement has many advantages. It is a natural way of exploring polyvagal states and the reciprocal effects on all layers of experience, particularly the physical body. Flowing movement while breathing can highlight the expansive nature of inhalation and the releasing or inward-drawing nature of exhalation. The combination of physical and breathing practices develops and maintains a keener sensitivity of breath rate (or speed) and volume as well as increasing clarity about how breath supports movement and how movement supports breath, noticing their reciprocity. It supports interoceptive awareness of changes in breath and its physiological manifestations (e.g., heartbeat), fostering the capacity to re-regulate and create resilience. Breath-movement coordination invites bottom-up sensitivity and awareness as well as promoting top-down regulation, thoughtfulness, intentionality, and planning.

A few general principles for connecting breath with movement are offered in Table 10.2 and can be kept in mind when developing movement-based variations for relevant specialized breathing practices. These guidelines offer general tips about how to combine breath and movement and suggestions for maintaining grounding, accessing expansion, and creating stability. Every offered breathing practice can be

Table 10.2 Combining breath and movement within specialized breathing practices

General principles for breath-movement combinations
- Inhale to support physical expansion (e.g., backbends, heart-opening shapes)
- Exhale to support physical contraction or curling inward (e.g., forward fold, rotations)
- Exhale to support a need for core stability (e.g., supine leg lift; moving to or out of a balance shape)
- Breathe into the front, sides, or back of the body depending on shape (e.g., back body in child)
- Breathe lightly (i.e., not moving excessive volume) to keep the breath subtle and movement settled
- Breathe rhythmically and slowly (lower rate; 5.5–10 bpm) to maintain harmonious movement and balanced posture
- Breathe low into the belly's midsection with ease (i.e., comfortable and natural diaphragmatic breath) to invite stability and ease
- Breathe nasally throughout to support dynamic, yet stable movement that is grounding and action that can endure
- Breathe quietly and smoothly, adjusting movement to the needs of the breath rather than allowing movement or exertion to dysregulate the breath

General principles for grounding during breath-movement combinations
- Maintain strong grounding through the feet and/or other body parts touching the floor, especially with more demanding breathing practices
- Maintain a visual focus on a point in the environment to prevent loss of balance or a drifting mind wile breathing with movement
- Maintain a stable breath that is grounding, not flighty—slow down movement to ease the breath as needed; slow down breath to calm and reground movement
- Reground with each exhalation, reconnecting to a sense of stillness in movement, breath, mind, and emotion
- Keep the mind grounded with a concentrated focus on linking breath and movement—a stable mind supports stillness in movement
- Invite a sense of intuitive breathing into the movement or shape to have a keen mental and emotional sense of the self-regulating link between the breath and movement
- Notice the link between breath rate, speed of movement, and mind state—calm one to settle all; vitalize one to energize all; create balance in one to support balance in all

(continued)

Table 10.2 (continued)

General principles for expansion during breath-movement combinations
- Find expansion with the inhalation and through the body's edges and periphery while maintaining optimal grounding and stability during movement
- Expand with each inhalation without sacrificing stability, balance, or grounding in the movement, physical shape, or mind
- Breathe in to support movements that open the body and movements that are expansive and open-hearted
- Breathe into the back and side bodies to find expansiveness and openness in vitality and body
- Breathe in to support activation or vitalization of the body
- Invite a sense of joyous breathing into the flow of postures and into physical activity in daily life

General principles for stability and balance during breath-movement combinations
- Maintain engagement in the core, perineum, and major muscles needed to initiate the movement—engaged muscles are less prone to injury during movement
- Maintain a stable breath tempo and volume—neither over- nor under-breathing—that matched the physical effort needed for the posture, movement, or daily activity
- Maintain a stable breath texture—reregulating the speed or type of movement if breath becomes choppy or labored
- Maintain a quiet, smooth, and rhythmic breath during all movement to invite harmony and balance in body and mind
- Continue to breathe diaphragmatically, drawing on the rhythm between core stabilizers and the diaphragm to stay stable and centered physically and affectively
- Continue to breathe nasally to retain a stable vital physical and mental presence
- Invite a resilient interaction between breath and movement that creates coherence—that invites ease within effort and allows for effort within ease
- Remember that breath can become rapid or slow depending on circumstances and movement and that self-regulation and rebalancing is possible by consciously controlling either the manner of breathing or moving

varied by adding movement or inviting the practice in a particular physical position of shape. Clinicians learn to be creative and offer an assortment of these variations to help keep breathwork fresh and dynamic.

10.2.2 Variations Based on Polyvagal State

As detailed in Chap. 4, polyvagal theory is useful in understanding patients in ways that guide discerning choices about using breath to shift nervous system states [1, 2]. Tailored uses of breath phases, breath qualities (rate, texture, sound, etc.), and nostril preferences allow for calming breath rhythms to address sympathetic nervous system arousal or, conversely, for vitalizing breathing that helps lift a collapsed breath or physical posture indicative of dorsal vagal disconnection. The details offered in Table 10.3 about how to cue and cultivate breath for shifting neural platforms are applicable to most practices offered in this chapter and Chap. 11. A review of Tables 4.11, 4.12, and 4.13 is also recommended.

It is worth noting that some of the specialized breathing practices are by their very nature either more up- or downregulating. They can nevertheless be varied along polyvagal lines by creating slight shifts in how a particular practice is executed in a given moment. For example, while bumblebee breathing is by nature calming, adding forceful movement or faster respiratory rates, it can be used to vitalize as well. While skull-shining breath is by nature activating and vitalizing, a slow-motion version can be used that is strengthening and maintains a sense of grounding and calming. This allows for a single breathing practice to be used in one way to meet a client's in-the-moment energy and then in another way to slowly shift its energy over the duration of its application to help transform the client's state of being with intention. Such gradual shifting is more helpful than meeting a client with a breathing practice that is completely counter to their present-moment experience.

Psychologically tailored breathing practice variations better support patient needs. Calming breathing cues enhance a greater sense of ease, calm, softening; freedom from desire or aversion; tranquility and peace. Alternatively, vitalizing

Table 10.3   Cuing suggestions for using breath to affect polyvagal state

Sampling of autonomically calming cuing tips
Cuing suggestions for grounding breathing
- Invite a soft, calm, calming, sweet, gentle, tender, light, easeful, loving, feathery, compassionate, kind breath
- Drop the breath into the belly or the mid-section of the torso
- Soften, lighten, relax, ease the breath
- Create ease, peace, lightness, comfort, effortlessness in the breath
- Attend closely to the exhalation
- Gently invite the exhalation to lengthen
- Ease up on the inhalation, let the inhalation move naturally
- Slow, lengthen, and lighten the breath without creating a sense of gasping for air
- Breathe increasingly slowly at a rhythm and volume that stays easeful
- Invite ease to balance effort
- Find a smooth and subtle texture
- Let the breath be silent, peaceful
- Use a mantra such as: "inhaling, I cultivate calm; exhaling, I cultivate grounding"

Sampling of autonomically vitalizing cuing tips
Cuing suggestions for energizing breathing
- Invite strong, energetic, robust, active, spirited, brave, decisive, lively, dynamic, determined, vigorous, resilient, buoyant breath
- Move the breath into the belly with intention, resolve, commitment, or determination
- Enliven, strengthen, invigorate, stimulate, refresh, revitalize the breath
- Create strength, determination, fortitude, willpower, resolve, courage in the breath
- Attend closely to the inhalation
- Encourage the inhalation to lengthen
- Ease up on the exhalation, let the exhalation move naturally
- Lengthen each breath with determination yet without creating a sense of gasping for air
- Breathe to create a sturdy rhythm and volume without forcing or chest breathing
- Let ease be balanced by effort
- Invite effort and discipline to balance ease
- Invite a sturdy but smooth texture
- Use a mantra such as: "Inhaling, I cultivate a sense of aliveness; exhaling, I maintain an open heart"

(continued)

Table 10.3 (continued)

Sampling of autonomically balancing cuing tips

Cuing suggestions for resilient breathing
- Invite a smooth, balanced, stable, steady, fluid, silky, smooth, natural, steady, even, uniform, sweet, tranquil, serene, unlabored breath
- Move the breath into the mid-section of the torse with compassion, attention, lovingkindness, open-heartedness, and no expectations
- Feel the rhythmic pulsation of the low rib basket
- Refresh, rejuvenate, harmonize, stabilize, soothe, steady, or revitalize the breath
- Create balance, stability, evenness, self-agency, clarity, or resolve in the breath
- Attend closely to the inhalation and exhalations—perhaps finding balance between the two
- Notice the texture of the inhalation and exhalation and invite the texture to even out if there is a difference
- Notice the sounds of the inhalation and exhalation and invite the sound to even out if there is a difference
- Notice the length of the inhalation and exhalation—perhaps inviting the lengths to become the same if they differ significantly
- Breathe to create a stable and steady rhythm and volume, balancing effort and ease
- Notice stillness in the movement of the breath
- Notice movement in the stillness of the breath
- Find a harmonious rhythm supported by a smooth vibrant texture
- Adapt rate and volume to the demands of the moment or movement
- Use a mantra such as Thich Nhat Hanh's *"breathing in, I know I am breathing in; breathing out, I know I am breathing out"*

cues can tailor breathing practices toward cultivating effort, energy, courage, strength, engagement, or determination. For individuals in sympathetic arousal, calming and grounding breathwork can bring vital and emotional balance; for clients prone to dorsal vagal disconnection, carefully energizing and expansive breathwork may be helpful. For all patients, balancing and stabilizing breathing, especially using breath awareness and observation, are a great introduction to breathwork if it is not yet clear which nervous system state predominates. By using polyvagal-informed variations of breathing practices, even practices that may look contraindicated may be recruited if properly adapted. For example, and as explored in Chap. 11, even a forceful breath such as *kapalabhati* can be offered in a manner that retains the breath's benefit of core strengthening while introducing a pace that does not aggravate sympathetic arousal. Clinicians are encouraged to use these variations thoughtfully and intentionally with all clients. It takes some practice to learn how to vary practices for individual clients—this is worth the effort, as polyvagal tailoring is an excellent way to introduce variation with clear intention and as an offering of self-regulation that can be generalized into daily life.

10.2.3 Variations to Support Practice Generalization to Daily Life

Amply addressed throughout all chapters, it merits repeating that clients are regularly reminded and taught how to bring breathwork from the session into daily life. For many (if not most) breathing practices, the real work and meaning of the practice emerges when it is applied in real-life settings. Thus, throughout work with clients, they are encouraged to bring their breathwork into relationships, work, and home lives. Generalization helps clients reap the benefits of natural and slow-paced breathing not only in a particularly well-suited and prepared context but also when it counts the most: when a challenge threatens to dysregulate the breath. Clinicians are encouraged to discuss with their clients how to apply each offered practice *or* the learning from the practice in daily life.

A Note of Encouragement …

The use of variations cannot be stressed enough. Breathwork becomes most meaningful when it is tailored, creative, and meaningful to each individual client. For each breathing practice presented in this chapter and Chap. 11, one specific variation is offered as an example. Helpful hints and comments about integrating movement or posture, polyvagal adjustments, and daily applications are interspersed. Clinician creativity in finding individualized variations needs to develop as part of auspicious breathwork practice and application. Clinicians are strongly encouraged to develop variations and adaptations from the start with each and every client, as well as in their own breathing practice and real-life application.

10.3 Discovering the Breath Phases

Early breathwork with the four phases of the breath focuses mostly on observation and awareness (see Chap. 8). Once students understand the four parts of their natural breath—recognizing inhalations, resting pauses at the top of the breath, exhalations, and resting pauses at the bottom of the breath—the rhythm of breath phases can be used to alter breathing and enhance well-being. Any of the four aspects of breath can be transformed. Examples include equalizing the inhalation and exhalation, extending the inhalation, extending the exhalation, extending the pause at the top (i.e., breath retention), and extending the pause at the bottom (i.e., breath suspension). Equalization and extension of inhalation and exhalation are practices that can happen relatively early in the practice arc; suspension and retention (as forms of breath *holding, not just pausing*) are more difficult and require slightly more experience with and understanding of breath and breathing, as well as reliable access to accurate interoception and neuroception and to engage commensurate self-regulation as needed.

10.3.1 Preliminary Comments About Discovering the Breath Phases

Although most patients intuitively understand the purposes of exhalations and inhalations, pauses are more confusing or alien to many. To review, if gaps at the top and bottom of the breath are lengthened deliberately and significantly, this represents a breath holding (or *kumbhaka*) practice. *Natural* breaks between inhalation and exhalation are not forced; they are just that—natural pauses. For some patients, pauses are barely perceptible; for others, they may be quite notable. Either way, pauses are not created—they happen on their own. When we work with phases of the breath, we draw on pauses *and* holds—each for different purposes.

Biochemically, suspension after inhalation facilitates perfusion of O_2 from the lungs to the blood and CO_2 from the blood into the lungs (external respiration); biomechanically, it maintains postural stability via air in the lungs and stabilizes intraabdominal pressure from the diaphragm contracting downward. Biochemically, retention after exhalation facilitates enhanced oxygenation of tissues, including the brain, and uptake of CO_2 into the blood (internal respiration); biomechanically, it maintains postural stability via intraabdominal pressure arising from contractions in the abdominal and pelvic floor muscles. Psychologically, the rests at the top and bottom of the breath provide a brief pause for the mind—a gap in our constant sense of arousal, thinking, feeling, and doing; a space for discernment. Along with exhalation, the *Yoga Sutras of Patanjali* tell us that regulation of the breath pauses stills the mind and its many fluctuations, worries, preoccupations, emotions, and distractions.

Review of the Four Breath Phases

Table 10.4 presents an overview of the biomechanics, biochemistry, psychology, and subtle energetics of all four breath phases. This information may help clinicians explain the breath phases to clients in the most applicable and tailored way. At different times and with different individuals, emphasis can be shifted to different manifestations and meanings of the various breath phases. This complexity offers many portals into discussions and applications of four-part breathing to create optimal accessibility to breath-phase-based practices in a client-tailored manner.

Biomechanics, Biochemistry, and Psychology of the Breath Phases

There are many ways to work with the four phases of the breath. Emphasis can be placed on making the phases equal (sometimes referred to as cadence breathing), differentially lengthening one phase over another (often related to polyvagal adjustments), emphasizing breath pauses for calming or creating longer breath holds, and more. This chapter sequences breath-phased-based practices by proceeding from the most accessible to the most challenging versions. That said, each client is different; what may *typically* be manageable for most, may be difficult for a particular individual. Vigilance, compassion, and observation always serve well—for clinician and client. As breathwork is now moving into breath control, it is important to remember there is always an option to return to freeing the breath—to calming and relaxation, observation and awareness, and subtle or natural breathing. Breathwork is not defined by breath control practices; it is defined by helping patients cultivate resilient, coherent, and natural breathing rhythms that result in adaptive and optimally functional breathing in all circumstances. The analysis of the breath phases (and their alterations) that follows can help guide decisions about which breaths to offer to whom and when.

Changing ratios of inhalation and exhalation has been scientifically explored and the most healthful effects (on various measures of health and well-being, e.g., heart

Table 10.4 The many wisdoms of four-part breathing

Inhalation	Retention after inhalation	Exhalation	Suspension after exhalation
Biomechanics of the four phases of breath			
• Diaphragm contracts into abdomen and low ribs lift • Intra-abdominal pressure supports posture and spinal stability • Decreasing pressure in lung invites air to flow in	• Postural stability is maintained • Inhaled air is retained in lungs	• Diaphragm relaxes upward • Intrathoracic pressure increases and air flows out • Core muscles engage and create stability and support intraabdominal pressure	• Core engagement continues to support postural stability • Residual volume of air is retained in the lungs
Biochemistry of the four phases of breath			
• Vagal brake lifts lightly and supports a sympathetic shift • Energy lifts • Nitric oxide increases • Air moves into lungs • Air is cleansed and purified	• Facilitates O_2 diffusion from lungs to blood	• Respiration stimulates the vagus nerve and creates a parasympathetic shift • Air moves out of the lungs • Airway are remoisturized and nasal passages are cleansed	• Arterial CO_2 increases and facilitates O_2 release into tissues • Oxygenation of tissues, brain, etc., is enhanced
Psychology of the four phases of breath			
• Receptivity without greed, aversion, or fear • Openheartedness with appreciation • Open-mindedness to possibilities • Gratitude for what we are receiving in the moment • A sense of fulfillment • A sense of being cared for	• Gratitude for what has been received • Metabolism of inputs • Stable, balanced affect and arousal • Beware of neediness or clinging—of hanging on rather than letting go • Inviting a sense of holding things lightly	• Willingness to let go and release • Groundedness based on faith in abundance • Non-clinging, non-grasping, non-attachment to needs or ego • Embracing the joy and ease of giving away • Open to sharing resources	• Trust in abundance • Faith in the presence of needed supports • Settled and grounded energy • Calm abiding in present-moment experience • Freedom from clinging, aversion, and fear
Subtle energies of the four phases of breath			
• Opening up to *prana vayu* and its inward and forward moving energies • Taking in nourishment and vitality for body, breath, and mind • Becoming receptive and open-hearted to taking in what is offered to us	• Welcoming balancing, peaceful energy of *samana vayu* • Integrating, digesting, and processing all that is taken in • Holding steady, taking in and letting go wisely and discerningly	• Embracing the downward energy of *apana vayu* • Letting go of what no longer serves • Grounding, settling, and calming • Feeling light and relieve, not weighted down by clinging	• Settling into integrating energy of *vyana vayu* • Distributing resources outward from the center to the periphery • Nourishing all layers of experience to create resilience and self-regulation

rate variability) are reportedly achieved via length ratios of 1:1.5–2 for the length of inhalation compared to the length of exhalation [3–5]. That is, the ideal exhalation is up to twice as long as the inhalation. However, it is important to understand this information in the context of individual clients. Specifically, the exhalation phase of the breath is calming and associated with the parasympathetic nervous system. Clients who are already hypoaroused, depressed, sluggish, or fully in dorsal vagal disconnection may not benefit from breathing practices that are focused on extending exhalation. In fact, it may be contraindicated for these patients. Extending exhalation, however, may be helpful for clients who are chronically upregulated and who need to access calming practices that support their progression toward energetic balance. Conversely, the inhalation phase is energizing or stimulating, as it is associated with the sympathetic nervous system response. Clients who are already upregulated, stressed, anxious, or generally in sympathetic arousal may not benefit from practices that extend or focus on inhalation; in fact, it may be contraindicated for them. However, for clients who are physically collapsed and emotionally disconnected, gentle activation via focus on or extension of inhalations can support energetic balance.

Equal breathing seeks to achieve 1:1 length ratios in length of inhalation versus exhalation. Instruction for equal breathing does not always attend to changes in minute ventilation as breath ratios change. Equal breathing typically focuses on lengthening the shorter of the two phases and often results in fewer breaths per minute, as low as 5 or 6 breaths per minute. As breath rate slows, perfusion is enhanced, leading to more time and alveolar surface area available for gas exchange [6]. Slower breath rate is correlated with greater cardiac-vagal baroreflex sensitivity (sensitivity of arterial pressure and pressure in the larger veins), which translates into more efficient and accurate regulation of blood pressure [7]. This enhanced sensitivity leads to greater healthful adaptation and heart rate variability [8]. Through creating slow-paced breathing, equal breathing can become calming for the nervous system and may allay anxiety and worry [9]. However, positive effects may not occur via this practice for all clients; some may increase breath volume to compensate for decreases in breath rate. This adjustment can lead to acute hyperventilation, most likely for the very clients who are already prone to over-breathing. Thus, care needs to be taken to use equal breathing with discernment and a clear understanding of clients' needs—and to keep an eye on clients while they breathe to notice how they are dealing with and reacting to instructions.

Breath pauses have positive effects on breath biochemistry and mechanics if applied thoughtfully and intentionally. As noted elsewhere, short breath suspensions increase CO_2 levels in the blood, which supports release of oxygen into the tissues for enhanced oxygenation. Breath suspensions increase nitric oxide production in the nose; this gas is then drawn into the airways and lungs with the next inhalation, promoting bronchodilation, vasodilation, and cerebral circulation (as cerebral capillaries also dilate) [10]. Long breath suspensions decrease O_2 levels in the blood and may cause temporary states of hypoxia, while maintaining high levels of blood CO_2, mimicking high-altitude training. Biomechanical effects explain extant evidence that breath suspension ameliorates chronic pain [11].

Psychologically, brief breath suspensions tend to be calming and less emotionally challenging than breath retentions because the diaphragm is in a relaxed position. However, for some individuals, the subtle energy of having released (or given away) their exhalation can lead to a mind state of need or grasping. For them, breath retention may be easier psychologically, but perhaps not as useful in the long term. Breath suspensions help develop top-down nervous system control as the cortex learns to override signals from the medulla oblongata to initiate inhalation. This capacity can sharpen mental focus and attention in general. Short, comfortable breath suspensions can be used to stop acute panic or asthma attacks and can become an empowering resource for individuals who suffer from these conditions by teaching them a strategy for preventing attacks when the first symptoms emerge [12].

Breath suspension begins with a focus on comfortable pauses, and over time, can increase to longer holds (including controlled or even maximum breath pauses). As pauses lengthen (and become breath holds), clients are observed for excessive effort, which may dysregulate biomechanics, biochemistry, and nervous system; interfere with attention and focus; and scatter peace of mind. Signs that clients are no longer benefitting from breath suspension include gasping for inhalation (suggestion intolerance of increasing CO_2 levels), visible abdominal spasms, significant negative changes in breath rhythms, and affective or mental dysregulation. Over time, extending suspensions and exhalations can increase CO_2 tolerance and foster slower, smoother breathing rhythms. It is notable that long breath holds that create spasms are a survival reflex (also called the diving response [13]) that can have positive effects on red blood cell counts (because increasing the number of red blood cells is invaluable as it is the only way to increase the amount of available hemoglobin; see Chap. 2) via spasms of the spleen that release (high nutritious fresh) red blood cells into the circulatory system.

Work with breath phases is kept at easeful levels with individuals with high blood pressure, tinnitus (and perhaps other ear issues), and glaucoma (and other eye issues, e.g., vitreous detachment), keeping pauses and extensions to lengths that invite awareness without effort to create changes. Suspensions beyond comfortable pauses are contraindicated for individuals who are pregnant, have uncontrolled high blood pressure and other cardiovascular diseases, seizure disorders, persistent mental illness, aneurysms, and respiratory disease (including COPD and long COVID-19).

Why the focus on breath *suspension* ***(i.e., the pause at the bottom of the breath) versus retention (the pause at the top of the breath)***
Breath retentions after the inhalation do not promote the release of nitric oxide and thus do not have the same benefits of creating vasodilation and bronchodilation and associated respiratory benefits. Breath retentions depend more on lung volume and work less with residual volume. They can result in rib flare, aggravating incomplete patterns of exhalation, especially with age. Breath retentions also have a less helpful effect on O_2 saturation (*not* creating hypoxia) and may not have the same benefits for exercise performance as breath suspensions. It has been argued that breath suspension is also more calming and accessible for most individuals because they arise in the context of a relaxed (rather than contracted diaphragm).

10.3.2 Breathing Practice: Equal Breathing

Focusing on both inhalation and exhalation phases of the breath, equal breathing is called *sama vritti* in Sanskrit. *Sama* can be translated as *equal* or *regular*; *vritti* is translated as *fluctuation*. The essence of this practice is equalization of the fluctuation of inhalations (*puraka* in Sanskrit) and exhalations (*rechaka* in Sanskrit). This equalization is most commonly taught as related to length of inspiration and expiration. However, it can be applied to any breath quality, including volume, texture and sound, location and space, and even resting pauses of inhalation and exhalation. Equal breathing can be utilized as a subtle breathing practice and in that application can lead to hyperventilation. Clinician vigilance is therefore recommended.

Sequencing Equal Breathing

Equal breathing is a subtle breathing practice for most clients. As such, it can be sequenced relatively early in a breathwork series overall, but after basic psychoeducation and facility with breath attunement practices. It is not ideal as the very first subtle breathing practice offered; most of the subtle breaths detailed in Chap. 9 are a better choice (e.g., feather breathing, hands-cupping-face). It is appropriate relatively early in a practice series, with care taken that the individual is equalizing length without inadvertently increasing volume, as this could lead to hyperventilation despite fewer breaths per minute. More experienced clients can add observation and equalization of volume, texture, and location, all of which require more sensitivity and interoception.

Equal breathing can be used at any logical point within a session when current intention matches the dynamics of equal breathing. It can be used for its calming and focusing effects at the beginning or end of a session, with intention or desired effect guiding which part of the session to choose. It can be explored within dynamic movement (e.g., in cat-cow, half sun salutation, and other short vinyasa style movements), during which equalization of inhalation and exhalation is translated physically into the length of the movement. Equal breathing is generally safe for home practice once other subtle breathing practices have been understood, both as a standalone practice and in the context of mindful movement. Adjusting equal breathing for polyvagal state is embedded in the key instructions.

Key Instructions and Cuing Tips for Equal Breathing

Equal breathing is integrated in a practice that has established calming and peacefulness, breath attunement, and thorough education about optimal functional breathing, as with other introductions of subtle breathing. When the client has established a natural breathing rhythm, equal breathing practice can begin. The instructions that follow are offered slowly and patiently, with significant pauses between steps to allow clients adequate time for exploration and interoception. Once a client has engaged in equal breathing repeatedly over the course of several sessions, the process may unfold more quickly. Equal breathing can be offered in any position and with movement, based on intention and client needs.

1. Begin with awareness of the natural breath cycle, sensing inhalations and exhalations and perhaps noting natural pauses as well—give ample time
2. Become familiar with the inhalation—start with observing texture, smoothness, sound, and volume
3. Explore the length of the inhalations via one of more of the following strategies:
   • Consciously counting (which can be helpful for beginners) and then calculating average length of each aspect of breath
   • Estimating length (especially for more seasoned students)
   • Using the letters of the alphabet
   • Reciting one's name or a brief mantra
4. Once the client has had time to meet the inhalation, explore the length of the exhalations using the same strategies
5. Choose how to equalize rate based on intention or need, using comfort in breath and arousal (PVT) as the guiding principle if possible
6. The changes offered in equalizing rate can be activating or calming or balancing—choose options for clients based on intention set earlier in practice and based on observation:
   • *Activating*: lengthening the inhalation to meet a longer exhalation *or* shortening the exhalation to meet the shorter inhalation
   • *Calming*: lengthening the exhalation to meet a longer inhalation *or* shortening the inhalation to meet a shorter exhalation
   • *Balancing*: meeting in the middle *or* slowing the breath rate to 5–6 breaths per minutes with balanced breathing
7. If unsure about how to equalize, start with equalizing rate of breath by lengthening the shorter part of the breath or shortening the longer part, or a little of both
8. End equal breathing by returning to a spontaneous rhythm of breath
9. Close the practice with natural optimal functional breathing, cuing calming as needed

Additional Notes for Clinicians

For more seasoned students, other breath qualities can be equalized, including volume, texture, and space/location, using similar cuing:

• First, draw awareness to natural manifestations, then to observation of differences in inhalation versus exhalatio
• Second, offer instructions to equalize the manifestation in the most intentional and beneficial way given client needs
   – *For volume*—notice if one aspect moves more air than the other; then equalize by deepening one or making the other shallower, depending on what best serves client needs for self-regulation based on observed polyvagal state
   – *For texture*—notice if the breath is smoother in one aspect or the other; if not, equalize texture by making the less smooth phase smoother

- *For sound*—notice if the breath is noisier in one aspect or the other; if not, equalize sound by making the noisier phase quiet
- *For location*—notice if aspects of the breath are noticeable in the same body location or space; if not—equalize by inviting the client to direct the inhalation and exhalation symmetrically or in a spatially evenly-distributed manner or in a spatial pattern of the *pancha vayus* (e.g., from the center to the edges, both downward, and so on)
- Throughout, remind clients to breathe
  - Nasally
  - Comfortably diaphragmatically
  - Lightly (i.e., not moving excessive volume) to keep the breath subtle
  - Rhythmically and slowly (lower rate; 5.5–10 bpm)
  - Quietly and smoothly

Recommended Observations to Help Guide Cuing
- *Rate*: notice any changes in breath qualities (e.g., volume, sound, space, or rest) as breath begins to become slower in rate (i.e., longer)—this may help identify struggles
- *Volume*: notice how breath changes in terms of amount of air moving in and out as breath equalizes (either in terms of length, space, or rest)
- *Texture and sound*: notice if there is a change in the texture of the breath as breath equalizes (either in terms of length, volume, space, or rest)
- *Space and location*: notice how the location changes where breath is felt most easily; notice if it is different how easy or hard it is to feel the breath in the body as breath equalizes (either in terms of length, volume, or rest)
- *Rests*: assess if there is a natural change in the presence of breath pauses as breath equalizes (either in terms of length, volume, space, or rest)

Sample Variation of Equal Breathing
Box breathing is a vitalizing version of equal breathing that is often recommended (somewhat undiscerningly) in yoga and clinical contexts. It is actually a very challenging breath flow because it requires equal cadence in inhalation, retention, exhalation, and suspension. The length of the count for the lingering in any given phase can be adjusted to clients' needs and nervous system state. Exploration of what is most adaptive for the client is recommended, rather than using a predetermined count of breathing for four or five beats per phase (a commonly-given instruction). The same context as recommended for equal breathing in general is established for box breathing, with extra vigilance to acute dysregulation, as breath pauses or holds are part of this equal breath rhythm. Working with the client on determining the length of the breath phases is key to making box breathing a supportive and useful breath. An indiscriminate or standard cadence can be dysregulating and defeats the purpose of this breath.

1. Start from natural breathing
2. Begin with an inhalation of an established count, breathing in and counting
3. Retain the breath for the established count, holding and counting
4. Exhale for the established count, exhaling and counting
5. Suspend the breath for the established count, holding and counting
6. Repeat for several rounds, returning to natural breathing if signs of dysregulation appear

10.3.3 Breathing Practice: Breathing with Extended Exhalation

In Sanskrit, this type of breathing is called *vishama vritti* with extended *rechaka*, where *vishama* is the opposite of *sama* (as in *sama vritti*), *meaning irregular or uneven fluctuations* of the breath. As a reminder, *sama vritti* refers to equal breathing—inhalation and exhalation (or all breath phases, as in box breathing) are matched to one another. In *vishama vritti*, inhalation and exhalation are deliberately disparate from one another, in this case extending the length of the exhalation. Extension of exhalation, practiced with care, represents subtle breathing that reduces volume of breath moved per breath cycle and decreases breath rate. It is a calming and grounding breath associated with increased parasympathetic activity, toning the vagus nerve, and putting the brakes on the sympathetic nervous system. However, overly extending the exhalation, as competitive individuals might seek to do, can obviate the typically calming effects of this breath.

Sequencing Extended Exhalation
Across a series of sessions, extended exhalation can be integrated once psychoeducation, breath attunement, and beginning subtle breathing practices (as detailed in Chap. 9) have been successfully introduced. This can happen relatively early in a beginner's practice as long as the client understands not to overdo the lengthening. Depending on client traits and needs, extended exhalation can be helpful at the beginning or end of a yoga or clinical session, especially at a time of day when clients may feel exhausted or tired and are in need of destressing and releasing (e.g., after a long workday). The intention or desired session effect further guides when during the session to use this breath—it can be useful when relaxation or calming is indicated (as long as lengthening is minimal to moderate only). Extended exhalation can be explored in the context of asanas that have dynamic holds during the lengthening exhalation (e.g., lowering the arms very slowly from extended mountain pose to arm by the side; gentle lowering out of bridge pose with a long exhalation, perhaps after an extended hold of the posture; moving extra slowly and deliberately through cat with a subsequent natural move through cow during inhalation). Extended exhalation is fine for home practice with clear parameters of when and how to use it (i.e., for calming and relaxing and not while already sluggish or depressed).

Key Instructions and Cuing Tips for Extended Exhalation
Extension of exhalation is offered in the context of a session that has already established calming, breath attunement, and subtle breathing. When the client has

established a natural breathing rhythm, breathing with extended exhalation can be invited. Extending the exhalation can be grounding, or it can be offered as a subtle breathing practice. The clinician needs to be clear about the current purpose and modify cuing accordingly, stressing calming and grounding if ease is desirable for the current nervous system state, and stressing the lengthening of the exhalation if the goal is subtle breathing that supports healthier breath biochemistry. This breath can be practiced in any position and during movement, chosen commensurate with intention and client need. The following instructions assume that the client is already familiar with equal breathing. If this is not the case, some additional guidance may be needed and can be drawn from the cuing for equal breathing.

1. Start with natural breath observation
2. Then invite measuring lengths of inhalation and exhalation with subsequent adjustment to support equal breathing (using the alphabet, numbers, or other strategies)
3. Then invite a conscious and deliberate lengthening in the exhalation—work to the point of comfort—the following inhalation should not be desperate or gasping
4. Be clear about the intention in cuing extension of the exhalation:
   - For grounding and calming, the extension is minimal and leads to no discomfort; cuing focuses on observing the calming and grounding nature of the gently and slowly (over time) lengthening exhalation
   - For subtle breathing, extension may be slightly longer, and attention paid to any signs of breath dysregulation (see instructions for basic nasal breathing variation in Chap. 9)
5. Transition the practice by coming back to an equal rhythm (1:1) in two ways:
   - By reducing length of exhalation, *or*
   - By *also* extending the inhalation and creating an even ratio that way—the latter may be a more challenging practice (depending on just how uneven the ratio was) as it requires a lower breath rate and may simply serve to increase breath volume; it may also lead to straining in the breath which is contraindicated—proceed with caution
6. Close the practice with natural optimal functional breathing, cuing calming as needed

Additional Notes for Clinicians
- Remind clients to breathe lightly (i.e., not moving excessive volume) and to not overeffort with the extension of the exhalation
- Remind clients to breathe slowly and easefully (i.e., reducing respiratory rate), including on the inhalation
- Caution clients that if the inhalation feels desperate or gasping, they are making the extension of the exhalation too long
- Remind students to breathe rhythmically, smoothly, and silently
- Remind students to breathe into the low rib basket and mid-section of the torso with ease (i.e., comfortably diaphragmatic)

Recommended Observations to Help Guide Cuing

- *Rate*: notice consciously and deliberately any changes in length of breath overall and note how lengthening the exhalation affects length of the inhalation
- *Volume*: notice how breath changes in terms of amount of air moving in and out as the exhalation extends in length—often, the longer the breath, the more air is moved in a single breath cycle—no the true goal for the practice
- *Texture and sound*: notice if there is a change in the texture as the exhalation extends; notice if texture suggests that breath is dysregulating; adjust length to re-regulate to a length that can support smoothness in texture
- *Space and location*: notice how location where breath is noticed most easily changes as the exhalation is extended; notice if ease changes with which breath is felt in the body
- *Rests*: notice if there is a natural change in pauses as the exhalation extends; in particular notice if there is spontaneous suspension that may lead to gasping at the point of inhalation; let that inform cuing to help decrease such gasping

Sample Variation of Extended Exhalation

Pausing for Recovery is an application of extended exhalation in daily life. Once the practice can be easily accomplished in session and predictably leads to grounding or calming, it can be taken into daily life as a method of emotional or stress recovery during challenge. Clients are encouraged to notice interoceptively and neuroceptively when they become emotionally reactive, sympathetically aroused, or tempted to disconnect. In those moments, they can invite a focus on their breathing, first locating the current breath manifestation in all its phases. Focus then shifts from noticing how the breath is emerging in the moment, by observing and tending to the exhalation. If the exhalation is choppy or raspy, it may be smoothed. If it is quick and shallow, it may be softened and lengthened. Creating calm, soft, smooth extension in the exhalation can help the individual shift from bottom-up reactivity to top-down self-regulation. The client can stay with this exhalation-focused breathing for as long as necessary.

10.3.4 Breathing Practice: Breathing with Extended Inhalation

This type of breathing is called *vishama vritti* with extended *puraka*, where *vishama* is the opposite of *sama* (as in *sama vritti),* meaning irregular or uneven fluctuations of the breath. In this *vishama vritti*, inhalation and exhalation are deliberately disparate from one another, by extending the length of the inhalation. Extension of the inhalation is activating and energizing; inhalation is associated with the sympathetic nervous system. This breath is helpful for individuals who are in an energetic slump (yet not exhausted) and need a quick pick-me-up. Some teachers joke that this breathing is better than a cup of coffee. Because of its activating or energizing nature, it does not have great utility for many clients—not being helpful for individuals who are already chronically sympathetically aroused and/or hyperventilating. This practice appears to be most helpful for individuals with a dorsal vagal nervous system default. It is essential to note the difference between dorsal vagal collapse and exhaustion or burnout from chronic hyperarousal. The latter clients do not tend to benefit from this practice. The careful discernment necessary about which individuals do and do not benefit from different ways of working with the phases of breath, especially with pauses and inhalations, may explain why B.K.S. Iyengar [14] has expressed concern about *vishama vritti* practices, promoting the use of *sama vritti* (or equal breathing) over breaths with disparate lengths and volumes in their phases. Carefully tailored choices need to be made about how to use breath phases, adapting the offering to the needs of each client.

Sequencing Extended Inhalation
Across a breathwork series, extended inhalation can be introduced (with clients who are appropriate for this practice) once clients are at ease with breath attunement, have a basic understanding of the psychoeducational information that guides their motivation and intention for breathwork, and know how to return themselves to a ventral vagal state via natural breathing or breathing with conscious exhalation. Expanded inhalation practice might be interspersed with subtle breathing practices as appropriate given clients' current-moment nervous system arousal.

Extended inhalation can be helpful at the beginning of a breathwork session, especially at a time of day when clients may feel slightly lethargic but not exhausted (e.g., at lunch time, to reenergize sluggish lymph systems and overworked minds or bodies). This practice can be explored in movements that coordinate dynamic muscular engagement with lengthening inhalation (e.g., raising the arms slowly against imaginary or actual resistance into an extended mountain pose with inhalation, with a subsequent natural release of the arms back down during exhalation; or moving with slow and deliberate muscular contraction and working into a cow shape with inhalation, with a subsequent natural move through cat during exhalation). For clients for whom this type of breathing is indicated, the practice is fine at home with clear parameters of when and how to use it (i.e., for energizing or activating, not while already anxious, hyper, or uneasy). It is important for clients to understand possible contraindications and how to spot hyperventilation if they practice this breath on their own. In other words, they need to have interoceptive and neuroceptive skills to prevent overdoing the lengthening and activation. Seasoned clients can use the practice with vigorous movement as long as they understand how to rebalance their vitality, mind, and emotions. Teaching clients recovery breathing is an excellent preventive measure.

Key Instructions and Cuing Tips for Extended Exhalation
Extension of inhalation is offered in the context of breathwork that has already established calming, breath attunement, and subtle breathing. When the client has established a natural breathing rhythm, breathing with extended inhalation can be

invited. Extension of the inhalation is activating and the clinician needs to double-check, based on what has already transpired in the session up to this point, that this remains an appropriate practice for the patient in this moment. This breath can be offered in any position and is particular helpful when grounded within a movement practice. Cuing assumes facility with equal breathing and is modified appropriately if this is not the case.

1. Start with natural breath awareness
2. Invite observing and measuring the lengths of inhalation and exhalation with subsequent adjustment to support equal breathing, as described above
3. Invite conscious and deliberate lengthening in inhalation—work to the point of comfort; exhalation should not be desperate
4. End the practice by coming back to an equal rhythm (1:1) in two ways:
   • By reducing length of inhalation, *or*
   • By also extending the exhalation and creating an even ratio that way—the latter may be a more challenging practice (depending on just how uneven the ratio was) as it requires a lower breath rate and decreases breath volume; it may lead to straining in the breath which is contraindicated—proceed with caution
5. Close the practice with natural optimal functional breathing, cuing calming as needed

Additional Notes for Clinicians
• Remind clients to breathe lightly (i.e., not moving excessive volume), not to overeffort with the extension of the inhalation
• Remind clients to breathe slowly overall (i.e., reducing respiratory rate), especially on the inhalation
• Caution clients that if the exhalation feels desperate, extension of the inhalation may be too long
• Notice if the pause after the inhalation evolves into a breath hold instead
• Remind students to breathe rhythmically, smoothly, and silently
• Remind students to breathe into the low rib basket and mid-section of the torso with ease (i.e., comfortably diaphragmatic)

Recommended Observations to Help Guide Cuing
• *Rate*: notice consciously and deliberately any changes in the length of the breath overall and note how lengthening the inhalation affects the length of the exhalation
• *Volume*: notice how the breath changes in terms of amount of air moving in and out as the inhalation extends in length—often the longer the breath, the more air is moved in a single breath cycle
• *Texture and sound*: notice if there is a change in the texture of the breath as the inhalation extends; notice if the texture or sound suggests that the breath is

dysregulating and adjust the length to reregulate the breath to a length that can support smoothness in texture
- *Space and location*: notice how the location where the breath is felt most easily changes as the inhalation is extended; notice if it is different how easy or difficult it is to feel the breath in the body
- *Rests*: notice if there is a natural change in the presence of pauses in the breath cycle as the inhalation extends, especially note if there is sudden breath retention

Sample Variation for Extended Inhalation

Extended Exhalation in Half Sun Salutes is an invigorating variation of this breath that adds arousal and movement to this practice. It may be helpful for moments of tiredness or listlessness (but not burnout) in the morning or at times of day after excessive sitting or inactivity. It combines a heart-opening physical movement flow with breath. The heart-opening is combined with lengthening inhalations to invite a sense of uplifting mental energy and increased vitality. This flow can be a wonderful gratitude practice by adding a focus on receiving the nurturance of the inhalation, with the heart space physically open.

The practice starts with a few moments of natural breath awareness. The instruction invites use of blocks so as not to overstretch the back of the body, to ensure that the flow is easeful. If a stronger physical flow is invited, physical warm-up is indicated first (e.g., six movements of the spine). For newer clients, this flow may be demonstrated by the clinician first, with appropriate physical guidance for each aspect of the movement.

1. Stand in mountain pose and breathe naturally, being aware of each inhalation as it travels in, perhaps noting the pause at the top of the breath; become aware of each exhalation as it travels out, perhaps aware of the pause at the bottom of the breath.
2. Breathe with awareness and appreciation for a few rounds of breath. Note the nurturing and uplifting energy of each inhalation, absorbing it into your tissue and letting it warm your heart and open your mind.
3. Lengthening your next inhalation and raise the arms forward and up, perhaps letting your gaze follow as you move into a slight spinal extension (or backbend). Perhaps linger here for a moment.
4. With your exhalation, dive forward maintaining a natural spine; let the hands come to rest on the blocks.
5. Lengthening and focusing on the inhalation, lift part-way up, hands resting on the blocks gaze moving slightly forward as you lift half-way, taking in the warmth and uplifting energy of the inhalation.
6. With the exhalation, release forward.
7. With a new long and open inhalation rise all the way up, heart lifting—receiving the warmth of the breath, the vitality of this moment, expansive and spacious as the inhalation lengthens and travels in slowly

8. With the exhalation, return the arms and hands to your sides and breathe naturally.
9. Repeat as desired.

This practice can also be offered seated on a chair with the same energetic, mental, and physical impact. It is a paced way of introducing extended inhalation and, when offered mindfully, can create more accessibility into extension than either a movement or a breathing practice alone. The meditative focus adds safety for the mind, regulates emotions, and makes most clients tolerant of the shifts in biochemistry.

10.3.5 Breathing Practice: Breathing with Breath Suspension

Four-part breathing is nothing new or modern; in fact, as noted earlier, it is the very essence of yogic breathing as reflected in the *Yoga Sutras of Patanjali*. Four-part breathing reminds us that breathing is not about breathing hard or deep. Instead, breathing is about setting the breath free, allowing it to unfold its essence with a rhythm that is slow and subtle; a cadence that honors preservation of vitality and energy through moderation in all we do. In the context of four-part breathing, *retention* refers to the pause at the top of the inhalation; *suspension* refers to the pause at the bottom of the exhalation. These pauses are natural and subtle (called *stambha* in Sanskrit); they are not an intentional holding of breath. *Intentional* lengthening of these transition periods is called *kumbhaka* and reflects a more advanced breathing practice of using breath holds for particular purposes in the body (biomechanically), breath and energy (biochemically), and mind or psyche (psychologically). Our primary focus here is on light to moderate breath suspension (*bahya kumbhaka* in Sanskrit). Four-part breathing practice begins with exploring natural pauses (*stambha*) and, after careful assessment and use of pauses, progresses to deliberately longer extensions or holding (*kumbakha*) of the bottom pause, creating longer breath suspension.

Cautions and Contraindications for Breath Suspension
Strong breath holds, much like forced breathing (see Chap. 11), are designed as stressors to cultivate greater capacity for adaptation and resilience. They cause vasoconstriction in blood vessels in the extremities (see the lobster claw caution in the *Kapalabhati* section in Chap. 11), are very vitalizing and upregulating, and can dysregulate respiratory biochemistry. They can have a profound impact on psychology—affecting clients mentally and emotionally—due to the challenges they present. They can be powerful practices of hormesis, inviting us to explore and relax into difficulty and creating new resilience.

Strong, effortful, or very long breath holds (lasting a minute or more) are not recommended in breathwork offered in healthcare contexts or therapeutic yoga settings. Focus in such settings is on short to moderate, sustainable breath holds. It serves to note that *strong breath holds* are contraindicated for several types of practitioners, including, but not necessarily limited to, individuals with the following conditions:

- Migraines
- Panic or acute anxiety disorders
- Cardiovascular disease, including hypertension
- Severe sleep apnea
- Pregnancy
- Type 1 diabetes
- Renal disease
- Seizures
- Glaucoma, retinal or vitreous detachment
- And perhaps other conditions

For clients with these concerns, care needs is taken with any type of breath hold (even holds typically considered short or moderate) via client observation, education about impacts and signs of dysregulation, and assurance of adequate self-awareness and interoceptive capacity. Client and clinician need to be prepared to return to attunement, natural breathing, and recovery breathing at the first signs of trouble (e.g., spasms in the abdomen, strain in neck muscles, sudden chest breathing, anxiety, and more; see Table 9.2). For individuals who have medical conditions listed earlier (or similar chronic or acute physical and mental health challenges), it is best to start with breath *pausing* practices withing a context of relaxation and breath attunement to invite a sense of ease and safety. Pauses are short and comfortable; they do not create air hunger or discomfort. Over time, especially if symptoms or conditions resolve, longer comfortable breath pauses may be introduced carefully and slowly, with constant check-ins with the client to prevent panic or breath dysregulation. It is helpful to monitor heart rate, and if it is easily dysregulated, breath holds are not indicated. If heart rate does not recover to baseline within 5–10 min, strong breath holds are best avoided.

Short breath pauses seem to be safe for individuals with coughing, wheezing, stress, sleep challenges, panic disorders, distraction, poor attention, and even asthma. As shown in Table 11.2 in Chap. 11, they can be used as rescue breathing and to prevent a full panic or asthma attack when used cautiously in the presence of a clinician who is available for co-regulation to support the client's return to a ventral vagal nervous system state.

Sequencing Breath Suspension

Short breath pauses are appropriate once clients are at ease with breath attunement practices focused on breath phases and have achieved comfort with subtle breathing practices offered in Chap. 9. Short breath pauses can be integrated with natural breath observation without prompting an increase in the pauses—simply focusing on whether pauses are naturally present. In that context, short breath pauses can be invited early in a session, depending on level of practice, with observation of pauses being most appropriate at the beginning, and significant lengthening better placed toward the middle of a session (allowing for adequate preparation *and* recovery time).

If the invited increase in the pause is minimal, both top and bottom pauses can be cued, using discernment and remaining vigilant about patients' ability and comfort levels. Lengthening of pauses is, of course, possible for retention and suspension. The recommendation here is to focus on suspension over retention because of the added benefits of suspension. Once facility is constant in session, clients can engage in home practice with short breath pauses. Breath pauses—at top and bottom—can be safely explored in movements that have four parts. For example, clients may move into cow with the inhalation, hold both shape and breath for a moment, then move into cat with the exhalation and hold both shape and the breath at the bottom. The length of inhalation, retention, exhalation, and suspension are translated physically into the length of the movement (e.g., move into and stay in cow [inhale] for the same amount of time as you move into and stay in cat [exhale]) and the length of the hold of the anchoring postures (i.e., the length in cow without movement; the length of cat without movement). Interestingly, this combination of four-part breathing with movement often is more accessible for clients than the breathing practice by itself.

Key Instructions and Cuing Tips for Breath Suspension

Breath holds and pauses, no matter how short, are predicated on a co-regulating relationship between clinician and client, prerequisite calming and breath attunement practices, and capacity for subtle breathing. Once the client manifests a natural breathing rhythm, focus on pauses and/or breath holds is added gradually. Breath holds can be very activating or very calming, depending on context and client nervous system state. Before proceeding with a premade plan for breath holds, clinician double-checks, based on what has already transpired in the session up to this point, that this remains an appropriate practice plan for the patient in this moment. Breath suspension can be accessed in any position and during movement. Familiarity with equal breathing is helpful; experience with breath observation of the four parts of breath is key. The following instructions invite the suspension to happen with manually closed nostrils. This is not appropriate for all clients and can be skipped. Most clients are able to suspend the breath for brief holds without closing the nostrils using their fingers. Obviously, if the suspension occurs in the context of movement, no fingers are used to create the suspension.

1. Start with natural breath observation, mostly with the purpose of supporting relaxation and accessing a ventral vagal state
2. Invite measuring the length of inhalation and exhalation and subsequent adjustment to support either equal breathing or extended exhalation breathing
3. Invite one or both of the following in sequence:
   • One of the subtle breathing practices (more challenging)
   • Observation of natural pauses (more calming)
4. Add a conscious or deliberately slightly longer natural pause at the bottom of breath and notice how this unfolds in the clients' experience

5. Invite possible lengthening from *breath pauses* to *breath holds*, only to the point to comfort (i.e., the inhalation should not be desperate or gasping); cue the following sequence:
   - Take a gentle breath in
   - Take a gentle breath out
   - Then gently pinch the nose shut with two fingers of the same hand (optional)
   - Hold for 3–5 s
   - Gently breathe in through the nose; nasal inhalation is key to benefit from the nitric oxide that was produced during breath suspension
   - Gently breathe in and out for about 10 s for recovery
   - Then repeat this process
   - As comfort develops, suspensions can become longer
   - Do this practice for no more than 10 min at a time
6. End the practice by returning to a spontaneous rhythm
7. Close the practice with natural optimal functional breathing, cuing calming as needed
8. If the practice was successful, it can be recommended for home practice
   - In the same way and for the same purposes as breathing with breath extension
   - Or for purposes of resetting biochemistry—in this case the practice is recommended hourly

Additional Notes for Clinicians
- Cue comfort during pauses, ensuring that clients understand that they should not be gasping for air when they begin to inhale again; there should be no (significant) sensation of discomfort—caution clients neither to overdo nor to overly strive for a particular length in the hold
- If the client's-controlled breath pause is known, suspension could start with half the length of CPB; if it is not known, a safe start for most people is approximately 3–5 s
- Remind clients to breathe lightly (i.e., not moving excessive volume) to keep the breath natural even with the pause or hold at the bottom
- Remind clients to breathe slowly (i.e., reducing respiratory rate) to keep breath optimal even with the pause or hold at the bottom
- Caution clients that if the breath feels gasping or desperate, they are pushing the pauses too long
  - Work up to longer suspensions gradually, with patience and acceptance
  - Use this as a reminder to clients to practice effort *and* ease
  - Remind clients to dwell in non-attachment to a specific outcome or goal
- Remind clients to breathe rhythmically, smoothly, and silently
- Remind clients to breathe into the low rib basket and mid-section of the torso with ease (i.e., comfortably diaphragmatic)

Recommended Observations to Help Guide Cuing

- *Rate*: notice how breath rate changes as breath pauses lengthen at the bottom
- *Volume*: notice how breath changes in terms of volume as breath pauses lengthen at the bottom
- *Texture and sound*: notice if there is a change in the texture of the breath as the breath pauses lengthen at the bottom
- *Space and location*: notice if location where the breath is felt most easily changes; notice if it is easier or harder to feel the breath in the body as the breath pauses lengthen at the bottom
- *Rests*: notice if there is an uncued increase in pauses at the top as the pause at the bottom is encouraged

Sample Variations of Breath Suspension

High-Altitude Simulation is a challenging version of breath suspension with movement, arising from Oxygen Advantage Training by Patrick McKeown [12]. It is a maximum breath hold—not a comfortable pause—and hence recommended for clients in good health and with significant breathwork experience. It is started after having established a natural and resilient breathing rhythm and starts with a natural inhalation.

1. Inhale naturally and exhale naturally. At the end of the exhalation, use the fingers to pinch the nose shut to ensure a full breath hold.
2. During breath suspension, start walking—slowly increasing pace and vigor of the movement; jogging is fine for some clients.
3. Keep suspending the breath—relax into contractions that may begin and attempt a maximum breath pause (i.e., a strong breath hold).
4. When air hunger becomes very strong, release the nostrils and breath; *breathe nasally only* (despite any urge to breathe in through the mouth) to draw in the nitic oxide that accumulated in the nose during the suspension. Reduce walking speed and come to a stop.
5. If possible, keep the breath subtle for a few rounds; then, recover a natural and resilient breath rhythm.
6. Repeat up to five times.

This practice is also a strong breath-hold practice for nasal clearing. It creates hypoxia and simulates high-altitude breathing. It can be a useful practice for athletes to enhance endurance.

10.4   Where We Go from Here

This chapter presented a toolbox for specialized breathing practices focused on the four phases of breath (i.e., four-part breathing). It established the importance of variation and adaptation, providing three paradigms for creating accessibility and adaptability in breathwork. It invited clinicians to reflect on how to add movement and posture considerations to breathing practices; it emphasized the importance of ensuring that polyvagal states and individual needs of clients are attended to (based on the comprehensive assessments collected about them before beginning breathwork per se); and it challenged clinicians to ponder how breathwork can be generalized into daily life.

All of the learning about adaptation and variation in the context of four-part breathing will next be applied to specialized breathing practices focused on alternate and single nostril breathing, breathing with sound, and breathing with force or against the grain of natural breath flow. These are practices of interest in Chap. 11 and round out the clinician's toolbox.

When the breath wanders, the mind is unsteady. But when the breath is calmed, the mind too will be still.—Yogi Swatmarama

References

1. Porges SW. Polyvagal theory: a science of safety. Front Integr Neurosci. 2022;16:871227. https://doi.org/10.3389/fnint.2022.871227.
2. Porges SW, Carter SC. Polyvagal theory and the social engagement system. In: Complementary and integrative treatments in psychiatric practice. American Psychiatric Association; 2017. p. 221–40.
3. Laborde S, Allen MS, Borges U, et al. Effects of voluntary slow breathing on heart rate and heart rate variability: a systematic review and a meta-analysis. Neurosci Biobehav Rev. 2022;138:104711. https://doi.org/10.1016/j.neubiorev.2022.104711.
4. Van Diest I, Verstappen K, Aubert AE, Widjaja D, Vansteenwegen D, Vlemincx E. Inhalation/exhalation ratio modulates the effect of slow breathing on heart rate variability and relaxation. Appl Psychophysiol Biofeedback. 2014;39:171–80. https://doi.org/10.1007/s10484-014-9253-x.
5. Adhana R, Gupta R, Dvivedii J, Ahmad S. The influence of the 2:1 yogic breathing technique on essential hypertension. Indian J Physiol Pharmacol. 2013;57(1):38–44. https://www.ncbi.nlm.nih.gov/pubmed/24020097
6. Zaccaro A, Piarulli A, Laurino M, et al. How breath-control can change your life: a systematic review on psycho-physiological correlates of slow breathing. Front Hum Neurosci. 2018;12:353. https://doi.org/10.3389/fnhum.2018.00353.
7. Noventi I, Sholihah U, Hasina SN, Wijayanti L. The effectiveness of mindfulness based stress reduction and sama vritti pranayama on reducing blood pressure, improving sleep quality and reducing stress levels in the elderly with hypertension. Bali Med J. 2022;11(1):302–5. https://doi.org/10.15562/bmj.v11i1.3108.
8. Bhavanani AB, Raj JB, Ramanathan M, Trakroo M. Effect of different pranayamas on respiratory sinus arrhythmia. J Clin Diagn Res. 2016;10(3):CC04–6. https://doi.org/10.7860/JCDR/2016/16306.7408.
9. Bentley TGK, D'Andrea-Penna G, Rakic M, et al. Breathing practices for stress and anxiety reduction: conceptual framework of implementation guidelines based on a systematic review of the published literature. Brain Sci. 2023;13(12):1612. https://doi.org/10.3390/brainsci13121612.

10. Kimberley B, Nejadnik B, Giraud GD, Holden WE. Nasal contribution to exhaled nitric oxide at rest and during breathholding in humans. Am J Respir Crit Care Med. 1996;153(2):829–36. https://doi.org/10.1164/ajrccm.153.2.8564139.

11. Reyes del Paso GA, Muñoz Ladrón de Guevara C, Montoro CI. Breath-holding during exhalation as a simple manipulation to reduce pain perception. Pain Med. 2015;16(9):1835–41. https://doi.org/10.1111/pme.12764.

12. McKeown P. Oxygen advantage: the simple, scientifically proven breathing techniques for a healthier, slimmer, faster, and fitter you. William Morrow; 2015.

13. Foster GE, Sheel AW. The human diving response, its function, and its control. Scand J Med Sci Sports. 2005;15(1):3–12. https://doi.org/10.1111/j.1600-0838.2005.00440.x.

14. Iyengar BKS. Light on pranayama. HarperCollins; 2013.

Specialized Intentional Breathwork

11

*To place you in my heart may turn you into a thought, I will not
do that. I will set you on my breath so you will become my life.*

Rumi

11.1 Overview: Diversity and Variation in Breathing

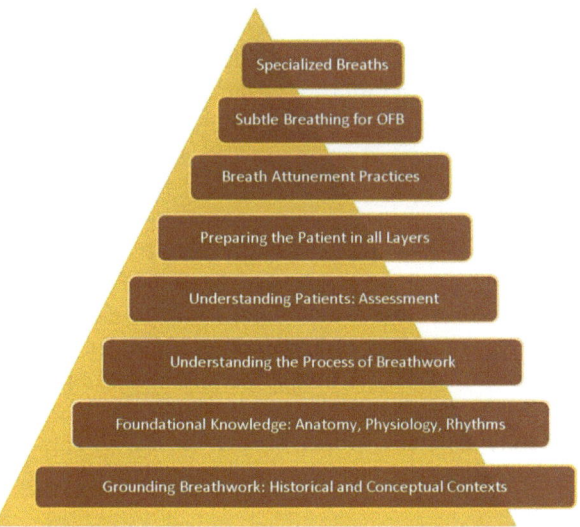

This chapter presents three essential categories of specialized breathing practices
that have specific purposes and can be tailored in a multitude of ways (summarized
in Table 10.1). This exploration builds upon breathing practices that draw on the

four phases of the breath (presented in Chap. 10), on subtle breathing, and on breath attunement practices. It introduces alternate and single nostril breathing practices and then shifts to more challenging practices that involve breathing with sound and/ or force. As was true for Chap. 10, all practices are used selectively based on patient needs and are meant to be adapted to specific contexts of clients' presentations and circumstances. These strategies are purposeful—they are not offered in a uniform way to all clients, nor simplistically by differentiating beginning or advanced practitioners (often the only tailoring offered). There are clients who have been engaging in yogic or other breathing practices for years—but choosing strategies that actually have served to perpetuate and reinforce dysfunctional breathing. For example, many individuals enjoy *kapalabhati* breathing and never realize that it perpetuates their chronic hyperventilation. It is essential to understand the client's complexity to select and apply specialized breathing strategies in the most patient-centered and appropriate way.

Similar to the four-part breathing-oriented practices of Chap. 10, the practices in this chapter have numerous variations that enhance resilience, coherence, and adaptability in the breath. Chap. 10 provided useful details about how to shape adaptations and variation via three specific foci: breathing with movement, breathing for polyvagal state, and generalizing breathing practices into daily life. These details are employed again in this chapter, applying them no to nostril breathing, breathing with sound, and breathing with force. An additional variation that is offered for these practices is an added focus within these breathing strategies on particular phases of the breath. For example, breathing with sound can be varied with emphasis on the inhalation or exhalation; breathing with force may be embedded in a context of four-part breathing. Offering variations that are carefully tailored to client needs becomes increasingly crucial as the demand characteristics of the offered therapeutic breathwork increase.

11.2   Learning Alternate and Single Nostril Breathing

The many variations of alternate and single nostril breathing make this practice enormously interesting, variable, and adaptive in terms of effects on nervous system, psychology, cardiovascular and respiratory health, and many other systems of human anatomy and physiology. Three primary types of practices detailed in this category involve either breathing while emphasizing the left nostril, the right nostril, or alternatingly the left and right nostril, making a switch either at the top or bottom of the breath.

11.2.1 Preliminary Comments About Nostril Breathing

Following are general comments that apply to all types of nostril breathing. After these comments, key instructions, impacts on various aspects of breath, sequencing, and variations are provided for each of the three main types of nostril breathing, namely:

- Alternating breathing between the two nostrils
- Breathing emphasizing the left nostril
- Breathing emphasizing the right nostril

Skill, creativity, and experience allow breathwork guides to adapt each of these practices in many different ways, depending on intention and client needs and abilities. Variations draw upon what was learned from optimal functional breathing, subtle breathing, and discovery of the four breath phases. Examples are offered further in the categories of variations via movement, polyvagal state, daily life, and integration of focus on the breath phases within the context of a specialized breathing practice.

Cautions and Guidance for Nostril Breathing

Generally speaking, nostril breathing might not be indicated during a severe head cold or sinus infections. Additionally, if a strong headache is present, this practice may be contraindicated. Nostril breathing, by definition, is a reduced or subtle breathing practice, as airflow is limited to one nostril at a time. Therefore, special care is needed with students who suffer from panic or anxiety or who have significant trauma histories. It is helpful to offer variations (e.g., imaginary nostril breathing) and empower patients to tune into their bodies and vitality, using interoception and neuroception, to make their own decisions about how to embrace this style of breathing.

Generally, alternate or single nostril breathing is practiced in an upright seat; a reclined seated posture may be possible as long as the incline is gentle. These practices are not recommended while fully supine because of the necessary use of the hands. Lying fully reclined places the strain of gravity on the lifted arm, which may lead to tightening in shoulders and neck, interfering with releasing and letting go and adding bracing or gripping. However, if nostril closure is practiced only in the imagination, a supine position is fine. If the arm becomes very heavy (even in a seated posture), it is possible to use props or support from the other arm (e.g., wrapped around the torso so the elbow of the lifted arm has support) to provide grounding for the lifted arm. If practiced at bedtime, it can be beneficial to practice lying on the right side in a half-open fetal position, with the right side of the head supported on a pillow and a pillow between the legs. The right hand is used to close the right nostril while resting the arm peacefully on the mattress.

Before moving into alternate or single nostril practices, it is helpful to demonstrate the hand position and action to be used in the practice, so as to not have to break concentration and focus when time comes to start using the fingers. Some clients find the gesture and fingering confusing. It is important to ensure that they understand the rhythm of the hand before starting the nostril breath of choice. Practicing first without involving the breath is generally a good idea, especially with the clinician demonstrating the fingering and the many possible options. The most typical gesture is shown in the following box. It is important to understand that other options are invited and that clients can create their own unique way of closing one nostril at a time. Experimentation is welcomed.

To make single or alternate nostril breathing happen biomechanically, a hand position or gesture is used to close either the right or left nostril. The traditional gesture is called *vishnu mudra* and involves curling the index and middle fingers toward the palm, and using thumb and ring finger either to close the right or the left nostril. It is fine to use the dominant hand, though in some traditions of yoga, only the right hand is used for this purpose.

Alternatively, index and middle finger can be stretched out and the tips of these fingers come to rest on the third eye—the space between and just above the eyebrows. Other fingering, based on a client's needs or preferences are also possible and options as well as creativity can override tradition to create accessibility. The fingering may feel a bit awkward at first, but with practice, it may get easier.

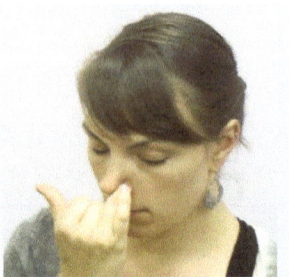

Illustration 11.1 *Vishnu mudra*

It is important not to distort the septum via excessive pressure from the fingers. Pressure exerted on the side of the nostrils is gentle and light. Restriction of air flow depends on where the fingers are placed on the nostrils. If they are very close to the opening, slightly more air can enter. If fingertips are placed into the hollow just above the opening, on the softer part of the nostril, restriction of air flow is more complete. Amount of pressure exerted by the fingertip can regulate how much air can travel in and out of a nostril. This fact can be highlighted to assure clients that they have control over whether the restriction is complete or partial. This capacity for airflow regulation is particularly helpful if the nostril through which the breath travels is congested. Clients can then exert less pressure on the closed nostril to allow some air to flow even through that side of the nose.

Some individuals may not be able to breathe only through one nostril (e.g., due to sinus blockages or other issues) or may feel triggered or panicked when closing one nostril. In this case, their chosen gesture is used, and the finger movement is made; however, this is done without actually depressing the active finger (i.e., without closing the nostril) and simply imagining the closure to encourage more flow of breath through the other nostril. The autonomic nervous system is somewhat overridden by the prefrontal cortex in this coordinated breathing, as breath flow and fingers control the breath in tandem or unison. This reality can make nostril breathing challenging for some clients and may require significant practice. To ease into nostril breathing practices, these clients may be offered breathing fully one-sided instead (rather than alternating nostrils). Alternate nostril breathing is also a powerful concentration practice and thus an excellent preliminary meditation practice.

Biomechanics, Biochemistry, and Psychology of Nostril Breathing

Since Kayser [1] first identified nostril dominance (i.e., the natural alternating closure of one nostril—see Chap. 2), the scientific literature has provided evidence of a natural nasal cycle in as many as 80% of humans. That means for the majority of clients, at any given moment, one nostril is likely more blocked than the other [2–4]. Natural, cyclical nostril blockage is due to swelling of the erectile tissue in one nostril but not in the other (or *more* swelling in one nostril than the other). The cycle has a periodicity that reportedly varies widely from individual to individual (from cycling every 30 min to 8 h) and is longer during sleep than awake hours [5, 6]. Most of the time, we are not aware that nostril dominance exists (i.e., that we are preferentially breathing more through one side of the nose), mainly because overall pressurization of the airstream does not change. However, if we are instructed to close one nostril and it happens to be the open one (i.e., the one we were relying on), we very quickly become aware of nostril dominance.

The science-based reality of nostril cycling warrants mentioning when offering nostril breathing to clients. It is useful to add that evidence exists that we can *shift* nasal dominance by persisting with breathing through the blocked nostril [6] or via a variety of other strategies (e.g., side-lying on the same side as the open nostril). This fact offers a portal to shift the nervous system from sympathetic to parasympathetic or vice versa, as the left nostril has been associated with parasympathetic arousal and the right nostril with sympathetic arousal [7–9]. Similarly, breathing through the left nostril is associated with increased activity in the right hemisphere and posterior cortex (associated with relaxation, rest, and recuperation) [10]; right-nostril breathing increases left-hemisphere activation [11, 12]. Clients can be encouraged to try breathing through the non-dominant nostril to see if the difference resolves or shifts after a few cycles if a good reason exists to do so (e.g., to support sleep via left nostril breathing). Of course, if this way of breathing to shift nostril dominance induces panic, the practice can be stopped immediately. However, giving clients the knowledge and agency that they can take measures to shift nasal dominance can be very empowering as it provides a method of nervous system self-regulation.

Nostril dominance occurs even during sleep and may be associated with duration of deep sleep [13]. Interestingly, some sleep research [14] has tied breathing through the right nostril to deep non-REM sleep and breathing through the left nostril to disrupted sleep, as experienced in sleep apnea. This finding contradicts yogic belief and much anecdotal evidence that the left nostril invites a cooler, calmer, more sleep-friendly breath; it will be necessary to track how knowledge evolves about this.

Nasal dominance can shift in relation to the following conditions:

- *Nervous system state*—the parasympathetic state is associated with the left nostril, sympathetic arousal with the right nostril
- *Hemispheric dominance*—the right nostril is open when the left hemisphere is more dominant and when the left nostril is open the right hemisphere is more dominant [15]
- *Outside temperature*—the right nostril opens when it is cold (attempting to heat the body); the left opens when it is hot (trying to cool the body) [16]
- *Mental state*—heated emotions are associated with the right nostril and depression with the left nostril [16]
- *Postural changes*—lying on the left side seems to open the right nostril, whereas lying on the right side tends to lead to left nostril dominance [6]; lying on the right is generally more conducive to easefulness and better for the heart because

it does not interfere as much with venous blood return to the heart; this aspect of science, unlike the sleep research mentioned above, aligns with ancient understandings about left versus right nostril functions

Alternate nostril breathwork has beneficial effects on brainwave activity, respiratory health, and cardiovascular functioning [17, 18]. It has been reported to increase heart rate variability [19, 20], aerobic fitness, and respiratory capacities (such as tidal volume, reserve volume, and vital capacity) [21]. It supports stress relief [22–24], reducing stress and perceptions of stress [25]. It has been shown to ease depression [26–28] and anxiety [29], enhancing overall emotional well-being [30].

Effects on biochemistry, biomechanics, and psychology differ depending on whether the nostrils alternate, or whether either the left or right nostril is closed. Alternating nostril breathing has a balancing effect on the nervous system; left nostril breathing is linked to the parasympathetic nervous system; and right nostril breathing activates the sympathetic side of the autonomic nervous system. As such, all nostril breathing practices have specific effects and can be tailored to the primary intention of the practice. Alternate nostril breathing is the default when it is uncertain whether the individual needs support in calming or vitalizing. Left nostril breathing is recruited for calming effects; right nostril breathing supports vitalization and increases energy and activation.

Sequencing of Nostril Breathing Practices

Within a breathing session, nostril breathing is preceded by natural breath attunement, perhaps tailored physical movement, and at least one of the subtle breathing practices covered in Chap. 9. Although it may appear that nasal congestion would be a contraindication for the practice, this is not necessarily the case. If clients have nasal congestion, the practices can be preceded by nasal clearing (see Table 7.15), although nostril breathing in and of itself can be clearing. It takes careful discernment about when nostril breathing needs to be abandoned in the case of congestion. Once clients seem settled into a state of concentrated focus and a natural, comfortable breath rhythm, the transition to nostril breathing can be made. It may be necessary to re-explain the hand rhythm at that moment (i.e., before actually starting nostril breathing) and the planned rhythm for the specific nostril breath (i.e., which nostril and any chosen variation). During this explanation, clients continue to breathe naturally.

The practice can be started with alternating nostrils or can initially focus only on one nostril at a time to increase accessibility. If students have specific energetic needs, single nostril breathing may be introduced first, with choice of nostril based on the client's need. Specifically, breathing in and out of *the left nostril only* may be beneficial for clients who need calming; breathing in and out of *the right nostril only* may be offered to clients in need of energizing. Notably, in the yogic tradition, nostrils typically alternate, even if the emphasis is placed on one specific energetic effect. In this case, inhalation occurs through the nostril of emphasis (i.e., left for calming; right for energizing), and exhalation is released through the other nostril. When balance is the goal (or when unsure of client need), alternating nostrils are used, inhaling left and exhaling right (more about all of the options below). Additional energetic variations can be accomplished via breath rhythms that alter breath qualities, such as rate, volume, and breath pauses, and sequencing needs to be adapted to patients' capacity. The introduction of other types of breath (e.g., extended exhalation or inhalation; breath holds) within nostril breathing is reserved for seasoned clients who have practiced alternate nostril breathing comfortably for a while.

Across sessions, nostril breathing is sequenced like subtle breathing practices—in the context of having received adequate psychoeducation, engaged in calming practices and breath attunement, physical preparation, ability to access natural breathing, and knowledge about recovery breathing. Beyond these cautions, nostril breathing is offered freely at any time in a session and a series, as guided by intention and intervention goals. The practice can be taken into daily life once the client has achieved facility and capacity for self-regulation in session. The most typical use of nostril breathing in daily life is to support sleep and to manage acute stress.

11.2.2 Breathing Practice: Channel Purifying Breath

In Sanskrit, this breath has two names: *nadi shodhana* or *anuloma viloma* (the latter is not to be confused with *viloma pranayama* or interrupted breathing, the final practice offered in this chapter). It is marked by alternating breathing through left and right nostrils, with a switch-over either at the top or bottom of the breath. Ancient yoga deems alternate nostril breathing the ultimate purifying breath, as it balances energy channels (specifically, the two major *nadis—ida* and *pingala*; see Table 11.1) and nervous system states. In traditional yoga, it is considered a breathing practice for uniting opposing tendencies (for example, stillness and movement, action and rest, male and female, creativity and logic), helping integrate conflicting or disparate ways of being to find balance and resilience. It is said to synchronize the two hemispheres of the brain, with the left nostril being associated with the right hemisphere and the right nostril with the left hemisphere of the brain (although, notably, the nostrils are wired neurologically to the olfactory bulb on the *same* side of the brain). Alternate nostril breathing is believed to balance the two branches of the autonomic

Table 11.1 The yogic energies of alternate nostril breathing by nostril

Calming energy of Ida Nadi	Activating energy of Pingala Nadi
Left nostril	*Right nostril*
Right brain activity	Left brain activity
Increased blood flow to right hemisphere	Increased blood flow to right hemisphere
Spatial and creative thinking	Verbal and linear thinking
Lunar—cooling	Solar—warming
Comforting, calming	Activating, energizing
Parasympathetic NS → decreased heart rate, lowered blood pressure, less anxiety	Sympathetic NS → increased cortisol, blood pressure, and heart rate
Tamas and *sattva*	*Rajas* and *sattva*
Supports sleep	Supports alertness

nervous system (sympathetic and parasympathetic) and has been shown to lower heart rate, reduce anxiety, support resilience and stress management, enhance concentration, and improve memory. Scientific explorations have provided evidence that alternate nostril breathing can help regulate blood pressure [31–33], enhance respiration [34], improve metabolism, and shift the organism toward sympathovagal balance with enhanced parasympathetic tone and heart rate variability [12, 35, 36].

Key Instructions and Cuing Tips for Channel Purifying Breath

After the preparations discussed earlier, fingering and breathing rhythms begin. If the breath patterns are offered for the first time, it is useful for the clinician to demonstrate fingering and rhythms while the client observes and then follows along in their imagination. Once clients seem to have understood, they attempt the finger work before coordinating it with breath. If a client has difficulty with finger coordination or compression of the nostril, the breath can be started in the imagination—either until the skills are learned or always. Breathing may start in the imagination first, taking a few rounds in that manner to help settle the rhythm and fingering into the client's nervous system. Actual restriction of a nostril can be added when appropriate. This unrushed approach tends to create greater ease and less confusion for clients. Whether imaginary or actual, after a few rounds of natural breathing and at the conclusion of a calm natural exhalation, alternate nostril breathing can proceed via the following steps.

1. Inhale through left nostril, while right nostril is closed (or imagined closed) via use of a chosen hand position (e.g., thumb for right-handed individuals; ring finger for left-handed individuals)
2. At the top of the breath (during the pause, which may naturally lengthen), release the right nostril while closing the left (e.g., ring finger for individuals using right hand; thumb for individuals using left hand)
3. Exhale through the right nostril, while the left nostril is closed
4. Inhale through the right nostril, keeping the left nostril closed
5. At the top of the breath (during the pause which may naturally lengthen), release the left nostril while closing the right (e.g., thumb for individuals using right hand; ring finger for individuals using left hand)
6. Vary ongoing cuing to create accessibility, using these possibilities:
   • Exhale through the left nostril, while the right nostril is closed
   • Inhale through the left nostril, keeping the right nostril closed
   • At the top of breath, switch sides …
   • One breath travels in through the left; the next breath travels in through the right …
   • In through the left; switch; out through the right; in through the right; switch; out through the left; in through the left; switch … and so the cycle goes
   • If you lose track, start again, closing the right nostril and breathing in through the left
   • Out and in, then switch sides—always at the top of the breathe—ut and in, switch sides

7. End the practice by coming back to a natural and spontaneous rhythm
8. Close the practice with natural optimal functional breathing, cuing calming or vitalizing as needed

Additional Notes for Clinicians
- Be careful not to talk the entire time in specifics but move to cues that support agency in each individual student, as breath rhythms and rates will vary widely
- Remind clients to maintain healthy biomechanics
  - Breath into the low rib basket and mid-section of the torso with ease (i.e., diaphragmatic)
  - Breath only through the nose, resist the urge to make up for the closed nostril with mouth breathing
- Maintain optimal functional breathing as much as possible—relinquish nostril breathing if the natural breath is lost
- Remind students to breathe lightly (i.e., no excessive volume) and slowly (lower rate; 5.5–10 bpm)
- Remind students to breathe rhythmically, smoothly, and quietly

Recommended Observations to Help Guide Cuing
- *Rate*: notice any changes in the length of the breath cycle overall or in the inhalations versus exhalation; notice if clogged nostrils affect the rate of breathing depending on which nostril is open versus closed
- *Volume*: notice changes in the amount of air moving in and out depending on which nostril is active; notice the impact of clogged or partially clogged nostrils
- *Texture and sound*: notice whether change in breath texture from side to side or with time, especially if one nostril is clogged or partially clogged; dysregulation in breath is most notable in texture and provides immediate biofeedback for any need for alterations to keep breath and nervous system regulated
- *Space and location*: notice how the location where the breath is felt most easily changes; notice whether there are changes in how easy or hard it is to feel the breath in the body with the focus being on the air traveling in and out of alternating (or just one) nostril
- *Rests*: notice the likely natural change in the presence of pauses in the breath cycle as the nostril change is initiated and accomplished

Sample Variation of Purifying Channel Breath
Energetic Alternate Breathing for Awakening is a vitalizing alternating nostril breath that integrates bottom-up signaling from the body with top-down control from the mind. It is a relatively straightforward practice that can be used safely once basic breathwork has been achieved in session and capacity for self-regulation is developing. The nice thing about the practice is that several breaths are taken through the same side and then through the other side. Alternating the nostrils does not happen within a single breath cycle but over the course of several cycles. This way of alternating the nostrils is much more accessible for many clients. This practice can be applied in daily life every morning upon awakening.

The practice starts with blocking one nostril, breathing in and out with a natural rhythm for ten rounds. Each breath is observed and counted to occupy the mind and create focus. After ten breaths, breathing returns to natural flow for a few moments. Then, the other nostril is blocked and ten rounds of single-nostril breathing are invited, again counting each breath for mindful presence. Then the practice moves into ten rounds of natural nasal breathing through both nostrils, again counting each breath. On completion of this set of 30 breaths, there is a moment of interoceptive attunement to feel the reverberation from the breath. From a recovered emotional and arousal state, the whole set is repeated at least once. The practice ends with gratitude for breath and life's abundance, as well as appreciation for this moment and all it contains.

An explanation and sample video of this breath is available from Yongey Mingyur Rinpoche at https://youtu.be/7ejGC3QiIqY?si=gOGVSgRkjB7kPYkG.

11.2.3 Breathing Practice: Moon Piercing Breath

Chandra bedha (also called *chandra bedhana*) is translated as moon piercing and is a calming, grounding breath. Traditionally, it is a practice of breathing in through the left nostril and out through the right nostril. However, modern variations have been developed. For example, nostril choices may be based on trying to find a reduced or subtle breath, breathing exclusively through either the right or the left nostril, depending on which side is blocked. The desired intention of the practice guides choice of exclusive use of the left nostril, if calming, cooling, and grounding are central. Another consideration can be current nostril dominance, sometimes choosing to breathe through the unblocked nostril only and, at other times, choosing only the blocked nostril. Specifically, the left nostril is the calming nostril. However, if it is severely blocked, such calming is not likely to be achieved. Nasal clearing practices can be used first, and then a decision can be made about what is most appropriate for the client in the moment.

Key Instructions and Cuing Tips for Moon Piercing Breath

The chosen nostril and associated breath rhythm can be started in the imagination first, taking a few rounds in that manner to help settle rhythm and fingering into the nervous system. Then, compression of the nostril can be added, if accessible. This option creates greater ease in the breath and less confusion or stress for most patients. Whether imaginary or actual, clients typically enter the practice after having settled into a natural breathing rhythm. Left nostril breathing begins at the end of a calming exhalation (i.e., it starts with an inhalation through the left nostril).

1. Inhale through the left nostril, while the right nostril is closed (or imagined closed) via use of a hand gesture
2. At the top of the breath, release the right nostril while closing the left
3. Exhale through the right nostril, while the left nostril is closed

4. At the bottom of the breath, close the right nostril and inhale again through the left nostril
5. At the top of the breath (during the pause which may naturally lengthen), release the right nostril while closing the left
6. Exhale through the right nostril, while the left nostril is closed
7. Switch fingering at the bottom of the breath to inhale again through the left nostril, keeping the right nostril closed
8. At top of breath switch ... and so the cycle goes—always inhaling left and exhaling right
9. Generic cues may be as follows—do this mostly if clients are struggling or drifting:
   - Inhale left; exhale right
   - If you lose track, start again, close the right nostril and breathe in through the left
   - In through the left; switch sides, out through the right; switch sides
10. End the practice by coming back to a spontaneous rhythm
11. Close the practice with natural optimal functional breathing, cuing calming or vitalizing as needed

Additional Notes for Clinicians
- Be careful not to talk the entire time in specifics but move to cues that support client agency, as breath rhythms vary widely
- Remind clients to maintain healthy
  - Breath into the low rib basket and mid-section of the torso with ease (i.e., diaphragmatic)
  - Breath only through the nose, resist the urge to make up for the closed nostril with mouth breathing
- Maintain optimal functional breathing—relinquish nostril breathing if the natural breath is lost
  - Remind students to breathe lightly (i.e., no excessive volume) and slowly (lower rate; 5.5–10 bpm)
  - Remind students to breathe rhythmically, smoothly, and quietly

Recommended Observations to Help Guide Cuing
- *Rate:* notice any changes in the length of the breath cycle overall or in the inhalations versus exhalation; notice if clogged nostrils affect the rate of breathing depending on which nostril is open versus closed
- *Volume:* notice the volume of air moving in and out depending on which nostril is active; notice the impact of clogged or partially clogged nostrils
- *Texture and sound:* notice if there is a change in breath texture, especially if one nostril is clogged or partially clogged; dysregulation is most notable in texture, which provides immediate biofeedback about necessary alterations to keep breath and nervous system regulated

- *Space and location:* notice where in the body breath is felt most easily; notice if there are changes in how easy or hard it is to feel the breath in the body with focus being on air traveling in and out of alternating nostrils
- *Rests:* notice natural changes in breath pauses as breath is channeled through one nostril only

Sample Variation of Moon Piercing Breath

Buteyko Variation of *Left Nostril Breathing* is a calming, left-nostril breath in which the breath flows *in and out* through only the left nostril, keeping the right nostril closed the entire time. This practice is a subtle breathing practice and can be offered relatively early during breathwork. The instructions are simple—following the same preparations as for moon-piercing breath. The right nostril is closed once a natural rhythm of breath has been established, and the individual breathes in and out through the left nostril for up to 3 minutes, monitoring for reactivity.

There will be air hunger, and as long as it is tolerable and does not cause acute hyperventilation, this reaction can simply be observed as breath flow remains smooth, quiet, light, and nasal. If excessive straining or gasping occurs, the client returns to a few rounds of nasal breathing through both nostrils until breath and nervous system have recovered. Then the practice is repeated a couple more times. Once the client can handle this breath rhythm well in session, this cooling and calming breath can be repeated regularly throughout the day as needed.

11.2.4 Breathing Practice: Sun Piercing Breath

Surya bedha (also called *surya bedhana*) means sun piercing and exemplifies an expansive, energizing breath. Traditionally, it is a practice of breathing in through the right nostril and out through the left nostril. However, as previously noted, modern variations have created more accessibility, by opening the door to single nostril breathing, wherein the breath travels in and out of the same nostril, making the practice less confusing [37]. Nostril choices may be based on trying to create a reduced or subtle breath, breathing exclusively through either the right or the left nostril, depending on which side is blocked. In the current case of an energizing intention, this may mean choosing the blocked nostril for breathing. This choice presents an initial challenge that can be dysregulating, until the nostril clears naturally from being used. Desired intentions for the practice may lead to exclusive use of the right nostril if activation, expansiveness, and vitalization are targeted.

Key Instructions and Cuing Tips for Sun Piercing Practice

The chosen breath rhythm for the right nostril can be started in the imagination, taking a few rounds to help settle the rhythm into the nervous system. Then, actual fingering can be added. This sequencing seems to create greater ease in the breath and less confusion or stress, especially helpful given that this breath is already somewhat upregulating in and of itself. As with all nostril breathing, natural breath is cultivated for several rounds first. Once a steady rhythm predominates, nostril breathing starts at the end of exhalation with inhalation through the nostril of emphasis, in this case, the right nostril. This approach is taken whether nostril breathing begins in the imagination or with actual nostril closure.

1. Inhale through the right nostril, while the left nostril is closed (or imagined closed) via use of a finger pressed to the bottom or side of the left nostril
2. At the top of the breath (during the pause, which may naturally lengthen), release the left nostril while closing the right
3. Exhale through the left nostril, while the right nostril is closed
4. At the bottom of the breath, close the left nostril and inhale through the right nostril
5. At the top of the breath, release the left nostril while closing the right
6. Exhale through the left nostril, while the right nostril is closed
7. Switch fingering at the bottom of the breath to inhale again through the right nostril, keeping the left nostril closed
8. At top of breath switch … and so the cycle goes—always inhaling right and exhaling left
9. Some generic cues may be as follows—used if clients are struggling or their attention is drifting:
   • Inhale right; exhale left
   • If you lose track start again, close the left nostril and breath in through the right
   • In through the right; switch sides, out through the left; switch sides
10. End the practice by coming back to a spontaneous breath rhythm
11. Close the practice with natural optimal functional breathing, cuing calming or vitalizing as needed

Additional Notes for Clinicians
• Be careful not to talk the entire time in specifics but move to cues that support client agency, as breath rhythms vary widely
• Remind clients to maintain healthy biomechanics
   – Breath into the low rib basket and mid-section of the torso with ease (i.e., diaphragmatic)
   – Breath only through the nose, resist the urge to make up for the closed nostril with mouth breathing
• Maintain optimal functional breathing—relinquish nostril breathing if the natural breath is lost
   – Remind students to breathe lightly (i.e., no excessive volume) and slowly (lower rate; 5.5–10 bpm)
   – Remind students to breathe rhythmically, smoothly, and quietly

Recommended Observations to Help Guide Cuing

- *Rate:* notice any changes in the length of the breath cycle overall or in the inhalations versus exhalation; notice if clogged nostrils affect the rate of breathing depending on which nostril is open versus closed
- *Volume:* notice the volume of air moving in and out depending on which nostril is active; notice the impact of clogged or partially clogged nostrils
- *Texture and sound:* notice if there is a change in breath texture, especially if one nostril is clogged or partially clogged; dysregulation is most notable in texture, which provides immediate biofeedback about necessary alterations to keep breath and nervous system regulated
- *Space and location:* notice where in the body breath is felt most easily; notice if there are changes in how easy or hard it is to feel the breath in the body with focus being on air traveling in and out of alternating nostrils
- *Rests:* notice natural changes in Breath phases as breath is channeled through one nostril only

Sample Variation of Sun Piercing Breath

The Buteyko-inspired practice offered for moon-piercing breath can, of course, be mirrored with right nostril breathing. The effect of this variation used with emphasis on the right nostril is activating and warming. For this reason, it tends to be more challenging for anyone who is already in a state of arousal. For the very reason that sun-piercing breathing is heating and linked to the sympathetic nervous system, fewer useful variations exist. Of course, the breath can be supplemented with specific attention to breath phases; it can be inspired by added movement, and it can be used in daily life as a quick pick-me-up. Because of its upregulating nature, it is particularly helpful with individual with dorsal vagal withdrawal and disconnection tendencies. However, right nostril breathing requires caution in all of these contexts. There is no single variation to highlight that is extra useful or extra special beyond any variations that make use of the warming and vitalizing effects of breath.

11.3 Breathing with Sound

Breathing with sound has a range of profound benefits, from regulating nervous system reactivity to supporting mental concentration and attention, to cardiovascular benefits, to increasingly efficient and auspicious respiration, to emotional calming and grounding. Sounding the breath can captivate the attention and support mental focus or one-pointedness. Sound in the back of the throat stimulates the vagus nerve (via contraction of the laryngeal muscles) and empowers the vagal brake, supporting movement into a parasympathetic (ventral vagal) state. Sounding the breath on the exhalation increases release of nitric oxide, a powerful vaso- and bronchodilator that not only enhances internal but also external respiration, increasing oxygenation of tissues and preventing accumulation of lactic acid that causes muscular pain after (significant or unusual) exertion.

Breathing with sound is a form of subtle breathing and helps promote optimal functional breath. It occurs during chanting, singing, sounding *om*, and some prayer or mantra practices. It is related to *udana vayu* because it stimulates the throat and has positive and transformative effects on the nervous system. Breath with sound promotes but is not in and of itself a form of optimal functional breathing or natural breathing—it is used with intention and purpose for short periods of time. Two types of breath with sound are explored, documenting their individual unique benefits and applications. We first turn to bumblebee breathing, a universally beneficial practice, and then explore *ujjayi*, a common breath promoted in yoga contexts.

11.3.1 Breathing Practice: Bumblebee Breath

Bumblebee breathing or *bhramari* is a breath that greatly serves our nervous system by stimulating the vagus nerve and respiratory and cardiovascular systems by generating nitric oxide and creating resistance in the back of the throat. It is an easily accessible breath that is calming and grounding for most, if not all, patients. It is universally salutary, easy to intone, and joyfully practiced in group settings. For some clients, there may be some self-consciousness when they first try this breath. However, hesitation is generally quickly transformed as clients can feel the positive reverberations of this breath in their body, vitality, and mind. Intoning and practicing this breath with the client can help break the ice.

Biomechanics, Biochemistry, and Psychology of Bumblebee Breath

Bhramari positively affects physiology and nervous system states in a variety of ways [38], most likely through calming secondary to the natural extension of exhalation, which also reduces breath rate [39]:

- It moves us into a parasympathetic nervous system state via stimulating somatosensory afferent fibers of the vagus nerve [40], enhancing sympathovagal tone [18] and subtle inner experience [41]
- It enhances pulmonary functioning and efficiency [42]
- It promotes cardiovascular health and has been shown to reduce heart rate and blood pressure [43, 44], even enhancing lipid profiles for some [17]
- Cardiovascular effects may be mediated by significant increases (15-fold) in nitric oxide that have been identified in the research on exhaled humming compared to silent exhalation [45, 46], especially with lower-frequency humming [47]
- Perhaps due to the antiviral, antifungal, and antibacterial effects of nitric oxide, humming has been shown to alleviate symptoms of rhinosinusitis [48]
- It reduces irritation, depression, and anxiety [49, 50]
- Humming may even bring relief to tinnitus [51, 52]

Some studies suggest that bumblebee breathing has positive effects on the brain via increased cognitive control [53] and reduced hyperreactivity [54]. Other benefits include strengthening of the tongue, which is pressed up against the hard palate during exhalation [55]; reducing mouth breathing, as it requires a complete mouth seal; and enhancing mindfulness and peacefulness as the sound concentrates the mind.

Sequencing Bumblebee Breathing

As is true for all specialized breathing practices, it is ideal to practice breath attunement, physical preparations, and natural breathing before offering bumblebee breathing, especially since it is a practice that increases the length of exhalation, decreases breath rate, and can function as a subtle breathing practice. That said, bumblebee breathing is generally a very safe breath as long as clients practice with mindfulness, taking care not to allow their breath to dysregulate and taking recovery breaks as needed. Bumblebee breathing is possible almost anytime during a session and is most helpfully embedded with a clear intention for its practice. It is generally initiated after having attuned to natural breathing via breath observation or a basic breathing practice (such as four-part breathing), or a subtle practice (such as feather breathing). Once clients have settled into a gentle and calm breath rhythm, bumblebee breathing is introduced.

Home practice of bumblebee breathing can be recommended relatively early in a client's practice with appropriate precautions and extant capacity to access natural breathing. Education about how to recognize hyperventilation and recover the breath is key to safe home practice, just as it is for all breathwork in daily life.

Key Instructions and Cuing Tips for Bumblebee Breathing

Once clients have settled into a gentle and calm breathing rhythm, bumblebee breathing is introduced. It is helpful to explain the overall breath rhythm and how to make the bumblebee sound before actually beginning the breath. The clinician might demonstrate the breath, and following the demonstration, can invite the client to join. Possible cuing options are as follows:

1. Find the natural rhythm of your breath and take a few rounds of breath while you invite your mind to begin to ponder the possibility of making a bumblebee (or extended *mmmmm*) sound on the exhalation
2. With your next natural exhalation begin to sound the *mmmmm* of the bumblebee breath
3. Invite the sound to be low and resonant
4. Notice if you can sense the vibration of the sound elsewhere in the body—perhaps in the throat, the chest, even the abdomen
5. Notice the effect of the humming on your physical and mental presence and experience
6. Gently nestle the tongue against the roof of the mouth; attempt to keep the tongue relaxed, while pressing upward, during the entire sounding of the exhalation
7. Invite the length of the exhalation to be natural; it is not necessary, especially in the beginning, to extend the exhalation with bumblebee breathing—though this may happen naturally
8. As you sound the bumblebee breath with the exhalation, begin to notice
   - If the exhalation changes/extends naturally/feels differently
   - If the transition between the exhalation and the bottom of the breath changes—for example, you might note that there is a moment during the

exhalation when the bumblebee sound stops, but the pause at the bottom has not yet begun
- If the pause at the bottom of the breath changes—work without a specific expectation here, simply notice
9. If the exhalation naturally begins to extend with the sound of the *m*, simply allow that
10. End the practice with a return to a spontaneous breath rhythm
11. Close the exercise when the client has recovered natural breathing.

Additional Notes for Clinicians
- If breathing becomes erratic or uncomfortable, cue natural breathing without sound for a few rounds; then, start bumblebee breathing again, without extending the exhalation
- Remind clients to maintain healthy biomechanics
  - Breath into the low rib basket and mid-section of the torso with ease (i.e., diaphragmatic)
  - Breath only through the nose
  - Let the tongue press gently on the hard palate of the mouth—do not let the tongue collapse downward as this may restrict airflow through the nose
- Maintain optimal functional breathing—relinquish nostril breathing if the natural breath is lost
  - Remind students to breathe lightly (i.e., no excessive volume) and slowly (lower rate; 5.5–10 bpm)
  - Remind students to breathe rhythmically, smoothly, and quietly.

Recommended Observations to Help Guide Cuing
- *Rate*: notice changes in the length of the breath, especially the exhalation, that arises with the humming; feel the impact of the throat constriction or sound on rate; notice if the sound of the humming stops before the exhalation is complete—there may be an extension of the exhalation
- *Volume*: notice how breath changes in terms of amount of air moving in and out; feel the impact of the constriction or sound on volume created by the humming; notice if there is a change in level of concentration with this breath and whether increased mental concentration has an effect on breath volume
- *Texture and sound*: notice changes in the texture and sound of the breath when humming; texture may change significantly due to the release of nitric oxide and its broncho- and vasodilating effects; experiment with different sounds and see how this affects the texture, vibration, and other breath characteristics
- *Space and location*: notice where the breath is felt, especially beyond the typical places; notice if there are changes in difficulty related to feeling breath in the body; notice the spaces and locations where vibration is created by the humming
- *Rests*: notice if there is a change in presence or length of pauses in the breath cycle; the bottom pause may change naturally; notice if there is a change in level of concentration with this breath and if increased mental concentration has an effect on breath rate and pauses

Sample Variation of Bumblebee Breathing

Bumblebee breathing lends itself beautifully to integration with a dynamic movement practice that recapitulates the rhythm of the breath. Integrated with movement, bumblebee breath often naturally begins to extend exhalation, creating well-being and uplifted mood. Movement can be added to bumblebee breathing from the beginning; in fact, the combination with movement makes this breath more accessible for some patients.

1. Take a few rounds of natural breath, seated or standing
2. Beginning with the next breath cycle, inhale naturally and exhale, inviting the sound of a bumblebee (as explained in the instructions above); take a few rounds of bumblebee breath until comfort is achieved with the sound and humming
3. Add movement as follows:
   - With the inhalation, open the arm wide out to the side at shoulder height
   - With the exhalation, intone the bumblebee sound and bring the arms toward each other in front of the body at shoulder height, drawing them in toward the heart with palms touching
   - Linger for a moment—perhaps extend the pause at the bottom of the breath
4. Repeat for several rounds and then return to natural breathing, ending the sound and the movement
5. Reflect on the experience and debrief

This particular movement with bumblebee breathing tends to lengthen the exhalation and the humming more than bumblebee breathing without movement. It also tends to be easier for clients to maintain focus and peacefulness. In many ways, bumblebee breathing with movement appears more accessible for some clients than the breath without movement.

11.3.2 Breathing Practice: Silent Ujjayi Breathing

Ujjayi breathing is almost ubiquitous in Western yoga classes and considered by many to be a quintessential breathing practice with *sound*. English-language labeling of the breath reflects this bias—ocean-sounding breath or Darth Vader breath. Interestingly, however, original *ujjayi* breathing does not have sound. It generates a conscious sensation of breath flow at the back of the throat, relaxes the tongue, and smooths the diaphragm. Silent *ujjayi* breathing vibrates the vagus nerve in the throat—similar to what occurs in humming and bumble bee breathing—and yet this is accomplished in silence. In a healthcare context, it seems preferable to practice *ujjayi* without sound to remind clients that optimally functional breathing is silent—quiet, slow, and subtle. It takes time, however, to develop this skill. Most likely, when first used, *ujjayi* does indeed create an ocean sound. This is perfectly fine; over time, however, as ease penetrates the practice, breath will quieten.

All too often people misunderstand *ujjayi* as a functional daily breath, especially since many yoga teachers contribute to this misunderstanding by asking students to maintain *ujjayi* throughout their mat practice. It is not; it has specific purposes, most importantly, the slowing of the breath and concentration of the mind. It has the benefits of sounded practices such as bumblebee and chanting (i.e., contracting the laryngeal muscles, massaging the vagus nerve), with the advantage of inviting the quiet concentration of an inner practice that can be accomplished in silence.

Biomechanics, Biochemistry, and Psychology of Silent Ujjayi Breathing

Silent *ujjayi* utilizes the glottis to slow the breath by controlling the opening through which the air travels. This constriction decreases the volume of air traveling through the throat at any given moment—a process that can be likened to a balloon whose opening is being pinched to control the outflow of the air, as opposed to letting the opening go and the air escaping rapidly and uncontrolled. It is important to ensure that contraction of the glottis is gentle and nasal breathing remains primary. If there is any sniffling or grunting noise during *ujjayi*, the individual is blocking their breath and interfering with oxygen uptake in the tissues. Learning control or tuning of the glottis can feel empowering for individuals who have little muscle control elsewhere in the body. It is accessible to most individuals, even those who have paralysis in other body parts. It is important to observe clients as they employ *ujjayi* for the first few times to note whether they are straining or bracing, especially in the jaws, around the temporomandibular joint. Relaxed muscles are key to success, as bracing and clenching will undo the calming and focusing functions of this breath.

Ujjayi slows the breath rate, increasing lengths of inhalation and exhalation. With the longer time requirement for each breath cycle, dormant regions of the lungs are infused with air; more time and alveolar surfaces become available for gas exchange, which should enhance respiratory biochemistry, although the findings about this potential benefit are mixed [56]. *Ujjayi* is thought to have promise for ameliorating breathing disorders, such as asthma and COPD; however, on occasion it has been known to trigger asthma attacks. Thus, it is crucial to proceed slowly and with awareness. *Ujjayi* has a calming effect on the nervous system via vagus nerve stimulation. It increases a sense of ease and peacefulness, has a relaxing and stress-reducing effect [41], and decreases anxiety [57], perhaps via a parasympathetic shift [58]. *Ujjayi* may increase attention and focus [59] and has shown promise in enhancing thyroid function [60, 61].

Sequencing Silent Ujjayi

Given its breath-rate-reducing effect, *ujjayi* can be sequenced in a similar manner as subtle breathing practice. It is embedded in a context of education, relaxation, breath attunement, and natural breathing. Capacity for interoception and recovery breathing is essential for clients who practice *ujjayi*, especially during home practice. Within a breathwork or yoga context, it is important not to make *ujjayi* a rote or habitual practice. Research findings about its utility are more mixed than for other practices. Perhaps when mindfulness is lost or sound becomes too loud or creates the physical stress of bracing, *ujjayi* loses some of its benefits. It is therefore important not to overuse *ujjayi* and to have a clear purpose for the practice. It is not usefully cued for the entirety of a session or a yoga class, and it is *not* a natural breath for daily life. When using *ujjayi*, it is important to observe clients to ensure that they do not overly restrict or sound the breath, offering it as a practice that increases breath sensitivity without inviting excessive breath restriction. Once mastered, silent *ujjayi* can be recommended for home practice. This recommendation comes with the caveat that clients understand that *ujjayi* is not a natural daily breath; it is used for a particular purpose for a limited time.

Key Instructions and Cuing Tips for Silent Ujjayi Breathing

It is useful to explain the overall work with the glottis before actually beginning the breath. Clients need to understand how to constrict the throat without bracing or straining. They can be taught to imagine fogging a mirror with their breath, starting this practice with an open mouth (and perhaps an actual mirror or a phone screen, as used in feather breathing). Then, the client is invited to perform the same sound and glottis action with the mouth closed. The teacher might need to demonstrate the breath and its possible initial sound; following this, the client joins. Most likely, on the first few attempts, *ujjayi* breathing does create significant sound. Over time, this can diminish as the client begins to relax into the practice. For some, this may take several sessions.

Once clients have settled into a gentle and calm breathing rhythm, *ujjayi* breathing can be introduced. Possible cuing options are as follows:

1. As you breathe, gently constrict or tone the throat, the area around the glottis—you will feel this in the same area where you feel a gargle or a cough
2. Perhaps imagine fogging a mirror; to begin with you can do this out loud with an open mouth
3. Then, attempt to maintain the constriction of the glottis but with the mouth closed and continue to breathe naturally and rhythmically through the nose
4. There may be a slight sound—perhaps a bit of a hissing or like sound of the ocean … for some people it may sound like Darth Vader …
5. Keep breathing with constriction at the throat … yet keep the breath rhythmic and light
6. Be sure not to overly tighten the jaws … notice if you are gripping and relax the muscles that can relax while continuing the light constriction of the throat …
7. Explore if you can engage the same sensation of constricted breath flow in the back of the throat while letting the sound become quieter and quieter … perhaps ultimately making no sound at all … no ocean, no Darth Vader … just silence …
8. If there is sound, can you make it so soft that only you can hear it?
9. End the practice with a return to a spontaneous breath rhythm
10. Close the exercise when the client has recovered natural breathing

Additional Notes for Clinicians

- If breath becomes erratic or uncomfortable, cue natural breathing without constriction of the glottis for a few rounds; then, start *ujjayi* again, monitoring for excessive sound
- Make sure jaws and face remain relaxed
- Invite patience and self-compassion if there is struggle
- Remind clients to maintain healthy biomechanics
  - Breath only through the nose, resist the urge to make up for constriction in the breath with mouth breathing
  - Breath into the low rib basket and mid-section of the torso with ease (i.e., diaphragmatic)
- Maintain optimal functional breathing—relinquish nostril breathing if the natural breath is lost
  - Remind students to breathe lightly (i.e., no excessive volume) and slowly (lower rate; 5.5–10 bpm)
  - Remind students to breathe rhythmically, smoothly, and as quietly as possible with the glottis constricted

Recommended Observations to Help Guide Cuing

- *Rate*: notice any changes in breath rate that arises with the toning of the throat muscles; feel the impact of the constriction on breath length
- *Volume*: notice if the volume of the inhalations or exhalations changes; feel the impact of the constriction on volume
- *Texture and sound*: notice changes in the texture of the breath when the glottis is constricted versus not; notice the range of sound possible with *ujjayi* breathing—this breath ideally is completely silent (although seldom cued that way) or quite loud, especially when learning this breathing practice
- *Space and location*: notice how the locations where the breath is felt most easily; notice if there are changes in how easy or hard it is to feel the breath in the body, when the focus is on the throat via toning and, if is exists, on sound
- *Rests*: notice if there is a change in presence or length of pauses in the breath cycle

Sample Variation of Silent Ujjayi Breathing

Ujjayi with Awareness of Breath Phases adds a challenging aspect to ujjayi breathing that integrates a four-part breathing focus with the constriction of this breath. The *ujjayi* action (and perhaps its gentle sound if present) accompanies the entire inhalation and exhalation and becomes silent, of course, during breath pauses. The client can pay attention to differences in the sensations of constriction in the throat with inhalation versus exhalation. Attention can also be drawn to the sensations in the throat during the breath pauses, differentiating sensations at the top versus bottom of the breath. This work is very subtle, and this added focus can hone mental concentration. It can also serve to make the breath more subtle, adding an even stronger shift in biochemistry. As a subtle or even suspension practice, all typical cautions apply. This combination of breaths is offered to seasoned practitioners who have a clear understanding of healthy breath dynamics, the capacity to self-regulate, and the interest in developing their breathing in daily life, especially in demanding contexts, including during athletic endeavors.

11.4   Breathing with Force

Forceful breaths are practices of hormesis—they can create extreme stress in several systems, including the respiratory, cardiovascular, and nervous systems—with the goal of stress inoculation and resilience-building [62]. They are for well-versed students with established optimal functional breathing skills and basic knowledge about hyperventilation and how to recover from such high-speed breathing. Medically vulnerable individuals do not use this type of breathing unless it is significantly modified, namely slowed (basically engaging the breath in slow motion for a very specific purpose) and lightened (i.e., with low volume) to reduce risk of hyperventilation and extreme vaso- and bronchoconstriction. If forceful breathing is used by these individuals (not something that this author advocates), beware of dizziness, lightheadedness, numbness or tingling, rapid and shallow breathing, shortness of breath, tachycardia, chest tightness, anxiety, and any other symptoms of acute hyperventilation (hypocapnia), combined with hypoxia. An extreme side effect of forced breathing that leads to hypocapnia *and* hypoxia is tetany, or carpopedal spasms that cause severe flexion in the finger and wrist joints (in the vernacular, this is called a "lobster claw"). Clients need to be alerted to these possible side effects and to discontinue forced breathing if they arise. Of course, the best course of action is not to teach breathing with such force that side effects develop or are considered "normal," as they are in some circles. If the *gentle* forced breathing described below (i.e., slow motion *kapalabhati* and gentle *viloma*) results in acute hyperventilation symptoms, immediate initiation of rescue breathing is warranted. Clinicians choosing to use these gentle variations of forceful breathing clinically need to be prepared to help clients rescue breathe. Two approaches, perhaps used in the offered sequence, are shown in Table 11.2.

11.4.1 Breathing Practice: Slow-Motion Skull Shining Breath

Kapalabhati or skull-shining breath is a challenging breathing practice even for advanced breathers. It generates heat in the body through forced exhalation and passive inhalation. The forced exhalation strongly recruits and strengthens the diaphragm and core muscles. Large amounts of CO_2 are blown off during very vigorous exhalations associated with typical *kapalabhati*. However, slow-motion *kapalabhati* engages the diaphragm and helps students develop interoception and diaphragmatic strength with a *forced but slow* rhythm that (*generally*) does not lead to hyperventilation. This is the only form of *kapalabhati* recommended in a healthcare setting, with new clients in a therapeutic yoga setting, and with individuals with patterns of hyperarousal or emotional and psychological challenges.

Table 11.2 Rescue breathing in the event of panic, hyperventilation, or hypoxia

Hyperventilation due to a physiological or psychological panic response to forceful breathing often is distinguished by a respiratory rate of over 20 breaths per minute (some forced breathing practice require even faster rates). The student will need help from the provider to calm this respiratory rate if they have moved into serious hyperventilation (i.e., hypocapnia, possibly accompanied by hypoxia) or panic.

- If severe, start with Option 1 and then follow up with Option 2.
- If mild, Option 1 can be used by itself.

Option 1: Reduced breathing using cupped hands
The typical recommendation is to breathe into a paper bag to increase the amount of CO_2 re-inhaled with each breath. The downside of this practice is that paper bags not only increase CO_2, but further reduce O_2 as no fresh air can move into the paper bag. Instead, it is helpful to use reduced breathing using cupped hands instead (see Chap. 9). This breathing practice pools CO_2 in the hands in sufficient amounts, while allowing enough fresh air into the hands to keep supplying an adequate amount of O_2.

- *First and foremost, the teacher needs to stay calm and regulated.*
- Invite a sense of safety and relaxation via a ventral vagal presence, especially via a calm and supportive tone of voice and prosody.
- Gently, without panic or excessive urgency, invite the student to cup their hands over the mouth and nose.
- Guide the student into a breath cadence of 3-second inhalations and 3-second exhalations into the cupped hands.
- Consider gestures or other means of demonstrating the cadence and volume of the suggested airflow and breath rate.
- Reassure the student that the breath will recover, and that the nervous system will re-regulate.
- Maintain comforting (not laser-like) eye contact with the student and breathe in the same cadence as the student to help them co-regulate with you.
- Once the student seems to be reregulating somewhat, increase the cadence to 4 s in and 4 s, then 5 s in and 5 s out.
- Perhaps add very short breath holds at the bottom of breath to bring the vagal brake back.
- Stay attuned to the student's and your own nervous system state, creating a calm environment.

Option 2: Breathing with very short breath suspensions
- This practice was detailed in Table 7.15 as a minimum breath hold practice. It can also be used as a recovery breath.
- The same context described for cupping as recovery needs to be created—safety and coregulation with the care provider are key.
- The client is then invited to try to return to a natural breath cycle—cupping may be needed first.
- Once a less dysregulated breath is available, and the client is able, very short (2–3 s) breath holds at the end of the exhalation are invited and repeated again and again until symptoms of panic and hyperventilation dissipate, breath rate returns to normal and client reports feeling recovered.

Biomechanics, Biochemistry, and Psychology of Skull-Shining Breath

Kapalabhati is a means of creating stress in several systems to develop resilience and stress inoculation via hormesis. It stimulates blood flow in the dormant areas of the lungs and stretches the airways (it is said to keep the sinuses clear and the lungs supple). These factors combine to result in increased alveolar ventilation (oxygenating the blood at a higher level than natural breathing) and vital capacity [49]. *Kapalabhati* has been shown to have stimulating, even exhilarating, effects [41]. It creates heat in the physical body, similar to *tummo* practices used by Tibetan monks to withstand extremely cold conditions [63].

Kapalabhati massages the internal organs in the abdomen via exaggerated movement of the diaphragm and abdominal wall that pushes abdominal organs upward and, as a result, is hypothesized to support metabolic health [64]. When the diaphragm's contraction is released, the organs drop into the lower portion of the belly, creating rapid expansion in the lungs. The air is thus sucked in for a passive inhalation. In this way, *kapalabhati* reverses the typical actions of the two active phases of breath; typically, inhalation is more active and shorter than exhalation. In *kapalabhati*, exhalation is the active phase of the breath; inhalation happens passively and is even shorter than exhalation.

Cautions for Skull-Shining Breath

Generally, *kapalabhati* is done seated or embedded within an asana (e.g., downward dog), never lying down flat. If a supine position is necessary or desirable, an incline is created for the torso (see Chap. 7 for options). This breath is always used with great discernment and care. It is not appropriate for:

- Pregnant women
- Individuals with high blood pressure or history of heart disease
- History of stroke
- History or current respiratory illnesses, including but not limited to asthma, emphysema, or collapsed lung
- Seizure disorder
- Tinnitus (and perhaps other ear issues)
- Glaucoma (and other eye issues such as vitreous detachment)
- Individuals with exhaustion or lack of vigor (e.g., individuals with cancer undergoing chemotherapy; individuals with autoimmune disorders)
- Individuals with acute panic disorder or severe anxiety
- Individuals with asthma or other respiratory illnesses
- Many other health and mental health conditions—anything that has impaired overall health.

Sequencing Skull-Shining Breath

Clients practicing this breath in its original form need to be optimal functional breathers who have demonstrated resilient, adaptive, and coherent breathing. If this is not the case, the danger of hyperventilation is too great, and recovery from fast breathing is too difficult. The slow-motion variation proposed here can be appropriate for clients who are newer to breathwork, but it is still not recommended for complete novices. Clinicians need to be discerning about recommending even slow-motion *kapalabhati* for home practice. If used in sessions, this type of breathing is appropriate later in a session, typically following other breathwork that has awakened awareness of lungs, rib basket, and core (especially pelvic floor) muscles. It needs to happen sufficiently early in a session to allow for recovery without feeling rushed or pressured for time. The practice is offered with a manageable number of exhalations (no more than 10–15) and allows for regular reregulation of the breath before initiating another cycle. *Kapalabhati* is practiced only on an empty stomach. Each use of this breath is debriefed to explore the client's experience and reaction.

Special Note: The inclusion of *kapalabhati* in this chapter is not an endorsement of its liberal or undiscerning use; it is included to encourage clinicians who are drawn to include more forceful practices to develop discernment, err on the side of caution, and constrain themselves to the gentle versions offered here.

Key Instructions and Cuing Tips for Skull-Shining Breath

It is helpful to ensure that the client has found a comfortable seat and is as relaxed and at ease as possible. Calming and breath attunement practices are best focused on first, followed by education about skull-shining breath and reassessment whether the breathing practice is appropriate for the client's nervous system at this moment in time. If there is any sign or hyperarousal, anxiety, or distress, the plan for the practice is abandoned and calming breathing is offered instead. It is important to stay visually connected to the client throughout.

1. Start with a breath attunement practice to prepare mind and body
2. Take a few rounds of natural, optimally functional breathing, centering the mind and gathering energy
3. Take a natural round of breath … then take a partial breath in
4. With the mouth closed, forcefully—but not very quickly—exhale, drawing the diaphragm up toward the lungs and drawing the abdominal wall inward strongly as if to push all the air out
5. Let the inhalation come in naturally and slowly—no need to take action … allow this to happen passively
6. Take a round or two of natural breathing … then repeat …
7. Exhale forcefully using the core muscles … drawing the pelvic floor inward and upward …
8. Let a passive inhalation follow as core muscles relax … and the vacuum creates in the lungs naturally sucks in air …
9. Find a steady rhythm … strong exhalation … passive inhalation
10. There is no need for this to be fast … take your time … be gentle…
11. Keep the breath smooth and comfortable … that is way more important than speed …
12. Try up to ten breaths like this … stopping if you feel yourself tightening or if the breath feels distressing …
13. Now let go of the effort and breathe naturally … softly … gently … until a natural easeful breath returns … perhaps engage in another cycle or two when the nervous system has fully recovered
14. Close and debrief the practice when a natural breath rhythm has been reestablished

Additional Notes for Clinicians
- Remember to breathe only nasally—there may be a strong urge to breath orally; stay vigilant
- Degree of force is adjusted to client needs and intentions (see above)
- Speed is slow and easy—if there is temptation to go faster, encourage slow movements of core muscles and diaphragm.
- Commentary or education may be offered based on the following observations:
  - Contraction of the diaphragm releases with exhalation
  - Core muscles create the force on the exhalation—supported by pelvic floor muscles
- Collaboratively and over time help clients work up to more breaths per cycle and more cycles per session
- Debrief each episode of *kapalabhati*, even if the client has used this breath before
- Be sure to help return clients to healthy biomechanics with patience and sufficient recovery time
  - Breath only through the nose
  - Breath into the low rib basket and mid-section of the torso with ease (i.e., diaphragmatic)
- Be sure to return clients to optimal functional breathing with patience and sufficient recovery time
  - Remind students to breathe lightly and slowly
  - Remind students to breathe rhythmically, smoothly, and quietly.

Recommended Observations to Help Guide Cuing
- *Rate*: notice the effect as the breath is forcefully expelled—does it speed breathing; can it be slowed
- *Volume*: notice how breath volume changes in inhalation versus exhalation—notice how this translates energetically and with regard to emotional and nervous system regulation
- *Texture and sound*: notice how texture and sounds are affected by the large difference in breath rate and volume on the exhalation versus inhalation; notice the intentionality of the exhalation and the passivity of the inhalation—how does this affect texture? How is it reflected in sound?
- *Space and location*: notice how the location changes where the breath is experienced; explore the effects on breath awareness and energy
- *Rests*: notice the changes in the pauses at the top and bottom of breath—are any pauses remaining? If so, how do they feel? How have they changed? If no, how has this changed the breath?

Variations and Intentions for Skull-Shining Breath
The only form of *kapalabhati* recommended in the context of working with breath in healthcare and therapeutic yoga is the slow-motion version provided. For advanced clients, more speed and vigor can be added, as well as more repetitions. However, this is not necessary or even appropriate for most patients.

11.4.2 Breathing Practice: Against-the-Grain Breathing

Viloma means breathing against the grain of typical breath patterns by interrupting the flow of either inhalation or exhalation (*vi* = against; *loma* = hair or natural flow). The most common *viloma* rhythm is to break either inhalation or exhalation into three segments, inhaling or exhaling one third of the way, pausing for a couple of seconds or less, inhaling or exhaling another third, pausing, and inhaling or exhaling the final third, followed by an extended or strong exhalation or inhalation. The focus in this chapter is on the against-the-grain patterns during inhalation only, with lengthened or slightly forceful exhalations. The exhalation may sound like a sigh, and many individuals release it through the mouth. However, it is possible to release even a longer or more forceful exhalation through the nose, and this is recommended in healthcare contexts. *Viloma*, combined with movement, can be a joyful and uplifting practice.

Biomechanics, Biochemistry, and Psychology of Against-the-Grain Breathing

Viloma, with its against-the-grain action during inhalation (the focus here), can be likened to a practice of physiological sighing. A physiological sigh is the spontaneous segmented drawing-in of breath, followed by strongly released exhalation and, most typically, breath suspension (called post-sigh apnea). Physiological sighing is triggered by the brainstem in response to respiration-related signals from mechanoreceptors and chemoreceptors that communicate changes in lung volume and pressure, signaling alveolar collapse via the vagus nerve [65]. These respiratory changes can arise in response to stress, strong emotion, sustained attention, paced breathing, or shallow breathing [66]. The subsequent sigh restores respiratory resilience, reverses alveolar collapse, and is helpful for normal pulmonary function and gas exchange [67, 68]. Sighing that occurs naturally can be stress-relieving and is prevalent in all mammals. It occurs more frequently while awakening from sleep and may have an arousal function [69, 70]. Physiological sighing should not be confused with the dysregulated sighing that is part of hyperventilation syndrome [71] (which does not tend to share the segmented nature of the inhalation). *Viloma* is claimed to increase lung elasticity, respiratory resilience, and lung capacity—all characteristics associated with long-term health [72, 73]. *Viloma* can be implemented as a mental concentration and emotional reset practice, especially if used with movement that invites focus and attention. It has been shown to have calming and stress-reducing effects [23], including reducing anxiety and improving mood [74]. Although the beneficial effects of *viloma* have not been amply scientifically explored, its nature as a physiological sigh (assuming it is practiced on the inhalation) suggests that anecdotal claims have some veracity because of *viloma's* overlap with the proven effects of physiological sighing.

Sequencing Against-the-Grain Breathing

Viloma breathing is generally not applied deliberately until optimal functional breathing has been established and the client has developed interoceptive skills. As with all specialized practices, *viloma* is embedded in a context of having established psychoeducation, breath attunement, and capacity to access natural and optimal breathing. *Viloma pranayama* is a relatively straightforward practice that introduces gentle force or control, especially when practiced with segmented inhalation and extended exhalation. *Viloma* may be useful in response to noticing stress, emotional dysregulation, or breathing that is becoming shallow. In such circumstances, it can be invited as a physiological sigh, with two or three segments on the inhalation and a natural, perhaps slightly longer or stronger, exhalation. It can be used as a reset practice in daily life to manage stress, invite ease, and reregulate breathing. Beware of confusing *viloma* with habitual dysfunctional sighing that is a symptom of hyperventilation syndrome. *Viloma* on the inhalation, in its function as a physiological sigh, is calming, grounding, and restorative.

Key Instructions and Cuing Tips for Against-the-Grain Breathing

Viloma can be practiced in any position (most typically upright but accessible while lying down) and during movement. It is embedded in breathwork in a thoughtful way that relies on client education, breath attunement, and capacity for spontaneous optimal breathing. It can support breath resilience and can be offered in sessions when the client seems stressed, emotional, or on the verge of disordered breathing.

1. Observe the breath for a few rounds to connect to the breath phases
2. Take a conscious round of breath in and out
3. With the next inhalation, draw a gentle but incomplete breath in ... pause for a beat or two ... take in a bit more breath
4. And release a slow, perhaps slightly longer or stronger breath out ...
5. Recover and breathe naturally
6. Repeat *viloma*, perhaps increasing the number of inhalation segments to three
7. Repeat as desired and then return to natural breathing
8. Close the session when the breath moves resiliently and quietly.

Additional Notes for Clinicians

- Commentary or education may be offered about the link between viloma and physiological sighing
- Collaboratively and over time, help clients use *viloma* as a stress-relief breath
- Debrief the first few episodes of *viloma*, ensuring that the breath is functional and helpful (and not reinforcing dysfunctional sighing and hyperventilation)
- Cue healthy biomechanics throughout
  - Preferably breathing only through the nose but acknowledging that some clients feel a strong urge to *exhale* orally; inhalation is always nasal
  - Breathing into the low rib basket and mid-section of the torso with ease (i.e., diaphragmatic)
- Be sure to return clients to optimal functional breathing with patience and sufficient recovery time
  - Remind students to breathe lightly and slowly
  - Remind students to breathe rhythmically, smoothly, and quietly

Recommended Observations to Help Guide Cuing
- *Rate*: notice the effect of the segmented inhalation; notice if the exhalation lengthens
- *Volume*: notice how breath volume changes during segmented inhalation; notices if the exhalation deepens (i.e., moves more volume)
- *Texture and sound*: notice how texture and sound are affected by the difference in actions on inhalation and exhalation—notice experience the textural effect of segmenting the inhalation, and the sound effect of the extended exhalation
- *Space and location*: notice if location changes where the breath is experienced; explore the effects on breath awareness and energy
- *Rests*: notice the changes in breath pauses, especially note if there is post-sigh apnea (i.e., spontaneous breath suspension)

Sample Variation of Against-the-Grain Breathing

Breath of Joy is a dynamic version of viloma on the inhalation or physiological sighing. It is an uplifting and joyful practice that is especially powerful when practiced in community. It is most commonly invited from standing but can work very well while seated on a chair. Although it can be practiced at any time during a session, it seems most helpful whenever there is a need for vitalization, invigoration, or stress release. The inhalation has three segments; the exhalation is strong and long. Ideally, breathing is nasal, although some clients cannot manage nasal exhalation and will spontaneously shift to oral exhalation. For them, nasal inhalation can be encouraged over time. Breath of joy is introduced after clients have successfully and repeatedly engaged in *viloma* on the inhalation without movement.

The flow requires significant arm movement. If full-range arm movements are challenging, arms can stay at shoulder height or move in any other accessible manner. The movement is practiced most safely for the low back after physical warm-up practices *and* with bent knees, with feet at least shoulder distance apart. The stance needs to feel resilient and adaptable—there is neither bracing nor collapsing. It is helpful to explain and demonstrate the flow and to invite clients to join whenever they understand the breath and movement combination.

1. *Inhalation Segment 1*—Stand with knees bent. Breathe in through the nose—breathe partway and pause briefly. With this first portion go the inhalation, raise the arms forward and up in front of the body, parallel to each other, with palms facing each other, and elbows remaining slightly bent.
2. *Inhalation Segment 2*: Restart the inhalation (i.e., invite the second segment); breathe partway and pause briefly. Simultaneously, lower the arms and then sweep them out to the sides and up.
3. Inhalation Segment 3: Restart and complete the inhalation via the third segment. Lift the arms forward and up, with palms facing each other.
4. *Exhalation*: With a strong and/or long exhalation, make an audible sound through the nose if possible—or the mouth if necessary. Bend the knees even more deeply as you dive forward and swing the arms down and behind you.
5. Repeat twice or up to as many as eight times (for a set of nine flows).

The three inhalation segments occur quickly in succession, with very brief pauses and feeling like one continuous inbreath. The exhalation combines with a forward fold movement and creates one fluid motion. The clinician observes the client carefully for healthful form and movement and debriefs the practice. A sample of this flow is provided at https://youtu.be/Ih6gBODwzIg.

11.5 Where We Go from Here

Ending the book with breath of joy was a deliberate choice. This breath is a breath shared in community; it is a breath that reminds us of the seed of joy that is alive in all of us. It invites us into gratitude and appreciation for our aliveness, our vitality—and its connection to our bodies, minds, relationships, and wisdom. We have come full circle together, and I thank you so much for taking this journey through breathwork with me. It has been a joy and challenge to shape these travels through such a vast and uneven terrain. There is no doubt that some roads and sights along the way were missed; there is no doubt that some directions will not serve you—but hopefully many will. From here on, you will forge your own path and will have the joy of continuing to learn, unlearn, and relearn all there is to know about breath and breathing—an endless and eternal topic and process that flows through all of us and connects us profoundly.

I wish you the resilience of an adaptive, resilient, and coherent breath as you apply the many offered pathways through your own unique journey into working with breath—in your own life and in your work with clients. Breathe lightly, slowly, softly, smoothly, and quietly. Invite moderation and discernment as you take in and expend energy. Each breath deserves our attention and deep appreciation for what it offers.

With gratitude for our connection of shared breath and with the joy of a shared passion—thank you!

Chris

Everything has a beginning, a middle, and an ending. Beginnings require energy and creativity; in the middle one needs to persist and follow through.
   Endings demand the courage to consciously bring matters to a close,
   enjoy what has been accomplished, and then let go.—Arnaud Maitland, Living without Regret, 2005, p. 58.

References

1. Kayser R. Die exakte messung der Luftdurchgangigkeit nase. Archives fur Laryngologie und Rhinologie. 1895;3:101.
2. Cingi C, Bayar Muluk N, Scadding GK, Mladina R. Challenges in rhinology. Springer Nature; 2021.
3. Pendolino AL, Lund VJ, Nardello E, Ottaviano G. The nasal cycle: a comprehensive review. Rhinology. 2018;1(1):67–76. https://doi.org/10.4193/RHINOL/18.021.

4. Susaman N, Cingi C, Mullol J. Is the nasal cycle real? How important is it? In: Cingi C, Bayar Muluk N, Scadding GK, Miadna R, editors. Challenges in rhinology. Springer Nature; 2020. p. 1–8.
5. Atanasov AT. Length of periods in the nasal cycle during 24-hours registration. Open J Biophys. 2014;4(3):93–6. https://doi.org/10.4236/ojbiphy.2014.43010.
6. Kahana-Zweig R, Geva-Sagiv M, Weissbrod A, Secundo L, Soroker N, Sobel N. Measuring and characterizing the human nasal cycle. PLoS One. 2016;11(10):e0162918. https://doi.org/10.1371/journal.pone.0162918.
7. Shannahoff-Khalsa DS, Kennedy B. The effects of unilateral forced nostril breathing on the heart. Int J Neurosci. 1993;73(1–2):47–60. https://doi.org/10.3109/00207459308987210.
8. Jain N, Srivastava RD, Singhal A. The effects of right and left nostril breathing on cardiorespiratory and autonomic parameters. Indian J Physiol Pharmacol. 2005;49(4):469–74. https://www.ncbi.nlm.nih.gov/pubmed/16579402
9. Jyothish U, Das S. Effect of left nostril breathing on postexercise recovery time. J Curr Res Sci Med. 2021;7(2):70–4. https://doi.org/10.4103/jcrsm.jcrsm_84_21.
10. Singh RB, Wilczyńska-Kwiatek A, Fedacko J, Pella D, De Meester F. Pranayama: the power of breath. Int J Disabil Hum Dev. 2009;8(2):141–54. https://doi.org/10.1515/IJDHD.2009.8.2.141.
11. Niazi IK, Navid MS, Bartley J, et al. EEG signatures change during unilateral yogi nasal breathing. Sci Rep. 2022;12(1):520. https://doi.org/10.1038/s41598-021-04461-8.
12. Telles S, Joshi M, Somvanshi P. Yoga breathing through a particular nostril is associated with contralateral event-related potential changes. Int J Yoga. 2012;5(2):102–7. https://doi.org/10.4103/0973-6131.98220.
13. Atanasov AT, Dimov DP. Nasal and sleep cycle—possible synchronization during night sleep. Med Hypotheses. 2003;61(2):275–7. https://doi.org/10.1016/S0306-9877(03)00169-5.
14. Kimura A, Chiba S, Capasso R, et al. Phase of nasal cycle during sleep tends to be associated with sleep stage. Laryngoscope. 2013;123(8):2050–5. https://doi.org/10.1002/lary.23986.
15. Farhi D. The breathing book: good health and vitality through essential breath work. Holt; 1996.
16. Devi NJ. Secret power of yoga. Harmony/Rodale; 2022.
17. Anuradha M, Natarajan DS, Jayanthi DC. Effect of Bhramari and Nadi Shodhana pranayama on lipid profile levels in diabetic women. Int J Yogic Hum Mov Sports Sci. 2023;8(2):290–3. https://doi.org/10.22271/yogic.2023.v8.i2e.1473.
18. Upadhyay J, Nandish NS, Shetty S, Saoji AA, Yadav SS. Effects of Nadishodhana and Bhramari Pranayama on heart rate variability, auditory reaction time, and blood pressure: a randomized clinical trial in hypertensive patients. J Ayurveda Integr Med. 2023;14(4):100774. https://doi.org/10.1016/j.jaim.2023.100774.
19. Ashwini D, Anandraj V. Effect of left and right nostril breathing on heart rate variability among healthy adult males: a cross-sectional study. Int J Physiol. 2020;8(2):34–8. https://doi.org/10.37506/ijop.v8i2.1239.
20. Malhotra V, Deep A, Javed D, et al. Slow frequency Anuloma Viloma pranayama modulates cardiac and neural oscillations in yoga practitioners. Mymensingh Med J. 2022;31(3):851–60. https://search.proquest.com/docview/2684097785
21. Baker JS, Bal BS, Supriya R, Kaur P, Paul M. Effects of Anulom Vilom pranayama and rope Mallakhamb training on respiratory parameters in young females with athletic backgrounds. Pedagog Phys Culture Sports. 2022;26(3):199–209. https://doi.org/10.15561/2664983 7.2022.0308.
22. Rung O, Stauber L, Loescher LJ, Pace TW. Assessment nostril breathing to reduce stress: an option for pregnant women survivors of intimate partner violence? J Holist Nurs. 2021;39(4):393–415. https://doi.org/10.1177/0898010120983659.
23. Solomon SG. Effect of Anuloma and Viloma pranayama on stress of nurses. Int J Adv Psychiatr Nurs. 2022;4(1):7–11. https://doi.org/10.33545/26641348.2022.v4.i1a.74.
24. Naik GS, Gaur GS, Pal GK. Effect of modified slow breathing exercise on perceived stress and basal cardiovascular parameters. Int J Yoga. 2018;11(1):53–8. https://doi.org/10.4103/ijoy. IJOY_41_16.

25. Mathur SK, Awasthi B, Gupta SK. Analyzing the impact of Nadi Shodhan pranayama (alternate nostril breathing) on health and stress management among generation Z. AIP Conf Proc. 2023:2782(1). https://doi.org/10.1063/5.0154420.

26. Annapoorna S, Wale GR. The effect of Anulom Vilom pranayama on levels of depression in geriatric population in selected areas of Hutti, Raichur District, Karnataka. Asian Pac J Nurs. 2019;6(2):87–90. https://mcmed.us/downloads/02201987-90.pdf

27. Kumar N, Pradhan B. Immediate role of two yoga-based breathing technique on state anxiety in patients suffering from anxiety disorder: a self as control pilot study. Int J Yoga Philos Psychol Parapsychol. 2017;5(1):18. https://doi.org/10.4103/ijny.ijoyppp_9_16.

28. Marshall RS, Basilakos A, Williams T, Love-Myers K. Exploring the benefits of unilateral nostril breathing practice post-stroke: attention, language, spatial abilities, depression, and anxiety. J Altern Complement Med. 2014;20(3):185–94. https://doi.org/10.1089/acm.2013.0019.

29. Khairy A, Hassanein A, Abdelkhalek W. Effect of Nadi Shodhana pranayama exercise on blood pressure and anxiety among preoperative patients. Mansoura Nurs J. 2022;9(2):375–86. https://doi.org/10.21608/mnj.2022.295602.

30. Bhattacharjee S, Sharma A, Chakraborty S, Chakraborty S, Chakaborty TR. Breath of relief by Nadi Shodhan yoga for hay fever, exploring holistic health benefits and emotional well-being. Intern J Yogic Hum Mov Sports Sci. 2024;9(1):122–7. https://doi.org/10.22271/yogic.2024. v9.i1b.1536.

31. Kalaivani S, Kumari MJ, Pal GK. Effect of alternate nostril breathing exercise on blood pressure, heart rate, and rate pressure product among patients with hypertension in JIPMER, Puducherry. J Educ Health Promot. 2019;8(1):145. https://doi.org/10.4103/jehp.jehp_32_19.

32. Raghuraj P, Telles S. Immediate effect of specific nostril manipulating yoga breathing practices on autonomic and respiratory variables. Appl Psychophysiol Biofeedback. 2008;33(2):65–75. https://doi.org/10.1007/s10484-008-9055-0.

33. Saravanan L, Anu S, Vairapraveena R, Rajalakshmi G. Impact of alternate nostril breathing exercises on vascular parameters in hypertensive patients - an interventional study. Natl J Physiol Pharm Pharmacol. 2019;9(3):210–4. https://doi.org/10.5455/njppp.2019.9.1237308012019.

34. Jahan I, Begum M, Akhter S, et al. Effects of alternate nostril breathing exercise on cardiorespiratory functions in healthy young adults. Ann Afr Med. 2021;20(2):69–77. https://doi.org/10.4103/aam.aam_114_20.

35. Pal GK, Agarwal A, Karthik S, Pal P, Nanda N. Slow yogic breathing through right and left nostril influences sympathovagal balance, heart rate variability, and cardiovascular risks in young adults. N Am J Med Sci. 2014;6(3):145–51. https://doi.org/10.4103/1947-2714.128477.

36. Sinha AN, Deepak D, Gusain VS. Assessment of the effects of pranayama/alternate nostril breathing on the parasympathetic nervous system in young adults. J Clin Diagn Res. 2013;7(5):821–3. https://doi.org/10.7860/JCDR/2013/4750.2948.

37. McKeown P. The breathing cure. Humanix; 2021.

38. Chetry D, Chhetri A, Rajak D, Rathore V, Gupta A. Exploring the health benefits of *bhramari pranayama* (humming bee breathing): a comprehensive literature review. Indian J Physiol Pharmacol. 2024;68:71–85. https://doi.org/10.25259/IJPP_325_2023.

39. Trivedi GY, Kathirvel S, Sharma K, Saboo B. Effect of various lengths of respiration on heart rate variability during simple Bhramari (humming). Int J Yoga. 2023;16(2):123–31. https://doi.org/10.4103/ijoy.ijoy_113_23.

40. Kuppusamy M, Kamaldeen D, Pitani R, Amaldas J, Shanmugam P. Effects of Bhramari Pranayama on health - a systematic review. J Tradit Complement Med. 2018;8(1):11–6. https://doi.org/10.1016/j.jtcme.2017.02.003.

41. Epe J, Stark R, Ott U. Different effects of four yogic breathing techniques on mindfulness, stress, and well-being. OBM Integr Complement Med. 2021;6(3):1–21. https://doi.org/10.21926/obm.icm.2103031.

42. Trivedi GY, Saboo B. Bhramari Pranayama—a simple lifestyle intervention to reduce heart rate, enhance the lung function and immunity. J Ayurveda Integr Med. 2021;12(3):562–4. https://doi.org/10.1016/j.jaim.2021.07.004.

43. Jain G, Rajak C, Rampalliwar S. Effect of Bhramari Pranayama on volunteers having cardio-vascular hyper-reactivity to cold pressor test. J Yoga Phys Ther. 2011;1(1):1000102. https://doi.org/10.4172/2157-7595.1000102.

44. Pramanik T, Pudasaini B, Prajapati R. Immediate effect of a slow pace breathing exercise Bhramari pranayama on blood pressure and heart rate. Nepal Med Coll J. 2010;12(3):154. https://www.ncbi.nlm.nih.gov/pubmed/21446363

45. Weitzberg E, Lundberg JON. Humming greatly increases nasal nitric oxide. Am J Respir Crit Care Med. 2002;166(2):144–5. https://doi.org/10.1164/rccm.200202-138BC.

46. Ushamohan BP, Rajasekaran AK, Belur YK, Ilavarasu J, Srinivasan TM. Nitric oxide, humming and Bhramari Pranayama. Indian J Sci Technol. 2023;16(5):377–84. https://doi.org/10.17485/IJST/v16i5.1212.

47. Maniscalco M, Sofia M, Weitzberg E, Carratu L, Lundberg JON. Nasal nitric oxide measurements before and after repeated humming maneuvers. Eur J Clin Investig. 2003;33(12):1090–4. https://doi.org/10.1111/j.1365-2362.2003.01277.x.

48. Eby GA. Strong humming for one hour daily to terminate chronic rhinosinusitis in four days: a case report and hypothesis for action by stimulation of endogenous nasal nitric oxide production. Med Hypotheses. 2006;66(4):851–4. https://doi.org/10.1016/j.mehy.2005.11.035.

49. Joshi BP. Psycho-physiological effects of some yogic practices on the selected parameters of human subjects. Int J Contemp Med Res. 2020;7(11):K1–3.

50. Srivastava S, Goyal P, Tiwari SK, Patel AK. Interventional effect of Bhramari Pranayama on mental health among college students. Int J Indian Psychol. 2017;4(2):29–33. https://doi.org/10.25215/0402.044.

51. Pandey S, Mahato NK, Navale R. Role of self-induced sound therapy: Bhramari Pranayama in tinnitus. Audiol Med. 2010;8(3):137–41. https://doi.org/10.3109/1651386X.2010.489694.

52. Shetty HN, Acharya D. Bhramari Pranayama in tinnitus: a systematic review. Indian J Otol. 2023;29(3):146–51. https://doi.org/10.4103/indianjotol.indianjotol_40_23.

53. Rajesh SK, Ilavarasu JV, Srinivasan TM. Effect of Bhramari Pranayama on response inhibition: evidence from the stop signal task. Int J Yoga. 2014;7(2):138–41. https://doi.org/10.4103/0973-6131.133896.

54. Rampalliwar S, Rajak C, Arjariya R, Poonia M, Bajpai R. The effect of Bhramari Pranayama on pregnant women having cardiovascular hyper-reactivity to cold pressor. Natl J Physiol Pharm Pharmacol. 2013;3(2):137. https://doi.org/10.5455/njppp.2013.3.128-133.

55. Rothenberg R. Restoring prana: a therapeutic guide to pranayama and healing through the breath for yoga therapists, teachers, and healthcare practitioners. Singing Dragon; 2020.

56. Mason H, Vandoni M, deBarbieri G, Codrons E, Ugargol V, Bernardi L. Cardiovascular and respiratory effect of yogic slow breathing in the yoga beginner: what is the best approach? Evid Based Complement Alternat Med. 2013;2013:743504. https://doi.org/10.1155/2013/743504.

57. Dwivedi N, Dwivedi S. Impact of Ujjayi Pranayama on anxiety. IAHRW Int J Soc Sci Rev. 2020;8(7–9):333–5. https://search.proquest.com/docview/2617209017

58. Mahour J, Verma P. Effect of Ujjayi Pranayama on cardiovascular autonomic function tests. Natl J Physiol Pharm Pharmacol. 2017;7(4):391–5. https://doi.org/10.5455/njppp.2017.7.1029809122016.

59. Niranjan P, Balaram P. Immediate effect of Ujjayi Pranayama on attention and anxiety among university students: a randomised self-control study. J Clin Diagn Res. 2022;16(2):VC01–4. https://doi.org/10.7860/JCDR/2022/51480.15934.

60. Baishya A, Metri K. Effects of yoga on hypothyroidism: a systematic review. J Ayurveda Integr Med. 2024;15(2):100891. https://doi.org/10.1016/j.jaim.2024.100891.

61. Varne SR, Balaji PA. Physiological effects of yoga and pranayama on serum adipokines, lipoprotein (a), thyrotropin levels, and blood pressure among obese hypothyroid patients with hypertension. Int Res J Ayurveda Yoga. 2023;6(8):9–14. https://doi.org/10.47223/IRJAY.2023.6802.

62. Singh UP. Evidence-based role of hypercapnia and exhalation phase in vagus nerve stimulation: insights into hypercapnic yoga breathing exercises. J Yoga Phys Ther. 2017;7(3):276. https://doi.org/10.4172/2157-7595.1000276.

63. Nestor J. Breath: the new science of a lost art. Riverhead Books; 2020.
64. Swathi PS, Raghavendra BR, Saoji AA. Health and therapeutic benefits of Shatkarma: a narrative review of scientific studies. J Ayurveda Integr Med. 2021;12(1):206–12. https://doi.org/10.1016/j.jaim.2020.11.008.
65. Li P, Yackle K. Sighing. Curr Biol. 2017;27(3):R88–9. https://doi.org/10.1016/j.cub.2016.09.006.
66. Vaschillo EG, Vaschillo B, Buckman JF, et al. The effects of sighing on the cardiovascular system. Biol Psychol. 2015;106:86–95. https://doi.org/10.1016/j.biopsycho.2015.02.007.
67. Vlemincx E, Van Diest I, Van den Bergh O. A sigh of relief or a sigh to relieve: the psychological and physiological relief effect of deep breaths. Physiol Behav. 2016;165:127–35. https://doi.org/10.1016/j.physbeh.2016.07.004.
68. Vlemincx E, Abelson JL, Lehrer PM, Davenport PW, Van Diest I, Van den Bergh O. Respiratory variability and sighing: a psychophysiological reset model. Biol Psychol. 2013;93(1):24–32. https://doi.org/10.1016/j.biopsycho.2012.12.001.
69. Severs LJ, Vlemincx E, Ramirez J. The psychophysiology of the sigh: I: the sigh from the physiological perspective. Biol Psychol. 2022;170:108313. https://doi.org/10.1016/j.biopsycho.2022.108313.
70. Vlemincx E, Severs L, Ramirez J. The psychophysiology of the sigh: II: the sigh from the psychological perspective. Biol Psychol. 2022;173:108386. https://doi.org/10.1016/j.biopsycho.2022.108386.
71. Maytum CK. Sighing dyspnea: a clinical syndrome. J Allergy. 1938;10(1):50–5. https://doi.org/10.1016/S0021-8707(38)90466-6.
72. Kannel WB, Hubert H, Lew EA. Vital capacity as a predictor of cardiovascular disease: the Framingham study. Am Heart J. 1983;105(2):311–5. https://doi.org/10.1016/0002-8703(83)90532-X.
73. Schünemann HJ, Dorn J, Grant BJB, Winkelstein WJ, Trevisan M. Pulmonary function is a long-term predictor of mortality in the general population: 29-year follow-up of the Buffalo Health Study. Chest. 2000;118(3):656–64. https://doi.org/10.1378/chest.118.3.656.
74. Balban MY, Neri E, Kogon MM, et al. Brief structured respiration practices enhance mood and reduce physiological arousal. Cell Rep Med. 2023;4(1):100895. https://doi.org/10.1016/j.xcrm.2022.100895.

Bibliography

Abel AN, Lloyd LK, Williams JS. The effects of regular yoga practice on pulmonary function in healthy individuals: a literature review. J Altern Complement Med. 2013;19(3):185–90. https://doi.org/10.1089/acm.2011.0516.

Achmad H, Ansar AW. Mouth breathing in pediatric population: a literature review. Ann Rom Soc Cell Biol. 2021;25(6):4431–55. https://search.proquest.com/docview/2596972859

Adhana R, Gupta R, Dvivedii J, Ahmad S. The influence of the 2:1 yogic breathing technique on essential hypertension. Indian J Physiol Pharmacol. 2013;57(1):38–44. https://www.ncbi.nlm.nih.gov/pubmed/24020097

Affairs IP. 2016 yoga in America study conducted by Yoga Journal and Yoga Alliance [Techreport]. 2016. https://www.yogajournal.com/page/yogainamericastudy

Al-Casey M, Al-Awadi RN. Oral health status, salivary physical properties and salivary Mutans Streptococci among a group of mouth breathing patients in comparison to nose breathing. J Coll Dent. 2013;25(Special):152–9. https://doi.org/10.12816/0015133.

Alghadir AH, Zafar H, Iqbal ZA. Effect of tongue position on postural stability during quiet standing in healthy young males. Somatosens Mot Res. 2015;32(3):183–6. https://doi.org/10.3109/08990220.2015.1043120.

Alire E, Brems C, Bell K, Chiswell A. The role of yoga in treating stress-related symptoms in dental hygiene students. Int J Yoga. 2020;13(3):213–22. https://doi.org/10.4103/ijoy.IJOY_5_20.

Annapoorna S, Wale GR. The effect of Anulom Vilom pranayama on levels of depression in geriatric population in selected areas of Hutti, Raichur District, Karnataka. Asian Pac J Nurs. 2019;6(2):87–90. https://mcmed.us/downloads/02201987-90.pdf

Ansari R. Kapalabhati pranayama: an answer to modern day polycystic ovarian syndrome and coexisting metabolic syndrome? Int J Yoga. 2016;9(2):163–7. https://doi.org/10.4103/0973-6131.183705.

Antosova M, Mokra D, Pepucha L, et al. Physiology of nitric oxide in the respiratory system. Physiol Res. 2017;66(Suppl 2):S159–72. https://doi.org/10.33549/physiolres.933673.

Anuradha M, Natarajan DS, Jayanthi DC. Effect of Bhramari and Nadi Shodhana pranayama on lipid profile levels in diabetic women. Int J Yogic Hum Mov Sports Sci. 2023;8(2):290–3. https://doi.org/10.22271/yogic.2023.v8.i2e.1473.

Arbo GD, Brems C, Tasker TE. Mitigating the antecedents of sports-related injury through yoga. Int J Yoga. 2020;13(2):120–9. https://doi.org/10.4103/ijoy.IJOY_93_19.

Arena M, Micarelli A, Guzzo F, et al. Outcomes of tongue-tie release by means of tongue and frenulum assessment tools: a scoping review on non-infants. Acta Otorhinolaryngol Ital. 2022;42(6):492–501. https://doi.org/10.14639/0392-100X-N2211.

Ashwini D, Anandraj V. Effect of left and right nostril breathing on heart rate variability among healthy adult males: a cross-sectional study. Int J Physiol. 2020; https://doi.org/10.37506/ijop.v8i2.1239.

Atanasov AT. Length of periods in the nasal cycle during 24-hours registration. Open J Biophys. 2014;4(3):93–6. https://doi.org/10.4236/ojbiphy.2014.43010.

Atanasov AT, Dimov DP. Nasal and sleep cycle—possible synchronization during night sleep. Med Hypotheses. 2003;61(2):275–7. https://doi.org/10.1016/S0306-9877(03)00169-5.

Badenoch B. The brain-savvy therapist's workbook. Norton; 2011a. https://search.proquest.com/docview/869981637

Badenoch B. Being a brain-wise therapist: a practical guide to interpersonal neurobiology. W.W. Norton; 2011b.

Badenoch B. The heart of trauma: healing the embodied brain in the context of relationship. Norton; 2018.

Baginski C. Restorative yoga: relax. Restore. Re-Energize. Alpha Books; 2020.

Baishya A, Metri K. Effects of yoga on hypothyroidism: A systematic review. J Ayurveda Integr Med. 2024;15(2):100891. https://doi.org/10.1016/j.jaim.2024.100891.

Baker JS, Bal BS, Supriya R, Kaur P, Paul M. Effects of Anulom Vilom pranayama and rope Mallakhamb training on respiratory parameters in young females with athletic backgrounds. Pedagog Phys Cult Sports. 2022;26(3):199–209. https://doi.org/10.15561/2664983 7.2022.0308.

Balban MY, Neri E, Kogon MM, et al. Brief structured respiration practices enhance mood and reduce physiological arousal. Cell Rep Med. 2023;4(1):100895. https://doi.org/10.1016/j.xcrm.2022.100895.

Banushi B, Brendle M, Ragnhildstveit A, et al. Breathwork interventions for adults with clinically diagnosedanxiety disorders: a scoping review. Brain Sci. 2023;13(2):256. https://doi.org/10.3390/brainsci13020256.

Barnes PM, Bloom B, Nahin RL. Complementary and alternative medicine use among adults and children: United States. Natl Health Stat Rep. 2007;12:1–23.

Barnett JE, Shale AL, Elkins G, Fisher W. Complementary and alternative medicine for psychologists: an essential resource. American Psychological Association; 2014.

Bentley TGK, D'Andrea-Penna G, Rakic M, et al. Breathing practices for stress and anxiety reduction: conceptual framework of implementation guidelines based on a systematic review of the published literature. Brain Sci. 2023;13(12):1612. https://doi.org/10.3390/brainsci13121612.

Bernardi L, Gabutti A, Porta C, Spicuzza L. Slow breathing reduces chemoreflex response to hypoxia and hypercapnia, and increases baroreflex sensitivity. J Hypertens. 2001;19(12):2221–9. https://doi.org/10.1097/00004872-200112000-00016.

Besco R, Sureda A, Tur J, Pons A. The effect of nitric-oxide-related supplements on human performance. Sports Med. 2017;42:99–117. https://doi.org/10.2165/11596860-000000000-00000.

Bhagat V, Simbak N, Husain R, Mat KC. A brief literature review retraining amygdala to substitute its irrational conditioned fear and anxiety responses with new learning experiences. Res J Pharm Technol. 2020;13(8):3987. https://doi.org/10.5958/0974-360X.2020.00705.2.

Bhanushali D, Tyagi R, Nityapragya NLR, Anand A. Effect of mindfulness meditation protocol in subjects with various psychometric characteristics at high altitude. Brain Behav. 2020;10(5):e01604. https://doi.org/10.1002/brb3.1604.

Bhattacharjee S, Sharma A, Chakraborty S, Chakraborty S, Chakaborty TR. Breath of relief by Nadi Shodhan yoga for hay fever, exploring holistic health benefits and emotional well-being. Int J Yogic Hum Mov Sports Sci. 2024;9(1):122–7. https://doi.org/10.22271/yogic.2024.v9.i1b.1536.

Bhavanani A, Ramanathan M, Balaji R, Pushpa D. Differential effects of uninostril and alternate nostril pranayamas on cardiovascular parameters and reaction time. Int J Yoga. 2014;7(1):60–5. https://doi.org/10.4103/0973-6131.123489.

Bhavanani AB, Raj JB, Ramanathan M, Trakroo M. Effect of different pranayamas on respiratory sinus arrhythmia. J Clin Diagn Res. 2016;10(3):CC04–6. https://doi.org/10.7860/JCDR/2016/16306.7408.

Bilo G, Revera M, Bussotti M, et al. Effects of slow deep breathing at high altitude on oxygen saturation, pulmonary and systemic hemodynamics. PLoS One. 2012;7(11):e49074. https://doi.org/10.1371/journal.pone.0049074.

Birdee G, Nelson K, Wallston K, et al. Slow breathing for reducing stress: the effect of extending exhale. Complement Ther Med. 2023;73:102937. https://doi.org/10.1016/j.ctim.2023.102937.

Birdee GS, Legedza AT, Saper RB, Bertisch SM, Eisenberg DM, Phillips RS. Characteristics of yoga users: results of a national survey. J Gen Intern Med. 2008;23:1653–8.

Blumer S, Eli I, Kaminsky-Kurtz S, Shreiber-Fridman Y, Dolev E, Emodi-Perlman A. Sleep-related breathing disorders in children—red flags in pediatric care. J Clin Med. 2022;11(19):5570. https://doi.org/10.3390/jcm11195570.

Boccio FJ. Mindfulness yoga. Wisdom Publications; 1993a. https://ebookcentral.proquest.com/lib/%5BSITE_ID%5D/detail.action?docID=3417477

Boccio FJ. Mindfulness yoga: the awakened union of breath, body, and mind. Wisdom Publications; 1993b.

Boccio FJ. Mindfulness yoga. Wisdom Publications; 2005. https://www.perlego.com/book/1397375/mindfulness-yoga-the-awakened-union-of-breath-body-and-mind-pdf

Bohr C, Hasselbalch K, Krogh A. Über einen in biologischer Beziehung wichtigen Einfluss, den die Kohlensäurespannung des Blutes auf dessen Sauerstoffbindung übt. Skandinavisches Archiv Für Physiologie. 1904;16(2):402–12. https://doi.org/10.1111/j.1748-1716.1904.tb01382.x.

Bondy D. Yoga for everyone: 50 poses for every type of body. Dorling Kindersley; 2019.

Bordoni B, Zanier E. Anatomic connections of the diaphragm: influence of respiration on the body system. J Multidiscip Healthc. 2013;6:281–91.

Bordoni B, Morabito B, Mitrano R, Simonelli M, Toccafondi A. The anatomical relationships of the tongue with the body system. Cureus. 2018;10(12):e3695. https://doi.org/10.7759/cureus.3695.

Borges U, Lobinger B, Javelle F, Watson M, Mosley E, Laborde S. Using slow-paced breathing to foster endurance, well-being, and sleep quality in athletes during the COVID-19 pandemic. Front Psychol. 2021;12:1–8. https://doi.org/10.3389/fpsyg.2021.624655.

Boyadzhieva A, Kayhan E. Keeping the breath in mind: respiration, neural oscillations, and the free energy principle. Front Neurosci. 2021;15:647579. https://doi.org/10.3389/fnins.2021.647579.

Bradley H, Esformes J. Breathing pattern disorders and functional movement. Int J Sports Phys Ther. 2014;9(1):28–39. https://www.ncbi.nlm.nih.gov/pubmed/24567853

Brashear RE. Hyperventilation syndrome. Lung. 1983;161:257–73. https://doi.org/10.1007/BF02713872.

Brems C. Psychotherapy: processes and techniques. Allyn & Bacon; 1999.

Brems C. Basic skills in psychotherapy and counseling. Brooks/Cole: Thomson Learning; 2001.

Brems C. A yoga stress reduction intervention for university faculty, staff, and graduate students. Int J Yoga Ther. 2015;25(1):61–77. https://doi.org/10.17761/1531-2054-25.1.61.

Brems C. Refinement of a multi-dimensional data collection tool for assessment, treatment planning, and outcomes tracking. Paper presented at: Symposium on yoga therapy and yoga research, Newport Beach, CA; June 2019.

Brems C. Yoga as a mind-body practice. In: Uribarri J, Vassalotti JA, editors. Nutrition, fitness, and mindfulness: an evidence-based guide for clinicians. Springer Nature; 2020. p. 137–55.

Brems C. Ancient wisdoms and science of yoga: a companion for 200-Hour Yoga Teacher Training for Healthcare and Allied Healthcare Settings. 2022.

Brems C. Yoga for mental health: cultivating emotional resilience and mental fortitude. Self-published; 2024.

Brems C. Ancient wisdom and modern science of yoga: a companion for 200-hour yoga teacher training for healthcare and allied healthcare settings. 2024.

Brems C, Rasmussen CH. A comprehensive guide to child psychotherapy and counseling. 4th ed. Waveland; 2019.

Brems C, Johnson ME, Warner TD, Roberts LW. Patient requests and provider suggestions for alternative treatments as reported by rural and urban care providers. Complement Ther Med. 2006b;14(1):10–9.

Brems C, Colgan D, Freeman H, et al. Elements of yogic practice: perceptions of students in healthcare programs. Int J Yoga. 2016;9:121–9. https://doi.org/10.4103/0973-6131.183710.

Brems C, Justice L, Sulenes K, et al. Improving access to yoga: barriers to and motivators for practice among health professions students. Adv Mind Body Med. 2015;29(3):6–13.

Brown KW, Ryan RM. The benefits of being present. J Pers Soc Psychol. 2003;84(4):822–48. https://doi.org/10.1037/0022-3514.84.4.822.

Brown KW, Ryan RM, Creswell JD. Mindfulness: theoretical foundations and evidence for its salutary effects. Psychol Inq. 2007;18:211–37.

Brown RP, Gerbarg PL. Non-drug treatments for ADHD: new options for kids, adults, and clinicians. Norton; 2012. https://www.vlebooks.com/vleweb/product/openreader?id=none&isbn=9780393707724

Brule D. Just breathe: mastering breathwork for success in life, love, business, and beyond. Atria/Enliven Books; 2017.

Burgess J, Ekanayake B, Lowe A, Dunt D, Thien F, Dharmage SC. Systematic review of the effectiveness of breathing retraining in asthma management. Expert Rev Respir Med. 2011;5(6):789–807. https://doi.org/10.1586/ers.11.69.

Carter J, Gerbarg PL, D'ambrosio C, et al. Multi-component yoga breath program for Vietnam veteran post traumatic stress disorder: randomized controlled trial. J Trauma Stress Disord Treat. 2013;2(3):10. https://doi.org/10.4172/2324-8947.1000108.

Chalupa DC, Morrow PE, Oberdörster G, Utell MJ, Frampton MW. Ultrafine particle deposition in subjects with asthma. Environ Health Perspect. 2004;112(8):879–82. https://doi.org/10.1289/ehp.6851.

Chambers D, Huang C, Matthews G. Basic physiology for anaesthetists. Cambridge University Press; 2019. https://doi.org/10.1017/9781108565011.

Chen Y, Huang X, Chien C, Cheng J. The effectiveness of diaphragmatic breathing relaxation training for reducing anxiety. Perspect Psychiatr Care. 2017;53(4):329–36. https://doi.org/10.1111/ppc.12184.

Cheng S, Butler JE, Gandevia SC, Bilston LE. Movement of the tongue during normal breathing in awake healthy humans. J Physiol. 2008;586(17):4283–94. https://doi.org/10.1113/jphysiol.2008.156430.

Chetry D, Chhetri A, Rajak D, Rathore V, Gupta A. Exploring the health benefits of bhramari pranayama (humming bee breathing): A comprehensive literature review. Indian J Physiol Pharmacol. 2024;68:71–85. https://doi.org/10.25259/IJPP_325_2023.

Choi JE, Waddell JN, Lyons KM, Kieser JA. Intraoral pH and temperature during sleep with and without mouth breathing. J Oral Rehabil. 2016;43(5):356–63. https://doi.org/10.1111/joor.12372.

Cingi C, Muluk NB, Scadding GK, Mladina R. Challenges in rhinology. Springer Nature; 2021. https://doi.org/10.1007/978-3-030-50899-9.

Clark B. Your body, your yoga. Wild Strawberry Productions; 2016.

Clark B. Your spine, your yoga: developing stability and mobility for your spine. Wild Strawberry Productions; 2018. https://www.vlebooks.com/vleweb/product/openreader?id=none&isbn=9780968766569

Colgan DD, Christopher M, Bowen S, et al. Mindfulness-based wellness and resilience intervention among interdisciplinary primary care teams: a mixed-methods feasibility and acceptability trial. Prim Health Care Res Dev. 2019;20:e91. https://doi.org/10.1017/S1463423619000173.

Colgan DD, Green K, Eddy A, et al. Translation, cross-cultural adaptation, and psychometric validation of the English version of the postural awareness scale. Pain Med. 2021;22(11):2686–99. https://doi.org/10.1093/pm/pnab200.

Coulter D. Anatomy of hatha yoga. Body and Breath; 2001.

Courtney R. Strengths, weaknesses, and possibilities of the Buteyko Breathing Method. Biofeedback. 2008;36(2):59–63. https://search.proquest.com/docview/208128464

Courtney R, Greenwood KM. Preliminary investigation of a measure of dysfunctional breathing symptoms: the self evaluation of breathing questionnaire (SEBQ). Int J Osteopath Med. 2009;12(4):121–7. https://doi.org/10.1016/j.ijosm.2009.02.001.

Cozolino L. Why therapy works: using our minds to change our brains. W.W. Norton; 2015.

Cozolino LJ. The neuroscience of psychotherapy: healing the social brain. 3rd ed. W.W. Norton; 2017.

Craig AD. How do you feel? An interoceptive moment with your neurobiological self. Princeton University Press; 2014.

Critchley HD, Nicotra A, Chiesa PA, et al. Slow breathing and hypoxic challenge: cardiorespiratory consequences and their central neural substrates. PLoS One. 2015;10(5):e0127082. https://doi.org/10.1371/journal.pone.0127082.

Csikszentmihalyi M. Flow: the psychology of optimal experience, Harper perennial modern classics. 1st ed. Harper Perennial; 2008.

Curley G, Kavanagh BP, Laffey JG. Hypocapnia and the injured brain: evidence for harm. Crit Care Med. 2011;39(1):229–30. https://doi.org/10.1097/CCM.0b013e3181ffe3c7.

Curley G, Laffey JG, Kavanagh BP. Bench-to-bedside review: carbon dioxide. Crit Care. 2010;14(2):220. https://doi.org/10.1186/cc8926.

Damasio AR. Self comes to mind: constructing the conscious brain. Vintage; 2012.

Dana D. The polyvagal theory in therapy: engaging the rhythm of regulation. Norton; 2018.

Dana D, Porges S. Clinical applications of the polyvagal theory: the emergence of polyvagal-informed therapies. Norton; 2018.

Davidovich E, Hevroni A, Gadassi LT, Spierer-Weil A, Yitschaky O, Polak D. Dental, oral pH, orthodontic and salivary values in children with obstructive sleep apnea. Clin Oral Investig. 2022;26(3):2503–11. https://doi.org/10.1007/s00784-021-04218-7.

del Paso GAR, de Guevara CML, Montoro CI. Breath-holding during exhalation as a simple manipulation to reduce pain perception. Pain Med. 2015;16(9):1835–41. https://doi.org/10.1111/pme.12764.

Devi NJ. Secret power of yoga. Harmony/Rodale; 2022.

Diest IV, Verstappen K, Aubert AE, Widjaja D, Vansteenwegen D, Vlemincx E. Inhalation/exhalation ratio modulates the effect of slow breathing on heart rate variability and relaxation. Appl Psychophysiol Biofeedback. 2014;39:171–80. https://doi.org/10.1007/s10484-014-9253-x.

Dittman KA, Freedman MR. Body awareness, eating attitudes, and spiritual beliefs of women practicing yoga. Eat Disord. 2009;17:273–92. https://doi.org/10.1080/10640260902991111.

Dwivedi N, Dwivedi S. Impact of ujjayi pranayama on anxiety. IAHRW Int J Soc Sci Rev. 2020;8(7–9):333–5. https://search.proquest.com/docview/2617209017

Eby GA. Strong humming for one hour daily to terminate chronic rhinosinusitis in four days: a case report and hypothesis for action by stimulation of endogenous nasal nitric oxide production. Med Hypotheses. 2006;66(4):851–4. https://doi.org/10.1016/j.mehy.2005.11.035.

Ekman P, Davidson RJ, Ricard M, Wallace BA. Buddhist and psychological perspectives on emotions and well-being. Curr Dir Psychol Sci. 2005;14(2):59–63. https://doi.org/10.1111/j.0963-7214.2005.00335.x.

Elliott S. Diaphragm mediates action of autonomic and enteric nervous systems. BMED Report. 2010. https://www.bmedreport.com/archives/8309

Elwy AR, Groessl EJ, Eisen SV, et al. A systematic scoping review of yoga intervention components and study quality. Am J Prev Med. 2014;47:220–32.

Epe J, Stark R, Ott U. Different effects of four yogic breathing techniques on mindfulness, stress, and well-being. OBM Integr Complement Med. 2021;6(3):1–21. https://doi.org/10.21926/obm.icm.2103031.

Esteve-Gibert N, Prieto P. Infants temporally coordinate gesture-speech combinations before they produce their first words. Speech Comm. 2014;57:301–16. https://doi.org/10.1016/j.specom.2013.06.006.

Fang Y, Jiang Z, Wang H. A novel sleep respiratory rate detection method for obstructive sleep apnea based on characteristic moment waveform. J Healthc Eng. 2018;2018:1902176. https://doi.org/10.1155/2018/1902176.

Farb N, Duabenmier J, Price CJ, et al. Interoception, contemplative practice, and health. Front Psychol. 2015;6:763. https://doi.org/10.3389/fpsyg.2015.00763.

Farhi D. The breathing book: good health and vitality through essential breath work. Holt; 1996.

Farhi D. Bringing yoga to life. HarperCollins Publishers; 2005.

Farhi D. Yoga mind, body & spirit: a return to wholeness. Owl Books; 2011. https://www.vlebooks.com/vleweb/product/openreader?id=none&isbn=9781429997430&uid=none

Farhi D, Leila S. Pathways to a centered body. Embodied Wisdom Publishing; 2022.

Feng H-Y, Zhang P-P, Wang X-W. Presbyphagia: dysphagia in the elderly. World J Clin Cases. 2023;11(11):2363–73. https://doi.org/10.12998/wjcc.v11.i11.2363.

Feuerstein G. The psychology of yoga: integrating eastern and western approaches for understanding the mind. Shambala; 2013.

Field T. Yoga clinical research review. Complement Ther Clin Pract. 2011;17:1–8.

Foster GE, Sheel AW. The human diving response, its function, and its control. Scand J Med Sci Sports. 2005;15(1):3–12. https://doi.org/10.1111/j.1600-0838.2005.00440.x.

Freeman H, Brems C, Michael P, Marsh S. Empowering a community from the inside out: evaluation of a yoga teacher training program for adults in custody. Int J Yoga Ther. 2019;29(1):19–29. https://doi.org/10.17761/2019-00015.

Freeman H, Vladagina N, Razmjou E, Brems C. Yoga in print media: missing the heart of the practice. Int J Yoga. 2017;10(3):160–6. https://doi.org/10.4103/ijoy.IJOY_1_17.

Gamboa A, Shibao C, Diedrich A, et al. Contribution of endothelial nitric oxide to blood pressure in humans. Hypertension. 2007;49(1):170–7. https://doi.org/10.1161/01.HYP.0000252425.06216.26.

Gard T, Noggle JJ, Park C, Vago DR, Wilson A. Potential self-regulatory mechanisms of yoga for psychological health. Front Hum Neurosci. 2014;8:770. https://doi.org/10.3389/fnhum.2014.00770.

Gard T, Taquet M, Dixit R, Holzel B, Dickerson B, Lazar S. Greater widespread functional connectivity of the caudate in older adults who practice kripalu yoga and vipassana meditation than in controls. Front Hum Neurosci. 2015;9:137. https://doi.org/10.3389/fnhum.2015.00137.

Garland EL, Farb NA, Goldin PR, Fredrickson BL. Mindfulness broadens awareness and builds eudaimonic meaning: a process model of mindful positive emotion regulation. Psychol Inq. 2015;26(4):293–314. https://doi.org/10.1080/1047840X.2015.1064294.

Gerritsen R, Band G. Breath of life: the respiratory vagal stimulation model of contemplative activity. Front Neurosci. 2018;12:1–25. https://doi.org/10.3389/fnhum.2018.00397.

Ghahjaverestan NM, Saha S, Kabir M, Gavrilovic B, Zhu K, Yadollahi A. Sleep apnea severity based on estimated tidal volume and snoring features from tracheal signals. J Sleep Res. 2022;31(2):e13490. https://doi.org/10.1111/jsr.13490.

Gil H, Fougeront N. Tongue dysfunction screening: assessment protocol for prescribers. J Dentofac Anom Orthod. 2015;18(4):408. https://doi.org/10.1051/odfen/2015026.

Gilbert C. Better chemistry through breathing: the story of carbon dioxide and how it can go wrong. Biofeedback. 2005;33(3):100–4. https://search.proquest.com/docview/208148631

Gilbert C, Chaitow L, Bradley D. Recognizing and treating breathing disorders. 2nd ed. Elsevier Health Sciences; 2013. https://doi.org/10.1016/C2011-0-05580-1.

Givens J. Essential pranayama: breathing techniques for balance, healing, and peace. Rockridge Press; 2020.

Goleman D, Davidson RJ. Altered traits. Avery; 2017.

Grant A. Think again. WH Allen; 2021.

Grassi M, Caldirola D, Vanni G, et al. Baseline respiratory parameters in panic disorder: a meta-analysis. J Affect Disord. 2012;146(2):158–73. https://doi.org/10.1016/j.jad.2012.08.034.

Grof S, Grof C. Holotropic Breathwork. 2nd ed. State University of New York Press; 2023.

Gu J, Strauss C, Bond R, Cavanagh K. How do mindfulness-based cognitive therapy and mindfulness-based stress reduction improve mental health and wellbeing? A systematic review and meta-analysis of meditation studies. Clin Psychol Rev. 2015;37:1–12.

Han MK. Breathing lessons: a doctor's guide to lung health. Norton; 2022.

Hartranft C. The yoga sutra of Patanjali: a new translation with commentary. Shambala Classics; 2003.

Haughey JP, Fine P. Effects of the lower jaw position on athletic performance of elite athletes. BMJ Open Sport Exerc Med. 2020;6(1):e000886. https://doi.org/10.1136/bmjsem-2020-000886.

Hayes M, Chase S. Prescribing yoga. Prim Care. 2010;37:31–47.

Herrero JL, Khuvis S, Yeagle E, Cerf M, Mehta AD. Breathing above the brain stem: volitional control and attentional modulation in humans. J Neurophysiol. 2018;119(1):145–59. https://doi.org/10.1152/jn.00551.2017.

Heyman J. Accessible yoga: poses and practices for every body. Shambhala; 2019. https://ebookcentral.proquest.com/lib/%5BSITE_ID%5D/detail.action?docID=6072130

Heyman J. Yoga revolution: building a practice of courage and compassion. Shambhala; 2021. https://ebookcentral.proquest.com/lib/%5BSITE_ID%5D/detail.action?docID=6792248

Heyman J. The teacher's guide to accessible yoga. Rainbow Mind; 2024.

Hodges PW, Cresswell AG, Daggfeldt K, Thorstensson A. In vivo measurement of the effect of intra-abdominal pressure on the human spine. J Biomech. 2001;34(3):347–53. https://doi.org/10.1016/S0021-9290(00)00206-2.

Hodges PW, Gandevia SC. Activation of the human diaphragm during a repetitive postural task. J Physiol. 2000;522(1):165–75. https://doi.org/10.1111/j.1469-7793.2000.t01-1-00165.xm.

Hof W. The Wim Hof method: activate your full human potential. Sounds True; 2020. https://www.vlebooks.com/vleweb/product/openreader?id=none&isbn=9781683644101

Hostetter AB, Alibali MW. On the tip of the mind: gesture as a key to conceptualization. 2004. https://escholarship.org/uc/item/0bq3923m

Hsu S-M, Tseng C-H, Hsieh C-H, Hsieh C-W. Slow-paced inspiration regularizes alpha phase dynamics in the human brain. J Neurophysiol. 2020;123(1):289–99. https://doi.org/10.1152/jn.00624.2019.

Hsu Y, Lan M, Huang Y, Kao M, Lan M. Association between breathing route, oxygen desaturation, and upper airway morphology. Laryngoscope. 2021;131(2):E659–64. https://doi.org/10.1002/lary.28774.

Hu Z, Sun H, Wu Y, et al. Mouth breathing impairs the development of temporomandibular joint at a very early stage. Oral Dis. 2020;26(7):1502–12. https://doi.org/10.1111/odi.13377.

Hylton H, Long A, Francis C, et al. Real-world use of the breathing pattern assessment tool in assessment of breathlessness post-COVID-19. Clin Med. 2022;22(4):376–9. https://doi.org/10.7861/clinmed.2021-0759.

Irving W. The stoic challenge: a philosopher's guide to becoming tougher, calmer, and more resilient. Norton; 2019.

Ito T, Caillet J-L, Perrier P. Stability in postural tongue control: response to transient mechanical perturbations. Paper presented at: Neuroscience 2018 - Annual Meeting of the Society for Neuroscience. 2018 Nov 3. https://explore.openaire.eu/search/result?id=dedup_wf_001::4b7dc2e691f4b89a5d0ad333f6670047

Iyengar BKS. Light on life. Rodale; 2006.

Iyengar BKS. Light on pranayama. HarperCollins; 2013.

Jahan I, Begum M, Akhter S, et al. Effects of alternate nostril breathing exercise on cardiorespiratory functions in healthy young adults. Ann Afr Med. 2021;20(2):69–77. https://doi.org/10.4103/aam.aam_114_20.

Jain G, Rajak C, Rampalliwar S. Effect of bhramari pranayama on volunteers having cardiovascular hyper-reactivity to cold pressor test. J Yoga Phys Ther. 2011; https://doi.org/10.4172/2157-7595.1000102.

Jain N, Srivastava RD, Singhal A. The effects of right and left nostril breathing on cardiorespiratory and autonomic parameters. Indian J Physiol Pharmacol. 2005;49(4):469–74. https://www.ncbi.nlm.nih.gov/pubmed/16579402

Jeter PE, Slutsky J, Singh N, Khalsa SB. Yoga as a therapeutic intervention: a bibliometric analysis of published research studies from 1967 to 2013. J Altern Complement Med. 2015;21:586–92.

Ji LL, Dickman JR, Kang C, Koenig R. Exercise-induced hormesis may help healthy aging. Dose Response. 2010;8(1):73–9. https://doi.org/10.2203/dose-response.09-048.Ji.

Johnson MC. Skill in action: radicalizing your yoga practice to create a just world. Shambhala; 2021.

Johnson MC. We heal together: rituals and practices for building community and connection. Shambhala; 2023.

Jones FP. Body awareness in action. Schocken Books; 1976.

Joshi BP. Psycho-physiological effects of some yogic practices on the selected parameters of human subjects. Int J Contemp Med Res. 2020;7(11):K1–3.

Jugé L, Knapman FL, Burke PGR, et al. Regional respiratory movement of the tongue is coordinated during wakefulness and is larger in severe obstructive sleep apnoea. J Physiol. 2020;598(3):581–97. https://doi.org/10.1113/JP278769.

Jung J-Y, Kang C-K. Investigation on the effect of oral breathing on cognitive activity using functional brain imaging. Healthcare. 2021;9(6):645. https://doi.org/10.3390/healthcare9060645.

Justice L, Brems C. Bridging body and mind: case series of a 10-week trauma-informed yoga protocol for veterans. Int J Yoga Ther. 2019;29(1):65–79. https://doi.org/10.17761/D-17-2019-00029.

Justice L, Brems C, Ehlers K. Bridging body and mind: considerations for trauma-informed yoga. Int J Yoga Ther. 2018;28(1):39–50. https://doi.org/10.17761/2018-00017R2.

Justice L, Brems C, Jacova C. Exploring strategies to enhance self-efficacy about starting a yoga practice. Ann Yoga Phys Ther. 2016;1(2):1–7. https://austinpublishinggroup.com/yoga-physical-therapy/fulltext/aypt-v1-id1012.pdf

Jyothish U, Das S. Effect of left nostril breathing on postexercise recovery time. J Curr Res Sci Med. 2021;7(2):70–4. https://doi.org/10.4103/jcrsm.jcrsm_84_21.

Kahana-Zweig R, Geva-Sagiv M, Weissbrod A, Secundo L, Soroker N, Sobel N. Measuring and characterizing the human nasal cycle. PLoS One. 2016;11(10):e0162918. https://doi.org/10.1371/journal.pone.0162918.

Kalaivani S, Kumari MJ, Pal GK. Effect of alternate nostril breathing exercise on blood pressure, heart rate, and rate pressure product among patients with hypertension in JIPMER, Puducherry. J Educ Health Promot. 2019;8(1):145. https://doi.org/10.4103/jehp.jehp_32_19.

Kannel WB, Hubert H, Lew EA. Vital capacity as a predictor of cardiovascular disease: the Framingham study. Am Heart J. 1983;105(2):311–5. https://doi.org/10.1016/0002-8703(83)90532-X.

Kasperk C. Hypercalcemic crisis and hypocalcemic tetany. Internist. 2017;58(10):1029–36. https://doi.org/10.1007/s00108-017-0311-3.

Kayser R. Die exakte messung der Luftdurchgangigkeit nase. Archives Fur Laryngologie Und Rhinologie. 1895;3:101.

Khairy A, Hassanein A, Abdelkhalek W. Effect of Nadi Shodhana pranayama exercise on blood pressure and anxiety among preoperative patients. Mansoura Nurs J. 2022;9(2):375–86. https://doi.org/10.21608/mnj.2022.295602.

Khalsa GDS, Stauth C, Borysenko J. Meditation as medicine: activate the power of your natural healing force. Simon & Schuster; 2011. https://www.vlebooks.com/vleweb/product/openreader?id=none&isbn=9781439117538

Khalsa SB, Cohen L, McCall T, Telles S. Principles and practice of yoga in health care. Handspring Publishing Limited; 2016. https://ebookcentral.proquest.com/lib/%5BSITE_ID%5D/detail.action?docID=30168027

Kimberley B, Nejadnik B, Giraud GD, Holden WE. Nasal contribution to exhaled nitric oxide at rest and during breathholding in humans. Am J Respir Crit Care Med. 1996;153(2):829–36. https://doi.org/10.1164/ajrccm.153.2.8564139.

Kimura A, Chiba S, Capasso R, et al. Phase of nasal cycle during sleep tends to be associated with sleep stage. Laryngoscope. 2013;123(8):2050–5. https://doi.org/10.1002/lary.23986.

King JC, Rosen SD, Nixon PG. Failure of perception of hypocapnia: physiological and clinical implications. J R Soc Med. 1990;83(12):765–7. https://doi.org/10.1177/014107689008301205.

Kolar P, Sulc J, Kyncl M, et al. Postural function of the diaphragm in persons with and without chronic low back pain. J Orthop Sports Phys Ther. 2012;42(4):352–62. https://doi.org/10.2519/jospt.2012.3830.

Krakauer LH, Guilherme A. Relationship between mouth breathing and postural alterations of children: A descriptive analysis. Int J Orofac Myol. 2000;26(1):13–23. https://doi.org/10.52010/ijom.2000.26.1.2.

Kumar N, Pradhan B. Immediate role of two yoga-based breathing technique on state anxiety in patients suffering from anxiety disorder: A self as control pilot study. Int J Yoga Philos Psychol Parapsychol. 2017;5(1):18. https://doi.org/10.4103/ijny.ijoyppp_9_16.

Kuppusamy M, Kamaldeen D, Pitani R, Amaldas J, Shanmugam P. Effects of Bhramari Pranayama on health - a systematic review. J Tradit Complement Med. 2018;8:11–7. https://doi.org/10.1016/j.jtcme.2017.02.003.

Laborde S, Allen MS, Borges U, et al. Effects of voluntary slow breathing on heart rate and heart rate variability: A systematic review and a meta-analysis. Neurosci Biobehav Rev. 2022;138:104711. https://doi.org/10.1016/j.neubiorev.2022.104711.

Laborde S, Allen MS, Borges U, et al. The influence of slow-paced breathing on executive function. J Psychophysiol. 2022;36(1):13–27. https://doi.org/10.1027/0269-8803/a000279.

Laborde S, Allen MS, Göhring N, Dosseville F. The effect of slow-paced breathing on stress management in adolescents with intellectual disability. J Intellect Disabil Res. 2017;61(6):560–7. https://doi.org/10.1111/jir.12350.

Laborde S, Hosang T, Mosley E, Dosseville F. Influence of a 30-day slow-paced breathing intervention compared to social media use on subjective sleep quality and cardiac vagal activity. J Clin Med. 2019;8(2):193. https://doi.org/10.3390/jcm8020193.

Laborde S, Iskra M, Zammit N, et al. Slow-paced breathing: influence of inhalation/exhalation ratio and of respiratory pauses on cardiac vagal activity. Sustain For. 2021;13(14):7775. https://doi.org/10.3390/su13147775.

Lasater JH. Restore and rebalance: yoga for deep relaxation. Shambhala; 2017.

Lasater JH. Yoga myths. Shambhala; 2020. https://www.vlebooks.com/vleweb/product/openreader?id=none&isbn=9780834843004

Lee K-J, Park C-A, Lee Y-B, Kim H-K, Kang C-K. EEG signals during mouth breathing in a working memory task. Int J Neurosci. 2020;130(5):425–34. https://doi.org/10.1080/00207454.2019.1667787.

Lehrer PM, Gevirtz R. Heart rate variability biofeedback: how and why does it work? Front Psychol. 2014;5:756. https://doi.org/10.3389/fpsyg.2014.00756.

Lehrer PM, Woolfolk RL. Principles and practice of stress management. 4th ed. Guilford Press; 2021.

Levine P. Waking the Tiger: healing trauma. North Atlantic Books; 1997.

Ley R. Panic attacks during relaxation and relaxation-induced anxiety: a hyperventilation interpretation. J Behav Ther Exp Psychiatry. 1988;19(4):253–9. https://doi.org/10.1016/0005-7916(88)90054-7.

Leyro TM, Versella MV, Yang M-J, Brinkman HR, Hoyt DL, Lehrer P. Respiratory therapy for the treatment of anxiety: meta-analytic review and regression. Clin Psychol Rev. 2021;84:101980. https://doi.org/10.1016/j.cpr.2021.101980.

Li P, Yackle K. Sighing. Curr Biol. 2017;27(3):R88–9. https://doi.org/10.1016/j.cub.2016.09.006.

Lin IM, Tai LY, Fan SY. Breathing at a rate of 5.5 breaths per minute with equal inhalation-to-exhalation ratio increases heart rate variability. Int J Psychophysiol. 2014;91:206–11. https://doi.org/10.1016/j.ijpsycho.2013.12.006.

Lipan MJ, Most SP. Development of a severity classification system for subjective nasal obstruction. JAMA Facial Plast Surg. 2013;15(5):358–61. https://doi.org/10.1001/jamafacial.2013.344.

Litchfield PM. Good breathing, bad breathing. 2006. https://www.breatheon.com/media/docs/Peter-Litchfield-on-goodbad-breathing-CapnoTrainer8.pdf

Lundberg JON, Farkas-Szallasi T, Weitzberg E, et al. High nitric oxide production in human paranasal sinuses. Nat Med. 1995;1(4):370–3. https://doi.org/10.1038/nm0495-370.

Lundberg JON, Weitzberg E. Nasal nitric oxide in man. Thorax. 1999;54(10):947–52. https://doi.org/10.1136/thx.54.10.947.

Lundberg JO. Nitric oxide and the paranasal sinuses. Anat Rec. 2008;291(11):1479–84. https://doi.org/10.1002/ar.20782.

Macefield G, Burke D. Paraesthesiae and tetany induced by voluntary hyperventilation: increased excitability of human cutaneous and motor axons. Brain. 1991;114(1):527–40. https://doi.org/10.1093/brain/114.1.527.

Mahour J, Verma P. Effect of Ujjayi Pranayama on cardiovascular autonomic function tests. Natl J Physiol Pharm Pharmacol. 2017;7(4):391–5. https://doi.org/10.5455/njppp.2017.7.1029809122016.

Maki B. The yogi's roadmap: the patanjali yoga sutra as a journey to self-realization. CreateSpace; 2013.

Malhotra V, Deep A, Javed D, et al. Slow frequency Anuloma Viloma pranayama modulates cardiac and neural oscillations in yoga practitioners. Mymensingh Med J. 2022;31(3):851–60. https://search.proquest.com/docview/2684097785

Malhotra V, Hulke SM, Bharshankar R, Chouhan S, Ravi N, Patrick KP. Effect of slow and deep breathing on brain waves in regular yoga practitioners. Mymensingh Med J. 2021;30(4):1163–7. https://search.proquest.com/docview/2579089112

Maniscalco M, Sofia M, Weitzberg E, Carratu L, Lundberg JON. Nasal nitric oxide measurements before and after repeated humming maneuvers. Eur J Clin Investig. 2003;33(12):1090–4. https://doi.org/10.1111/j.1365-2362.2003.01277.x.

Marshall RS, Basilakos A, Williams T, Love-Myers K. Exploring the benefits of unilateral nostril breathing practice post-stroke: attention, language, spatial abilities, depression, and anxiety. J Altern Complement Med. 2014;20(3):185–94. https://doi.org/10.1089/acm.2013.0019.

Martel J, Ko Y-F, Young JD, Ojcius DM. Could nasal nitric oxide help to mitigate the severity of COVID-19? Microbes Infect. 2020;22(4–5):168–71. https://doi.org/10.1016/j.micinf.2020.05.002.

Mason H, Vandoni M, deBarbieri G, Codrons E, Ugargol V, Bernardi L. Cardiovascular and respiratory effect of yogic slow breathing in the yoga beginner: what is the best approach? Evid Based Complement Alternat Med. 2013;2013:743504. https://doi.org/10.1155/2013/743504.

Mather M, Thayer JF. How heart rate variability affects emotion regulation brain networks. Curr Opin Behav Sci. 2018;19:98–104. https://doi.org/10.1016/j.cobeha.2017.12.017.

Mathur SK, Awasthi B, Gupta SK. Analyzing the impact of Nadi Shodhan pranayama (alternate nostril breathing) on health and stress management among generation Z. AIP Conf Proc. 2023;2782(1):020154. https://doi.org/10.1063/5.0154420.

Maytum CK. Sighing dyspnea: a clinical syndrome. J Allergy. 1938;10(1):50–5. https://doi.org/10.1016/S0021-8707(38)90466-6.

McCall MC. How might yoga work? An overview of potential underlying mechanisms. J Yoga Phys Ther. 2013;3(1):1. https://doi.org/10.4172/2157-7595.1000130.

McCall MC. In search of yoga: research trends in a western medical database. Int J Yoga. 2014;7:4–8.

McKeown P. Buteyko instructor training manual. Oxygen Research Institute; 2020.

McKeown P. The breathing cure. Humanix; 2021.

McKeown P. Oxygen advantage: the simple, scientifically proven breathing techniques for a healthier, slimmer, faster, and fitter You. William Morrow; 2015.

McKeown P, O'Connor-Reina C, Plaza G. Breathing re-education and phenotypes of sleep apnea: a review. J Clin Med. 2021;10(3):471. https://doi.org/10.3390/jcm10030471.

Meuret AE, Ritz T, Wilhelm FH, Roth WT, Rosenfield D. Hypoventilation therapy alleviates panic by repeated induction of dyspnea. Biol Psychiatry Cogn Neurosci Neuroimaging. 2018;3(6):539–45. https://doi.org/10.1016/j.bpsc.2018.01.010.

Meuret AE, Rosenfield D, Hofmann SG, Suvak MK, Roth WT. Changes in respiration mediate changes in fear of bodily sensations in panic disorder. J Psychiatr Res. 2009;43(6):634–41. https://doi.org/10.1016/j.jpsychires.2008.08.003.

Michelis ED. A history of modern yoga. Continuum; 2004. https://doi.org/10.5040/9781472548436.

Miller R. Yoga nidra: the iRest meditative practice for deep relaxation and healing. Sounds True; 2022.

Miller WR, Rollnick S. Motivational interviewing. 3rd ed. Guilford Press; 2013.

Missri JC, Alexander S. Hyperventilation syndrome: a brief review. JAMA J Am Med Assoc. 1978;240(19):2093–6. https://doi.org/10.1001/jama.1978.03290190071038.

Mitchell AJ, Bacon CJ, Moran RW. Reliability and determinants of self-evaluation of breathing questionnaire (SEBQ) score: a symptoms-based measure of dysfunctional breathing. Appl Psychophysiol Biofeedback. 2016;41(1):111–20. https://doi.org/10.1007/s10484-015-9316-7.

Mitchell J. Yoga biomechanics. Handspring; 2019. https://www.perlego.com/book/2789657/yoga-biomechanics-stretching-redefined-pdf

Morton L, Cogan N, Kolacz J, et al. A new measure of feeling safe: developing psychometric properties of the neuroception of psychological safety scale (NPSS). Psychol Trauma. 2022; https://doi.org/10.1037/tra0001313.

Myers TW. Anatomy trains. 4th ed. Elsevier; 2022.

Naik GS, Gaur GS, Pal GK. Effect of modified slow breathing exercise on perceived stress and basal cardiovascular parameters. Int J Yoga. 2018;11(1):53–8. https://doi.org/10.4103/ijoy. IJOY_41_16.

Nardi AE, Freire RC, Zin WA. Panic disorder and control of breathing. Respir Physiol Neurobiol. 2008;167(1):133–43. https://doi.org/10.1016/j.resp.2008.07.011.

Nelson N. Diaphragmatic breathing: the foundation of core stability. Strength Cond J. 2012;34(5):34–40. https://doi.org/10.1519/SSC.0b013e31826ddc07.

Nestor J. Breath: the new science of a lost art. Riverhead Books; 2020.

Niazi IK, Navid MS, Bartley J, et al. EEG signatures change during unilateral yogi nasal breathing. Sci Rep. 2022;12(1):520. https://doi.org/10.1038/s41598-021-04461-8.

Niranjan P, Balaram P. Immediate effect of Ujjayi Pranayama on attention and anxiety among university students: a randomised self-control study. J Clin Diagn Res. 2022;16(2):VC01–4. https://doi.org/10.7860/JCDR/2022/51480.15934.

Nivethitha L, Mooventhan A, Manjunath NK. Effects of various prāṇāyāma on cardiovascular and autonomic variables. Anc Sci Life. 2016;36(2):72–7. https://doi.org/10.4103/asl.ASL_178_16.

Noble DJ, Hochman S. Hypothesis: pulmonary afferent activity patterns during slow, deep breathing contribute to the neural induction of physiological relaxation. Front Physiol. 2019;10:1176. https://doi.org/10.3389/fphys.2019.01176.

Nosetti L, Zaffanello M, di Valserra FDB, et al. Exploring the intricate links between adenotonsillar hypertrophy, mouth breathing, and craniofacial development in children with sleep-disordered breathing: unraveling the vicious cycle. Children. 2023;10(8):1426. https://doi.org/10.3390/children10081426.

Noventi I, Sholihah U, Hasina SN, Wijayanti L. The effectiveness of mindfulness based stress reduction and sama vritti pranayama on reducing blood pressure, improving sleep quality and reducing stress levels in the elderly with hypertension. Bali Med J. 2022; https://doi.org/10.15562/bmj.v11i1.3108.

Okuro RT, Morcillo AM, Ribeiro MÂGO, Sakano E, Conti PBM, Ribeiro JD. Mouth breathing and forward head posture: effects on respiratory biomechanics and exercise capacity in children. J Bras Pneumol. 2011;37(4):471–9. https://doi.org/10.1590/S1806-37132011000400009.

O'Sullivan PB, Beales DJ, Beetham JA, et al. Altered motor control strategies in subjects with sacroiliac joint pain during the active straight-leg-raise test. Spine. 2002;27(1):E1–8. https://doi.org/10.1097/00007632-200201010-00015.

Pal GK, Agarwal A, Karthik S, Pal P, Nanda N. Slow yogic breathing through right and left nostril influences sympathovagal balance, heart rate variability, and cardiovascular risks in young adults. N Am J Med Sci. 2014;6(3):145–51. https://doi.org/10.4103/1947-2714.128477.

Palmer BF, Clegg DJ. Respiratory acidosis and respiratory alkalosis: core curriculum 2023. Am J Kidney Dis. 2023;82(3):347–59. https://doi.org/10.1053/j.ajkd.2023.02.004.

Pandey S, Mahato NK, Navale R. Role of self-induced sound therapy: Bhramari Pranayama in tinnitus. Audiol Med. 2010;8(3):137–41. https://doi.org/10.3109/1651386X.2010.489694.

Panksepp J, Biven L. The archaeology of mind. 1st ed. Norton; 2012. http://bvbr.bib-bvb.de:8991/F?func=service&doc_library=BVB01&local_base=BVB01&doc_number=025768872&sequence=000001&line_number=0001&func_code=DB_RECORDS&service_type=MEDIA

Paris-Alemany A, Proy-Acosta A, Adraos-Juárez D, Suso-Martí L, Touche RL, Chamorro-Sánchez J. Influence of the craniocervical posture on tongue strength and endurance. Dysphagia. 2021;36(2):293–302. https://doi.org/10.1007/s00455-020-10136-9.

Park LC, Braun T, Siegel T. Who practices yoga? A systematic review of demographic, health-related, and psychosocial factors associated with yoga practice. J Behav Med. 2015;38:460–71.

Parkes MJ. The limits of breath holding. Sci Am. 2012;306(4):74–9. https://doi.org/10.1038/scientificamerican0412-74.

Patel K. The complete guide to postural training. Bloomsbury; 2015.

Patel S, Jose A, Mohiuddin SS. Physiology, oxygen transport and carbon dioxide dissociation curve. StatPearls Publishing; 2022. https://www.ncbi.nlm.nih.gov/books/NBK539815/

Paul M, Garg K. The effect of heart rate variability biofeedback on performance psychology of basketball players. Appl Psychophysiol Biofeedback. 2012;37(2):131–44. https://doi.org/10.1007/s10484-012-9185-2.

Payne L, Gold T, Goldman E. Yoga therapy and integrative medicine: where ancient science meets modern medicine. Basic Health Publications; 2015.

Payne P, Crane-Gondreau MA. The preparatory set: a novel approach to understanding stress, trauma, and the bodymind therapies. Front Hum Neurosci. 2015;9:178.

Pendolino AL, Lund VJ, Nardello E, Ottaviano G. The nasal cycle: a comprehensive review. Rhinology. 2018;1(1):67–76. https://doi.org/10.4193/RHINOL/18.021.

Pham V, O'Connell J. Sit up straight. Scribner; 2022.

Pleil JD. Breath biomarkers in toxicology. Arch Toxicol. 2016;90(11):2669–82. https://doi.org/10.1007/s00204-016-1817-5.

Popov. Human exhaled breath analysis. Ann Allergy Asthma Immunol. 2011;106(6):451–6. https://doi.org/10.1016/j.anai.2011.02.016.

Porges S. The polyvagal theory: neurophysiological of emotions, attachment, communication, and Self-regulation. Norton; 2011.

Porges S. The pocket guide to the polyvagal theory: the transformative power of feeling safe. Norton; 2017.

Porges SW. The polyvagal theory: new insights into adaptive reactions of the autonomic nervous system. Cleve Clin J Med. 2009;76(Suppl 2):S86–90. https://doi.org/10.3949/ccjm.76.s2.17.

Porges SW. Polyvagal theory: a science of safety. Front Integr Neurosci. 2022;16:871227. https://doi.org/10.3389/fnint.2022.871227.

Porges SW, Carter SC. Polyvagal theory and the social engagement system. American Psychiatric Association; 2017. p. 221–40.

Porter K. Natural posture for pain-free living. Inner Traditions International; 2013.

Pramanik T, Pudasaini B, Prajapati R. Immediate effect of a slow pace breathing exercise Bhramari pranayama on blood pressure and heart rate. Nepal Med Coll J. 2010;12(3):154. https://www.ncbi.nlm.nih.gov/pubmed/21446363

Prescott SL, Liberles SD. Internal senses of the vagus nerve. Neuron. 2022;110(4):579–99. https://doi.org/10.1016/j.neuron.2021.12.020.

Radwan L, Maszczyk Z, Koziej M, et al. Respiratory responses to chemical stimulation in patients with obstructive sleep apnoea. Monaldi Arch Chest Dis. 2000;55(2):96–100. https://www.ncbi.nlm.nih.gov/pubmed/10949866

Raghurai P, Telles S. Immediate effect of specific nostril manipulating yoga breathing practices on autonomic and respiratory variables. Appl Psychophysiol Biofeedback. 2008;33(2):65–75. https://doi.org/10.1007/s10484-008-9055-0.

Rajesh SK, Ilavarasu JV, Srinivasan TM. Effect of Bhramari Pranayama on response inhibition: evidence from the stop signal task. Int J Yoga. 2014;7(2):138–41. https://doi.org/10.4103/0973-6131.133896.

Rampalliwar S, Rajak C, Arjariya R, Poonia M, Bajpai R. The effect of Bhramari Pranayama ón pregnant women having cardiovascular hyper-reactivity to cold pressor. Natl J Physiol Pharm Pharmacol. 2013;3(2):137. https://doi.org/10.5455/njppp.2013.3.128-133.

Ratey JJ. A user's guide to the brain: perception, attention, and the four theaters of the brain. Pantheon; 2001.

Razmjou E, Freeman H, Vladagina N, Freitas J, Brems C. Popular media images of yoga: limiting perceived access to a beneficial practice. Media Psychol Rev. 2017; http://mprcenter.org/review/popular-media-images-of-yoga-limiting-perceived-access-to-a-beneficial-practice/

Recinto C, Efthemeou T, Boffelli PT, Navalta JW. Effects of nasal or oral breathing on anaerobic power output and metabolic responses. Int J Exerc Sci. 2017;10(4):506–14. https://www.ncbi.nlm.nih.gov/pubmed/28674596

Reich W. Character analysis. 3rd ed. Orgone Inst. Press; 1949.

Riley KE, Park CL. How does yoga reduce stress? A systematic review of mechanisms of change and guide to future inquiry. Health Psychol Rev. 2015;9:379–96. https://doi.org/10.1080/17437199.2014.981778.

Rinpoche YM, Swanson E. Joyful wisdom. Three Rivers Press; 2009. https://ebookcentral.proquest.com/lib/%5BSITE_ID%5D/detail.action?docID=6068276

Ritz T, Meuret AE, Bhaskara L, Petersen S. Respiratory muscle tension as symptom generator in individuals with high anxiety sensitivity. Psychosom Med. 2013;75(2):187–95. https://doi.org/10.1097/PSY.0b013e31827d1072.

Rosen R. The yoga of breath: a step-by-step guide to pranayama. Shambala; 2002.

Rosen R. Pranayama beyond the fundamentals: an in-depth guide to yogic breathing. Shambala; 2006.

Rosenberg S. Accessing the healing power of the vagus nerve. North Atlantic Books; 2017.

Ross A, Friedmann E, Bevans M, Thomas S. National survey of yoga practitioners: mental and physical health benefits. Complement Ther Med. 2013;21:313–23. https://doi.org/10.1016/j.ctim.2013.04.001.

Rossman ML. Guided imagery for self-healing. 2nd ed. New World Library; 2000. http://www.books24x7.com/marc.asp?bookid=12914

Rothenberg R. Restoring prana: a therapeutic guide to pranayama and healing through the breath for yoga therapists, teachers, and healthcare practitioners. Singing Dragon; 2020. https://search.proquest.com/docview/2357879855

Rowley J. Recognising and treating breathing disorders: a multidisciplinary approach. N Z J Physiother. 2014;42:110. https://search.proquest.com/docview/1548421934

Rung O, Stauber L, Loescher LJ, Pace TW. Assessment nostril breathing to reduce stress: an option for pregnant women survivors of intimate partner violence? J Holist Nurs. 2021;39(4):393–415. https://doi.org/10.1177/0898010120983659.

Russo L, Giustino V, Toscano RE, et al. Can tongue position and cervical ROM affect postural oscillations? A pilot and preliminary study. J Hum Sport Exerc. 2020;15(3):840–7. https://doi.org/10.14198/jhse.2020.15.proc3.35.

Russo MA, Santarelli DM, O'Rourke D. The physiological effects of slow breathing in the healthy human. Breathe. 2017;13(4):298–309. https://doi.org/10.1183/20734735.009817.

Saccomanno S, Pirino A, Bianco G, Paskay LC, Mastrapasqua R, Scoppa F. Does a short lingual frenulum affect body posture? Assessment of posture in the sagittal plane before and after laser frenulotomy: a pilot study. J Biol Regul Homeost Agents. 2021;35(3 Suppl. 1):185–95. https://doi.org/10.23812/21-3suppl-21.

Sakakibara M, Hayano J. Effect of slowed respiration on cardiac parasympathetic response to threat. Psychosom Med. 1996;58(1):32–7. https://doi.org/10.1097/00006842-199601000-00006.

Sansbury BE, Hill BG. Regulation of obesity and insulin resistance by nitric oxide. Free Radic Biol Med. 2014;73:383–99. https://doi.org/10.1016/j.freeradbiomed.2014.05.016.

Saravanan L, Anu S, Vairapraveena R, Rajalakshmi G. Impact of alternate nostril breathing exercises on vascular parameters in hypertensive patients - an interventional study. Natl J Physiol Pharm Pharmacol. 2019;9(3):210–4. https://doi.org/10.5455/njppp.2019.9.1237308012019.

Scaer R. 8 keys to brain-body balance. Norton; 2012.

Schiffmann E. Yoga: the spirit and practice of moving into stillness. Gallery Books; 2013.

Schmalzl L, Crane-Godreau MA, Payne P. Movement-based embodied contemplative practices: definitions and paradigms. Front Hum Neurosci. 2014;8:205. https://doi.org/10.3389/fnhum.2014.00205.

Schmalzl L, Powers C, Blom EH. Neurophysiological and neurocognitive mechanisms underlying the effects of yoga-based practices: towards a comprehensive theoretical framework. Front Hum Neurosci. 2015;9:235. https://doi.org/10.3389/fnhum.2015.00235.

Schünemann HJ, Dorn J, Grant BJB, Winkelstein WJ, Trevisan M. Pulmonary function is a long-term predictor of mortality in the general population: 29-year follow-up of the Buffalo Health Study. Chest. 2000;118(3):656–64. https://doi.org/10.1378/chest.118.3.656.

Schwartz A. Applied polyvagal theory in yoga: therapeutic practices for emotional health. Norton; 2024.

Scoppa F, Pirino A. Is there a relationship between body posture and tongue posture? Glosso-postural syndrome between myth and reality. Acta Medica Mediterr. 2019;35:1897–907. https://doi.org/10.19193/0393-6384_2019_4_296.

Scott JB, Kaur R. Monitoring breathing frequency, pattern, and effort. Respir Care. 2020;65(6):793–806. https://doi.org/10.4187/respcare.07439.

Sebanz N, Bekkering H, Knoblich G. Joint action: bodies and minds moving together. Trends Cogn Sci. 2006;10(2):70–6. https://doi.org/10.1016/j.tics.2005.12.009.

Sengupta P. Health impacts of yoga and pranayama: a state-of-the-art review. Int J Prev Med. 2012;3:444–58.

Severs LJ, Vlemincx E, Ramirez J-M. The psychophysiology of the sigh: I: the sigh from the physiological perspective. Biol Psychol. 2022;170:108313. https://doi.org/10.1016/j.biopsycho.2022.108313.

Sevoz-Couche C, Laborde S. Heart rate variability and slow-paced breathing: when coherence meets resonance. Neurosci Biobehav Rev. 2022;135:104576. https://doi.org/10.1016/j.neubiorev.2022.104576.

Shaffer F, Meehan ZM, Zerr CL. A critical review of ultra-short-term heart rate variability norms research. Front Neurosci. 2020;14:594880. https://doi.org/10.3389/fnins.2020.594880.

Shah S, Shirodkar S, Deo M. Effectiveness of core stability and diaphragmatic breathing vs. core stability alone on pain and function in mechanical non-specific low back pain patients: a randomised control trial. Int J Health Sci Res. 2020;10(2) https://www.ijhsr.org/IJHSR_Vol.10_Issue.2_Feb2020/36.pdf

Shannahoff-Khalsa DS, Kennedy B. The effects of unilateral forced nostril breathing on the heart. Int J Neurosci. 1993;73(1–2):47–60. https://doi.org/10.3109/00207459308987210.

Shao R, Man ISC, Lee TMC. The effect of slow-paced breathing on cardiovascular and emotion functions: a meta-analysis and systematic review. Mindfulness. 2024;15(1):1–18. https://doi.org/10.1007/s12671-023-02294-2.

Shetty HN, Acharya D. Bhramari pranayama in tinnitus: a systematic review. Indian J Otol. 2023;29(3):146–51. https://doi.org/10.4103/indianjotol.indianjotol_40_23.

Shieh W-Y, Wang C-M, Cheng H-YK, Imbang TI. Noninvasive measurement of tongue pressure and its correlation with swallowing and respiration. Sensors. 2021;21(8):2603. https://doi.org/10.3390/s21082603.

Shimizu A, Maeda K, Nagami S, et al. Low tongue strength is associated with oral and cough-related abnormalities in older inpatients. Nutrition. 2021;83:111062. https://doi.org/10.1016/j.nut.2020.111062.

Siegel DJ. Aware. Penguin; 2018.

Siegel DJ, Bryson TP. Whole-brain child: 12 revolutionary strategies to nurture your child's developing mind. Scribe Publications; 2012.

Singh RB, Wilczyńska-Kwiatek A, Fedacko J, Pella D, Meester FD. Pranayama: the power of breath. Int J Disabil Hum Dev. 2009;8(2):141–54. https://doi.org/10.1515/IJDHD.2009.8.2.141.

Singh UP. Evidence-based role of hypercapnia and exhalation phase in vagus nerve stimulation: insights into hypercapnic yoga breathing exercises. J Yoga Phys Ther. 2017;7(3):1000276. https://doi.org/10.4172/2157-7595.1000276.

Singleton M. Yoga body: the origins of modern posture practice. Oxford University Press; 2010. https://doi.org/10.1093/acprof:oso/9780195395358.001.0001.

Sinha AN, Deepak D, Gusain VS. Assessment of the effects of pranayama/alternate nostril breathing on the parasympathetic nervous system in young adults. J Clin Diagn Res. 2013;7(5):821–3. https://doi.org/10.7860/JCDR/2013/4750.2948.

Skaggs SA, McCarthy M, Shelledy DC. Physical assessment. In: Shelledy DC, Peters JI, editors. Respiratory care: patient assessment and care plan development. Jones & Bartlett Learning; 2022. p. 151–202.

Smikowski J, Dewane S, Johnson ME, Brems C, Bruss C, Roberts LW. Community-based participatory research for improved mental health. Ethics Behav. 2009;19(6):461–78. https://doi.org/10.1080/10508420903274971.

Smith L, Gasser M. The development of embodied cognition: six lessons from babies. Artif Life. 2005;11(1–2):13–29. https://doi.org/10.1162/1064546053278973.

Sokoloff A, Burkholder T. Tongue structure and function. In: McLoon LK, Andrade F, editors. Craniofacial muscles. Springer; 2012. p. 207–27. https://doi.org/10.1007/978-1-4614-4466-4_12.

Solomon SG. Effect of Anuloma and Viloma pranayama on stress of nurses. Int J Adv Psychiatr Nurs. 2022;4(1):7–11. https://doi.org/10.33545/26641348.2022.v4.i1a.74.

Spicuzza L, Gabutti A, Porta C, Montano N, Bernardi L. Yoga and chemoreflex response to hypoxia and hypercapnia. Lancet. 2000;356(9240):1495–6. https://doi.org/10.1016/S0140-6736(00)02881-6.

Srinivasan T. Entrainment and coherence in biology. Int J Yoga. 2015;8(1):1–2. https://doi.org/10.4103/0973-6131.146040.

Srivastava S, Goyal P, Tiwari SK, Patel AK. Interventional effect of Bhramari Pranayama on mental health among college students. Int J Indian Psychol. 2017;4(2) https://doi.org/10.25215/0402.044.

Stanley J. Every body yoga. Workman; 2017.

Stephen MJ. Breath taking. Grove/Atlantic; 2021.

Sterios P. Gravity and grace. Sounds True; 2019. https://doi.org/10.2307/j.ctv16km193.

Stern D. The interpersonal world of the infant. Basic; 1985.

Stewart MG, Witsell DL, Smith TL, Weaver EM, Yueh B, Hannley MT. Development and validation of the nasal obstruction symptom evaluation (NOSE) scale. Otolaryngol Head Neck Surg. 2004;130(2):157–63. https://doi.org/10.1016/j.otohns.2003.09.016.

Stone L. Just breathe: building the case for email apnea. 2008. https://www.huffpost.com/entry/just-breathe-building-the_b_85651

Stone M. The inner tradition of yoga. Shambhala; 2008. http://bvbr.bib-bvb.de:8991/F?func=service&doc_library=BVB01&local_base=BVB01&doc_number=028969209&sequence=000002&line_number=0001&func_code=DB_RECORDS&service_type=MEDIA

Stühlinger MC, Abbasi F, Chu JW, et al. Relationship between insulin resistance and an endogenous nitric oxide synthase inhibitor. JAMA. 2002;287(11):1420–6. https://doi.org/10.1001/jama.287.11.1420.

Sulenes K, Freitas J, Justice L, Colgan DD, Shean M, Brems C. Underuse of yoga as a referral resource by health professions students. J Altern Complement Med. 2015;21(1):53–9. https://doi.org/10.1089/acm.2014.0217.

Sullivan MB, Erb M, Schmalzl L, Moonaz S, Taylor JN, Porges S. Yoga therapy and polyvagal theory: the convergence of traditional wisdom and contemporary neuroscience for self-regulation and resilience. Front Hum Neurosci. 2018;12:67–82. https://doi.org/10.3389/fnhum.2018.00067.

Sullivan MB, Moonaz S, Weber K, Taylor JN, Schmalzl L. Toward an explanatory framework for yoga therapy informed by philosophical and ethical perspectives. Altern Ther Health Med. 2018;24(1):38–46. https://www.ncbi.nlm.nih.gov/pubmed/29135457

Surlya BK, Jain DM. To evaluate the effect of om mantra chanting along with Anulom Vilom Pranayama on medical and paramedical students. Sch Int J Anat Physiol. 2021;4(3):38–43. https://doi.org/10.36348/sijap.2021.v04i03.005.

Susaman N, Cingi C, Mullol J. Is the nasal cycle real? How important is it? In: Cingi C, Bayar Muluk N, Scadding GK, Miadna R, editors. Challenges in rhinology. Springer Nature; 2020. p. 1–8. https://doi.org/10.1007/978-3-030-50899-9_1.

Svatmarama S, Akers BD. Hatha yoga pradipika (translated). YogaVidya.com. 2002. https://www.vlebooks.com/vleweb/product/openreader?id=none&isbn=9780989996648&uid=none

Swathi PS, Raghavendra BR, Saoji AA. Health and therapeutic benefits of Shatkarma: a narrative review of scientific studies. J Ayurveda Integr Med. 2021;12(1):206–12. https://doi.org/10.1016/j.jaim.2020.11.008.

Tavel ME. Hyperventilation syndrome: a diagnosis usually unrecognized. Intern Med Prim Healthc. 2017;2(1):1–4. https://doi.org/10.24966/IMPH-2493/100006.

Taylor AG, Goehler LE, Galper DI, Innes KE, Bourguignon C. Top-down and bottom-up mechanisms in mind-body medicine: development of an integrative framework for psychophysiological research. Explore. 2010;6:29–41. https://doi.org/10.1016/j.explore.2009.10.004.

Telles S, Gupta RK, Yadav A, Pathak S, Balkrishna A. Hemisphere specific EEG related to alternate nostril yoga breathing. BMC Res Notes. 2017;10(1):306. https://doi.org/10.1186/s13104-017-2625-6.

Telles S, Joshi M, Somvanshi P. Yoga breathing through a particular nostril is associated with contralateral event-related potential changes. Int J Yoga. 2012;5(2):102–7. https://doi.org/10.4103/0973-6131.98220.

Tellhed U, Daukantaitė D, Maddux RE, Svensson T, Melander O. Yogic breathing and mindfulness as stress coping mediate positive health outcomes of yoga. Mindfulness. 2019;10(12):2703–15. https://doi.org/10.1007/s12671-019-01225-4.

Terraciano T, Loeckenhoff C, Zonderman A, Ferrucci L, Costa P. Personality predictors of longevity: activity, emotional stability, and conscientiousness. Psychosom Med. 2008;70:621–7.

Thelen E. Motor development: a new synthesis. Manch Sch. 1995;50(2):79–95. https://search.proquest.com/docview/38713200

Thribhuvanan L, Saravanakumar MS. Influence of mode of breathing on pharyngeal airway space and dento facial parameters in children: a short clinical study. Bull Natl Res Cent. 2022;46(1):1–7. https://doi.org/10.1186/s42269-022-00802-3.

Timmons BH, Ley R. Behavioral and psychological approaches to breathing disorders. Springer; 1994.

Todd S, Walsted ES, Grillo L, Livingston R, Menzies-Gow A, Hull JH. Novel assessment tool to detect breathing pattern disorder in patients with refractory asthma. Respirology. 2018;23(3):284–90. https://doi.org/10.1111/resp.13173.

Tortora GJ, Derrickson BH. Principles of anatomy and physiology. 16th ed. Wiley; 2023.

Trabalon M, Schaal B. It takes a mouth to eat and a nose to breathe: abnormal oral respiration affects neonates' oral competence and systemic adaptation. Int J Pediatr. 2012;2012:1–10. https://doi.org/10.1155/2012/207605.

Trayhurn P. Oxygen—a critical, but overlooked, nutrient. Front Nutr. 2019;6:10. https://doi.org/10.3389/fnut.2019.00010.

Trevisan ME, Boufleur J, Soares JC, Haygert CJP, Ries LGK, Corrêa ECR. Diaphragmatic amplitude and accessory inspiratory muscle activity in nasal and mouth-breathing adults: a cross-sectional study. J Electromyogr Kinesiol. 2015;25(3):463–8. https://doi.org/10.1016/j.jelekin.2015.03.006.

Trivedi GY, Kathirvel S, Sharma K, Saboo B. Effect of various lengths of respiration on heart rate variability during simple Bhramari (humming). Int J Yoga. 2023;16(2):123–31. https://doi.org/10.4103/ijoy.ijoy_113_23.

Trivedi GY, Saboo B. Bhramari pranayama—a simple lifestyle intervention to reduce heart rate, enhance the lung function and immunity. J Ayurveda Integr Med. 2021;12(3):562–4. https://doi.org/10.1016/j.jaim.2021.07.004.

Tsakiris M, Jiménez AT, Costantini M. Just a heartbeat away from one's body: interoceptive sensitivity predicts malleability of body-representations. Proc R Soc B Biol Sci. 2011;278(1717):2470–6. https://doi.org/10.1098/rspb.2010.2547.

Tu W, Zhang N. Neural underpinning of a respiration-associated resting-state fMRI network. eLife. 2022;11:e81555. https://doi.org/10.7554/eLife.81555.

Uithol S, van Rooij I, Bekkering H, Haselager P. Understanding motor resonance. Soc Neurosci. 2011a;6(4):388–97. https://doi.org/10.1080/17470919.2011.559129.

Uithol S, van Rooij I, Bekkering H, Haselager P. What do mirror neurons mirror? Philos Psychol. 2011b;24(5):607–23. https://doi.org/10.1080/09515089.2011.562604.

Upadhyay J, Nandish NS, Shetty S, Saoji AA, Yadav SS. Effects of Nadishodhana and Bhramari Pranayama on heart rate variability, auditory reaction time, and blood pressure: a randomized clinical trial in hypertensive patients. J Ayurveda Integr Med. 2023;14(4):100774. https://doi.org/10.1016/j.jaim.2023.100774.

Ushamohan BP, Rajasekaran AK, Belur YK, Ilavarasu J, Srinivasan TM. Nitric oxide, humming and Bhramari Pranayama. Indian J Sci Technol. 2023;16(5):377–84. https://doi.org/10.17485/IJST/v16i5.1212.

Vago DR, Silbersweig DA. Self-awareness, self-regulation, and self-transcendence (S-ART): a framework for understanding the neurobiological mechanisms of mindfulness. Front Hum Neurosci. 2012;6:296. https://doi.org/10.3389/fnhum.2012.00296.

van der Kolk B. The body keeps the score. Penguin; 2014.

van Dixhoorn J, Folgering H. The Nijmegen Questionnaire and dysfunctional breathing. ERJ Open Res. 2015;1(1):1. https://doi.org/10.1183/23120541.00001-2015.

Varne SR, Balaji PA. Physiological effects of yoga and pranayama on serum adipokines, lipoprotein (a), thyrotropin levels, and blood pressure among obese hypothyroid patients with hypertension. Int Res J Ayurveda Yoga. 2023;6(8):9–14. https://doi.org/10.47223/IRJAY.2023.6802.

Vaschillo EG, Vaschillo B, Buckman JF, et al. The effects of sighing on the cardiovascular system. Biol Psychol. 2015;106:86–95. https://doi.org/10.1016/j.biopsycho.2015.02.007.

Vladagina N, Freeman H, Razmjou E, et al. Media images of yoga poses: increasing injury instead of access. Paper presented at: 144th Annual American Public Health Association Meeting and Exposition. 2016 Oct.

Vlemincx E, Abelson JL, Lehrer PM, Davenport PW, Diest IV, den Bergh OV. Respiratory variability and sighing: A psychophysiological reset model. Biol Psychol. 2013;93(1):24–32. https://doi.org/10.1016/j.biopsycho.2012.12.001.

Vlemincx E, Diest IV, den Bergh OV. A sigh of relief or a sigh to relieve: the psychological and physiological relief effect of deep breaths. Physiol Behav. 2016;165:127–35. https://doi.org/10.1016/j.physbeh.2016.07.004.

Vlemincx E, Severs L, Ramirez J-M. The psychophysiology of the sigh: II: the sigh from the psychological perspective. Biol Psychol. 2022;173:108386. https://doi.org/10.1016/j.biopsycho.2022.108386.

Vukojević B, Vater C, Laborde S. The role of resonance frequency in slow-paced breathing: systematic review. Curr Issues Sport Sci. 2024;9(2):80. https://doi.org/10.36950/2024.2ciss080.

Ward L, Stebbings S, Sherman K, Cherkin D, Baxter GD. Establishing key components of yoga interventions for musculoskeletal conditions: a delphi survey. BMC Complement Altern Med. 2014;14(196):1. https://doi.org/10.1186/1472-6882-14-196.

Watkins A, Wilber K. Wicked and wise: how to solve the world's toughest problems. Urbane; 2015.

Weitzberg E, Lundberg JON. Humming greatly increases nasal nitric oxide. Am J Respir Crit Care Med. 2002;166(2):144–5. https://doi.org/10.1164/rccm.200202-138BC.

White G. Yoga beyond belief. North Atlantic Books; 2007.

Wielgosz J, Schuyler BS, Lutz A, Davidson RJ. Long-term mindfulness training is associated with reliable differences in resting respiration rate. Sci Rep. 2016;6(1):27533. https://doi.org/10.1038/srep27533.

Wilber K. Integral psychology. Shambhala; 2000.

Wilber K. Integral meditation: mindfulness as a path to grow up, wake up, and show up in your life. Shambhala; 2016. https://ebookcentral.proquest.com/lib/%5BSITE_ID%5D/detail.action?docID=6057496

Wimbarti S, Self PA. Developmental psychology for the clinical child psychologist. In: Walker CE, Roberts MC, editors. Wiley; 1992. p. 33–46.

Witkiewitz R, Roos CR, Colgan DD, Bowen S. Advances in psychotherapy evidence-based practice. Hogrefe; 2017.

Yildiz S, Grinstead J, Hildebrand A, et al. Immediate impact of yogic breathing on pulsatile cerebrospinal fluid dynamics. Sci Rep. 2022;12(1):10894. https://doi.org/10.1038/s41598-022-15034-8.

You M, Laborde S, Ackermann S, Borges U, Dosseville F, Mosley E. Influence of respiratory frequency of slow-paced breathing on vagally-mediated heart rate variability. Appl Psychophysiol Biofeedback. 2024;49(1):133–43. https://doi.org/10.1007/s10484-023-09605-2.

You M, Laborde S, Zammit N, Iskra M, Borges U, Dosseville F. Single slow-paced breathing session at six cycles per minute: investigation of dose-response relationship on cardiac vagal activity. Int J Environ Res Public Health. 2021;18(23):12478. https://doi.org/10.3390/ijerph182312478.

You M, Laborde S, Zammit N, et al. Emotional intelligence training: influence of a brief slow-paced breathing exercise on psychophysiological variables linked to emotion regulation. Int J Environ Res Public Health. 2021;18(12):6630. https://doi.org/10.3390/ijerph18126630.

Zaccaro A, Piarulli A, Laurino M, et al. How breath-control can change your life: a systematic review on psycho-physiological correlates of slow breathing. Front Hum Neurosci. 2018;12:353. https://doi.org/10.3389/fnhum.2018.00353.

Zhao Z, Zheng L, Huang X, Li C, Liu J, Hu Y. Effects of mouth breathing on facial skeletal development in children: a systematic review and meta-analysis. BMC Oral Health. 2021;21(1):108. https://doi.org/10.1186/s12903-021-01458-7.

Index